Manual
of
ICU PROCEDURES

Manual
of
ICU PROCEDURES

Editor

Mohan Gurjar

MD PDCC FICCM

Associate Professor
Department of Critical Care Medicine
Sanjay Gandhi Postgraduate Institute of Medical Sciences
Lucknow, Uttar Pradesh, India

Foreword

Arvind Kumar Baronia

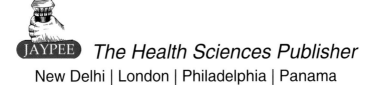

JAYPEE *The Health Sciences Publisher*
New Delhi | London | Philadelphia | Panama

Jaypee Brothers Medical Publishers (P) Ltd.

Headquarters
Jaypee Brothers Medical Publishers (P) Ltd.
4838/24, Ansari Road, Daryaganj
New Delhi 110 002, India
Phone: +91-11-43574357
Fax: +91-11-43574314
E-mail: jaypee@jaypeebrothers.com

Overseas Offices

J.P. Medical Ltd.
83, Victoria Street, London
SW1H 0HW (UK)
Phone: +44-20 3170 8910
Fax: +44 (0)20 3008 6180
E-mail: info@jpmedpub.com

Jaypee-Highlights Medical Publishers Inc.
City of Knowledge, Bld. 237, Clayton
Panama City, Panama
Phone: +1 507-301-0496
Fax: +1 507-301-0499
E-mail: cservice@jphmedical.com

Jaypee Medical Inc.
The Bourse
111, South Independence Mall East
Suite 835, Philadelphia, PA 19106, USA
Phone: +1 267-519-9789
E-mail: jpmed.us@gmail.com

Jaypee Brothers Medical Publishers (P) Ltd.
17/1-B, Babar Road, Block-B
Shaymali, Mohammadpur
Dhaka-1207, Bangladesh
Mobile: +08801912003485
E-mail: jaypeedhaka@gmail.com

Jaypee Brothers Medical Publishers (P) Ltd.
Bhotahity, Kathmandu, Nepal
Phone: +977-9741283608
E-mail: kathmandu@jaypeebrothers.com

Website: www.jaypeebrothers.com
Website: www.jaypeedigital.com

Inquiries for bulk sales may be solicited at: jaypee@jaypeebrothers.com

Manual of ICU Procedures

First Edition: **2016**

ISBN: 978-93-5152-422-9

Printed at Sanat Printers, Kundli

Dedicated to

*All men and women (including our patients)
who, over the years, have contributed to develop
standards for procedures, which being done
in critically ill patients, to improve safety with
better skills.*

Contributors

A Ebru Salman MD
Associate Professor
Department of Anesthesiology
and Reanimation
Atatürk Training and Research Hospital
Ankara, Turkey

Abhishek Kumar MD
Chief Intensivist
Patel Hospital
Jalandhar, Punjab, India

Abraham Samuel Babu MPT
Assistant Professor
Department of Physiotherapy
School of Allied Health Sciences
Manipal University
Manipal, Karnataka, India

Aditya Kapoor DM FACC
Professor
Department of Cardiology
Sanjay Gandhi Postgraduate
Institute of Medical Sciences
Lucknow, Uttar Pradesh, India

Afzal Azim MD PDCC FICCM
Additional Professor
Department of Critical Care Medicine
Sanjay Gandhi Postgraduate
Institute of Medical Sciences
Lucknow, Uttar Pradesh, India

Amit Keshri MS
Assistant Professor
Unit of Neuro-otology
Department of Neurosurgery
Sanjay Gandhi Postgraduate
Institute of Medical Sciences
Lucknow
Uttar Pradesh, India

Amol Kothekar MD IDCC
Assistant Professor
Intensive Care Medicine
Department of Anesthesia
Critical Care and Pain
Tata Memorial Hospital
Mumbai
Maharashtra, India

Anju Dubey MD
Assistant Professor
Department of Transfusion Medicine
All India Institute of Medical Sciences
Rishikesh, Uttarakhand, India

Ankur Bhatnagar MS MCh
Associate Professor
Department of Plastic Surgery
Sanjay Gandhi Postgraduate
Institute of Medical Sciences
Lucknow, Uttar Pradesh, India

Anupam Wakhlu MD DM
Associate Professor
Department of Rheumatology
King George's Medical University
Lucknow, Uttar Pradesh, India

Armin Ahmed MD PDCC
Senior Research Associate
Department of Critical Care Medicine
Sanjay Gandhi Postgraduate
Institute of Medical Sciences
Lucknow, Uttar Pradesh, India

Arun G Maiya PhD PT
Dr TMA Pai Endowment Chair in Exercise
Science and Health Promotion
Professor
Department of Physiotherapy
School of Allied Health Sciences
Manipal University
Manipal, Karnataka, India

Arun K Srivastava MS MCh
Associate Professor
Department of Neurosurgery
Sanjay Gandhi Postgraduate
Institute of Medical Sciences
Lucknow, Uttar Pradesh, India

Arun Sharma MD PDCC
Consultant
Critical Care Medicine
Santokba Durlabhji Memorial Hospital
Jaipur, Rajasthan, India

Atul P Kulkarni MD
Professor and Head
Division of Critical Care
Department of Anesthesia
Critical Care and Pain
Tata Memorial Hospital
Mumbai, Maharashtra, India

Atul Sonker MD
Additional Professor
Department of Transfusion Medicine
Sanjay Gandhi Postgraduate
Institute of Medical Sciences
Lucknow, Uttar Pradesh, India

Banani Poddar MD
Professor
Department of Critical Care Medicine
Sanjay Gandhi Postgraduate
Institute of Medical Sciences
Lucknow, Uttar Pradesh, India

Barnali Banik MD
Clinical Fellow
Department of Hematology
Peter MacCallum Cancer Center
Melbourne, Australia

Basant Kumar MS MCh
Associate Professor
Department of Pediatric Surgical
Superspecialty
Sanjay Gandhi Postgraduate
Institute of Medical Sciences
Lucknow, Uttar Pradesh, India

Bhaskar P Rao MD PDCC
Assistant Professor
Department of Anesthesiology
All India Institute of Medical
Sciences, Bhubaneswar
Odisha, India

Bhuwan Chand Panday MD
Consultant
Department of Anesthesia
Sir Ganga Ram Hospital
New Delhi, India

Biju Pottakkat MS MCh PDF FICS
Additional Professor and Head
Department of Surgical
Gastroenterology Jawaharlal
Institute of Postgraduate
Medical Education and Research
Puducherry, India

Devendra Gupta MD PDCC
Additional Professor
Department of Anesthesiology
Sanjay Gandhi Postgraduate
Institute of Medical Sciences
Lucknow, Uttar Pradesh, India

Devesh Dutta MD FNB
Consultant
Department of Anesthesiology
Fortis Escorts Heart Institute
New Delhi, India

Devesh K Singh MS MCh
Senior Resident
Department of Neurosurgery
Sanjay Gandhi Postgraduate
Institute of Medical Sciences
Lucknow, Uttar Pradesh, India

Dharmendra Bhadauria MD DM
Assistant Professor
Department of Nephrology and
Renal Transplantation
Sanjay Gandhi Postgraduate
Institute of Medical Sciences
Lucknow, Uttar Pradesh, India

Divyesh Patel MD IDCCM
Consultant Intensivist
Deenanath Mangeshkar Hospital
Pune, Maharashtra, India

Eti Sthapak MS
Assistant Professor
Department of Anatomy
Era's Lucknow Medical College and Hospital
Lucknow, Uttar Pradesh, India

Fahri Yetisir MD
Associate Professor
Department of General Surgery
Atatürk Training and Research Hospital
Ankara, Turkey

Gaurav Srivastava MD
Clinical Fellow
Department of Hematology
Peter MacCallum Cancer Center
Melbourne, Australia

Girija Prasad Rath MD DM
Additional Professor
Department of Neuroanesthesiology
All India Institute of Medical Sciences
New Delhi, India

Harsh Vardhan MD DM
Assistant Professor
Department of Nephrology
Indira Gandhi Institute of Medical Sciences
Patna, Bihar, India

Hemanshu Prabhakar MD
Additional Professor
Department of Neuroanesthesiology
All India Institute of Medical Sciences
New Delhi, India

Hemant Bhagat MD DM
Associate Professor
Department of Anesthesia and Intensive Care
Postgraduate Institute of
Medical Education and Research
Chandigarh, India

Hira Lal MD
Additional Professor
Department of Radiodiagnosis
Sanjay Gandhi Postgraduate
Institute of Medical Sciences
Lucknow, Uttar Pradesh, India

Indu Lata MD MNAMS
Associate Professor
Department of Maternal and
Reproductive Health
Sanjay Gandhi Postgraduate
Institute of Medical Sciences
Lucknow, Uttar Pradesh, India

Jayantee Kalita MD DM
Professor
Department of Neurology
Sanjay Gandhi Postgraduate
Institute of Medical Sciences
Lucknow, Uttar Pradesh, India

Jugal Sharma MD
Senior Resident
Department of Cardiology
Sanjay Gandhi Postgraduate
Institute of Medical Sciences
Lucknow, Uttar Pradesh, India

JV Divatia MD FICCM FCCM
Professor and Head
Department of Anesthesia,
Critical Care and Pain
Tata Memorial Hospital
Mumbai, Maharashtra, India

Jyoti Narayan Sahoo MD PDCC
Consultant Intensivist
Department of Critical Care Medicine
Apollo Health City
Hyderabad, Telangana, India

Kamal Kataria MS
Research Associate
Department of Trauma Surgery
JPN Apex Trauma Center
All India Institute of Medical Sciences
New Delhi, India

Kamal Kishore MD
Associate Professor
Department of Anesthesiology
Sanjay Gandhi Postgraduate
Institute of Medical Sciences
Lucknow, Uttar Pradesh, India

Kapil Dev Soni MD
Assistant Professor
Critical and Intensive Care
JPN Apex Trauma Center
All India Institute of Medical Sciences
New Delhi, India

Kirti M Naranje MD
Assistant Professor
Department of Neonatology
Sanjay Gandhi Postgraduate
Institute of Medical Sciences
Lucknow, Uttar Pradesh, India

Kranti Bhavana MS DNB
Assistant Professor
Department of Otorhinolaryngology
All India Institute of Medical
Sciences, Patna
Bihar, India

Kundan Kumar MD DNB DM
Senior Resident
Department of Gastroenterology
Sanjay Gandhi Postgraduate
Institute of Medical Sciences
Lucknow, Uttar Pradesh, India

Kuntal Kanti Das MS
Assistant Professor
Department of Neurosurgery
Sanjay Gandhi Postgraduate
Institute of Medical Sciences
Lucknow, Uttar Pradesh, India

Manish Gupta MD FNB EDIC
Senior Consultant and Head
Department of Critical Care Medicine
Max Superspecialty Hospital
New Delhi, India

Manish Paul MD
Clinical Observer
Department of Critical Care Medicine
Sanjay Gandhi Postgraduate
Institute of Medical Sciences
Lucknow, Uttar Pradesh, India

Mohan Gurjar MD PDCC FICCM
Associate Professor
Department of Critical Care Medicine
Sanjay Gandhi Postgraduate
Institute of Medical Sciences
Lucknow, Uttar Pradesh, India

MS Ansari MS MCh
Additional Professor
Department of Urology
Sanjay Gandhi Postgraduate
Institute of Medical Sciences
Lucknow, Uttar Pradesh, India

Namita Mehrotra MD
Assistant Professor
Department of Radiodiagnosis
Sanjay Gandhi Postgraduate
Institute of Medical Sciences
Lucknow, Uttar Pradesh, India

Narendra Agrawal MD DM
Consultant
Hemato-oncology and
Bone Marrow Transplantation
Rajiv Gandhi Cancer Institute
and Research Center
New Delhi, India

Neeta Bose MD
Associate Professor
Department of Anesthesia
Gujarat Medical Education and
Research Society Medical College
Vadodara, Gujrat, India

Neha Singh MD
Assistant Professor
Department of Anesthesiology
Institute of Medical Sciences and SUM Hospital
Bhubaneswar, Odisha, India

Nikhil Kothari MD PhD
Assistant Professor
Department of Anesthesiology
Critical Care and Pain Medicine
All India Institute of Medical Sciences
Jodhpur, Rajasthan, India

Nirvik Pal MD
Resident
Department of Anesthesiology
Washington University
St Louis, Missouri, USA

Nishant Verma MD
Assistant Professor
Department of Pediatrics
King George's Medical University
Lucknow, Uttar Pradesh, India

Nitin Garg MD FNB EDIC
Senior Consultant and Head
Department of Critical Care Medicine
Rockland Hospital
New Delhi, India

Oskay Kaya MD
Associate Professor
Department of General Surgery
Dışkapı Yıldırım Beyazit Research
and Training Hospital
Ankara, Turkey

Pradeep Bhatia MD
Professor and Head
Department of Anesthesiology
Critical Care and Pain Medicine
All India Institute of Medical Sciences
Jodhpur, Rajasthan, India

Pralay K Sarkar MD DM MRCP (UK) FCCP
Assistant Professor
Division of Pulmonary and
Critical Care Medicine
Department of Medicine
Baylor College of Medicine
Ben Taub General Hospital
Houston, Texas, USA

Prasad Rajhans MBBS MD FICCM
Chief Intensivist
Deenanath Mangeshkar Hospital, Pune
Consultant in Emergency
Medical Services
Symbiosis International University
Pune, Maharashtra, India

Prashant Saxena MD EDIC FCCP
Consultant
Department of Pulmonology,
Critical Care and Sleep Medicine
Saket City Hospital
New Delhi, India

Praveer Rai MD DM
Additional Professor
Department of Gastroenterology
Sanjay Gandhi Postgraduate
Institute of Medical Sciences
Lucknow, Uttar Pradesh, India

Puja Srivastava MD
Senior Resident
Department of Clinical Immunology
Sanjay Gandhi Postgraduate
Institute of Medical Sciences
Lucknow, Uttar Pradesh, India

Puneet Goyal MD DM
Associate Professor
Department of Anesthesiology
Sanjay Gandhi Postgraduate
Institute of Medical Sciences
Lucknow, Uttar Pradesh, India

Puneet Khanna MD
Assistant Professor
Department of Anesthesiology
All India Institute of Medical Sciences
New Delhi, India

Rabi N Sahu MS MCh
Additional Professor
Department of Neurosurgery
Sanjay Gandhi Postgraduate
Institute of Medical Sciences
Lucknow, Uttar Pradesh, India

Raj Kumar Mani MD
Director Critical Care
Pulmonology and Sleep Medicine
Saket City Hospital
New Delhi, India

Rajanikant R Yadav MD
Assistant Professor
Department of Radiodiagnosis
Sanjay Gandhi Postgraduate
Institute of Medical Sciences
Lucknow, Uttar Pradesh, India

Rajendra Kumar BPT
Physiotherapist Grade I
Department of Critical Care Medicine
Sanjay Gandhi Postgraduate
Institute of Medical Sciences
Lucknow, Uttar Pradesh, India

Rakesh Garg MD
Assistant Professor
Department of Anesthesiology
All India Institute of Medical Sciences
New Delhi, India

Rakesh Lodha MD
Additional Professor
Department of Pediatrics
All India Institute of Medical Sciences
New Delhi, India

Ravinder Kumar Pandey MD
Additional Professor
Department of Anesthesiology
All India Institute of Medical Sciences
New Delhi, India

Ravindra M Mehta MD FCCP
Chief
Critical Care and Pulmonology Apollo
Hospitals
Bengaluru, Karnataka, India

Richa Misra MD
Assistant Professor
Department of Microbiology
Sanjay Gandhi Postgraduate
Institute of Medical Sciences
Lucknow, Uttar Pradesh, India

Ritesh Agarwal MD DM
Associate Professor
Department of Pulmonary Medicine
Postgraduate Institute of
Medical Education and Research
Chandigarh, India

RK Singh MD PDCC
Additional Professor
Department of Critical Care Medicine
Sanjay Gandhi Postgraduate
Institute of Medical Sciences
Lucknow, Uttar Pradesh, India

Rohan Aurangabadwalla MD
Pulmonologist
Apollo Hospitals
Bengaluru, Karnataka, India

Samir Mohindra MD DM
Associate Professor
Department of Gastroenterology
Sanjay Gandhi Postgraduate
Institute of Medical Sciences
Lucknow, Uttar Pradesh, India

Sandeep Sahu MD PDCC FACEE
Associate Professor
Department of Anesthesiology
Sanjay Gandhi Postgraduate
Institute of Medical Sciences
Lucknow, Uttar Pradesh, India

Sanjay Dhiraaj MD
Additional Professor
Department of Anesthesiology
Sanjay Gandhi Postgraduate
Institute of Medical Sciences
Lucknow, Uttar Pradesh, India

Sanjay Singhal MD
Graded Chest Specialist and Intensivist
Command Hospital
Lucknow, Uttar Pradesh, India

Sanjeev Bhoi MD
Additional Professor
Department of Emergency Medicine
JPN Apex Trauma Center
All India Institute of Medical Sciences
New Delhi, India

Sanjeev K Bhoi MD DM
Assistant Professor
Department of Neurology
Sanjay Gandhi Postgraduate
Institute of Medical Sciences
Lucknow, Uttar Pradesh, India

Saswata Bharati MD FIPM
Ex-Assistant Professor
Department of Anesthesiology
Calcutta National Medical College
Kolkata, West Bengal, India

Saurabh Saigal MD IDCC PDCC EDIC
Assistant Professor
Department of Trauma and
Emergency Medicine
All India Institute of Medical Sciences
Bhopal, Madhya Pradesh, India

Saurabh Taneja MD FNB
Consultant
Department of Critical Care Medicine
Sir Ganga Ram Hospital
New Delhi, India

Sumit Ray MD FICCM
Senior Consultant
Department of Critical Care Medicine
Sir Ganga Ram Hospital
New Delhi, India

Sushma Sagar MS FACS
Additional Professor
Department of Trauma Surgery
JPN Apex Trauma Center
All India Institute of
Medical Sciences
New Delhi, India

Usha K Misra MD DM
Professor and Head
Department of Neurology
Sanjay Gandhi Postgraduate
Institute of Medical Sciences
Lucknow, Uttar Pradesh, India

V Darlong MD
Additional Professor
Department of Anesthesiology
All India Institute of Medical Sciences
New Delhi, India

Vandana Agarwal MD FRCA
Associate Professor
Department of Anesthesia,
Critical Care and Pain
Tata Memorial Hospital
Mumbai, Maharashtra, India

Vijai Datta Upadhyaya MS MCh
Associate Professor
Department of Pediatric Surgical
Superspecialty
Sanjay Gandhi Postgraduate
Institute of Medical Sciences
Lucknow, Uttar Pradesh, India

Vikas Agarwal MD DM
Additional Professor
Department of Clinical Immunology
Sanjay Gandhi Postgraduate
Institute of Medical Sciences
Lucknow, Uttar Pradesh, India

Virendra K Arya MD
Visiting Professor
Department of Anesthesia and
Perioperative Medicine
Winnipeg Regional Health Authority
University of Manitoba, Canada
Additional Professor
Cardiac Anesthesia Unit
Advanced Cardiac Center
Department of Anesthesia
and Intensive Care
Postgraduate Institute of Medical
Education and Research
Chandigarh, India

Vishal Shanbhag MD IDCCM
Intensivist
Kasturba Medical College
Manipal University, Manipal, India
Physician and Specialist
Critical Care Medicine
Hamad Medical Corporation
Doha, Qatar

Vivek Ruhela MD
Senior Resident
Department of Nephrology and
Renal Transplantation
Sanjay Gandhi Postgraduate
Institute of Medical Sciences
Lucknow, Uttar Pradesh, India

VN Maturu MD
Senior Resident
Department of Pulmonary Medicine
Postgraduate Institute of
Medical Education and Research
Chandigarh, India

Zafar Neyaz MD
Associate Professor
Department of Radiodiagnosis
Sanjay Gandhi Postgraduate
Institute of Medical Sciences
Lucknow, Uttar Pradesh, India

Foreword

I am confident that the first edition of *Manual of ICU Procedures* will serve as a single source of valuable information to the students and practitioners of critical care. The 61 procedures described in this manual represent the core-competency of intensive care services. All the contributors have provided actionable guidance on how to perform the ICU procedures safely and successfully. Dr Mohan Gurjar has done a marvelous job by maintaining the uniformity in content, style and standard of information for each chapter, beginning with basic principles and progressing to more complex issues. This manual holds a great potential for its extensive educational value.

Arvind Kumar Baronia MD
Professor and Head
Department of Critical Care Medicine
Sanjay Gandhi Postgraduate Institute of Medical Sciences
Lucknow, Uttar Pradesh, India

Preface

As specialty, critical care medicine is now entering in its adulthood, there is a lot of scope for improvement in teaching and training in this field. Critical care medicine is a unique specialty, where the sickest patients are being managed with a wide spectrum of procedures. In fact, there is need of hour to have a book with a compilation of all common procedures being done in critically ill patients for education and training purpose, despite easily available information on individual topic in current era.

Manual of ICU Procedures has 61 chapters, covering almost all relevant procedures, including simple as well as more complex, done in critically and acutely ill patients.

The book has five different sections, such as airway and respiratory procedures, vascular and cardiac procedures, neurological procedures, gastrointestinal/abdominal/genitourinary related procedures; while section miscellaneous covers a few other procedures. This book will be helpful to various clinicians across specialty including critical care physicians, emergency physicians, anesthetists, pulmonologists, pediatricians, general physicians and general surgeons.

The splendid chapters are written by experts with their vast experience and knowledge from various specialties, keeping in mind that it is also intended for the trainee students to help them to understand the procedures. Most of the chapters outline somewhat similar with headings such as introduction, indication, contra-indication, applied anatomy, technique and equipment, preparation, steps of procedure, the post-procedure care, and complication/problem associated with the procedure.

All the procedures described in the book may not be necessarily done by critical care physicians depend upon the local ICU policy, but understanding these procedures will lead towards the optimal management of critically ill patients. As ever-evolving fast information and technology, changes may happen in procedure's technique and equipment, author advice to keep updated on these issues in the future. Readers should also be aware that complications and problems for each procedure are highlighted briefly in the chapter, which may not cover exhaustive list. This is highly recommended by the author that being nature of patients, procedures are supposed to learn under supervision as per local policy, to achieve better skills while taking utmost care for safety to the patient.

The highlighted feature of the book is that procedures are described step by step along with images. I hope that the book will serve as a ready resource in any ICU and emergency room and for all clinicians who are dealing with critically ill patients.

So, have a great satisfaction from treating the sickest patients with better understanding and skill for a safe procedure.

Mohan Gurjar

Acknowledgments

The concept of *Manual of ICU Procedures* is the result of feedbacks from students in critical care medicine about the urgent need of such a book. My inspiration to write a book comes from (Late) Mr NL Verma, a great teacher of Physics in Rajasthan University. With this thought and initial guidance from Professor Amit Agarwal, I met Shri Jitendar P Vij (Group Chairman) of M/s Jaypee Brothers Medical Publishers (P) Ltd, New Delhi, India, who obliged me by accepting this project.

At the beginning of the project, Professor Arvind K Baronia and Dr Afzal Azim helped me with careful selection of the content of the book as well as developing format for the chapters.

I am indebted to all contributors, from various institutes and specialties, without their contribution, the book was not possible. They kept patience with me while making changes in the chapter for improvement and provided good quality images.

I would also like to sincerely thank the production team at M/s Jaypee Brothers Medical Publishers (P) Ltd, New Delhi, India, for their effort to make the book in present form.

Throughout this project, I received much-needed moral support from my colleagues, friends, staffs and students of my department and Sanjay Gandhi Postgraduate Institute of Medical Sciences (SGPGIMS), Lucknow, Uttar Pradesh, India.

I owe for blessings from my parents Dr Ganga Bishan Gurjar and Dr Gulab Gurjar, and also best wishes from my sister Divya Kasana.

Finally, I acknowledge the tolerance and support of my wife Dr Sheetal Gurjar and daughters Ishani and Bhavya during this endeavor, without whom the book could never have been completed.

Acknowledgments

Contents

Section 2 Vascular and Cardiac Procedures

Section 3 Neurological Procedures

Section 4   Gastrointestinal/Abdominal/Genitourinary Procedures

Section 5 Miscellaneous

SECTION 1

Airway and Respiratory Procedures

1

Bag-Mask Ventilation

Ravinder Kumar Pandey, Rakesh Garg, V Darlong

INTRODUCTION

The adequate oxygenation is paramount in a critically ill patient. In such patients, ventilatory assistance with patent airway may be required for optimizing the oxygenation.[1] Effective bag and mask ventilation is an important skill required in such cases. It may not only provide optimal ventilation till the establishment of definite airway but also prove to be life-saving where endotracheal intubation has failed and surgical or other definitive airway management technique has been explored.[2-4] Hence, positive-pressure ventilation using bag-mask-valve device provides positive-pressure ventilation and thus may be life-saving. Though bag and mask ventilation appears to be simplest as well as single most important emergency airway management technique but it has been reported that in 2–5% of patients, bag and mask ventilation is difficult even by experienced anesthesiologists.[5,6] Hence, a good knowledge and understanding of the airway anatomy, airway equipment, skill and regular practice is paramount for effective and successful bag and mask ventilation. The learning curve for bag and mask ventilation has been studied in interns and the authors reported a failure rate of less than 20% after 25 attempts of bag and mask ventilation.[7] This emphasizes the need for training and regular practice to maintain such an important skill of bag and mask ventilation using bag-mask-valve device.

INDICATION

The bag and mask ventilation may be life-saving in critically ill patients.[8] Broadly, the bag and mask ventilation is required for any patient requiring ventilatory assistance to maintain oxygenation till a definitive airway with mechanical ventilation using ventilator is initiated. The indications include:[8,9]
- Preoxygenation prior to securing definitive airway
- Failed tracheal intubation as rescue measure
- During cardiopulmonary resuscitation
- *Respiratory failure:*
  - Failure of ventilation: Central nervous diseases
  - High spinal trauma
  - Neuromuscular diseases
- *Failure of oxygenation:*
  - Increased metabolic demand, sepsis
  - Lung diseases with desaturation

CONTRAINDICATION

Bag-mask ventilation is contraindicated only in a selected group of patients like complete upper airway obstruction or severe facial trauma (due to inadequate mask seal and risk of aspiration due to bleeding). Before initiating bag and mask ventilation, any visible foreign body in oral cavity should be removed. The technique of bag-mask ventilation requires caution in patients with suspected cervical spine instability and should be avoided in patients with full stomach as well as those planned for rapid sequence intubation (RSI).[10-12]

APPLIED ANATOMY AND PHYSIOLOGY

The upper airway comprises of nose oral cavity and pharynx.[2,5,8,9] The pharynx may be further divided into nasopharynx, oropharynx and laryngopharynx. Any insult of these anatomical structures may compromise the passage of airway to glottis and then to lungs. The provision of artificial airway may bypass these structures to maintain passage of the air/oxygen to lungs. The lower airway is made up of trachea, bronchus and its divisions till alveoli. It provides smooth passage of air from upper airway till alveolar capillary membrane for its diffusion into the blood and then to body tissues. Any abnormality in these structures may again compromise the oxygenation of the tissues and cells. Not only these internal complex but also the supportive structures like ribcage (ribs and muscles) and diaphragm may also hamper the transfer of oxygen from outside into the blood.

There are anatomical differences in the airway of children and adults and are important for airway management.[13] The occiput of children is large and when laid supine may lead to neck flexion leading to airway obstruction. The tongue is relatively larger with respect to oral cavity and can cause airway obstruction. Even a trivial trauma in the airway or tongue can lead to edema which may cause airway obstruction. The epiglottis is large and floppy; larynx is more anterior and more angulated. All these airway differences in children make their airway more prone for obstruction and lead to difficult airway management including bag and mask ventilation. Children also have high respiratory rate and oxygen metabolism. They have lesser functional residual capacity and increased chest wall compliance leading to their faster desaturation as compared to adults in cases of any airway compromise.

Ventilation is the movement of air in and out of the lungs. Inspiration is an active process and requires the work of muscles including intercostal muscles and diaphragm. But in cases of labored breathing, certain accessory muscles are also activated to maintain optimal ventilation. On the other hand, exhalation is passive process and may sometimes be an issue in conditions like obstructive lung disease.

The hypoxemia/hypoxia may happen due to inadequate alveolar oxygenation, alveolocapillary diffusion abnormalities, increased dead space, ventilation-perfusion mismatch, or inadequate supply of oxygenated blood to cells. In presence of such problems, supplementing with high concentration of oxygen may temporarily prevent hypoxia at tissue levels till the definitive measures are taken care of. During airway management, oxygen reserves may further be increased with preoxygenation. The preoxygenation can be accomplished by providing 100% oxygen with tight-fitted mask for approximately three minutes or by providing eight vital capacity breaths with 100% oxygen.[14] Bag-valve-mask (BVM) assembly attached with a reservoir and attached to oxygen source may deliver more than 90–100% of inspired oxygen concentration and may be used for preoxygenation. The oxygen source should deliver oxygen with at least a flow of 12–15 L/min.

TECHNIQUE AND EQUIPMENT

The BVM assembly was proposed by a German engineer, Dr Holger Hesse and Danish anesthetist, Henning Ruben in 1953.

The bag and mask ventilation may be required both for conscious and unconscious patient.[14] The unconscious patient should follow basic resuscitation protocols including bag and mask ventilation followed by accomplishment of definitive airway. The adequacy of breathing should be assessed by "look, listen and feel".[15] Patient should be exposed and looked for chest rise (both sides), or any abnormal pattern in breathing movement. The rate, rhythm, quality and depth of breathing movements should be assessed. Listen for any abnormal breath sound like gurgling, gasping, crowing, wheezing, snoring and stridor. Also, auscultation of chest needs to be done for checking the air entry on both sides and for assessing any abnormal breath sound like rhonchi or crepts. Feel for the air movements at the external nares. These assessments should be done in addition to other signs of inadequate oxygenation like presence of cyanosis. The sign of inadequate breathing includes:

- Minimal or uneven chest movements
- Abdominal breathing and noises
- Rate of breathing, too rapid (more than 30 breaths/min) or too slow (less than 10 breaths/min)
- Shallow and labored breathing (use of accessory muscles of breathing)
- Retractions (pulling in of the muscles) above the clavicles and between and below the ribs
- Nasal flaring (widening of the nostrils of the nose with respiration)
- Prolonged inspiration (indicating a possible upper airway obstruction) or
- Prolonged expiration (indicating a possible lower airway obstruction)
- Patient is not able to speak full sentences.

The effective technique of bag and mask ventilation requires appropriate equipment, patient preparation including their positioning and most importantly is appropriate technique using airway adjuncts, if required. A good seal is required along with maintenance of a patent airway. Mask holding can be done by either one-hand technique or two-hand technique (see below). Certain adjuncts like oral or nasal airway may aid in maintaining a patent airway. This is achieved by providing a support to oral structures, especially tongue and thus making the hypopharynx patent for airflow.

Cricoid Pressure (Sellick's Maneuver)

Sellick's maneuver provides external force to the anterior cricoid ring. This compresses the esophagus against the vertebra and prevents air entry into the stomach and also prevents regurgitate entering the airway during positive-pressure ventilation.[16,17] The cricoid ring can be found by palpating the Adam's apple and then identifying the ring just inferior to it. During this maneuver, one person will provide artificial ventilation and the second person will place his two fingers on this ring and firmly press it backward while maintaining the patient's ventilation.[18,19]. However, there are also conflicting reports and some controversies on whether cricoid pressure is really effective. Nevertheless, cricoid pressure is currently recommended and should be performed when possible during resuscitation and all RSIs.[20,21] The excessive force must not be applied so as to avoid tracheal compression leading to airway obstruction. It should be noted that this technique will cause discomfort in the conscious patient and should be limited to those patients who are unconscious. This maneuver should be avoided if the patient is vomiting or begins to vomit.

Bag and Mask Ventilation in Children

The pediatric airway is always challenging due to some anatomical differences as compared to adult airway. This imposes some difficulty in airway management with regards to effective ventilation.[22,23] Children have large occiputs which may make the neck flexed and thus may obstruct the airway. Also, too much extension may cause airway obstruction. To overcome such issues, a roll may be inserted under the shoulder on the back. Children have a relatively large tongue that may fall back into the oropharynx, which can cause airway obstruction. Otherwise innocuous materials like edema, secretions, vomitus or foreign body may obstruct the relatively narrow airway of the children. Any nasal secretions or obstructions may functionally obstruct the airway as infants are obligate nasal breathers.

Usually, airway suctioning is not required for newborns as suctioning may itself delay and hamper adequate oxygenation.[24] This may also cause trauma leading to airway edema in a narrow airway and thus may cause further airway obstruction. But presence of blood clots, vernix, or particulate meconium needs to be cautiously removed without causing undue trauma.

The availability of various sizes of mask makes selection of appropriate mask easier. Some of us prefer circular mask with cushioned rim, as it appears to have better seal with lesser trauma especially to eyes and nose. The adequacy of tidal volume needs to be judged with visible chest rise. As per American Heart Association (AHA) guideline (2010) ventilation rate should be 10–12 per minute irrespective of children age (i.e. same for both children and infant).[25]

Equipment

The following equipment are required for initiating the bag and mask ventilation (Fig. 1):
- *Bag-valve-mask with reservoir:* These are available in various sizes, types and with additional features. The sizes available include newborn, infant, child and adult (Fig. 2). Bag-valve-mask (BVM) comprises of self-inflating bag, a non-rebreathing unidirectional valve, oxygen reservoir, ports for attachment of oxygen and a mask (Fig. 3). The unidirectional valve functions in both spontaneous and mechanical positive-pressure ventilation. The assembly is connected to an oxygen source which delivers oxygen with a minimum flow rate of 12-15 L/min. This technique allows delivery of 90% oxygen.[15] Otherwise, only room air with 21% oxygen is entrained and thus reduces the delivered fraction of oxygen. Facemasks are available in various designs,

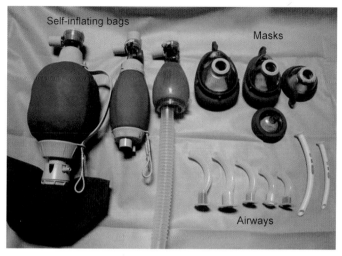

Fig. 1 Equipment required for initiating the bag and mask ventilation

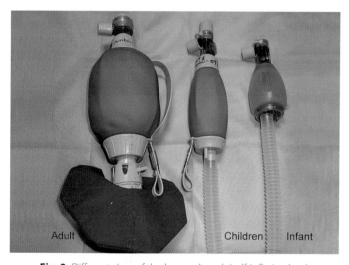

Fig. 2 Different sizes of the bag and mask (self-inflating bag)

sizes and construction materials. The masks are available in both opaque and transparent material but transparent one has a benefit of observing the patient mouth for any secretions or vomitus. The face mask size should be appropriately chosen based on patient size, i.e. the mask is chosen so as to cover the patient's face, i.e. mouth and nose with upper margin over the bridge of nose and lower margin over the chin. The BVM has standard 15/22 respiratory fitting to ensure a proper fit with other respiratory equipment like face masks and endotracheal tubes. The working of BVM includes delivery of oxygen on squeezing the bag through the mask. At this point, the inlet is closed by diaphragm valve. When the squeeze of the bag is released, a passive expiration by the patient will occur. While the patient exhales, oxygen enters the reservoir to be delivered to the patient when next time the bag is squeezed.

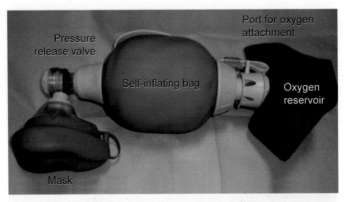

Fig. 3 Parts of the self-inflating bag

In certain bag-mask-valve assemblies, especially in assemblies for infants, there is provision of an adjustable positive end expiratory pressure (PEEP) valve for better positive-pressure ventilation.

- *Airway adjuncts:* Airways like nasal pharyngeal airway (NPA), oral pharyngeal airway (OPA) (Fig. 1) of appropriate sizes along with lubricant (lignocaine jelly). The NPA is inserted into nasopharynx through nares and provides a patent airway. The OPA is inserted into the oral cavity and thus prevents falling back of the tongue and keeps the airway patent. The patient tolerance is better with NPA as compared to OPA. OPA elicits gag reflex and thus the risk of aspiration. On the other hand, NPA should be avoided in patients with fracture base of the skull. The oral airways should be used where gag reflex is absent and/or patient is unconscious as it may illicit coughing, vomiting, and laryngospasm in patients with intact reflexes. In semiconscious patients, the use of nasal airway is desirable. The selection of airway size is also important for both the nasal and oral airway as inappropriate size may further obstruct the airway or may not be of any help.[26] The size is chosen by keeping the OPA adjacent to the face so that it should correspond from angle of mouth to angle of mandible (Figs 4 and 5). The OPA may be inserted by two techniques. In one technique, OPA is inserted into the oral cavity with its concavity facing toward head and rotating it by 180 degrees when resistance to its further insertion is met and then pushing it further. The other technique requires tongue depressor. Here, the tongue is depressed and OPA inserted directly into the oral cavity. The size of NPA is measured from tip of the nose to the tragus of the ear (Figs 6 and 7). The NPA is lubricated and inserted into the more patent nares while facing posteriorly keeping it perpendicular to the face.

PREPARATION

The patient may require bag and mask ventilation to assist the ventilation in cases where equipment for definitive airway is being arranged or in cases where the airway is difficult and conventional technique of securing the airway has failed. To buy time, till the expertise and special equipment like fiberoptic bronchoscopy is being arranged, bag and mask ventilation may be used as rescue technique to maintain oxygenation. The assessment mandating the different

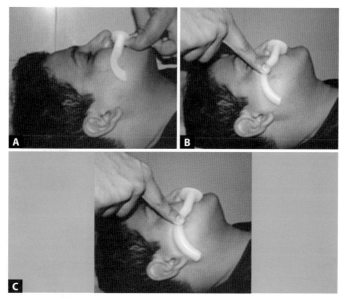

Figs 4A to C Adequacy of oropharyngeal airway size: (A) Small; (B) Correct; (C) Large

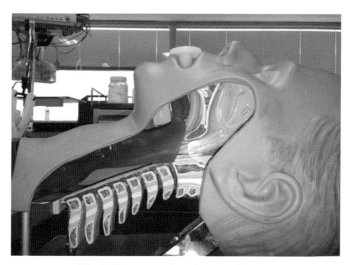

Fig. 5 Placement of oropharyngeal airway

modality of airway assistance has been discussed above. Appropriately done bag and mask ventilation is usually effective. Certain anatomical features give an indication of difficult bag and mask ventilation. These predictors include presence of beard, edentulous patient, a body mass index greater than 26 kg/m², age older than 55 years, and a history of snoring.[14] Other predictors of difficult mask ventilation include oropharyngeal malproportion (Mallampati class III or IV) and limited jaw protrusion.[14]

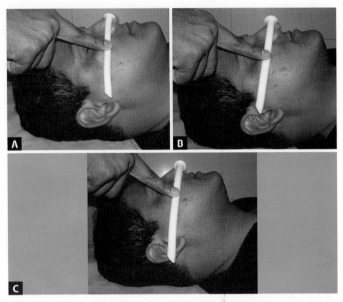

Figs 6A to C Adequacy of nasopharyngeal airway size; (A) Small; (B) Correct; (C) Large

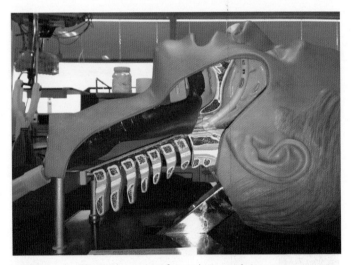

Fig. 7 Placement of nasopharyngeal airway

Apart from BVM assembly and airway adjuncts, other accessory things required for bag and mask ventilation include:
- Oxygen source with an oxygen connecting tubing
- Suction machine and suction catheters
- Universal precaution equipment including eyeglasses, gowns, masks, gloves (Fig. 4). These should preferably be used during patient airway management
- *Monitoring:* Cardiorespiratory monitor, pulse oximeter and capnograph.

PROCEDURE

The key to effective ventilation should follow manual opening of the airway, proper positioning of head and neck, placing an OPA/NPA and effective facemask seal.

- *Universal precautions:* The standard precautions like gloves, mask, and gown (Fig. 8) should be donned.
- *Patient position:* The "sniffing" position (flexion at lower cervical spine and extension at upper cervical spine) is considered the conventional position for ventilation (Fig. 9). It should be avoided in patients with cervical spine instability.[26,27] For optimal position, especially in obese patients, the ear level should be in line with the sternal notch (ear-to-sternal notch position). This position is considered better indicator of optimal alignment of oropharyngeal-laryngeal axis. This may require placement of towel below the shoulder and the back, especially in obese patients. A head tilt may additionally be required.
- *Open the airway:* The opening of the airway may require head-tilt chin-lift maneuver or the jaw thrust. The head-tilt needs to be avoided in patients of cervical spine injuries.
- *Suction:* The oral cavity should be looked for any visible foreign body. If visible, remove the foreign body and perform suctioning for secretions or blood.
- *Airway adjunct:* In cases of airway obstruction due to tongue fall, placement of an airway adjunct like OPA or NPA is required. Use OPA in patients who are unresponsive and do not have a gag reflex. In case of conscious patient with airway obstruction due to tongue fall, placement of an NPA is desirable but should be avoided in events of head injury.
- *Mask holding:*
  - The selection of an appropriate size mask as described above should be made.
  - In one-hand technique, the mask is placed over the face with index and thumb encircling the mask and rest of the three fingers holding the mandible so as to make a tight seal (one-hand EC technique) (Fig. 10).

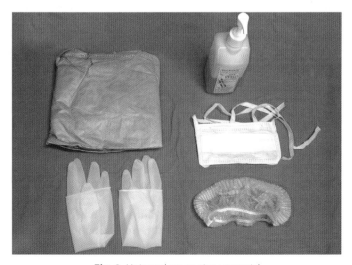

Fig. 8 Universal precautions material

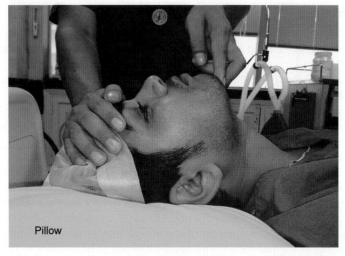

Fig. 9 Head and neck position in a volunteer (pillow below head and head tilt)

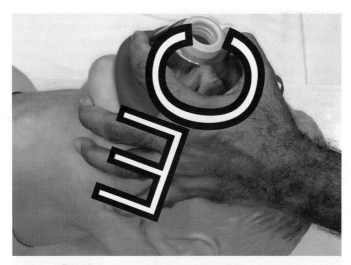

Fig. 10 Technique of mask holding ("EC" technique)

The excessive pressure should be avoided as downward pressure may lead to tongue fall and pressure at submandibular area may also compromise the airway by pushing the tongue against the palate. After optimal mask holding, bag is squeezed with the other hand to observe visible chest rise. In case of difficult ventilation, a two-hand technique can be used (Figs 11 and 12).[27] In this technique, one person holds the mask with both the hands and the other person squeezes the bag for ventilation. The mask holding includes encirclement using thumb and index finger of the both the hands around the mask (Fig. 10). The rest of the three fingers support the mandible and provide jaw thrust while maintaining a good tight seal. The other technique of the mask holding is using the thenar eminences of both the hands over

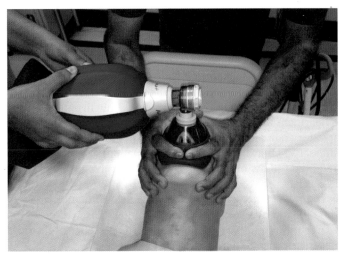

Fig. 11 Two-hand technique of mask holding ("encircling" method)

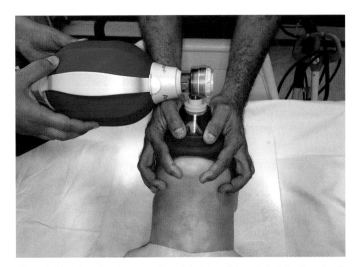

Fig. 12 Two-hand technique of mask holding ("thumb holding" method)

the mask and rest of the fingers lift up the mandible (Fig. 12). Here as well, the other person squeezes the bag to provide mechanical ventilation.

- *Ventilation:*
  - Ensure the bag is attached to oxygen source with oxygen turned on to a flow of 15 L/min. Allow the reservoir to fill with oxygen prior to the first ventilation. After achieving adequate mask seal, self-inflating bag is squeezed so as to have visible chest rise. Also, look for any gastric distension. In that case, patient needs to be repositioned, so that air does not go to stomach. During resuscitation, squeeze it over 1 second and wait for expiration to happen which is a passive procedure. For optimal and effective ventilation, good mask seal and adequate bag squeezing

is required. However, over and aggressive bag-mask ventilation causes stomach inflation and increases the risk of aspiration. The goal is to achieve adequate gas exchange while keeping the peak airway pressures low. Squeezing the bag forcefully and abruptly creates a high-peak airway pressure and is more likely to inflate the stomach.

- For effective ventilation, tidal volume required is 6–7 mL/kg per breath.[28] The respiratory rate is kept at 10–12 breaths/min in patients with functioning heart. On the other hand, for patients with cardiopulmonary arrest, respiratory rate required is 8–10 breaths per minute. In case of respiratory distress, BVM may be used to assist the patient respiratory efforts. If PEEP is required (adults only) connect the PEEP valve firmly to the expiratory flow diverter.

- *Assessment of adequacy of ventilation:* Effective ventilation and oxygenation should be judged by chest rise, breath sounds, pulse oximeter (SpO_2), and exhaled CO_2 monitoring (capnography).[29,30] The presence of gastric distension indicates gastric insufflation during BMV.

- *Pearls:*
  - Avoid pushing the mask downward for better seal.
  - Change of mask of different size may sometimes give a better seal.
  - Dentures may leave in place for better mask seal. Be careful for their dislodgement.
  - Patients with facial hair, beard, apply some water-soluble jelly for better seal.
  - Two-handed technique may be used in cases of ineffective mask ventilation with one-hand technique.

In case of ineffective bag and mask ventilation, laryngeal mask airway (LMA) may be required for optimal ventilation till a definitive control of airway is done.

Procedure Steps for Children

- *Open and clean the airway.*
  - Careful head extension: Excessive extension of neck needs to be avoided to prevent obstruction of the airway.
  - The mouth is opened and gentle suction of the oral cavity is done once or twice.
- Make a mask seal.
- Ventilation is initiated to target a visible chest rise for optimal ventilation. Observe any gastric inflation.
  - In case of ineffective ventilation: Recheck an optimal mask seal if leak is observed.
  - Patient positioning needs adjustment with optimal jaw thrust and avoiding excessive downward pressure or over the mandible.
  - OPA, NPA or LMA may be inserted if the problem of ineffective ventilation persists.
- The effectiveness of ventilation is confirmed by observing:
  - Increase in heart rate to more than 100 beats/min
  - Visible chest rise
  - Rise in saturation.

COMPLICATION/PROBLEM

The main concerns of bag and mask ventilation remain ineffective ventilation. This may lead to gastric insufflation, increased risk of regurgitation and aspiration. Other complications include damage to cornea due to pressure on the eyes and may lead to blindness due to ischemia. Other soft tissue injuries to nose, lips may also occur. The systemic body changes may also occur due to excessive or underventilation. The risk of barotrauma and cardiovascular effects like vagal response and hypotension are also associated with inappropriate bag and mask ventilation.

Problems and Troubleshooting

In cases of ineffective BMV, check:
- *Equipment:*
  - Supply of oxygen
  - Appropriateness of bag and valve mechanism
  - Adequacy of size and seal of the mask
  - Need of airway adjunct like OPA, NPA and LMA
- *Patient:*
  - Clinical differential diagnosis
  - Position:
    - Ear-sternal notch position
    - Chin lift, jaw thrust
- *Technique:* Need of two-person technique.

REFERENCES

1. Kallstrom TJ. AARC Clinical Practice Guideline: Oxygen therapy for adults in the acute care facility—2002 revision and update. Respir Care. 2002;47:717.
2. Levitan R. Mask ventilation, rescue ventilation, and rescue intubation. In: Levitan R (Ed). The Airway Cam Guide to Intubation and Practical Emergency Airway Management. Wayne, PA: Airway Cam Technologies, Inc. 2004. p. 49.
3. McGee J, Vender J. Nonintubation management of the airway: Mask ventilation. In: Hagberg C (Ed). Benumof's Airway Management, 2nd edition. Philadelphia: Mosby. 2007. p. 345.
4. Yentis SM. Predicting difficult intubation—worthwhile exercise or pointless ritual? Anaesthesia. 2002;57:105.
5. Kheterpal S, Han R, Tremper KK, Shanks A, Tait AR, O'Reilly M, et al. Incidence and predictors of difficult and impossible mask ventilation. Anesthesiology. 2006;105: 885-91.
6. Langeron O, Masso E, Huraux C, Guggiari M, Bianchi A, Coriat P, et al. Prediction of difficult mask ventilation. Anesthesiology. 2000;92:1229-36.
7. Komatsu R, Kasuya Y, Yogo H, Sessler DI, Mascha E, Yang D, et al. Learning curves for bag-and-mask ventilation and orotracheal intubation: an application of the cumulative sum method. Anesthesiology. 2010;112:1525-31.
8. Ortega R, Mehio AK, Woo A, Hafez DH. Positive-pressure ventilation with a facemask and a bag-valve device. N Engl J Med. 2007;357:e4.
9. Sagarin MJ, Barton ED, Chng YM, Walls RM. Airway management by US and Canadian emergency medicine residents: a multicenter analysis of more than 6,000 endotracheal intubation attempts. Ann Emerg Med. 2005;46:328.

10. Gausche M, Lewis RJ, Stratton SJ, Haynes BE, Gunter CS, Goodrich SM, et al. Effect of out-of-hospital pediatric endotracheal intubation on survival and neurological outcome: a controlled clinical trial. JAMA. 2000;283(6):783-90.

11. Schneider R, Murphy M. Bag/mask ventilation and endotracheal intubation. In: Walls R, Murphy M (Eds). Manual of Emergency Airway Management, 2nd edition. Philadelphia: Lippincott Williams & Wilkins. 2004. pp. 43-51.

12. McGee J, Vender J. Nonintubation management of the airway: mask ventilation. In: Hagberg C (Ed). Benumof›s Airway Management, 2nd edition. Philadelphia: Mosby. 2007. p. 345.

13. Chua C, Schmolzer GM, Davis PG. Airway maneuvers to achieve upper airway patency during mask ventilation in newborn infants: historical prospective. Resuscitation. 2012;83:411-6.

14. Pandit JJ, Duncan T, Robbins PA. Total oxygen uptake with two maximal breathing techniques and the tidal volume breathing technique: a physiologic study of preoxygenation. Anesthesiology. 2003;99:841-6.

15. The American Heart Association in Collaboration with the International Liaison Committee on Resuscitation. Guidelines 2000 for Cardiopulmonary Resuscitation and Emergency Cardiovascular Care. Part 6: Advanced cardiovascular life support: Section 3: Adjuncts for oxygenation, ventilation and airway control. Circulation. 2000;102:95.

16. Sellick BA. Cricoid pressure to control regurgitation of stomach contents during induction of anaesthesia. Lancet. 1961;2:404.

17. Petito SP, Russell WJ. The prevention of gastric inflation—a neglected benefit of cricoid pressure. Anaesth Intensive Care. 1988;16:139.

18. Levitan RM. The Airway Cam Guide to Intubation and Practical Emergency Airway Management. Wayne, Pa: Airway Cam Technologies, Inc. 2004. pp. 49-54.

19. Brimacombe JR, Berry AM. Cricoid pressure. Can J Anaesth. 1997;44:414.

20. Dutton R, McCunn M. Anesthesia for trauma. In: Miller R (Ed). Miller's Anesthesia, 6th edition. Philadelphia: Elsevier. 2005. pp. 2451-95.

21. Suresh M, Munnur U, Wali A. The patient with a full stomach. In: Hagberg C (Ed). Benumof's Airway Management, 2nd edition. Philadelphia: Mosby. 2007. p. 756.

22. American Heart Association Guidelines for Cardiopulmonary Resuscitation and Emergency Cardiovascular Care. Circulation. 2005;112:51-7.

23. Grein AJ, Weiner GM. Laryngeal mask airway versus bag-mask ventilation or endotracheal intubation for neonatal resuscitation. Cochrane Database Syst Rev. 2005;2:CD003314.

24. Carrasco M, Martell M, Estol PC. Oronasopharyngeal suction at birth: effects on arterial oxygen saturation. J Pediatr. 1997;130:832-4.

25. Travers AH, Rea TD, Bobrow BJ, Edelson DP, Berg RA, Sayre MR, et al. Par 4: CPR overview: 2010 American Heart Association Guidelines for Cardiopulmonary Resuscitation and Emergency Cardiovascular Care. Circulation. 2010;122(18 Suppl 3): S676-84.

26. Meier S, Geiduschek J, Paganoni R, Fuehrmeyer F, Reber A. The effect of chin lift, jaw thrust, and continuous positive airway pressure on the size of the glottic opening and on stridor score in anesthetized, spontaneously breathing children. Anesth Analg. 2002;94:494.

27. Joffe AM, Hetzel S, Liew EC. A two-handed jaw-thrust technique is superior to the one-handed "EC-clamp" technique for mask ventilation in the apneic unconscious person. Anesthesiology. 2000;113:873-9.

28. Dörges V, Ocker H, Hagelberg S, Wenzel V, Schmucker P. Optimisation of tidal volumes given with self-inflatable bags without additional oxygen. Resuscitation. 2000;43:195.

29. Maneker AJ, Petrack EM, Krug SE. Contribution of routine pulse oximetry to evaluation and management of patients with illness in a pediatric emergency department. Ann Emerg Med. 1995;25:36.

30. Lee WW, Mayberry K, Crapo R, Jensen RL. The accuracy of pulse oximetry in the emergency department. Am J Emerg Med. 2000;18:427.

2

Endotracheal Intubation

Pradeep Bhatia

INTRODUCTION

Endotracheal intubation is the most commonly performed procedure in the intensive care unit (ICU), in which a tube is placed into the trachea to maintain an open airway, to allow the free flow of air to and from the lungs in unconscious patients and in trauma patients who cannot maintain a patent, protected airway; and also to support ventilation, who are unable to breathe adequately on their own. Airway control is vital to improve pulmonary gas exchange during hemodynamic instability and respiratory failure, as well as to protect the patient from aspiration. Oral or nasal airways are often used to keep the airway patent temporarily during preparation for endotracheal intubation. Oxygen, anesthetics or some medications can also be delivered through the tube.

INDICATION

- Cardiac arrest
- Respiratory arrest
- Airway obstruction
- Imminent risk of upper airway obstruction (e.g. upper airway burns)
- Facial injuries associated with compromised airway
- Altered mental status for protection from aspiration
- Head injury [Glasgow coma scale (GCS <8)]
- Need to control and remove pulmonary secretions
- Need for invasive ventilation in respiratory failure with inadequate oxygenation (which is not corrected by oxygen supplementation through mask/nasal cannula) or inadequate ventilation and hypercarbia
- Severe hemodynamic instability and shock
- General anesthesia with muscle relaxants.

CONTRAINDICATION

For Both Oral and Nasal Intubations

- Patients with an intact gag reflex
- Partial transection of the trachea (can lead to complete transection)
- Patients with high-risk of laryngospasm during intubation (e.g. children with epiglottitis)

- Caution with unstable cervical spine that requires in-line cervical stabilization makes endotracheal intubation difficult (relative contraindication)
- Severe airway trauma or obstruction providing very small area to place the endotracheal tube (ETT) as attempts to intubate may worsen the condition resulting in severe respiratory obstruction. Emergency cricothyrotomy/tracheostomy is indicated in such cases (relative contraindication).

For Nasal Intubation

- Basilar skull fracture and cerebrospinal fluid (CSF) rhinorrhea
- Nasal polyp, abscess, adenoids or foreign body
- Bleeding disorders
- Previous nasal surgery is only relative contraindication.

APPLIED ANATOMY

The upper airway (Fig. 1) starts at the nostrils/oral cavity, to the hypopharynx and larynx. The high vascular areas of nasal and septal mucosa, the little's area and the Kiesselbach's plexus may bleed profusely during nasal route intubation especially in presence of bleeding disorder. The epiglottis is attached to the base of the tongue by a median and two lateral glossoepiglottic folds. The larynx is a 5–7 cm long structure. Its upper boundary starts at the tip of the epiglottis, opposite the third to fourth cervical vertebra. Its lower end is at the lower border of the cricoid cartilage, which lies at the level of sixth cervical vertebra. The structural rigidity of the larynx is provided by the three median cartilages: the epiglottis, thyroid cartilage and cricoid cartilage along with the hyoid bone. The six smaller cartilages of the larynx (3 pairs) are functionally involved with the movements of the vocal cords (Fig. 2). These are the arytenoids, the corniculates and the cuneiforms. The arytenoid cartilages are pyramid-shaped and articulate with the superior margin of the cricoid lamina. On their summit, are the corniculate cartilages; on their anterior aspect, the cuneiform cartilages. The vocal ligaments are attached posteriorly to the apex of the arytenoids and corniculates. The cuneiforms extend laterally, between the layers of the vocal cords, from the anterior aspect of the arytenocorniculate complex. The trachea is a membranous and D-shaped cartilaginous tube, with incomplete cartilaginous ring and extends from the lower part of the larynx, at the level with the sixth cervical vertebra, up to the upper border of the fifth thoracic vertebra, where it ends by dividing into the two bronchi, one for each lung. It is about 11 cm long and its diameter is greater in the male (25–27 mm) than in the female (21–23 mm).

TECHNIQUE AND EQUIPMENT

In 1885, Joseph O'Dwyer, an American pediatrician and obstetrician, inserted metal tubes between the vocal cords in patients with diphtheria and in patients requiring surgery. The first direct laryngoscopy was performed in 1895 by Alfred Kirstein with an external light source. In 1913, Chevalier Jackson designed a laryngoscope and was the first to perform intubation with it. Laryngoscope was later modified by Magill, Miller and Macintosh.[1,2]

The traditional and most commonly used method of intubation is oral intubation using direct laryngoscopy. Nasal intubation in ICU is better tolerated

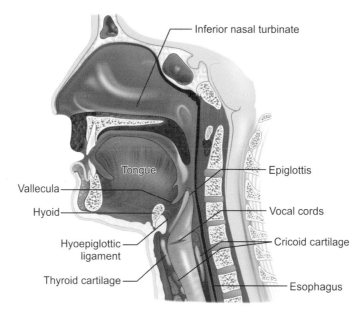

Fig. 1 Upper airway anatomy

Source: With permission from http://www.airwaycam.com

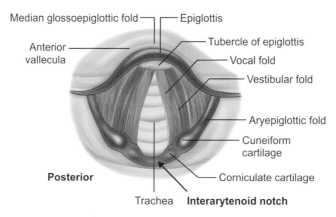

Fig. 2 Laryngoscopic view of glottis

Source: With permission from http://www.airwaycam.com

than oral tube, requires less sedation and leaves the oral cavity clear to maintain oral hygiene. The disadvantages of nasal intubation are—it is more difficult than oral intubation and may result in bleeding due to the rich blood supply to the nasal mucosa. A nasal tube may create a false passage beneath nasal mucosa, or in patients with basal skull fractures, into the cranium. If kept for a long time, nasal tube may be associated with infection of the paranasal air sinuses. Other methods of intubation include blind nasal intubation, intubation using video laryngoscope, intubating laryngeal mask airway (LMA) and fiberoptic techniques.

Equipment

Most commonly used ETTs are made out of polyvinyl chloride and have a radiopaque line that helps verify the tube position by X-ray. To make it easier to pass through the vocal cords and to give you a better vision ahead of the tip, ETTs tip have a cut called a bevel. Some ETTs have an additional opening at the tip called a Murphy's, which provides an alternative channel for gas flow, if the main opening of the ETT gets blocked or placed against the tracheal wall. The ETT cuff forms a seal against tracheal wall that prevents gas leaking during positive pressure ventilation and also prevents aspiration of secretions and regurgitated gastric contents. There are two types of cuff. High-volume, low-pressure cuffs have a lower risk of tracheal wall ischemia and necrosis compared to low-volume high-pressure cuffs, particularly if used for a prolonged period of time. In long-term ventilated patients, subglottic secretions can accumulate above the cuff of the ETT that provides medium for bacterial growth and increases the risk of ventilator-associated pneumonia (VAP). Especially designed tubes are available that permits frequent or continuous elimination of subglottic secretions to decrease the risk of VAP.

PREPARATION

Adjunct Equipment

- Intravenous access
- Electrocardiography (ECG), pulse oximeter and end-tidal carbon dioxide (EtCO$_2$) monitors
- Suction machine and catheters
- Oropharyngeal, nasopharyngeal airways (Figs 3 and 4, respectively)
- Non-rebreathing mask
- Oxygen source (15 L/minute flow)
- Bag valve mask
- Appropriate size ETTs (*Adults:* 7.5 mm; *Children:* Size roughly equal to the diameter of little finger) (Fig. 5) and a 10-cc syringe
- Stylet, Magill's forceps, Bougie (Figs 6 to 8, respectively)
- Laryngoscope blades, different types (Figs 9A to C)
- Adhesive tape.

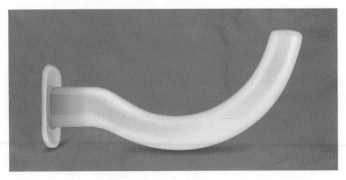

Fig. 3 Oropharyngeal airway
Source: Fexicare

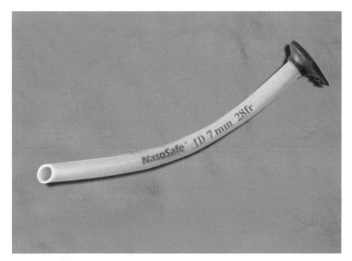

Fig. 4 Nasopharyngeal airway
Source: Fexicare

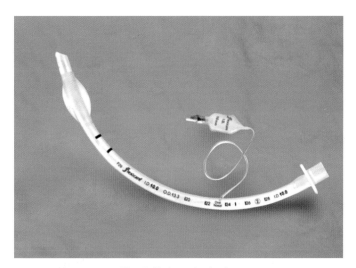

Fig. 5 Endotracheal tube
Source: Fexicare

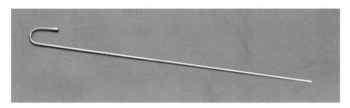

Fig. 6 Stylet
Source: Fexicare

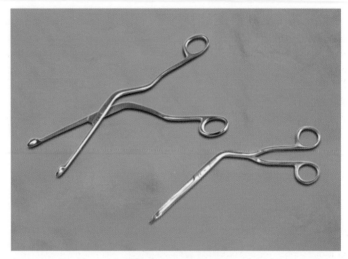

Fig. 7 Magill forceps
Source: Fexicare

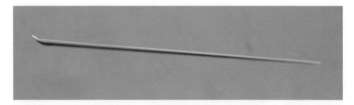

Fig. 8 Bougie
Source: Fexicare

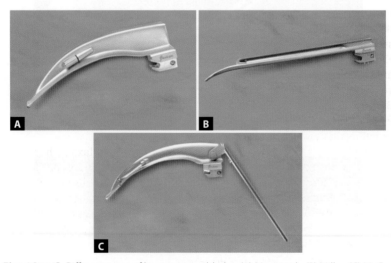

Figs 9A to C Different types of laryngoscope blades. (A) Macintosh; (B) Miller; (C) McCoy
Source: Fexicare

Assess Airway

Carefully observe for the landmarks, swelling or any deformity. Assess tongue size, dental obstruction and the degree of neck mobility. Remove dentures.

Mallampati classification is generally performed to assess upper airway access. This test is performed while the patient is in the sitting position, awake and cooperative. This may not always be possible in the ICU settings.
Ask the patient to open mouth and protrude tongue.

Class I: Visualization of the soft palate, fauces, uvula and pillars. No anticipated difficulty.

Class II: Visualization of the soft palate, fauces, uvula. No anticipated difficulty.

Class III: Visualization of the soft palate and base of the uvula. Anticipate moderate difficulty.

Class IV: Soft palate is not visible. Anticipate severe difficulty.

A seven-item simplified score (MACOCHA score) for identifying patients with difficult intubation in the ICU and related complications is developed.[3] The main predictors of difficult intubation are related to patient (Mallampati score III or IV, obstructive sleep apnea syndrome, reduced mobility of cervical spine, limited mouth opening); pathology (severe hypoxia, coma); and operator (nonanesthesiologist).

Drugs

The patient in ICU may be restless, agitated and delirious and may require sedation/short anesthesia and relaxant for intubation. The commonly used drugs for intubation in ICU are:

- Propofol (2–2.5 mg/kg) causes bradycardia, myocardial depression and reduced systemic vascular resistance and is usually avoided in critically ill patients with potential hemodynamic instability.
- Etomidate (0.2–0.6 mg/kg) possesses the best hemodynamic profile of all the induction agents, has rapid onset and short half-life but may cause suppression of adrenocortical function.
- Ketamine (1–2 mg/kg) produces a state of dissociative anesthesia, profound analgesia, and amnesia but causes hallucinations, delirium, nausea and vomiting. Ketamine has been advocated for intubation in ICU.[4]
- Besides anesthetic agents mentioned above, midazolam (0.05 mg/kg), fentanyl (1–2 mg/kg) and dexmedetomidine (1 mg/kg) are also used for sedation/analgesia during endotracheal intubation.
- Succinylcholine (1 mg/kg) is a depolarizing muscle relaxant, has a rapid onset and short duration of action and is recommended for intubation in ICU settings provided there are no contraindications to its use like the possibility of cannot ventilate—cannot intubate situation and the risk of hyperkalemia.
- Rocuronium (0.6 mg/kg) is a nondepolarizing muscle relaxant and compared to succinylcholine, it has fewer side effects but is associated with less optimal intubation conditions and has a longer duration.
- The use of muscle relaxants for intubation is reported to be associated with fewer complications, including in patients with difficult airways.[5]

Monitoring

Electrocardiogram (heart rate, rhythm, ST changes), blood pressure, pulse oximetry and $EtCO_2$.

PROCEDURE

Position of the Patient

- Maintain cervical spine stability, if necessary.
- The patient should lie supine with a pillow under the head.
- To visualize the larynx, all the three anatomic axes (oral, pharyngeal and laryngeal) should be aligned, which is done by extension of atlanto-occipital joint and flexion of lower cervical joints so that the ETT passes from the lips to the glottis opening in almost a straight line.
- *Unless contraindicated*, (i.e. suspected cervical injury) elevate the patient's head by approximately 10 cm with pads or a pillow under the occiput and extend the head into the sniffing position so as to align the oral, pharyngeal and laryngeal axes (Figs 10A to C).

Procedure

- The operator should wear gloves, a gown and goggles
- Stand at the supine patient's head end
- Preoxygenate with 100% oxygen to prevent arterial desaturation during intubation, if possible, should be done
- *Use artificial airways, if needed:* Oropharyngeal, nasopharyngeal during bag-mask ventilation
- Open the patient's mouth and remove foreign material, if any, manually or by suction. Perform chin lift and jaw thrust maneuver
- Separate lips and pull the upper jaw to open the patient's mouth
- Hold a laryngoscope in the left hand and gently insert the blade of laryngoscope into the mouth of the patient being careful not to break a tooth, directing the blade toward the right tonsil
- On reaching the right tonsil, sweep the laryngoscope blade to the midline and keep the tongue to the left to view the epiglottis
- Advance the laryngoscope blade up to the angle between the base of the tongue and the epiglottis
- Lift the laryngoscope upward and forward, without changing the angle of the blade, to expose the vocal cords. Often an assistant applies backward, upward rightward pressure (the BURP maneuver) on the cricoid cartilage to get the full view of the glottis
- Hold the ETT in the right hand keeping its concavity toward the right side. Insert the tube through the mouth opening
- Continue inserting the tube till it passes through the vocal cords which is approximately at 20–22 cm mark on the ETT
- Remove stylet
- Inflate the cuff with 5–10 mL air using a syringe allowing minimal leak on manual ventilation (cuff pressure should be kept between 20–30 cm H_2O, using a cuff pressure manometer to prevent tracheal ischemic changes).

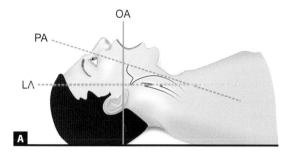

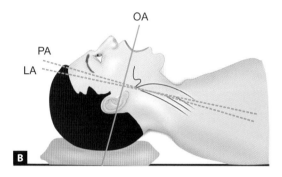

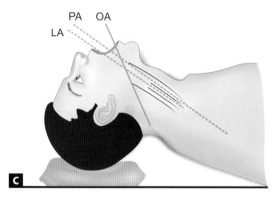

Figs 10A to C Alignment of three axes (LA, Laryngeal axis; PA, Pharyngeal axis; OA, Oral axis) for intubation

- Ventilate manually
- Confirm the correct placement of the ETT by:
  - Directly visualizing the passage of the tube through the vocal cords
  - Condensation of water vapors in the tube with respirations
  - Movement of the chest with respirations
  - Bilaterally auscultating the chest
  - Auscultation over the stomach to rule out the gurgling sound
  - End-tidal CO_2 monitoring
  - Improving oxygen saturation

- Clinical improvement of the patient
- Chest X-ray anteroposterior (AP) view in a semierect or supine position keeping the patient's head in the neutral position and confirm that the tip of the ETT is 2 cm above the carina
- Secure tube (3 methods—Twill tape, adhesive tape and tube fastener devices that prevents the formation of lip ulcers and has better access to the oral cavity to optimize oral care) (Fig. 11).

Difficult Intubation

An intubation is called difficult, if normally trained anesthesiologists need more than three attempts or more than 10 minutes for a successful endotracheal intubation. Intubations in the ICU are more likely to be difficult than intubations in theater. In the ICU settings; it is often difficult to visualize the glottis due to space constraints, uncooperative patient and the accompanying comorbidities. Multiple attempts of endotracheal intubation, often required in ICU, may increase the risk of airway edema, trauma, hemorrhage and vomiting leading to difficulty in intubation.

Alternatives

Alternatives to conventional laryngoscopy and orotracheal intubation include and should be considering in case of difficult/failed intubation:
- Nasotracheal intubation
- Endotracheal intubation using the videolaryngoscope/bronchoscope
- Esophageal tracheal combitube (ETC)
- Laryngeal mask airway
- Tracheostomy
- Cricothyrotomy (for an emergency).

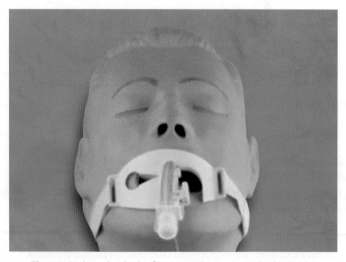

Fig. 11 Endotracheal tube fixation with commercial tube holder
Source: Fexicare

POST-PROCEDURE CARE

Once the position of the ETT is confirmed, it should be reassessed periodically because the ETT can migrate over time as a consequence of coughing, suctioning and movement. The clinical examination to confirm the correct ETT placement like chest auscultation for breath sounds, symmetrical chest expansion and palpable tube cuff in the suprasternal notch may be inaccurate in the ICU settings. Hence, daily chest X-rays are done at many centers to verify tube position. However, studies suggest a more restrictive approach (e.g. chest radiographs only in response to a change in clinical condition) to decreases the number of chest radiographs without worsening clinical outcomes.

Routine change of ETT every 1–2 weeks, to decrease the incidence of complications (given here) is not recommended as the process itself may lead to silent aspirations and nosocomial pneumonia.

COMPLICATION/PROBLEM

Tracheal intubation procedure in ICU settings is more complex compared to that done in the operation theater (OT). In the OT, intubation is associated with a low rate of complication as it is done by a trained anesthesiologist, generally in a stable patient with good physiological reserve. Conversely, high incidence of failure and complications are associated with intubation in the ICU, where airway tools may not be readily available. In ICU settings, intubation is done often by a junior doctor with little or no training of intubation, as an emergency, in a critically ill patient with precarious hemodynamic and respiratory status. There is under-evaluation of the airways and suboptimal response to preoxygenation. In addition, many drugs used during intubation are associated with adverse hemodynamic effects.[6]

Following complications may occur during intubation in ICU:

- Injury to teeth, soft tissue (lips, pharyngeal tissue), arytenoid cartilages, larynx and related structures
- Nasal intubation may be associated with damage to turbinates, bleeding and nasopharyngeal mucosal perforation
- Airway edema, bleeding, tracheal and esophageal perforation, laryngospasm causing a complete airway obstruction
- Barotrauma due to absence or malfunction of pressure release valve, pneumothorax, subcutaneous emphysema
- Endotracheal tube obstruction by a foreign body, dry respiratory secretions or blood clots causing collapsed lung
- Severe hypoxia because of central respiratory dysfunction, deranged chest wall mechanics, or intrapulmonary ventilation/perfusion abnormalities that may induce hypoxic arrhythmias on intubation
- Endobronchchial intubation (ETT inserted too far)
- Esophageal intubation, if remain undiagnosed, will result in gastric distension and regurgitation on attempting ventilation (possibly leading to hypoxemia, hypercapnia and death), vomiting and aspiration
- Bradycardia, sympathetic stimulation resulting in hypertension and tachycardia [dangerous in a patient with intermittent hemodialysis (IHD)] cardiac arrhythmias

- Cardiovascular collapse due to hypovolemia, vasodilatation, myocardial depression and suppression of sympathetic response by anesthetic drugs used for intubation, and due to the negative effects of positive pressure ventilation on venous return, prophylactic intravenous crystalloid administration may prevent, these adverse cardiovascular effects
- Endotracheal tube cuff damage that may result in inadequate seal and leak
- Microorganisms may colonize and multiply on the inner surface of the ETT and subsequently develop biofilms. These biofilms are resistant to antibiotic penetration may act as source of pulmonary infection and development of VAP.

To decrease complications related to endotracheal intubation in the ICU, Samir Jaber et al.[7] developed an intubation care bundle management system based on a review of the ICU airway literature.

Intubation Care Bundle Management[7]

Preintubation

- Presence of two operators
- Fluid loading (isotonic saline 500 mL or starch 250 mL) in absence of cardiogenic pulmonary edema
- Preparation of long-term sedation
- Preoxygenation for 3 minutes with noninvasive positive pressure ventilation (NIPPV) in case of acute respiratory failure [fraction of inspired oxygen (FiO_2) 100%, pressure support ventilation level between 5 and 15 cm H_2O to obtain an expiratory tidal volume between 6 and 8 mL/kg and positive end-expiratory pressure (PEEP) of 5 cm H_2O].

During Intubation

- *Rapid sequence induction:* Etomidate 0.2–0.3 mg/kg or ketamine 1.5–3 mg/kg combined with succinylcholine 1–1.5 mg/kg in absence of allergy, hyperkalemia, severe acidosis, acute or chronic neuromuscular disease, burn patient for more than 48 hours and medullar trauma.
- Sellick's maneuver (cricoid pressure of 20–44 N to occlude the esophagus, preventing regurgitation and subsequent aspiration of gastric contents during intubation).

Postintubation

- Immediate confirmation of tube placement by capnography
- Norepinephrine, if diastolic blood pressure remains below 35 mm Hg
- Initiate long-term sedation
- *Initial "protective ventilation":* Tidal volume 6–8 mL/kg of ideal body weight, PEEP 5 cm H_2O and respiratory rate between 10 and 20 cycles/minutes, FiO_2 100% for a plateau pressure less than 30 cm H_2O.

The implementation of an endotracheal intubation care bundle management in the ICU may reduce the incidence of life-threatening complications occurring within the first hour after intubation from 34–21%. Severe hypoxemia and cardiovascular collapse incidences, which were the main life-threatening complications after intubation, were reduced by half in the intervention group compared to the control group.[7]

REFERENCES

1. Szmuk P, Ezri T, Evron S, Roth Y, Katz J. A brief history of tracheostomy and tracheal intubation, from the Bronze Age to the Space Age. Intensive Care Med. 2008;34(2):222-8.
2. Burkle CM, Zepeda FA, Bacon DR, Rose SH. A historical perspective on use of the laryngoscope as a tool in anesthesiology. Anesthesiology. 2004:100(4):1003-6.
3. Jaber S, Amraoui J, Lefrant JY, Arich C, Cohendy R, Landreau L, et al. Clinical practice and risk factors for immediate complications of endotracheal intubation in the intensive care unit: a prospective, multiple-center study. Crit Care Med. 2006;34(9):2355-61.
4. Jabre P, Combes X, Lapostolle F, Dhaouadi M, Ricard-Hibon A, Vivien B, et al. Etomidate versus ketamine for rapid sequence intubation in acutely ill patients: A multicentre randomised controlled trial. Lancet. 2009;374:293-300.
5. De Jong A, Molinari N, Terzi N, Mongardon N, Arnal JM, Guitton C, et al. Early Identification of Patients at Risk for Difficult Intubation in the Intensive Care Unit: development and validation of the MACOCHA score in a multicenter cohort study. Am J of Respir Crit Care Med. 2013;187(8):832-9.
6. Divatia JV, Khan PU, Myatra SN. Tracheal intubation in the ICU: Life saving or life threatening? Indian J Anaesth. 2011;55(5):470-5.
7. Jaber S, Jung B, Corne P, Sebbane M, Muller L, Chanques G, et al. An intervention to decrease complications related to endotracheal intubation in the intensive care unit: a prospective, multiple-center study. Intensive Care Med. 2010;36(2):248-55.

3
Laryngeal Mask Airway Insertion

Neeta Bose

INTRODUCTION

The laryngeal mask airway (LMA) is a novel device that is an intermediate between tracheal intubation and a facemask. It is blindly inserted into the pharynx, forming a low-pressure seal around the laryngeal inlet and permitting gentle positive-pressure ventilation. It allows oxygenation and ventilation and also the administration of inhaled anesthetics, with minimal stimulation of the airway.[1,2]

INDICATION

- Prehospital airway management
- Cardiac arrest [American Heart Association (AHA) 2010 guidelines indicate that supraglottic devices like the LMA can be used instead of intubation]
- During elective ventilation for short duration instead of bag-mask ventilation
- *Difficult airway:* LMA is an important part of difficult airway algorithm
- As a rescue device after a failed attempt at intubation
- In a situation of cannot be intubated, but can be ventilated, LMA can be used instead of bag-mask ventilation[3]
- In *cannot ventilate, cannot intubate (CVCI)* situation, when a surgical airway is indicated, LMA insertion can easily be attempted quickly, while preparing for cricothyroidotomy[4]
- In "CVCI" situations, one can ventilate through the LMA and also it forms a passage for intubation
- Fastrach LMA and LMA CTrach are useful, especially in patients with cervical spine injury.

CONTRAINDICATION

Absolute Contraindications
(In Emergency as well as Elective Settings)
- No mouth opening
- Severe upper airway obstruction.

Relative Contraindications (In the Elective Setting)

- Increased risk of aspiration (prolonged bag-valve-mask ventilation, morbid obesity, symptomatic hiatus hernia, second or third trimester pregnancy, patients who have not fasted before ventilation, upper gastrointestinal bleed, acute abdominal or thoracic surgery, multiple or massive injury)
- Abnormal anatomy for supraglottic airway
- Need for high airway pressures [in all but the Pro-Seal LMA (PLMA), pressure cannot exceed 20 cm H_2O for effective ventilation]
- Patients with low pulmonary compliance and pulmonary fibrosis.

APPLIED ANATOMY

The basic design of any LMA is that it forms the mirror image of the laryngeal inlet (Fig. 1).

The design of the laryngeal mask is such that the distal part facing the larynx forms a seal around the laryngeal inlet (Fig. 4) and side walls of the mask faces toward the pyriform fossa.[5]

TECHNIQUE AND EQUIPMENT

The LMA was designed by Dr Archie Brain in 1981. He had developed the LMA in search of and easier to use and more effective device than the facemask and less invasive than an endotracheal tube (ETT). The LMA was available for commercial use in the United Kingdom in 1988 and within 12 months it was in use in more than 500 British hospitals.[5] The LMA family and their chronological order of clinical use is as follows: Classic LMA (1988), Flexible LMA (1991), Intubating LMA (1997), Disposable (Unique) (1998), Pro-Seal LMA (2000); Pediatric or PLMA (2004), LMA CTrach (2006), LMA Supreme (Disposable PLMA) (2007).

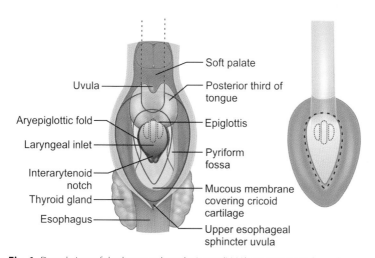

Fig. 1 Dorsal view of the laryngeal mask airway (LMA) superimposed on pharynx

Advantages and Disadvantages of LMA

Advantages

- More secure than facemask and reduces potential damage to eyes and facial nerve
- Rapidity and ease of placement, particularly for the inexperienced operators; blind, rapid and atraumatic insertion versus ETT
- Hemodynamic stability on induction and during
- Lesser drugs for maintenance and airway tolerance; no muscle relaxant required—useful in myasthenia gravis, etc. Emergence is smooth due to lesser coughing
- Due to no tube in situ, there is lesser incidence of sore throat
- Less impact on mucociliary clearance than an ETT, hence lower incidence of retention of secretions, atelectasis, pulmonary infection[6]
- *Bailey's maneuver:* Device is inserted behind an ETT while patient is still deeply anesthetized. ETT is removed then and patient is allowed to emerge from anesthesia with LMA device in place.

Disadvantages

- Inability to seal the larynx and protect against aspiration, gastric insufflations and air leak with positive-pressure ventilation[7]
- Magnitude of insufflation depends on airway pressure and position of LMA. In a large series, it has been shown that positive-pressure ventilation with the LMA is both safe and effective, with no episodes of gastric dilatation in 11,910 patients.[8]

Classic Laryngeal Mask Airway

Laryngeal mask airway has a curved tube which is connected to an elliptical mask at an angle of 30° (Fig. 2). An inflatable cuff surrounds the inner rim of the mask.

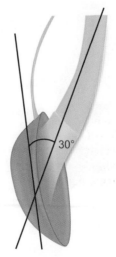

Fig. 2 30° angle between the shaft and the mask

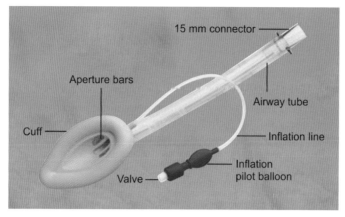

Fig. 3 Parts of the classic laryngeal mask airway
Source: LMA International

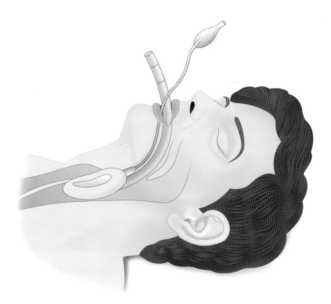

Fig. 4 Laryngeal mask airway (LMA) positioned at the laryngeal inlet

A self-sealing pilot balloon is attached to the proximal wider end of the mask via an inflation tube. At the junction of the tube and the mask, there are two vertical bars. They prevent obstruction of the tube by keeping the epiglottis off the lumen. There is black line running longitudinally on the posterior side of the tube. There is a 15-mm connector at the proximal end of the tube. The LMA is made from silicone (Fig. 3).

The shape of the LMA is such that it forms a seal around the larynx and is a mirror image of the hypopharynx (Fig. 4). The walls of the long axis of the mask facing toward the pyriform fossa.[5]

LMA Sizes and Cuff Inflation

Generally, the size 4 is for adult females and size 5 for males up to 100 kg. There is a new size 6 for adult patients over 100 kg (Table 1).

LMA Insertion Technique

- *Standard technique:* Details as described here under procedure
- *180° technique:* Another technique is to insert the LMA with the laryngeal aperture pointing cephalad and rotate it 180° as it enters the hypopharynx.[9,10] This method may be as satisfactory as the standard technique especially in pediatric patients.
- *Partial inflation technique:* Inflate the cuff partially or fully before insertion.[11,12] This may be useful for an inexperienced user, but there may be possibility of malpositioning.[13]
- *Thumb insertion technique:* This is useful when standing at the head end is difficult or impossible. The LMA is held with the thumb in the position occupied by the index finger, while using the standard technique. The LMA is advanced with the thumb entering the mouth, rest of the fingers are stretched over the patient's face. The thumb is advanced to the fullest and before removing, the tube is pushed into its final position with the other hand. Maintaining pressure with the finger on the tube in the cranial direction, advance the mask until definite resistance is felt at the base of hypopharynx; note flexion of the wrist.
- *Laryngoscopic-guided LMA insertion:* Insertion by the standard method versus laryngoscopic-guided method does not have any significant difference as regards to the ease of insertion, hemodynamic instability, local trauma and sore throat. Although, ease of insertion is greater in the classical technique with less incidence of blood tinge, it is inferred that the laryngoscopic-guided LMA insertion is reasonable option in situations like doubling over of the LMA, increased pharyngeal tone, tonsillar hypertrophy, high-arched palate and large floppy epiglottis.[14]
- *Laryngeal mask airway insertion in prone position:* In one study, as opposed to the traditional approach, classic LMA (cLMA) has been used successfully in patients who need controlled ventilation during short, moderate and even long duration surgeries in prone position, involving 100 patients, without

Table 1 Laryngeal mask airway sizes and corresponding weight of patients

LMA size	Patient selection guidelines	Maximum cuff inflation volume (mL)
1	Neonates/infants up to 5 kg	4
1½	Infants 5–10 kg	7
2	Infants/children 10–20 kg	10
2½	Children 20–30 kg	14
3	Children 30–50 kg	20
4	Adults 50–70 kg	30
5	Adults 70–100 kg	40
6	Adults over 100 kg	50

compromising the safety.[15] It requires experience and appropriate patient selection to introduce LMA in prone position, especially in the setting of ambulatory surgery to induce and maintain anesthesia.[16]

Variants of LMA

LMA Classic Excel

This is an improved version of the cLMA. It has an epiglottic elevating bar and a removable connector for easy insertion of the endotracheal tube (ETT) through the LMA. This improved design facilitates intubation and can be used up to 60 times. It is latex-free and has a soft silicone cuff, hence less of throat irritation and stimulation, allowing intubation up to a size 7.5 ETT.

Flexible LMA

The LMA flexible (Fig. 5) has the original LMA cuff design along with a wire-reinforced tube, which is narrower and longer. Due to its flexibility it can be diverted away from the surgical field without its lumen getting occluded, thereby useful for head and neck, mouth, throat and nasal surgeries. It is not possible to intubate through this device as the airway tube is longer and narrower. While insertion, a stylet is required in the airway tube to stiffen it. A single-use disposable version is also available.

Pro-Seal LMA

The PLMA has four main parts: cuff, inflation line with pilot balloon, airway tube and the drain tube (gastric access) (Fig. 6). Modifications in the Pro-Seal as compared to the cLMA are (Figs 7A to D):
- The airway tube is reinforced and flexible; this minimizes kinking
- Larger and deeper bowl with no aperture bars; hence chances of migration of the epiglottis into the distal lumen become less

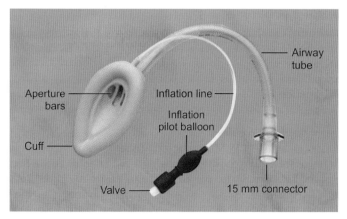

Fig. 5 Flexible laryngeal mask airway (LMA)
Source: LMA International

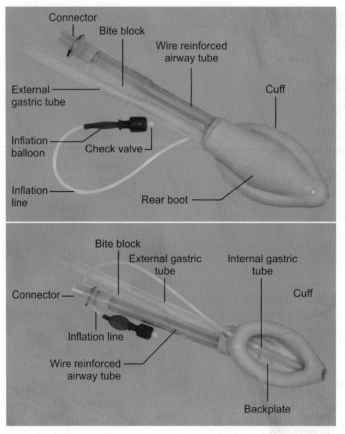

Fig. 6 Parts of the Pro-Seal laryngeal mask airway
Source: LMA International

- There is availability of double cuff, second one being the posterior extension of the cuff around the mask. The second cuff improves the sealing property of the device
- Drainage tube/esophageal conduit runs along the airway tube and exits at the mask tip, hence providing access to the esophagus to minimize chances of aspiration
- Integral silicone bite-block prevents bite-induced airway obstruction and tube destruction
- Anterior pocket/slot for seating an introducer or finger during insertion (Fig. 8).

Advantages of the modifications
- The correct position of PLMA is such that the opening faces the glottis and the drainage tube tip is positioned behind the cricoid, at the beginning of the esophagus. Hence, the respiratory and gastrointestinal tracts remain functionally separate and this is an important advantage of the PLMA in comparison to cLMA

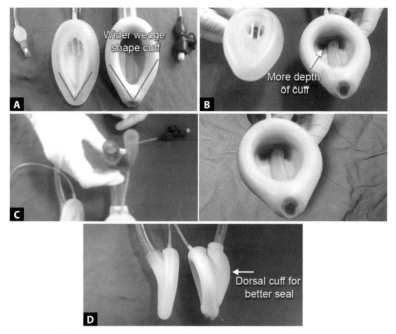

Figs 7A to D Differences between classic and Pro-Seal laryngeal mask airway. (A) Wider wedge shaped cuff; (B) Depth of the cuff is more; (C) Large bore gastric channel; (D) Dorsal cuff for better seal

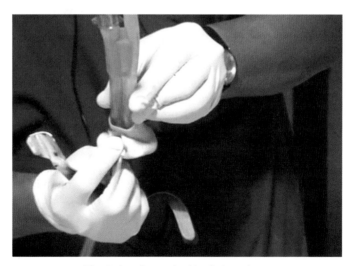

Fig. 8 Anterior pocket/slot for introducer

- The dual-tube arrangement forms a better seal and there are lesser chances of malplacement
- An orogastric tube can be inserted through the drain tube
- Channeling of regurgitated stomach contents away from the respiratory tract[17]
- During controlled ventilation, there is lesser chances of stomach inflation

- The presence of drainage tube in the design makes it possible for diagnosis of mask misplacement quickly
- Due to the built in bite block, lesser chances of airway obstruction/tube damage
- Can be used for spontaneous as well as controlled ventilation, hence suitable for laproscopic surgeries.

Pro-Seal LMA drawbacks
- Less suitable for intubation due to the narrow airway tube
- It is more difficult to insert than the cLMA.

Size selection for Pro-Seal LMA (Table 2)

Table 2 All sizes of Pro-Seal laryngeal mask airway

PLMA size	Patient size	Maximal cuff inflation volume (mL)	Max diameter orogastric tube
1½	5–10 kg	7	10
2	10–20 kg	10	10
2½	20–30 kg	14	14
3	30–50 kg	20	16
4	50–70 kg	30	16 Fr (5.5 mm)
5	70–100 kg	40	18 Fr (6.0 mm)

Note: Sizes 1½–2½ have no dorsal cuff[18]

LMA Supreme

The LMA supreme (Fig. 9) is a disposable device. The tube is elliptical in cross-section and the shape is in perfect fit with the oropharyngeal anatomy, with the distal end placed at the laryngeal inlet. Intubation is not possible due to this elliptical shape. The two lateral grooves in the tube prevent its kinking on flexing. The cuff has molded fins which prevent epiglottis from downfolding and the tip of the cuff is reinforced to avoid folding during insertion. The drain tube is a separate tube, which forms a channel with the upper esophageal sphincter and a well-lubricated orogastric tube can be negotiated through the drain tube to empty stomach contents. It is easy to insert and does not move along with head movement. The built-in bite-block prevents damage.

Fastrach Intubating LMA

The Fastrach intubating LMA (FT-LMA) was designed by Dr Archie Brain in 1997, following difficulty in passing the ETT through the cLMA, for this purpose he had used the magnetic resonance imaging (MRI) scans of adult airways.[19,20] The FT-LMA can provide ventilation through the airway lumen and an ETT can be passed through the same to negotiate into the trachea.

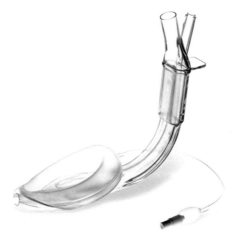

Fig. 9 Laryngeal mask airway (LMA) supreme
Source: LMA International

In comparison to the cLMA, the FT-LMA has following differentiating features:
- The airway tube is rigid, anatomically curved and silicone coated. This allows insertion with patient's head in neutral position/any position viz sitting position trapped in car, thus great advantage in suspected neck injury
- An integrated metal guiding handle
- Airway tube is shorter and wider than cLMA
- Oxygenation possible simultaneously with intubation
- There is an epiglottic elevating bar (versus the vertical bars in cLMA) for lifting the epiglottis, for smooth entry of ETT
- The mask aperture has a guiding ramp[19]
- Specially designed noncurved ETT with atraumatic tip should be used (Parker-flexi tip) (Fig. 10)
- *Chandy's maneuver:* Gentle lifting of device 2–5 mm for intubation provides good alignment of the trachea and the ETT
- Airway tube is not transparent so check inside for particulate matter. Extra care should be taken to clean the tube with soft nylon bristle brush
- Single use LMA Fastrach is also available.

Due to the above-mentioned features, the mask aligns well with the glottis opening and also provides a conduit for ETT. The reusable ETTs are available in size 3, 4 and 5. Disposable versions are also available. Contraindications for Fastrach LMA are lack of skill and non-fasted patient.

LMA CTrach

Laryngeal mask airway CTrach is similar to intubating LMA (ILMA), with facility of continuous video endoscopy of the distal end.[21,22] It comprises of anatomically shaped LMA, epiglottic elevating bar, fiberoptic channels and detachable LCD viewer. The larynx can be viewed directly and one can visualize the process of endotracheal intubation through the LMA. The fiberoptic channels are two in number, one for light conduction and the other for conveying the image. The insertion of the CTrach is similar to the LMA Fastrach, but once it is placed

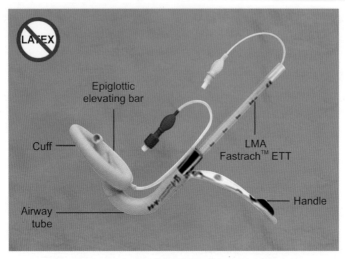

Fig. 10 Components of FasTrach laryngeal mask airway
Source: LMA International

in situ, the viewer is switched on to obtain an image of the larynx. The entry of the ETT into the larynx can be visualized and after intubation, the viewer and the mask are removed leaving.

PREPARATION

- The airway assessment for difficult esophagogastroduodenoscopy (EGD) insertion permits the provider to make appropriate airway management plans. "RODS" is a mnemonic that can identify the problem patients when EGD is being considered.
  - Restricted mouth opening—depending on the EGD, a minimum oral access may be needed, for example, at least 2 cm mouth opening is required to insert a LMA Fastrach[23]
  - Obstruction—one cannot bypass any upper airway obstruction at the level of larynx or below
  - Disrupted or distorted airway—the placement and the seal of the EGD may be difficult[24]
  - Stiff lungs and stiff cervical spine—ventilation may become impossible due to increased airway resistance (e.g. asthma) or decreased pulmonary compliance (e.g. pulmonary edema). In deformities where the neck is in fixed flexion, seal may not be possible.[24] There may be difficulty in LMA insertion in patients of restricted neck movement (e.g. ankylosing spondylitis).[25]
- *Performance test (preuse check):* Before use of LMA, the following steps have to be carried out to check for usefulness:
  - *Visual test:* Examine for transparency of the tube; cut/tear on the surface; aperture for intact structure.
  - *Inflation/Deflation:* Carefully deflates the cuff to see whether it remains flattened or not (do not use the device, if it gets spontaneously inflated even slightly). The cuff should be inflated from the fully deflated state to 50% more air than the maximum capacity and watch for any leak.

PROCEDURE

Standard Technique of LMA Insertion

Standard technique of LMA insertion is described in details as here; while other modified techniques are briefly described under technique heading.

- Midline or slightly diagonal approach with the cuff fully deflated into a smooth "spoon-shape" and wrinkle-free distal edge (Fig. 11), which could be done with the help of a cuff-deflator or by pressing with fingers to flatten the cuff.
- Head should be extended and the neck flexed (sniffing position).[26] This position is best maintained during insertion by using the noninserting hand to stabilize the occiput (Fig. 12). LMA insertion can be done without the sniffing position,[27] but lesser chances of success.[28,29] The jaw may be pulled down by an assistant to open the mouth.
- The index finger is placed at the junction of the mask and the tube and it is held like a pen (Fig. 13). The black line faces the patient's upper lip; the cuff tip is placed along the hard palate. In the patient with restricted mouth opening an alternative method is to pass the LMA behind the molar teeth into the pharynx and later maneuver the tubular part toward the midline.[30]
- The LMA is inserted with the index finger and sliding it against the hard palate. If there is any resistance, it may be due to tip infolding or impaction on the posterior pharynx or some irregularity. In this case, finger may be placed posterior to the mask to relieve the obstruction. If at any time during insertion the mask fails to stay flattened or starts to fold back, is should be withdrawn and reinserted.
- As the mask tip encounters the posterior pharyngeal wall (which can be perceived as a change of direction), the other fingers are withdrawn and the index finger is advanced further downward, along with slight pronation of the forearm (Fig. 14). If this maneuver is not successful, the tube is held with the other hand and straightened; it is then pushed down quickly and gently till a resistance is encountered.

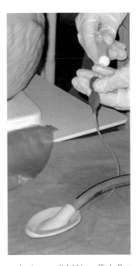

Fig. 11 Laryngeal mask airway (LMA) cuff deflated into spoon shape

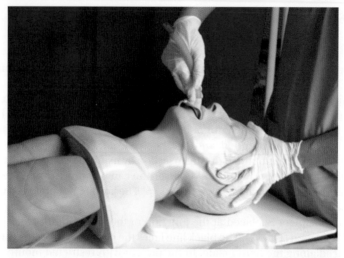

Fig. 12 To assist the laryngeal mask airway (LMA) introduction, the middle finger is pressed onto the jaw

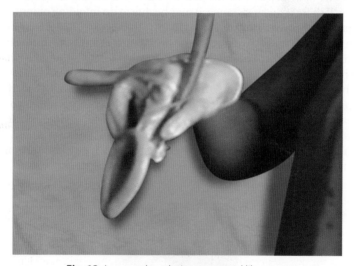

Fig. 13 Laryngeal mask airway grasped like a pen

- The position of the black line on the shaft should be in the midline, facing the upper lip (Fig. 15).
- There can be problems while passing the LMA around the angle at the back of the tongue; this is due to wrong approach. The inserting finger should continuously press against the palate (Fig. 16).
- When initial insertion is unsuccessful, a number of maneuvers may be helpful which include inserting the LMA from the corner of the mouth and then pulling the tongue forward; a jaw thrust; repositioning the head; can be done.[14,31-33]

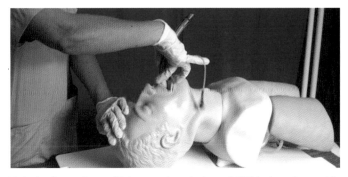

Fig. 14 Index finger along with laryngeal mask airway (LMA) being advanced forward

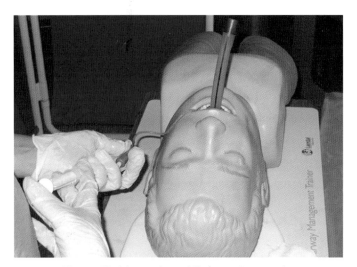

Fig. 15 Black line in the middle facing the upper lip

- When properly placed, the mask rests on the floor of the hypopharynx. The side of the mask faces the pyriform fossa and the upper part of the cuff lies behind the base of the tongue (Fig. 1). The epiglottis tip may lie in the bowl of the mask or near the proximal cuff, depending on the angle at which the mask has deflected.[34]

Ideal Position

- *Distal cuff:* In hypopharynx
- *Sides:* Facing pyriform fossa
- *Post-cuff and back plate:* Resting against posterior pharyngeal wall
- *Proximal cuff:* Base of the tongue
- *Tube:* Goes along posterior oropharynx, soft palate, hard palate and teeth
- *Epiglottis:* Flattened between proximal cuff lies abuts base of the tongue.

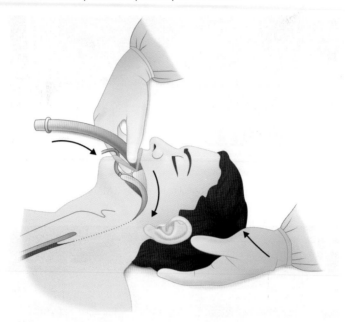

Fig. 16 Maintain pressure against the palate

Tracheal Intubation with LMA Classic

The LMA can be used as a passage through which an ETT, stylet or fiberscope is passed.[35,36]

Blind

Intubation can be done blindly through the LMA, success rate being variable depending upon technique, time, patient's head manipulation, operator's experience, number of attempts and the tracheal tube used.[37,38]

Epiglottis downfolding can be a major problem while going in blind, hence fiberoptic assessment is recommended. If downfolding occurs, maneuvers like moving the LMA up and down without cuff deflation or withdrawing the mask about 5 cm, followed by reinsertion, along with the jaw thrust may help.[39]

A well-lubricated ETT is introduced in the LMA; it is rotated 15–90° anticlockwise as it is advanced to prevent the bevel from catching on the bars. After crossing the bars, the bevel is turned clockwise and with slight extension of the neck, the tip passes anterior to the arytenoids. The ETT is then advanced and on meeting resistance, the head is flexed to allow the tube to advance into the trachea. Alternately, LMA can be introduced by preloading the lubricated ETT inside, with the tip at the level of the bars so that the tube can pass smoothly through the aperture.

If the ETT does not enter the trachea, neck flexion and extension at atlanto-occipital joint may be helpful. The LMA cuff can be deflated and the pushed a little farther into the hypopharynx. A stylet, bougie or exchange catheter can be introduced into the LMA, over which the ETT can be inserted.[40-42]

Fiberscope Guided

The LMA classic can be used to aid fiberoptic-guided intubation. A lubricated endotracheal tube is loaded over the fiberscope and then advanced through the LMA. A bougie or guide can be inserted with the help of the fiberscope through the LMA, after which it can be removed to be replaced with a tracheal tube and it can be inserted into the trachea [43,44]

POST-PROCEDURE CARE

Confirming Placement

- Confirm the position of the LMA by auscultation for breath sounds and absence of sounds at the epigastrium, observing chest rise with ventilation and placing an end-tidal carbon dioxide ($EtCO_2$) to look for color change
- Make sure the black line on the tube lies on the patient's midline (Fig. 16)
- Assess for ability to generate up to 20 cm of water pressure without a leak.

Fixation

- To prevent biting of the patient, a bite-block or a roll of gauze can be inserted
- The LMA can be secured with a tape, similar to what is used for ETTs (Fig. 17).

Sterilization

- Only disposable varieties of LMA are supplied in sterile pack
- All other LMA and accessories should be sterilized by autoclaving at 135°C for 3–4 minutes
- Only steam autoclaving is recommended
- Ensure complete dryness and deflate the cuff before autoclaving (no air or moisture should remain in the cuff)

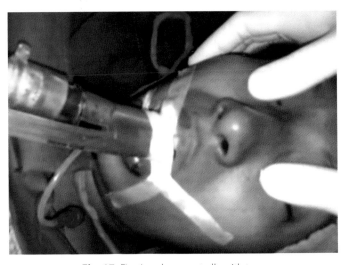

Fig. 17 Fixation done centrally with tape

- Allow to cool to room temperature before use
- The recommendation for PLMA is up to 40 sterilizations.[18]

COMPLICATION/PROBLEM

- Functional—Failure (0.3–4%)
  - Malposition (20–30%)
  - Inadequate seal (<5%)
  - Gastric insufflation (0.5%)
  - Regurgitation (0.1–8%)
  - Aspiration (0.01%)
- Pathophysiological—Hemodynamic changes
- Airway morbidity—Sore throat (10%)
  - Dysphagia (4–24%)
  - Dysarthria (4–40%)
  - Ear pain (1%)
  - Coughing (<2%)
- More sore throat with larger LMA and on spontaneous breathing
- More discomfort with more cuff volume
- Insertion in prone position does not appear to increase morbidity.

ACKNOWLEDGMENTS

I would heartily acknowledge the cooperation and help extended by my ex-colleagues, Dr Hemlata Kamat (Professor and Head), Dr Madhvi Choudhari (Associate Professor), Dr Hitendra Kanzariya (IIIrd year Resident), especially for the photographs, which were taken at our Institute, Shri Krishna Hospital, Karamsad, Gujarat, by our team. I also acknowledge the help extended by colleagues from the Difficult Airway Gujarat group, Dr Apex Patwa and Dr Amit Shah, to help with some photographs. Without the help of the above-mentioned people, it would not possible to go ahead with this chapter.

REFERENCES

1. Brain AI. The laryngeal mask: a new concept in airway management. Br J Anaesth. 1983;55(8):801-5.
2. Maltby JR, Loken RG, Watson NC. The laryngeal mask airway: clinical appraisal in 250 patients. Can J Anaesth. 1990;37(5):509-13.
3. Miller RD. Miller's Anesthesia, 6th edn. Philadelphia, Pa: Elsevier Churchill Livingstone; 2005. pp. 1625-8.
4. Walls RM. Manual of Emergency Airway Management. Philadelphia, Pa: Lippincott Williams and Williams. 2004. pp. 97-109.
5. Brain AI. The development of the laryngeal mask: a brief history of the invention, early clinical studies and experimental work from which the laryngeal mask evolved. Eur J Anaesthesiol Suppl. 1991;4:5-17.
6. Keller C, Brimacombe J. Bronchial mucous transport velocity in paralyzed anaesthetized patients: a comparison of the laryngeal mask airway and cuffed tracheal tube. Anesth Analg. 1998;86(6):1280-2.
7. Brimacombe J. The advantages of the LMA over the tracheal tube or facemask: a meta-analysis. Can J Anaesth. 1995;42(11):1017-23.
8. Verghese C, Brimacombe JR. Survey of Laryngeal Mask Airway Usage in 11,910 Patients: Safety and Efficacy for Conventional and Nonconventional Usage. Anesth Analg. 1996;82(1):129-33.

9. Payne FB, Wilkes NC. A prospective study of two insertion techniques of the laryngeal mask airway. Anesthesiology. 1996;85:A2.
10. Soh CR, Ng AS. Laryngeal mask airway insertion in paediatric anaesthesia: comparison between the reverse and standard techniques. Anaesth Intensive Care. 2001;29(5): 515-9.
11. Matta BF, Marsh DS, Nevin M. Laryngeal mask airway: a more successful method of insertion. J Clin Anesth. 1995;7(2):132-5.
12. Wakeling HG, Butler PJ, Baxter PJC. The laryngeal mask airway: a comparison between two insertion techniques. Anesth Analg. 1997;85(3):687-90.
13. Ferson D. Laryngeal mask airway: its role in anesthetic practice (ASA Refresher course), Dallas: ASA. 1999.
14. Koay CK, Yoong CS, Kok P. A randomized trial comparing two laryngeal mask airway insertion techniques. Anaesth Intensive Care. 2001;29(6):613-5.
15. Vijay Kumar, K Lalitha, Talib Lone. The use of classic laryngeal mask airway inserted in prone position for controlled ventilation: a feasibility study. Indian J Anaesth. 2008; 52(6):813-7.
16. Ng A, Raitt DG, Smith G. Induction of anesthesia and insertion of a laryngeal mask airway in the prone position for minor surgery. Anesth Analg. 2002;94(5):1194-8.
17. Brain AI, Verghese C, Strube PJ. The LMA 'ProSeal': a laryngeal mask with an oesophageal vent. Br J Anaesth. 2000;84:650-4.
18. Cook TM, Lee G, Nolan JP. The ProSeal™ laryngeal mask airway: a review of the literature. Can J Anesth. 2005;52(7):739-60.
19. Brain AI, Verghese C, Addy EV, Kapila A. The intubating laryngeal mask: Development of a new device for intubation of the trachea. Br J Anaesth. 1997;79(6):699-703.
20. Brain AI, Verghese C, Addy EV, Kapila A, Brimacombe J. The intubating laryngeal mask. II: a preliminary clinical report of a new means of intubating the trachea. Br J Anaesth. 1997;79:704-9.
21. Liu EH, Goy RW, Chen FG. The LMA CTrach, a new laryngeal mask airway for Endotracheal intubation under vision: evaluation in 100 patients. Br J Anaesth. 2006;96(3):396-400.
22. Brimacombe J. Intubating LMA for airway intubation. In: Brimacombe J (Ed). Laryngeal Mask Anesthesia. Philadelphia: Saunders. 2005. pp. 469-504.
23. Teoh WH, Lim Y. Comparison of the single use and reusable intubating laryngeal mask airway. Anaesthesia. 2007;62(4):381-4.
24. Buckham M, Brooker M, Brimacombe J, Keller C. A comparison of the reinforced and standard laryngeal mask airway: ease of insertion and the influence of head and neck position on oropharyngeal leak pressure and intracuff pressure. Anaesth Intensive Care. 1999;27(6):628-31.
25. Olmez G, Nazarogle H, Arslan SG, Özyılmaz MA, Turhanoğlu AD. Difficulties and failure of laryngeal mask insertion in a patient with ankylosing spondylitis. Turk J Med. 2004;34:349-52.
26. Asai T, Morris S. The laryngeal mask airway: its features, effects and role. Can J Anaesth. 1994;41:930-60.
27. Pennant JH, Pace NA, Gajraj NM. Role of the laryngeal mask airway in the immobile cervical spine. J Clin Anesth. 1993;5:226-30.
28. Brimacombe J, Berry A. Laryngeal mask airway insertion. A comparison of the standard versus neutral position in normal patients with a view to its use in cervical spine instability. Anaesthesia. 1993;48:670-1.
29. Asai T, Neil J, Stacey M. Ease of placement of the laryngeal mask during manual in-line stabilization. Br J Anaesth. 1998;80:617-20.
30. Maltby JR, Loken RG, Beriault MT, Archer DP. Laryngeal mask airway with mouth opening less than 20 mm. Can J Anaesth. 1995;42:1140-2.
31. Aoyama K, Takenaka I, Sata T, Shigematsu A. The triple air way manoeuvre for insertion of the laryngeal mask airway in paralyzed patients. Can J Anaesth. 1995;42:1010-6.

32. Fukatome T. Correct positioning of the epiglottis for application of the brain laryngeal mask airway. Anaesthesia. 1995;50:818-9.

33. Dingley J, Asai T. Insertion methods of the laryngeal mask airway. A survey of current practice in Wales. Anaesthesia. 1996. pp. 596-9.

34. DuPlessis MC, Barr AM, Verghese C, Lyall JR. Fiberoptic bronchoscopy under general anaesthesia using the laryngeal mask airway. Eur J Anaesth. 1993;10:363-5.

35. Zagnoev M, McCloskey J, Martin T. Fiberoptic intubation via the laryngeal mask airway. Anesth Analg. 1994;78:813-4.

36. Sartore DM, Kojima RK. Laryngeal mask airway-assisted, wire-guided fiberoptic tracheal intubation. Anesthesiology. 1994;81(6):1550-1.

37. Rabb MF, Minkowitz HS, Hagberg CA. Blind intubation through the laryngeal mask airway for management of the difficult airway in infants. Anaesthesiology. 1996;84:1510-1.

38. Benumof JL. Laryngeal mask airway and the ASA difficult airway algorithm. Anaesthesiology. 1996;84:686-99.

39. Murashima K, Fukutome T. Jaw thrust manoeuvre for repositioning the epiglottis down folded by the ILM. Anaesthesia. 2000;55:921-2.

40. Brimacombe J, Berry A. Placement of a Cook airway exchange catheter via the laryngeal mask airway. Anaesthesia. 1993;48:351-2.

41. Ahmed AB, Nathanson MH, Gajraj NM. Tracheal intubation through the laryngeal mask airway using a gum elastic bougie: the effect of head position. J Clin Anesth. 2001;13:427-9.

42. Higgs A, Clark E, Premraj K. Low-skill fibreoptic intubation: use of the Aintree catheter with the classic LMA. Anaesthesia. 2005;60:915-20.

43. Cook TM, Silsby J, Simpson TP. Airway rescue in acute upper airway obstruction using a ProSeal laryngeal mask airway and an Aintree catheter: a review of the Pro-Seal laryngeal mask airway in the management of the difficult airway. Anaesthesia. 2005;60:1129-36.

44. Walburn MB, Corner J, Ryder IG. Fiberoptic intubation through a laryngeal mask airway facilitated by a guidewire. Anaesthesia. 2000;55:1027-8.

4

Fiberoptic Intubation

Amol Kothekar, JV Divatia

INTRODUCTION

Fiberoptic intubation with preserved spontaneous breathing is considered the safest and most effective technique for elective intubation in patients with an anticipated difficult airway. Difficult intubation might be encountered in intensive care unit (ICU) patients due to various reasons. Most importantly ICU patients are never optimized compared to operation theater (OT) patients and reversing patient and postponing intubation is not an option. So anticipation is the key. Every intensivist should be aware of indication/contraindications and comfortable with procedure of fiberoptic bronchoscopic (FOB) intubation. FOB gives easy access to upper and lower airway without need of general anesthesia. Hence, use of FOB has been extended to confirm endotracheal (ET) tube as well as double lumen tube placement, visualization of trachea in preoperative or postextubation stridor, and to diagnose ET blockage by secretions, kinking of tube or cuff herniation. Successful FOB intubation requires time, skill, and preparation. It is a combination of art and science with approach tailored to particular patient and situation.

INDICATION

- Difficult airway
  - History of difficult intubation
  - Anticipated difficult intubation
    - Limited mouth opening
    - Thyromental distance less than 4 cm
    - Large tongue
    - Involvement of base of tongue with tumor with inability to protrude tongue
    - Restricted neck extension due to any cause
    - Compression of airway due to infection, tumor, edema, hematoma
    - Previous tracheostomy or prolonged intubation
- Unanticipated failed intubation
- Morbid obesity
- When awake intubation in a conscious patient is preferred
  - High risk of aspiration
  - Movement of neck not desirable like cervical spine instability or fracture
  - Known difficult mask ventilation

- – Morbid obesity
- – Self-positioning
- – Patients with airway obstruction
- To prevent dental damage
  - – Fragile or protuberant teeth
  - – Expensive dental restorations
- Fiberoptic bronchoscopic for tube exchange (To change ET tube to a new one)
- To minimize incidence and severity of hypoxia in patients requiring high positive end-expiratory pressure (PEEP) and fraction of inspired oxygen (FIO_2)
- To prevent accidental esophageal intubation in esophagectomy with a gastric pull-up
- Unstable cervical spine
- Fiberoptic bronchoscopic-guided extubation
  - – Failed previous extubation with suspicion of upper airway obstruction like tracheomalacia and tracheal stenosis
  - – Uncooperative patient.

CONTRAINDICATION

- Airway bleeding
- Copious secretions
- Inexperienced operator
- Uncooperative patient
  - – Awake FOB intubations
  - – Fiberoptic bronchoscopic-guided extubation
- Unprepared airway
- Faulty setup
- High-grade stenosis of any part of the airway.

APPLIED ANATOMY

Beginners are recommended to go through basic anatomy of airway before attempting FOB. Knowledge of airway is essential for identifying anticipated difficult intubation and also for the procedure of FOB intubation. For transtracheal (translaryngeal) injection of local anesthetics (LA), cricothyroid membrane is commonly punctured. It is easily identified between thyroid cartilage and cricoid cartilage (Fig. 1).

TECHNIQUE AND EQUIPMENT

Nasotracheal intubation using fiberoptic choledochoscope was first reported by Murphy on a patient with Still's disease way back in 1967. FOB intubation has evolved from work by Stiles and colleagues in 1972.

Fiberoptic bronchoscopic intubation can be done via nasal or oral route. It can be done in an awake (conscious) patient or under general anesthesia. FOB intubation in awake patient is preferred over FOB intubation under anesthesia as airway patency and spontaneous ventilation are better preserved with awake patient. In uncooperative, intoxicated patients and children, FOB intubation under anesthesia can be performed. Such intubations should be

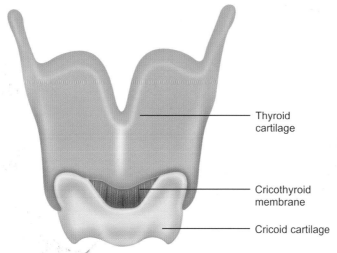

Fig. 1 Location of cricothyroid membrane

preferably done by experienced person in presence of emergency airway cart with standby preparation of surgical airway and preferably standby surgeon.

Equipment

Fiberoptic bronchoscopic has two parts, control section and an insertion cord. Light source is connected to FOB via a cable.

- *Control section body:* It is held by nondominant hand of endoscopist. It has following parts:
  - *Eyepiece:* Can be either viewed directly or attached to a camera for display on monitor. It has a black mark at 12 o'clock position. Vertical movement of tip of insertion cord (vide infra) occurs in the direction of black mark. There is a subtle difference between direct view through eyepiece and indirect view through a camera and monitor. When viewed through monitor, the black mark remains in its original position but the image rotates in the direction of rotation. This happens because when scope is rotated; there is equal rotation of camera. Movement of scope will occur in vertical direction parallel to black mark.

    When viewed through naked eye at eyepiece, rotation of FOB causes equal movement of the black mark from the 12 o'clock position in the direction of rotation. However, image does not rotate. This is important to note because change in orientation of black mark cause change in plane of movement of FOB. User needs to understand that movement of scope will occur only toward or away from black mark.

    Video monitor gives advantage of supervision which is extremely useful for teaching FOB intubation. Also it avoids bad posturing. If video monitor is used white balance should be confirmed and black mark should be at 12 o'clock position (Figs 2A and B).
  - *Diopter ring for focusing:* This ring is rotated to get optimum focus of near structures.

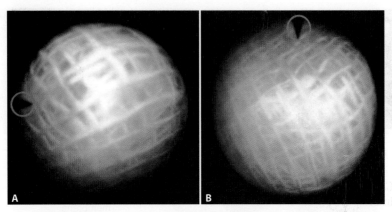

Figs 2A and B Orientation of fiberoptic bronchoscopic through camera

- *Control lever:* It allows movement of tip of insertion cord only in one plane. Moving the lever down moves the tip up (anteriorly) and moving the lever up moves the tip down (posteriorly) (Figs 3A to C). This movement corresponds with black mark seen on eyepiece. Moving the lever down moves the tip toward black mark and moving the lever up moves the tip away from black mark. Movement to right and left side (90° to black mark) are not possible with FOB. For this combination of lateral rotation (clockwise and anticlockwise), and lever movement is used. FOB should be rotated with simultaneous movement of wrist and shoulder of the operator. Ensure FOB is not twisted when such movement is done.
  - *Working channel port:* This is a multipurpose port. Each FOB can have one or two working channels. It can be used for suction, instillation of LA and oxygen delivery. Suction valve is used to control suction function. This allows suction through the working channel when the valve is pressed.
- *Insertion cord:* It contains multiple fiberoptic bundles for light and image transmission. It also contains wires from the control lever for vertical movement of tip and also the working channel. Usual length of FOB insertion cord is around 60 cm. FOB is most vulnerable at junction of body and cord. Acute bends in FOB especially at this site should be strictly avoided.

Handling and Care

Fiberoptic bronchoscope should be mounted on a cart. The cart should contain the FOB, a light source, camera control unit, LA and airway adjuvant used to aid FOB intubation. The cart should be easily movable to various places like operation theater, ward, the ICU and the emergency department. This cart can be clubbed with difficult airway kit.

Sterilization/Disinfection: Bronchoscope is heat-sensitive endoscope, hence cannot be sterile by steam. Centers for Disease Control (CDC) and Prevention recommends proper cleaning and, at least high-level disinfection between two patients. Steps are discussed further.

- *Leak testing:* As per manufacturer's recommendations. Further steps should be done only if leak test is passed.

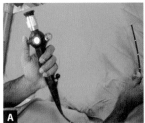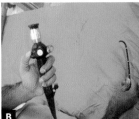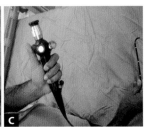

Figs 3A to C Fiberoptic bronchoscopic lever and tip movement

- *Cleaning:* External surfaces should be cleaned with water and detergent. Internal channels should be cleaned with a brush and flushed with water and a detergent. Cleaning will reduce microbial contamination by 10,000–1,000,000 times).
- *Disinfection:* Immerse endoscope in disinfectant. Inject disinfectant into each working channel. Remove air pockets in working channels.
- *Rinsing:* Use sterile or filtered water to rinse all channels of the endoscope and the external surface.
- *Drying:* Use alcohol followed by dry air to dry out the external surface of the scope and inner channels.
- *Storage:* Promote drying. Do not allow recontamination. Can be hung vertically.

Disinfection will destroy all microorganisms, however, a few spores might survive. Various agents can be used for disinfection like 2.4% glutaraldehyde, 0.55% ortho-phthalaldehyde (OPA), and 7.5% hydrogen peroxide. However, compatibility of FOB with the particular chemical should be checked with manufacturers.

PREPARATION

- Fiberoptic cart should be on the nondominant side of the endoscopist, usually the left side. The FOB is connected to the light source and the light is turned on. Focus is adjusted by pointing tip of FOB toward an object (preferably printed words) and rotating focus lens till a clear image is obtained. After this, light may be turned off until the time of intubation.
- Endoscopist should stand on head end of table/bed. Bed should be lowered as low as possible. Also foot stool can be taken depending on endoscopist's height. This helps in avoiding acute bends in scope. Remember, FOB is very precious instrument and acute bends especially at neck can damage scope.
- Universal sterile precautions should be taken. FOB should be held in left (nondominant) hand with arm by the side of body. Endoscopist should stand comfortable without bending at back (Fig. 4).
- Prewarming of FOB in lukewarm water can prevent fogging. However, caution should be employed since FOB might get damaged due to excess heat and hence readers are recommended to follow manufacturer's recommendations. ET tube should be mounted on FOB before intubation (Fig. 5). Prewarming of ET softens it and improves its pliability due to thermoplastic nature of material. Defogging solution as per manufacturer recommendation may also be applied to the optical tip of the FOB to prevent fogging.

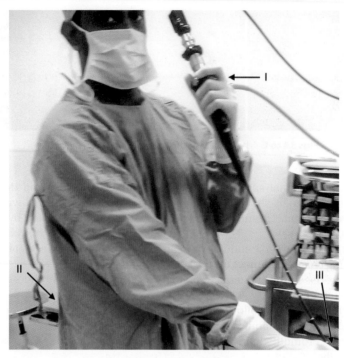

Fig. 4 Method of holding fiberoptic bronchoscopic. (I) Fiberoptic bronchoscopic held in non-dominant hand by side of body; (II) No bending at back; (III) Keep fiberoptic bronchoscopic straight without bends

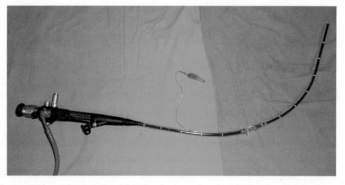

Fig. 5 Fiberoptic bronchoscopic with ET tube mounted on it for intubation. Universal connecter of endotracheal tube can be removed (optional) to provide extra length of fiberoptic bronchoscopic as a margin of safety

- *Ancillary equipment:* Fiberoptic bronchoscopic intubation can be assisted by various devices including intubating oral and nasopharyngeal airways and facemasks. These adjuvants increase the ease of FOB intubation. Examples of ancillary equipment: The Berman II intubating airway, the ovassapian fiberoptic intubating airway, the Patil fiberoptic airway, the

Williams airway intubator, face mask with an endoscopy port, bronchoscopy Swivel adapter face mask.

- *Preparation of the patient*
  - *Awake versus anesthetized patient:* Fiberoptic intubation is easier in a conscious patient because the muscles of the tongue and neck prevent the tongue from falling back into the pharynx, and spontaneous ventilation keeps the airway open. A conscious patient can assist the operator in locating the glottis by deep breathing and phonating, especially when the airway anatomy is distorted. Hence, awake (conscious) FOB intubation is preferred in ICU patients.
  - *Psychological preparation of the patient*
    - Explain the procedure to the patient
    - Reassure the patient
    - Explain the need for patient cooperation (deep breathing, phonation)
    - Explain that the patient will not be able to speak once ET tube is in situ
    - If time permits, visit the patient before the scheduled time.
  - *Pharmacological preparation of the patient*
    - *Antisialagogue:* Glycopyrrolate (preferably intramuscular, half an hour before for planned intubation) is preferred over atropine due to minimal cardiac and central nervous system (CNS) effects
    - *Sedation*
      - Sedation or opioids should be avoided in case of airway compromise or poor general condition of the patient
      - If there no such concerns, conscious sedation during intubation can be given
      - Midazolam provides sedation and amnesia. Airway protective reflexes remain intact, but the patient may react more vigorously to instrumentation of the airway or can become uncooperative
      - Opioids produce profound analgesia and depress airway reflexes. This allows airway instrumentation while the patient is still capable of following verbal commands. However, they can cause respiratory depression
      - A combination of fentanyl (1.5 µg/kg) and midazolam (30 µg/kg), is commonly used
      - Dexmedetomidine may help to produce sedation and amnesia without the potential for respiratory depression and loss of airway reflexes
      - Sedation should be titrated to the effect.
  - *Topical preparation*
    - Antisialagogue should be given before topical preparation. Excess secretions will wash out or dilute the LA solution
    - Local anesthetic can be sprayed either prior to procedure or by "spray-as-you-go" technique during procedure
    - Absorption is most rapid from alveoli, followed by tracheobronchial tree and pharynx. LA from respiratory tract mucosal surfaces enters circulation more rapidly compared to neuraxial or peripheral nerve blocks. Therefore, half of the "allowable systemic dose" should be used
    - Addition of vasoconstrictors to LA is not beneficial
    - *Additional preparation for nasotracheal intubation:* Deviated nasal septum is ruled out and the more patent nostril is selected. Xylometazoline

drops shrink mucosa and decrease the chances of bleeding. Lignocaine gel provides topical anesthesia and lubrication
- *Additional preparation for orotracheal intubation:* Fiberoptic broncho-scopic must be inserted through a bite block to avoid biting by patient. Patient should be explained to protrude his tongue, if required.

PROCEDURE

In Spontaneous Breathing Patient

- *Position of patient:* Supine.
- *Local anesthesia*
  - *Prior to procedure:* Oropharyngeal application of a 4% solution or a 10% aerosolized lignocaine spray. Alternatively gargles with viscous lignocaine, or nebulization of 4 mL 4% lignocaine can be tried. Cricothyroid mem-brane is punctured with a needle or cannula and larynx and trachea is anesthetized with 4% lidocaine (Translaryngeal injection technique). This gives excellent anesthesia, preventing cough and laryngeal spasm. Hence, this technique is suited for novices.
  - *Spray-as-you-go technique:* It involves spraying LA through the working channel of FOB. Vocal cords are directly visualized and sprayed with LA. One has to wait for minimum of 30 seconds prior to advancement of FOB. Almost all awake ET intubations can be done with this technique. This technique is of particular importance for patients at high risk for aspiration since airway reflexes are abolished late during procedure. This technique is suited for experienced operators.
  Note: Most adult FOBs have working channels of diameter 2–2.5 mm. This can cause nonuniform spread of LA. Injection of LA through an epidural catheter inserted earlier through working channel might be used to overcome this issue. For best result, tip of epidural catheter should be outside working channel.
  Topical preparation can be supplemented with bilateral superior laryngeal and lingual nerve blocks.
- *Nasotracheal intubation:* It is easier than orotracheal route since there are no sharp turns to take for FOB. Minimal cooperation from patients is required and patients need less sedation to tolerate tube. However, chances of sinus infections are more with nasal tube especially when kept for long-term. There are higher chances of bleeding with nasotracheal intubation and once bleeding starts, FOB becomes difficult to impossible.
  - Putting ET tube first in nasopharynx and then advancing FOB through tube reduces possibility of nasal secretions blocking view through the objective lens. However, manipulation of FOB may become more difficult.
  - Fiberoptic bronchoscopic with mounted ET tube is advanced through nares in to nasopharynx under vision. Care is taken not to force FOB blindly as this may cause bleeding. [FOB is passed through caudal most part (around lower turbinate) of nasal cavity] Once FOB is advanced further into oropharynx, epiglottis is seen. One can ask patient to phonate (say "Eeee") to easily identify vocal cords. This step is usually not mandatory.
  - Using up and down lever and lateral rotation of FOB, area of interest (epiglottis, cords, trachea, and carina) is kept in center of view and FOB is slowly advanced further (Figs 6A to F).

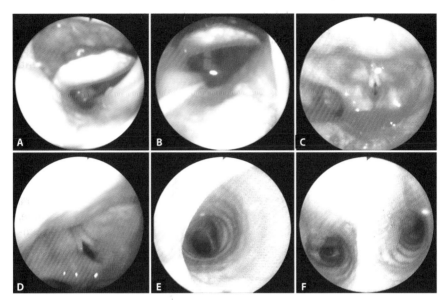

Figs 6A to F Bronchoscopic views. (A) Epiglottis and vocal cords. Note presence of Ryle's tube; (B) Epiglottis and vocal cords. Closer view; (C) Adducted vocal cords. Note presence of bleeding; (D) Adducted vocal cords; (E) Carina seen through tip of ET tube this confirms ET tube tip; (F) Carina

- Once FOB is close to carina, ET tube is pushed using FOB as a stylet.
- Make sure that ET tube is well below glottis. Inflation of cuff of the ET in the larynx may cause recurrent laryngeal nerve palsy. This also increases chances of accidental extubation.

Fiberoptic Intubation in Anesthetized Patient

It should be reserved for uncooperative, intoxicated patients and children. It should be done by operators who are experienced and confident. This can be clubbed with rapid sequence induction. It requires one assistant to hold FOB ready, opening mouth and give jaw thrust or to retract tongue. An intubating airway helps for easier insertion. Avoiding muscle relaxants and keeping spontaneous breathing intact, reduces apnea time. This is best done in operative room with inhalational agents. Standby preparation of surgical airway is desirable.

Fiberoptic Intubation through the Laryngeal Mask Airway

Laryngeal mask airway (LMA) is one of the most important accessories in difficult intubation cart. Advantages of LMA like ease and speedy insertion without using direct laryngoscopy or muscle relaxants can be clubbed with direct visualization of the larynx through FOB. Combination of FOB and LMA improves the success rate of intubation. This is used for oral intubations.

- Initially LMA is placed, and ventilation confirmed. A well-lubricated FOB (with a premounted ET) is advanced through the LMA. The ET tube is then advanced over the FOB under vision into the trachea.

- For short duration intubations (short surgeries) LMA can be placed in situ along with ET tube. After surgeries, ET tube is removed first and LMA later when patient regains airway reflexes.
- For long-term intubations (ICU intubation) LMA is removed and ET tube is kept in situ. Since length of ET tube is short for such use, utmost care should be taken to prevent displacement of ET tube from trachea into larynx or complete extubation. Removal of universal connecter of LMA during removal increases margin of safety. Following adjuvant can help for such intubations.

Aintree intubation catheter (AIC) can be used in following steps:
- Laryngeal mask airway is inserted
- Aintree intubation catheter mounted on FOB is inserted through LMA
- Fiberoptic bronchoscopic passed beyond vocal cords and carina is visualized
- Aintree intubation catheter is pushed in and FOB is removed
- Laryngeal mask airway is removed while taking care not to displace AIC
- Endotracheal tube is threaded over AIC with or without laryngoscope.

Alternately tube-in-tube method can be used:
- Laryngeal mask airway is inserted
- Endotracheal tube (without connecter) mounted on FOB is inserted through LMA
- Fiberoptic bronchoscopic passed beyond vocal cords and carina is visualized
- Endotracheal is pushed in and FOB is removed
- Smaller endotracheal tube without connecter is put in series with the existing ET tube
- Laryngeal mask airway is removed over smaller ET while taking care not to displace larger ET.

   Other options are LMA Fastrach (Intubating LMA) or a split and sealed LMA.

Fiberoptic Intubation through Special Oral Airways

Various intubating airways can be used to aid FOB intubation.
- *The Berman II intubating airway:* It is an oropharyngeal airway with an opening on its side throughout the length of the airway. The FOB is introduced through this longitudinal groove or slit. Once the FOB is in the trachea, the airway can be separated from the FOB and removed from the patient's mouth. It is available in different sizes. Since it is not flexible, FOB inside airway cannot be maneuvered. So, if glottic opening is not seen at the end of airway, airway is partially withdrawn to align with glottic opening.
- The ovassapian fiberoptic intubating airway is available in only one size which accommodates an ET up to 8.5 mm in inner diameter (ID). The distal half of the airway is wide, giving additional space for maneuvering the tip of the FOB.
- *The Patil fiberoptic airway:* This allows anterior-posterior maneuvering of the FOB. However, it is available in only one size, and has to be removed before insertion of ET tube.

Procedure of Fiberoptic Bronchoscopic-guided Tube Exchange

- Adequate starvation for elective tube exchange
- Suction of gastric contents

- Route (oral vs nasal) selected
- The new ET is selected and mounted on FOB
- Fiberoptic bronchoscopic is placed near vocal cords by the side of the existing ET tube
- Thorough suction of posterior pharynx is done
- The existing ET is removed and the new tube is advanced over the FOB into the trachea. This is the preferred method because airway control is not lost. There may be a small chance of losing the view due to secretions or coughing during removal of existing tube
- Alternatively existing tube is removed first followed by insertion of FOB in trachea followed by new ET tube. Use only when FOB cannot be inserted in trachea along with existing ET.

Procedure of Fiberoptic Bronchoscopic-guided Extubation

Criteria for weaning should be fulfilled. Airway is adequately prepared. FOB is advanced through ET tube. Position of tip of FOB outside ET tube is confirmed by visualization of trachea. Both FOB and tube are slowly removed and careful inspection of subglottic and glottic airway is done. If any abnormality (stricture, severe collapse of trachea) is seen, FOB is reinserted immediately followed by ET tube.

POST-PROCEDURE CARE

Care of Patient

- Securing tube
- Confirmation of tube placement with end-tidal carbon dioxide ($ETCO_2$)
- Reassurance to patient
- Sedation/anesthesia
- Ventilation.

Care of Scope

- Light source and camera should be removed
- Leak test and stepwise cleaning as described earlier.

COMPLICATION/PROBLEM

- *Hypoxia:* It occurs commonly during fiberoptic intubation. It can be prevented by giving 100% O_2 and maintaining spontaneous respiration as far as possible. Cardioscope and pulse oximetry and blood pressure monitoring should be done to pick up hypoxia earlier. Capnography monitoring is desirable to monitor respiration and confirm tube position.
- *Myocardial ischemia:* Combination of hypoxia, tachycardia and hypertension due to sympathetic stimulation places patient for risk of myocardial ischemia.
- *Raised intracranial pressure (ICP):* Fiberoptic bronchoscopic is the quickest and least traumatic method of intubation. Adequate airway preparation will reduce magnitude of rise in ICP during intubation.

- *Barotrauma:* During FOB, use through ET tube during mechanical ventilation there is increase in peak airway pressure due to increase in resistance. Peak airway pressure, visible chest rise and expired tidal volume should be monitored. Suctioning should be done only intermittently to prevent loss of PEEP leading to atelectasis and hypoxia. Postprocedure X-ray chest should be done for FOB use in mechanically ventilated patient.

Troubleshooting

Problem	Prevention	Solution
Secretions blocking view	Proper dose and time of antisialagogue	Suction
Bleeding blocking view	Be gentle while insertion. Avoid trauma	Suction. Wipe-off blood. If problem persists, abandon and go for alternative method
		Never attempt FOB in a bleeding airway
Inadequately prepared airway	Antisialagogue Give time for local to act	Give local anesthetic and give time for it to act
Fogging of the FOB	Prewarming, anti-fog solution to lens. Oxygen through working channel	Remove FOB. Redo preventive measures
Obstruction by base of tongue or epiglottis (under anesthesia)	Jaw thrust by assistant	Jaw thrust, tongue retraction
Lack of experience	Practice elective easy FOB intubations first before actually doing in real emergency	Do not attempt FOB in emergency if you are not used to it
Difficulty in identifying landmarks	Only awake FOB if such case is anticipated	Ask the patient to phonate. This may ease in visualizing cords

Abbreviation: FOB, fiberoptic bronchoscopic.

Hang-up: Sometimes ET tube gets struck at some level above trachea after successful insertion of FOB into trachea leading to failed or delayed intubation. When there is difference in size between two devices, it causes a cleft leading to "hang-up". When this happens actually there is entrapment of the epiglottis, corniculate/arytenoid cartilages, the aryepiglottic folds, or the vocal folds. This can occur with any stylet-guided techniques (FOB, retrograde wire, lighted stylet and bougie). Chances of hang-up increase when there is large difference between outer diameter of stylet (FOB, retrograde wire, lighted stylet and bougie) and ID of tube. Hang-up can be minimized by selecting larger stylet and smaller tube. When one encounters "hang-up"; ET tube should be withdrawn by few centimeters and rotated by 15° each time either clockwise or anticlockwise and reinserted. This step can be repeated, if required.

To summarize, difficult airway can be encountered in ICU. Anticipation is the key. ICU patients are physiologically more prone to complications of difficult airway including hypoxia and death. FOB in a spontaneously breathing patient is gold standard for anticipated difficult airway. One needs to practice few FOB intubations in elective scenario before attempting it in emergency situation. Never attempt FOB in bleeding airway or in an uncooperative patient.

SUGGESTED READING

1. Delinger RP. Fiberoptic bronchoscopy in adult airway management. Crit Care Med. 1990;18(8):882-7.
2. Rosenblatt WH, Sukhupragarn W. Airway management. In: Barash PG, Cullen BF, Stoelting RK, Cahalan MK, Stock MC (Eds). Handbook of Clinical Anesthesia. 6th edition. Lippincott Williams & Wilkins. 2009.
3. Rutala WA, Weber DJ. The Healthcare Infection Control Practices Advisory Committee (HICPAC). Guideline for disinfection and sterilization in healthcare facilities;2008. Available from http://www.cdc.gov/hicpac/pdf/guidelines/Disinfection_Nov_2008.pdf [Accessed October 2013].
4. Wheeler M, Ovassapian A. Fiberoptic endoscopy-aided techniques. In: Hagberg CA (Ed). Benumof's Airway management: Principles and practice, 2nd edition. St. Louis, Mosby. 2007. pp. 399-438.

5

Video Laryngoscopy

Manish Paul, Banani Poddar

INTRODUCTION

The anatomy of the larynx does not permit direct visualization. It is often essential for the clinician to view the larynx at the bedside or in the examination room. The video laryngoscope essentially brings the 'eye' of the clinician right above the larynx. The equipment, a fiber-optic or digital scope, can be inserted via the nasal or the oral route. The image is generally a magnified view of the larynx and the adjoining structures as seen on a monitor, permitting a detailed examination.[1] The procedure can also be recorded.[2] The use of this equipment will enable the intensive care unit (ICU) physician to further the care of critically ill patients at the bedside. The images so obtained can also be useful in training medical and paramedical staff employed in patient care. Their proper use will also reduce expensive diagnostics and procedures requiring exposure of the patient to radiation (fluoroscopy and X-rays) and avoid transport of critically ill patients to the radiology suite. Despite the initial cost of procurement such equipment will prove economically viable.

INDICATION

Video laryngoscope finds use in various settings and locations within and outside the hospital.[3-5] It is an important aid to perform tracheal intubation and also for bedside assessment of laryngeal dysfunction.[6,7]

- Important indications for use in ICU and emergency room for tracheal intubation
  - Mandibular fracture
  - Partially obstructing laryngeal lesions such as supraglottitis
  - Awake intubation (anticipated difficult airway)
  - Cervical spine injuries or cervical instability
  - Patients unable to extend the neck
  - Trismus
  - Craniofacial trauma.
- Diagnostic and therapeutic indications when video laryngoscopy is used for assessing laryngeal structure and function
  - Stridor
  - Subglottic stenosis
  - Airway obstruction by any tumor or mass

- – Vocal cord palsy
- – Foreign body.
- Other common indications in the ICU
  - – Endotracheal tube (ETT) exchange
  - – Insertion of other devices in a patient who is already intubated
    - - Nasogastric tube
    - - Transesophageal echocardiography (TEE) probe
    - - Esophageal dilatation bougie
  - – Visualization of laryngeal function.

CONTRAINDICATION

Contraindications to video laryngoscopy include the following:
- Highly obstructive lesions
- Maxillofacial trauma with orofacial bleed
- Operator unfamiliar with the equipment.

TECHNIQUE AND EQUIPMENT

Historical aspect: Control of airway during surgical procedures using a tube was first reported by William MacEwen, a Glasgow surgeon, in 1878.[8] The tube so designed was essentially placed blindly through the larynx prior to induction of chloroform anesthesia with the patient being awake. Later in 1895, Alfred Kirstein developed the "autoscope" for direct laryngoscopy at Berlin, Germany.[9] His equipment was basically a handle containing an electric bulb to which a short esophagoscope was attached. Almost half a century later in 1940s Miller and Macintosh modified his design to make the laryngoscopy blades which are still in vogue in the present era. The idea of using optical instruments to improve the view of the larynx or to enable a view of the glottis around the base of the tongue is not new and was pursued before the introduction of the instrument now known as the video laryngoscope. In 1992, Bumm P, an otorhinolaryngologist, presented an endoscopic or indirect laryngoscopic method for tracheal intubation in which a conventional Macintosh blade was combined with a rigid 30° or 70° endoscope. Earlier in the late 1980s, the endoscopic Bullard laryngoscope was initially studied and described scientifically. In 1983, the Swiss anesthetist, Bonfils, introduced an optic intubation stylet that consisted of a rigid endoscope with its tip bent at an angle of 40°; this is still being used in anesthesia practice.

The commonly available devices used nowadays are as listed in Table 1.

Table 1 Examples of commercially available devices

Stylets	*Guide channels*	*Traditional modifications*
1. Bonfils	1. AirTraq	1. Coopdech VLP-100
2. Rigid/flexible laryngoscope	2. Pentax AWS	2. Storz DCI
	3. Res-Q-Scope II	3. Storz C-Mac
		4. McGrath
		5. GlideScope

Equipment

A good video laryngoscope should have the following characteristics:
- Easy to handle by an operator skilled in traditional direct laryngoscopy
- Suitable and adaptable for different types of endotracheal intubations, i.e. oral/nasal and adult/pediatric
- Permits the use of special-purpose tubes such as double-lumen endobronchial tubes
- A large separate screen for teaching purposes and for sharing of information among the medical team
- Should be inexpensive (*Caution:* Cost of acquisition can be high for both reusable and disposable devices)
- Should be lightweight, low profile, and easy to maneuver.
- Antifog capability is surprisingly important.

Advantages

- Eye and airway need not line-up
- Better view when mouth opening or neck mobility is limited
- Others can see and help
- Permits sharing of medical information among the team
- Higher success rate of tracheal intubation, especially in difficult airway scenario.

Disadvantages

- Variable learning curve; may take longer to intubate
- Passage of tube may be difficult despite great view; stylet often necessary
- Fogging and secretions may obscure view
- Loss of depth perception
- More complicated
- Expensive
- Greater processing time and expense.

PREPARATION

- *Assessment:* The operator must be able to assess the likely difficulties in intubation for which a formal assessment of the airway is essential. At this stage the operator must also decide whether to go for an awake intubation or that under anesthesia. Laboratory work-up solely for the procedure is generally not essential.
- *Anesthesia:* If the laryngoscopy is only for a diagnostic purpose, lignocaine 4% spray may be used locally in the oropharynx. While, if a decision for awake intubation is made, anesthesia should be provided to the following three regions prior to and during the procedure: nasal cavity (if nasal intubation is to be performed), pharynx and larynx.
  - Nasal cavity is prepared by having the patient inhale phenylephrine 1% or oxymetazoline 0.05% nasal spray. The alpha adrenergic action causes vasoconstriction of the nasal mucosa and makes it dry enabling easy

manipulation for nasal intubation. Anesthesia is provided by lightly coating nostrils with lidocaine 4% jelly. Anxiolysis may be provided by a small dose of benzodiazepine like midazolam if not contraindicated.

– Pharyngeal anesthesia is delivered by nebulizer. 3–4 mL of 4% lidocaine is nebulized.

– Laryngeal anesthesia can be delivered in any one of the following ways:

- 1 mL of 4% lidocaine is applied via the fiber-optic scope channel when the scope is positioned directly above the larynx.

- A cotton ball soaked in lidocaine 4% can also be used to apply the anesthesia to the larynx. The soaked cotton ball is held with Jackson laryngeal forceps. With the tongue grasped, the cotton ball is applied transorally to the epiglottis, hypopharynx, and vocal fold mucosal surfaces.

- Alternately, a bilateral superior laryngeal nerve block can be performed. To perform this block the hyoid bone is located. The operator inserts the needle 1 cm below each greater cornu (where the internal branch of the superior laryngeal nerve penetrates the thyrohyoid membrane). A "pop" is felt as the needle penetrates the membrane. 2–3 mL 2% lignocaine is infiltrated.

- Tracheal anesthesia, though not necessary, can be delivered. 2–4 mL of lidocaine 2% can be injected transtracheally. The same dose could be delivered by nebulization with 4% solution of lignocaine topical.

- Glycopyrrolate may be administered intravenously to reduce secretions prior to the procedure.

- Equipment required for the procedure:
  - Video laryngoscope
  - Lignocaine 4% and 2%
  - Glycopyrrolate 0.2 mg (to be administered intravenously before start of the procedure)
  - Endotracheal tubes (assorted of different sizes)
  - Warmed saline
  - Syringes 10 mL, 5 mL and 2 mL
  - Oral airways of multiple sizes
  - Carbon dioxide detector (if intubation is planned)
  - Antifog solution or an alcohol pad
    Suction apparatus with suction catheters
  - Oxygen with appropriate delivery device (self-inflating bag, Mapleson D circuit)
  - Airway devices like laryngeal mask airway (LMA) may also be kept ready.

PROCEDURE

Positioning

If the patient is undergoing awake video laryngoscopy then he/she should be seated with the head of bed elevated almost 90°. For the procedure under sedation, the traditional supine position with the head in a sniffing position suffices.

Specific Procedural Features of Commonly Used Devices

1. *Using the GlideScope Video Laryngoscope (GVL) (Fig. 1):* A four step technique is adopted.
   - *Introduce the laryngoscope:* With the patient appropriately positioned (as described earlier), the operator uses the left hand to introduce the GVL into the midline of the oral pharynx and gently advances it until the blade tip is past the posterior portion of the tongue. This step is done using direct vision. In other words, the operator is looking directly into the patient's mouth, as is the case for direct laryngoscopy.
   - After the scope has been inserted the appropriate positioning for visualization is guided by the imagery on the monitor. In contrast to conventional laryngoscopy which necessitates lateral mobilization of the tongue the same is not required in using GVL, which is essentially a midline equipment. The optimization of the view on the monitor is done by a combination of advancement and withdrawal of the blade with increasing tilt on the blade to place the tip in the vallecula or the posterior surface of the epiglottis. The operator must attempt to place the image of the glottis in the mid upper third of the video display.
   - *Introduce the ETT (if intubation is planned):* Usually, the video image of the glottis is a Cormack-Lehane grade I or II view and the operator is immediately tempted to insert the ETT and attempt to navigate it through the glottic aperture while continuously visualizing the video screen. In fact, it is better to maintain the laryngoscopic position in the mouth with the left hand but focus the eyes from the video screen back to the patient's open mouth. After the glottis has been visualized the operator takes a standard ETT with a stylet in situ, the combination having been already modified into a "j" shape in his right hand. This is inserted under direct vision till the distal end of the ETT is judged to be near the tip of the laryngoscope blade.

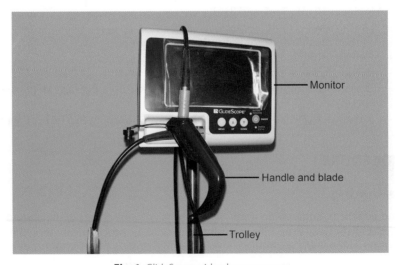

Fig. 1 GlideScope video laryngoscope

- *Intubate (if intubation is planned):* The operator now returns to the view on the monitor and the tube is advanced with the stylet in situ through the glottic aperture. Post placement of the tube the stylet is withdrawn and the ETT is connected to an appropriate device/equipment to maintain ventilation.

2. *Using the McGRATH Video Laryngoscope Series 5 (Fig. 2):*
   - The tip of the laryngoscope blade is inserted inside the oral cavity above the tongue keeping it in the center and angulating it upwards till the epiglottis is visualized. While taking care that there is no contact with the teeth, a direct vision along the superior surface of the blade or the view of the image on the screen is used to guide the tip of the blade towards the larynx.
   - The tip of the blade is further guided into the vallecula applying further rotation and/or minimal force along the long-axis of the handle to view the glottis.
   - Once the glottis is visualized, intubation can be performed with an appropriate ETT prepared with a stylet in situ and the distal end curved making a "j" shape. If a malleable introducer is used, it is recommended that a "hockey stick" curve be made at a point about 5 cm from the tip of the tracheal tube.

3. *Using the PENTAX-AWS:*
   - The patient is positioned as described in the earlier techniques. The manufacturer, however recommends that excessive extension of the neck is not required when using this equipment. The PENTAX-AWS is then prepared by attaching the disposable blade to the scope. Antifogging liquid is applied to the scope window. Lubricant is applied to the outer surface of the ETT. Finally the tube is inserted into the slot provided in the blade.
   - Intubation is performed as described below:
     - After turning the monitor on, the laryngoscope is held between fingers and thumb (not in the palm as with a Macintosh) and introduced

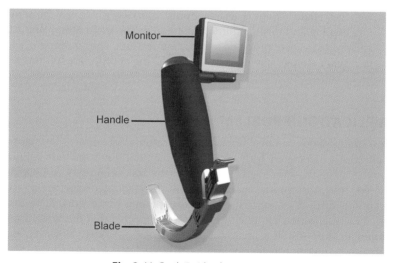

Fig. 2 McGrath 5 video laryngoscope
(*Courtesy:* Aircraft Medical Limited, UK)

under direct vision into the mouth in the midline. The laryngoscope is then rotated around its long-axis (while watching the view on the screen). This will move the tip of the blade towards the larynx. The tip of the blade must be passed under the epiglottis and the epiglottis is lifted with the help of the tip of the blade (as would be done with a traditional straight blade). When the blade is under the epiglottis the target symbol on the screen should be lined up with the laryngeal inlet. This may require a rocking motion (continued rotation in the long-axis of the scope) to line up vertically, and a clockwise/anticlockwise rotation, to line up horizontally.

- While holding the scope steady with the left hand the tube is advanced slowly with the right hand while viewing the screen. If the tube needs redirecting to ensure that it continues towards the larynx, this can only be achieved by further rotation of the scope (using the vertical and horizontal techniques described earlier). Once the tube has entered the trachea to a suitable depth, as viewed on the screen, the tube is stabilized in position with the right hand as the left hand is used to rotate the laryngoscope back out of the mouth along the curvature of the tongue.

4. *Using the C-Mac Video Laryngoscope:*
   - A rigid blade video laryngoscope manufactured by Karl Storz Endoscopy—the equipment is provided with blades ranging from size zero to four along with an additional "D" size blade. The size zero and one are Miller blades while those ranging from one to four are Macintosh blades (Fig. 3). The D blade is a recent innovation of the manufacturer (Fig. 3). The idea behind the development was management of difficult airway. It shows a pronounced angulation of 40°. The distal part of the blade is further bent at 20°. The light unit is located closer to the distal end of the blade, thus ensuring a clearer view (Fig. 4). One may need to use a preshaped stylet with the D blade.
   - The equipment has a fiber-optic cable to connect the main monitor with the blade. There is an electronic interface which can be removed for cleaning and disinfection of the handle. The main motor unit can be enclosed in a cover provided by the manufacturer. The equipment also has facility for storage of videos in SD card using appropriate buttons on the main unit.

COMPLICATION/PROBLEM

Video laryngoscopy shares most complications of direct laryngoscopy. Complications associated with airway management could include injuries to the larynx, pharynx, esophagus, and brain (the last, secondary to hypoxia). It is believed that most injuries associated with direct laryngoscopy are a result of use of undue force to visualize the laryngeal opening. Since video laryngoscopy makes the visualization of the glottis easy it is expected that the force used will be minimal, thus resulting in reduced incidence of injury. However, palatal perforation,[10] anterior tonsillar pillar injury, lingual nerve injury (due to stylet)[11] and palatopharyngeal arch injury[12] have been reported.

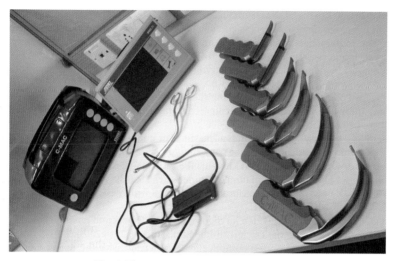

Fig. 3 The various components of the C-MAC
(*Courtesy:* Karl Storz Endoscopy India Pvt. Ltd.)

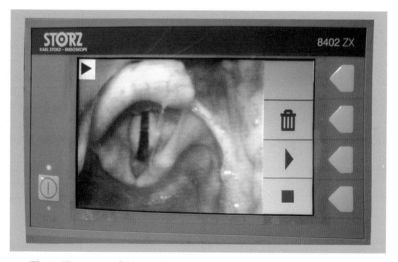

Fig. 4 The screen of C-MAC showing the glottis as viewed with the D blade
(*Courtesy:* Karl Storz Endoscopy India Pvt. Ltd.)

REFERENCES

1. Kaplan MB, Ward DS, Berci G. A new video laryngoscope—an aid to intubation and teaching. J Clin Anesth. 2002;14(8):620-6.
2. Stone RE. Video laryngoscopy. Otolaryngol Clin North Am. 1995;28(4):731-5.
3. Sakles JC, Mosier JM, Chiu S, Keim SM. Tracheal intubation in the emergency department: a comparison of GlideScope° video laryngoscopy to direct laryngoscopy in 822 intubations. J Emerg Med. 2012;42(4):400-5
4. Chen JC, Shyr MH. Role of video laryngoscopy in the management of difficult intubations in the emergency department and during prehospital care. Tzu Chi Med J. 2012;24:100-3.

5. Lakticova V, Koenig SJ, Narasimhan M, Mayo PH. Video laryngoscopy is associated with increased first pass success and decreased rate of esophageal intubations during urgent endotracheal intubation in a medical intensive care unit when compared to direct laryngoscopy. J Intensive Care Med. 2015;30(1):44-8.
6. Cantarella G. Value of flexible video laryngoscopy in the study of laryngeal morphology and functions. J Voice. 1988;1(4):353-8.
7. Ellis SF, Pollak AC, Hanson DG, Jiang JJ. Videolaryngoscopic evaluation of laryngeal intubation injury: incidence and predictive factors. Otolaryngol Head Neck Surg. 1996;114:729-31.
8. Batra YK, Mathew PJ. Airway management with endotracheal intubation (including awake intubation and blind intubation). Indian J Anaesth. 2005;49(4):263-8.
9. Reinhard M, Eberhardt E. Alfred Kirstein (1863–1922)—pioneer in direct laryngoscopy. Anasthesiol Intensivmed Notfallmed Schmerzther. 1995;30(4):240-6.
10. Williams D, Ball DR. Palatal perforation associated with McGrath video laryngoscope. Anaesthesia. 2009;64:1141-51.
11. Magboul MM, Joel S. The video laryngoscopes blind spots and possible lingual nerve injury by the Gliderite rigid stylet. Middle East J Anesth. 2010;20(6):857-60.
12. Thong SY, Goh SY. Reported complications associated with the use of GlideScope video laryngoscope: how can they be prevented? OA Anaesth. 2013;1(1):1.

6

Double Lumen Endotracheal Tube Placement

Kamal Kishore

INTRODUCTION

Double lumen tube (DLT) was developed way back in 1950 by Carlens to isolate the lungs during thoracic surgery. This tube had high flow resistance and carinal hook which posed difficulty in passing through glottis in some patients. Robertshaw introduced a modified right and left sided DLT with wide bore lumen without hook in 1960. Further in 1980, disposable DLTs were introduced and the modification continued in the form of adding the radiographic markers and bright blue, low volume and low pressure endobronchial cuffs.

INDICATION

Patient-related Indications

- Confine infection to one lung
- Confine bleeding to one lung
- Separate ventilation to one lung
  - Bronchopleural fistula
  - Tracheobronchial disruption
  - Large cyst or bulla
- Severe hypoxemia due to unilateral lung disease.

Procedure-related Indications

- Lung resection
- Thoracoscopy
- Bronchoalveolar lavage
- Esophageal surgery
- Repair of thoracic aortic aneurism.

CONTRAINDICATION

It should not be placed in certain situations:
- Difficult airway

- Small patients
- Airway bleeding or tumor or growth.

APPLIED ANATOMY

Trachea starts at the level of cricoid cartilage (C6) and divides into two bronchus right and left at the level of sternomanubrial joint (T5). There are certain differences in both the bronchus which should be kept in mind while inserting DLT.

- The right bronchus is more in line to the trachea as compared to that of left. The right one makes an angle of 25° from carina while left bronchus makes an angle of 45°
- The right bronchus is divided into three lobar branches (upper, middle and lower) whereas left bronchus is divided into upper and lower lobe branches only
- The orifice for the right upper lobe branch is 1.25 cm away from carina while that of left upper lobe is 5.0 cm away from carina.

TECHNIQUE AND EQUIPMENT

Double Lumen Tube

Double lumen tubes are essentially two endotracheal tubes fused together and have two curves at 90° of each other. The longer tube is endobronchial tube with a blue, low volume cuff (1–3 mL) and the smaller tube is endotracheal tube with transparent, high volume cuff (5–10 mL) (Fig. 1). There are two separate pilot balloons to inflate the bronchial and tracheal cuffs respectively (Fig. 2). The blue colored endobronchial cuff helps to determine the position of bronchial lumen with fiberoptic bronchoscope. The modern DLTs are made up of polyvinyl chloride and the left sided DLT should have bronchial tip smaller than the inner diameter of left sided bronchus.

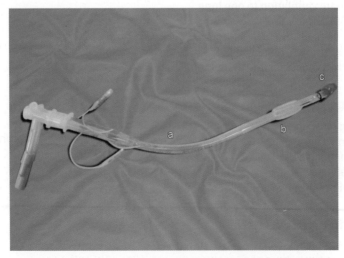

Fig. 1 Double lumen tube. (a) Proximal curvature; (b) Bronchial cuff; (c) Tracheal cuff

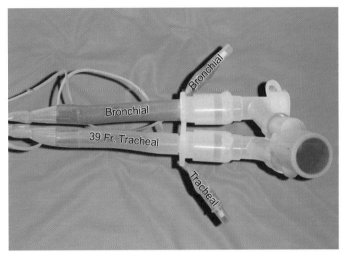

Fig. 2 Two separate lumens (bronchial and tracheal) with respective pilot balloons

Type of Double Lumen Tube

The right sided DLT contains an orifice in the bronchial cuff to ventilate the right upper lobe but anatomical variations among individuals create difficulty in ventilating right upper lobe with right sided DLT. Therefore, many physicians, however, use left sided DLT regardless of lung pathology and ventilation strategy.

Size Selection

Choosing an appropriate size of DLT is of paramount importance. Many studies have done using various methods of imaging to determine the appropriate size of DLT.[1] Chest radiograph and CT scan are valuable tools not only for determining the proper size of DLT but also assessing the anatomical variability in tracheobronchial tree and it should be reviewed before placing the DLT. A properly sized DLT must have a bronchial tip 1–2 mm smaller than the bronchial diameter to accommodate the bronchial cuff. Various sizes of DLT are available and there is no single predictor in determining the size of tube. A general formula in determining the tube size is:

- A woman shorter than 160 cm should be intubated with a 35-Fr tube
- A woman taller than 160 cm should be intubated with a 37-Fr tube
- A man shorter than 170 cm should be intubated with a 39-Fr tube
- A man taller than 170 cm should be intubated with a 41-Fr tube.

For smaller adults and children smaller size tubes (32 Fr and 28 Fr) should be used. In one study it was shown that the mean diameter of cricoid ring is similar to main stem bronchus.[2] Therefore, if the tube cannot be advanced easily through that part of airway, it is probably too large and should be changed for a smaller one.

PREPARATION

- Obtain consent
- Be sure the patient has a freely running intravenous catheter

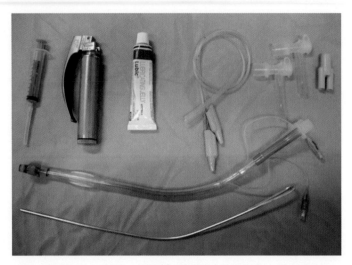

Fig. 3 Equipment needed for double lumen tube insertion

- Fiberoptic bronchoscope is functional
- *Appropriate size DLT with stylet:* Check the integrity of both the cuffs of DLT and apply the lubricant on the outer surface. Both cuffs are deflated before the procedure
- *Other adjunctive equipment (Fig. 3):* Availability of all appropriate resuscitation equipment including laryngoscope, single lumen endotracheal tube, soft tipped airway clamp, flexible suction tubing, bronchoscope adapters, lubricant jelly and Y-type adapter, syringe 10 mL
- *Monitoring:* Including but not limited to noninvasive blood pressure, electro-cardiogram and pulse oximeter.

PROCEDURE (FOR LEFT SIDED DOUBLE LUMEN TUBE)

- Preoxygenate the patient and induce anesthesia
- Hold the DLT in dominant hand with endobronchial (longer) tube pointing forward (up)
- Carryout direct laryngoscopy and insert the endobronchial tube through vocal cords
- Once the endobronchial cuff has passed the cords, remove the stylet and turn the tube to 90° in counter clockwise (for left sided DLT) (Figs 4A to C)
- Gently advance the tube until resistance is experienced
- In average size adults, depth, measured at the teeth, for a properly positioned DLT will be approximately 12 + (patient height/10) cm (not appropriate for patients with height less than or equal to 155 cm).[3] In general, to the 27–29 cm marking at the level of the teeth
- Inflate the endotracheal cuff and attach the tube to the anesthesia circuit
- Confirm the equal chest rise, presence of bilateral breath sounds and end-tidal carbon dioxide is present

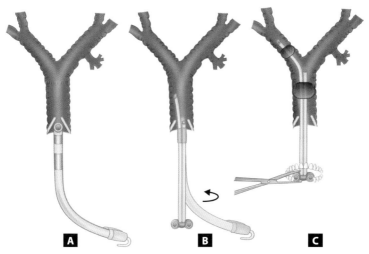

Figs 4A to C Blind method for placement of a left-sided double-lumen endotracheal tube (DLT). (A) The DLT is passed with direct laryngoscopy beyond the vocal cords; (B) The DLT is rotated 90° to the left (counterclockwise); (C) The DLT is advanced to an appropriate depth (in general, to the 27–29 cm marking at the level of the teeth)

Source: Reproduced with permission from Slinger PD, Campos JH. Miller's anesthesia. Ronald D. Miller (Ed) Anesthesia for Thoracic Surgery, 7th edition. Copyright Elsevier, 2010. pp. 1819-88.

- Confirm proper placement of DLT
  - *Functional confirmation:* Inflate the endobronchial cuff and occlude the bronchial lumen of DLT with soft tipped airway clamp. Breath sounds should be absent on left side of lung and present over right side. Move the clamp on the tracheal lumen and breath sound are now absent on right side and present on left side. Check in all lung fields to avoid segmental ventilation
  - There may be misplacement of DLT in the trachea in the form of both the lumen of DLT are: (1) Too far in on left side; (2) Too far out in the trachea; (3) Too far in on right side. Stepwise approach for identification of misplacement of DLT is described in Table 1. The described methods and measures to correct it should be taken into account to align the DLT in the right position, but correct position of DLT should always be confirmed with fiberoptic bronchoscope.
    - *Fiberoptic confirmation (preferred method):* The fiberoptic broncho-scopy is first performed through tracheal lumen to ensure that endobronchial portion of DLT is in left bronchus and its blue cuff is not herniating over carina after inflation. Also the tracheal lumen ends at least 2 cm above carina. Further observation with the fiberoptic bronchoscope is made through the endobronchial lumen to check for patency of the tube and determination of margin of safety. The orifices of both the left upper and lower lobes must be identified to avoid distal impaction in the left lower lobe and occlusion of the left-upper lobe.[4]

Table 1 Stepwise approach for identification of misplacement of double lumen tube and measures to correct it

		Breath Sounds			
Step 1	Both cuff inflated and bronchial lumen clamped	L – R +	L + R –	L + R +	L – R +
Step 2	Both cuff inflated and tracheal lumen clamped	L + R –	L – R – (or very diminished over both side)	L – R – (or very diminished over both side)	L – R – (or very diminished over both side)
Position of the double lumen tube		Correct position	Too far in (L)	Too far out	Too far in (R)
Remedial procedure		None	Pull the tube out a bit	Push the tube in a bit	Reposition the tube to left side

- Tape the tube in position
- Displacement of the DLT during patient positioning with subsequent inadequate lung isolation is a common problem. Therefore, clinicians should always confirm the position of DLT with bronchoscope after final position of the patient.

POST-PROCEDURE CARE

- Confirm the position of the tube after every position change
- At time of extubation, first suction each lumen of the tube then dilate the cuffs and gently pull the tube out while giving the positive pressure breath
- Once the need of DLT is over and patient still need ventilation, then exchange DLT with single lumen tube following proper laryngoscopy
- A properly sized airway exchange catheter may facilitate re-intubation.
- Sometimes airway edema resulting from long-standing DLT or surgery may pose difficulty during re-intubation.

COMPLICATION/PROBLEM

- Failed intubation
- Malposition of DLT leading to inadequate lung isolation or hypoxia
- Traumatic injury to the airway may cause:
  - Hoarseness
  - Sore throat
  - Arytenoid dislocation
  - Vocal cord rupture or paralysis
  - Tracheal or bronchial laceration or rupture[5]
  - Pneumothorax
  - Hemorrhage
Tracheal or bronchial mucosal tissue pressure necrosis due to cuff.

REFERENCES

1. Eberle B, Weiler N, Vogel N, Kauczor HU, Heinrichs W. Computed tomography-based tracheobronchial image reconstruction allows selection of the individually appropriate double-lumen tube size. J Cardiothorac Vasc Anesth. 1999;13:532.

2. Seymour AH. The relationship between the diameters of the adult cricoid ring and main tracheobronchial tree: a cadaver study to investigate the basis for double lumen tube selection. J Cardiothorac Vasc Anesth. 2003;17(3):299-301.

3. Bahk JH,Oh YS. Prediction of double-lumen tracheal tube depth. J Cardiothorac Vasc Anesth. 1999;13(3):370-1.

4. Slinger PD, Compos JH. Anesthesia for thoracic surgery. In: Miller R (Ed). Miller's Anesthesia, 7th edition. Philadelphia: Elsevier. 2007.

5. Sagawa M, Donjo T, Isobe T, Notake S, Nakai M, Sugita M, et al. Bilateral vocal cord paralysis after lung cancer surgery with a double-lumen endotracheal tube: a life-threatening complication. J Cardiothorac Vasc Anesth. 2006;20(2):225-6.

7

Cricothyroidotomy

Kapil Dev Soni, Sanjeev Bhoi

INTRODUCTION

Managing a difficult airway is always a challenging task for acute care physicians. Its frequency varies between 0.4 and 14% based on the clinical scenarios. A difficult airway can encountered during difficult mask ventilation, difficult intubation or difficulty in obtaining surgical airway even with experienced hands. Although, the definition of difficult airways differs considerably across the literature but cricothyroidotomy remains integral part of difficult airway management. Cricothyroidotomy is described as creation of an opening in cricothyroid membrane for an airway access. Its usage has declined over the years, as a result of emergence of less invasive newer adjuncts such as - laryngeal mask airways and other supraglottic devices. In emergency department, the cricothyroidotomy rate varies from 0.6% to 0.9%. Though, an uncommon procedure; it is an integral part of the armamentarium for unexpected difficult airways. It is been used more often in prehospital or trauma settings.

INDICATION

- The absolute indication of cricothyroidotomy is the "cannot intubate cannot oxygenate (CICO) scenario"
- Below are the conditions which might require use of cricothyroidotomy as the rescue measures:
  - Tracheal injuries
  - Maxillofacial injuries
  - Massive hemorrhage inside oral cavity
  - Traumatic foreign body inside oral cavity
  - Acute airway obstruction
  - Edema of the glottis (as seen with anaphylaxis or inhalation injuries)
  - Trismus
- Trauma is by far the most frequent scenario.[1]

CONTRAINDICATION

- *Absolute contraindications:* Achieving a secured airway with lesser invasive means.

- Relative contraindications which might preclude cricothyroidotomy or make the procedure technically difficult:
  - Tracheal disruption
  - Massive cervical swelling
  - Subcutaneous emphysema
  - Obesity with loss of landmarks
  - Young pediatric patients (Age younger than 10–12 years).

Although, the pediatric patients have relatively increased incidence of postoperative complications from surgical cricothyroidotomy, it can be performed, if airway cannot be secured by any other means in CICO scenario.

APPLIED ANATOMY

Anatomical landmarks are located at anterior midline of the neck (Fig. 1). It consists of hyoid bone, thyrohyoid membrane, thyroid notch, thyroid cartilage, cricothyroid membrane, cricoid cartilage and tracheal rings in cranial to caudal direction. Thyroid cartilage (Adam's apple) is by far the most important cartilage of larynx and is the most prominent landmark in anterior triangle of neck. It is triangular in shape and contains vocal cords. It continues with cricoid cartilage which is a complete ring shaped structure and forms the narrowest part of airways in pediatric population. Further on, cricoid cartilage is attached to tracheal rings which are deficient posteriorly and separates esophagus by a strip of muscles.

Cricothyroid membranes bridges the gap between thyroid and cricoid cartilage. On surface, it is marked by a depression between the above two and delineated laterally by cricothyroid muscles. The average size of the membrane varies between 8.2 mm wide and 10.4 mm high. Based on this size the cricothyroidotomy tube's outer measurement should not exceed 8 mm.

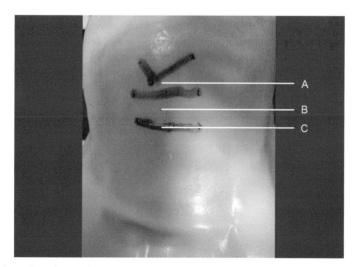

Fig. 1 Thyroid cartilage (Adam's apple) is most prominent part in anterior neck. This landmark is easily palpable even in most difficult airways. The depression between end of thyroid cartilage and cricoid marks the cricothyroid membrane. (A) Thyroid cartilage; (B) Cricothyroid membrane; (C) Cricoid cartilage

Commercial kits generally use 6 mm tube which allows easy insertion, reduced risk of cartilage fracture and provides adequate ventilation.

Elliott DS[2] studied ability of 18 anesthesiologists to accurately determine location of the cricothyroid membrane during an emergency on 6 adult humans within a 10-second period. He found that the subjects were correct only 30% of the time. This demonstrates poor accuracy of trained doctors to perfectly identify location of the membrane and highlights the need of continuous training.

TECHNIQUE

In 1909, Dr Chevalier Jackson started cricothyroidotomy in patients of laryngeal infections. He was treating children presented with airway obstruction for acute infections such as diphtheria. It was termed "high tracheostomy". Later on, as the technique was used more frequently, he observed an increase number of patients suffering from chronic laryngeal stenosis. He criticized the procedure[3] and paved the way for low tracheostomy.

The cricothyroidotomy did not gain wide acceptance until 1975 when Brantigan and Grow, presented their work in a case series of 655 patients of elective cricothyroidotomy for prolonged mechanical ventilation postcardiac surgery.[4] They demonstrated lower rate of complications (6.1%) with no case of chronic subglottic stenosis. They also reviewed the Chevalier Jackson's paper and attributed his higher rate of complications to inflammatory process or poor technique. They recommended routine use of cricothyroidotomy instead of tracheostomy for prolonged mechanical ventilation. However, study was criticized for lack of proper follow-up. Following this publication, role of cricothyroidotomy was revisited and its use was explored in both emergency as well as elective settings. Further on, O'Connor JV et al validated the above findings by performing cricothyroidotomy on 49 patients requiring prolonged ventilatory support following cardiac surgery.[5] On the contrary, Sise MJ et al.[6] observed high morbidity and mortality in a prospective study of cricothyroidotomy in 76 critically ill patients for long-term tracheal access. Rate of major complication was 7% and majority consist of subglottic stenosis. Later on, the use of cricothyroidotomy was expanded by Van Hasselt EJ et al. who performed cricothyroidotomies instead of tracheostomies in 61 adult patients over a period of two years for vide array of indications including severe trauma, respiratory problems and sepsis.[7]

In literature, numerous techniques of cricothyroidotomy have been described. They vary in use of equipment and rapidity to achieve definitive airway. Following are the common techniques being used:
- Needle cricothyroidotmy
- Standard
- Rapid four step
- Seldinger techniques
- Ultrasound-guided cricothyroidotomy.

PREPARATION

- *Prerequisite:* Proper informed consent should be sought, if time permits.
- *Precaution:* Performer should practice standard precautions, i.e. wear mask, sterile gloves, gown preparation and drape the area with antiseptics such as povidone or chlorhexidine.

- All the standard monitors such as pulse oxymeter, heart rate, noninvasive blood pressure instrument should be placed on the patient. End-tidal carbon dioxide monitor should be kept ready to check proper placement of definitive airway.
- *Drugs required:* Normally cricothyroidotomy is performed as an emergency procedure for difficult airway so it is advisable to avoid sedatives as much as possible. However, short-acting sedatives such as midazolam can be administered if patient is belligerent because of hypoxia and it is hampering the cricothyroidotomy.
- *Instruments required:* Standard surgical procedure needs the following instruments: oxygen source with tubing, intravenous tubing, scalpel, tracheal hook, tracheal dilator, tracheostomy tube and 14 or 16 gauge intravenous cannula.
- However, additional tools or modification of the available equipment may be needed depending upon the technique.

PROCEDURE

- *Position:* Patient is placed in supine position with neck extended except in trauma setting with high suspicion of cervical spine injury
- *Techniques:* The most common techniques and their steps will be described sequentially.

Needle Cricothyroidotomy[8] (Figs 2 to 5)

- Place the patient in supine position.
- Oxygen tubing is cut on proximal end to create a hole. The distal end is connected to oxygen source with high pressure (min. 50 psi).
- A needle catheter of 12 or 14 gauge is connected to 12-mL syringe with saline.
- Neck is prepared with antiseptic solutions.
- Cricothyroid membrane is identified after locating depression between thyroid and cricoid cartilage. After palpating cricothyroid membrane, trachea is stabilized by placing thumb and fingers of nondominant hand over the trachea to prevent unwanted movement during the procedure.
- Skin is punctured over the lower half of cricothyroid membrane, directing the needle at 45° caudally and continuously aspirating while advancing the needle.
- Tracheal access will be marked by air bubbles in syringe. Immediately stop the advancement of the needle and withdraw the stylet while sliding the catheter downward. Any further advancement of the needle may produce posterior wall perforation.
- Attach the proximal end of oxygen tubing to catheter. Ventilate by placing your finger on the triway (connected to oxygen tubing) for 1 second and releasing for next 4 seconds to allow passive exhalation.
- *Limitation:* Adequate oxygenation can only be achieved for 30–45 minutes depending on the lung compliance. With passage of time, it would lead to accumulation of carbon dioxide in blood.

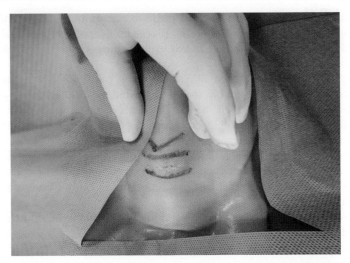

Fig. 2 Use of nondominant hand to stabilize the trachea during the procedure. Trachea is held between thumb and fingers to prevent displacement. This is important step as patient will be belligerent due to hypoxia. Placement of incision can produce fatal complications if there are exaggerated movements of neck

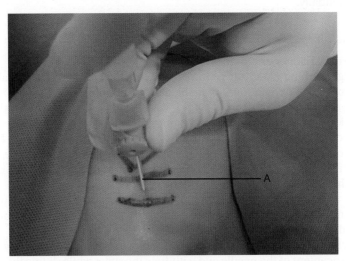

Fig. 3 Insertion of over the needle catheter into the cricothyroid membrane. The needle should be wide-bore short length. Correct placement is confirmed by presence of air bubbles during aspiration via saline-filled syringe connected to the needle. (A) Over the needle catheter

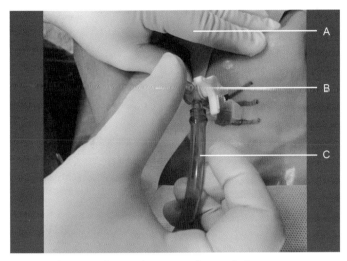

Fig. 4 Attachment of oxygen tubing and provision of jet ventilation as a rescue measure through needle cricothyroidotomy. Inspiration is provided for 1 second by occluding the open port of triway whereas expiration is passive by releasing the port open for four seconds. (A) Nondominant hand stabilizing trachea; (B) Thumb controlling the inspiration and expiration; (C) Oxygen tubing

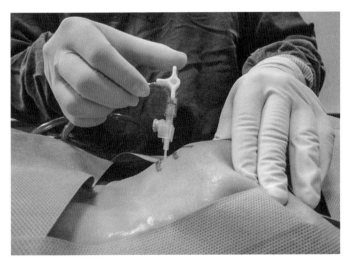

Fig. 5 Attachment of oxygen tubing and provision of jet ventilation as a rescue measure through needle cricothyroidotomy. This maneuver is only a temporizing procedure to tackle life-threatening hypoxia. This should be followed by placement of definitive airway

Standard[9] (Figs 6 to 11)

- *Position:* Patient is placed supine keeping the neck in neutral position.
- Antiseptic solutions are applied over the neck.
- Essential equipment are assembled.

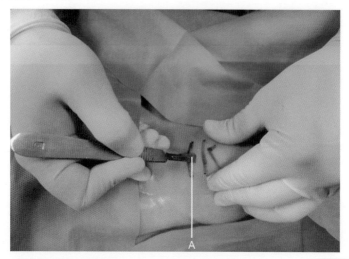

Fig. 6 An open-surgical cricothyroidotomy. Use of scalpel to make incision over cricothyroid membrane. The incision should be wide enough to accommodate a proper size tracheostomy tube. (A) Scalpel making an incision

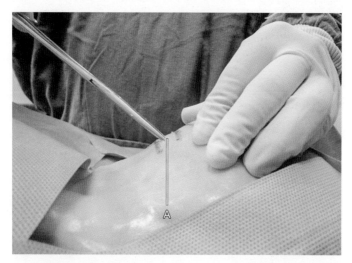

Fig. 7 Use of forceps to dilate the opening made by scalpel. It is important to dilate skin and underlying cricothyroid membrane together. (A) Incision is being widened

- *Thyroid cartilage immobilization:* Trachea is stabilized by placing thumb and forefingers on either side. This maneuver prevents excessive movement of thyroid cartilage during the procedure.
- *Palpation of cricothyroid membrane:* Palpate the thyroid cartilage and move caudally till it meets a depression between distal end of thyroid cartilage and cricoid ring. This is the surface landmark of cricothyroid membrane.
- *Placement of incision:* Incise the overlying skin and underlying subcutaneous tissue with scalpel in longitudinal direction. A horizontal incision, of approximately 1 cm is placed ove the lower half of cricothyroid membrane. This prevents injury to the vocal cords.

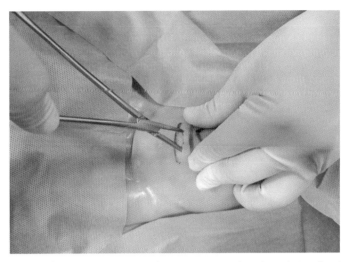

Fig. 8 Widening of incision in transverse plane to accommodate desired size of tracheostomy tube. Maximum size of tube which the area can accommodate is 6 mm internal diameter

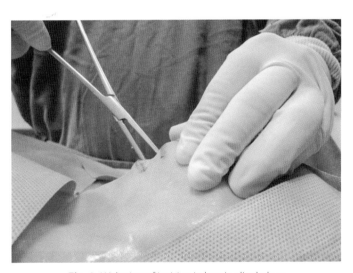

Fig. 9 Widening of incision in longitudinal plane

- *Stabilization of trachea:* Tracheal hook is placed and gentle traction is applied upward to avoid displacement of thyroid cartilage.
- *Dilation of cricothyroid membrane incision:* Dilate the stoma with curved hemostats. The incision is expanded further with Trousseau dilator and enlarged longitudinally.
- *Placement of tracheostomy tube:* The tracheostomy tube is placed in the opening without removing dilator and hook.
- The cuff of the tracheostomy tube is inflated and proximal end is connected to an oxygen source.
- Correct placement of tracheostomy tube is confirmed by monitoring the end-tidal carbon dioxide curve indicating tracheal placement of tube.

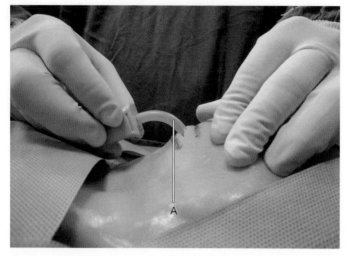

Fig. 10 Insertion of tracheostomy tube through the opening created in cricothyroid membrane. It should be inserted following its curvature. (A) Tracheostomy tube

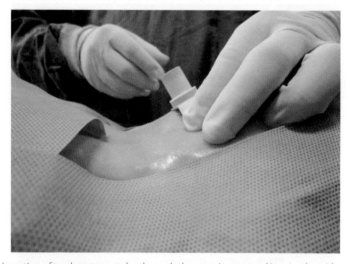

Fig. 11 Insertion of tracheostomy tube through the opening created in cricothyroid membrane. Once inserted the correct placement of airway is checked by clinical auscultation and confirmed by end-tidal carbon dioxide graph

Rapid Four-Step Technique[10]

- Cricothyroid membrane is palpated
- Both skin as well as cricothyroid membrane are incised via horizontal incision, placed in one stroke
- Tracheal hook is inserted under cricoid cartilage and traction applied caudally in contrast to standard technique where it is applied on thyroid cartilage

- Tracheostomy tube is inserted quickly into the opening and hook removed with confirmation of tube placement
- Above procedure can be modified by using Bougie-guided tracheostomy tube placement. Bougie is placed directly into the trachea through the incision opening and tracheostomy tube is rail loaded over it.

Seldinger Technique[11] (Figs 12 and 13)

- Commercial cricothyroidotomy kits contains following instruments: 6-mL syringe, 18 gauge needle with catheter, guidewire, tissue dilator, modified airway catheter and tracheostomy tape.
- Stabilize the larynx by holding the trachea with thumb and forefingers. Identify the cricothyroid membrane by palpating the depression between thyroid and cricothyroid cartilage.
- Insert the needle connected to a saline-filled syringe and advance caudally at an angle of 45° with continuous aspiration.
- As soon as bubbles appear, disconnect the syringe, remove the needle, leaving the distal tip of catheter in the trachea. Thread the guidewire into the trachea through the catheter and withdraw the catheter.
- Place an incision on the skin and cricothyroid membrane while retaining the guidewire in situ. Advance the dilator unit over the guidewire dilating the skin, subcutaneous tissue, and cricothyroid membrane.
- Withdraw the dilator and guidewire from the trachea holding the modified airway catheter inside the trachea. Connect to the oxygen source and confirm the position through end-tidal carbon dioxide.
- Secure with the tape.

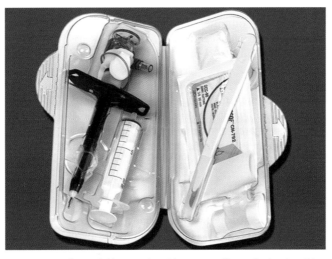

Fig. 12 A commercially available cricothyroidotomy set (Portex® cricothyroidotomy kit)
Source: Smith Medical

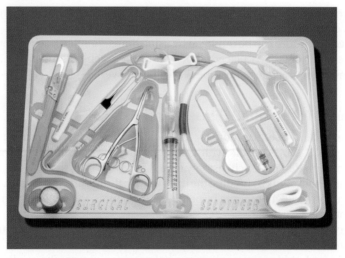

Fig. 13 A commercially available cricothyroidotomy set
(Melker emergency cricothyroidotomy set)
Source: Cook Medical

Ultrasound-Guided Cricothyroidotomy[12]

- A high frequency linear transducer is used to locate cricothyroid membrane. Equipment which are needed are similar to standard operating technique. It includes 6.0 endotracheal tube, no. 20 scalpel and 12 mL saline-filled syringe.
- Linear transducer is placed longitudinally in the midline with marker pointing toward headend. The cricothyroid membrane is focused in the center of the screen.
- After locating the membrane, horizontal incision is placed through it under ultrasound guidance with scalpel.
- The scalpel is rotated 90° once it pierces cricothyroid membrane thereby widening the incision.
- A Bougie is placed alongside scalpel into the incision so as to use it as a guide. Scalpel is removed once the Bougie is correctly inserted.
- The 6.0 tracheostomy tube is rail loaded over the Bougie. The Bougie is withdrawn after inflating the cuff of tracheostomy tube.
- The tube placement is confirmed clinically, and by end-tidal carbon dioxide curve.

POST-PROCEDURE CARE

- Once the definitive airway has been placed, it is of utmost importance to check correct placement. This can be confirmed by five-point auscultation, elevation of bilateral chest, with end-tidal carbon dioxide measurement and its graphical representation being most specific.
- The tracheostomy tube should be properly strapped to prevent displacement during transportation and movement.

- X-ray chest (anteroposterior view) should be done to confirm and document the correct placement of tube.
- Since the diameter of tube remains smaller, it is predisposed to obstruction with secretions and blood clots. Frequent suctioning of tube is recommended to prevent fatal complications.

COMPLICATION/PROBLEM

- Bleeding episodes
- Laceration of the thyroid cartilage, cricoid cartilage or tracheal rings
- Perforation of the posterior tracheal wall
- False passage insertion
- Infections

REFERENCES

1. Fortune JB, Judkins DG, Scanzaroli D, McLeod KB, Johnson SB. Efficacy of prehospital surgical cricothyrotomy in trauma patients. J Trauma. 1997;42:835.
2. Elliott DS, Baker PA, Scott MR, Birch CW, Thompson JM. Accuracy of surface landmark identification for cannula cricothyroidotomy. Anaesthesia. 2010;65(9):889-94.
3. Jackson C. Tracheotomy. Laryngoscope. 1909;18:285.
4. Brantigan CO, Grow JB. Cricothyroidotomy: elective use in respiratory problems requiring tracheotomy. J Thorac Cardiovasc Surg. 1976;71:72.
5. O'Connor JV, Reddy K, Ergin MA, Griepp RB. Cricothyroidotomy for prolonged ventilatory support after cardiac operations. Ann Thorac Surg. 1985;39(4):353-4.
6. Sise MJ, Shackford SR, Cruickshank JC, Murphy G, Fridlund PH. Cricothyroidotomy for long-term tracheal access. A prospective analysis of morbidity and mortality in 76 patients. Ann Surg. 1984;200(1):13-7.
7. Van Hasselt EJ, Bruining HA, Hoeve LJ. Elective cricothyroidotomy. Intensive Care Med. 1985;11(4):207-9.
8. Committee on Trauma, American College of Surgeons. ATLS: Advanced Trauma Life Support Program for Doctors. 8th edition. Chicago: American College of Surgeons. 2008.
9. Roberts JR, Hedges JR. Clinical Procedures in Emergency Medicine. 2nd edition. Philadelphia: WB Saunders. 1991. pp. 40-59.
10. Brofeldt BT, Panacek EA, Richards JR. An easy cricothyrotomy approach: the rapid four-step technique. Acad Emerg Med. 1996;3:1060-3.
11. Schaumann N, Lorenz V, Schellongowski P, Staudinger T, Locker GJ, Burgmann H, et al. Evaluation of Seldinger technique emergency cricothyroidotomy versus standard surgical cricothyroidotomy in 200 cadavers. Anesthesiology. 2005;102(1):7.
12. Curtis K, Ahern M, Dawson M, Mallin M. Ultrasound-guided, Bougie-assisted cricothyroidotomy: a description of a novel technique in cadaveric models. Acad Emerg Med. 2012;19(7):876-9.

8

Percutaneous Tracheostomy

Devendra Gupta

INTRODUCTION

Tracheostomy is a common critical care procedure performed in patients of medical intensive care units (ICUs), in about 24% of patients.[1,2] Advancement in technique of bedside percutaneous dilatational tracheostomy (PCDT) has replaced the surgical tracheostomy in intensive care. It is a well established bedside procedure in critically ill patient that every intensivist needs to know.

Percutaneous dilatational tracheostomy, first designated by Toye and Weinstein in 1969, has so much evolved over the last three decades that has change the practice of tracheostomy ICU.[3] Though the technique may be performed blind, however, the trachea should be visualized through intubating fiberoptic laryngoscope or bronchoscope passed down the tracheal tube.

INDICATION

- Need for prolonged mechanical ventilation (time is not well defined in literature; in general if need for translaryngeal intubation is anticipated for more than 10–14 days at one time point, then consider for PCDT).
- Nonemergency airway obstruction
- Facilitate weaning from ventilation and sedation
- Prevent aspiration
- Management of secretions

CONTRAINDICATION

It is a subject of intense debate over absolute and relative contraindications.

Absolute

- Emergency surgical airway management
- Preexisting infection or malignancy
- Unstable cervical spine injury
- Uncertainty of anatomical landmarks
- Pediatric patients

Relative

- Enlarged thyroid
- Previous surgery at tracheostomy site
- Preadolescent children
- Bleeding diathesis
- Preexisting tracheomalacia
- Morbid obesity

APPLIED ANATOMY

The thyroid notch is the most prominent point on the laryngeal prominence of the thyroid cartilage. If finger is placed over thyroid notch and move down along with body of thyroid cartilage, a space between the lower border of the thyroid cartilage and upper border of the cricoid cartilage can be felt called as cricothyroid space (Fig. 1).

The length of trachea varies between 10 cm and 13 cm depending on the height of the individual. The cartilages of trachea are C-shaped. These are total 18–22 in numbers and, with an average of two rings per cm. In coronal section the diameter may vary from 2.0 cm to 2.5 cm whereas it is 1.5–1.8 cm sagitally in adults. On average it is 2.0–2.5 cm deep from skin at the level of the second tracheal ring. Important step is to identify thyroid cartilage (most prominent cartilage in midline of the neck), followed by the cricothyroid membrane and cricoids cartilage and the tracheal rings. It is essential that the tracheal puncture be made inferior to the cricoid cartilage landmark.

Trachea enters the superior mediastinum through the suprasternal notch. The innominate artery, or brachiocephalic trunk, cross from left to right anterior

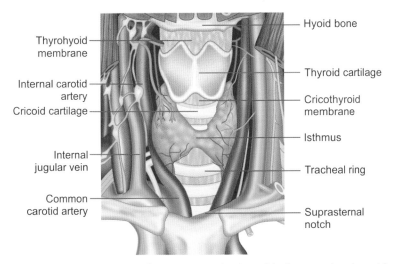

Fig. 1 Anatomy relevant to tracheostomy: anterior view of the larynx and trachea with neighboring structure

Source: Adapted from Figure 2.1 Anatomy of the Larynx and Trachea, Principles and Practice of Percutaneous Tracheostomy, SP Ambesh, Jaypee Brothers Medical Publishers (P) Ltd.

to the trachea at superior thoracic inlet and lie just beneath the sternum. Trachea has a close relationship with the mediastinal pleura, azygos vein and vagus nerve laterally on right side and the aortic arch and major left side arteries on the left side.

TECHNIQUE AND EQUIPMENT

Tracheostomy has various advantages over endotracheal intubation, including lower airway resistance, smaller dead space, decreased need for sedation, more efficient suction, improved oral hygiene thus reduced risk of ventilator associated pneumonia and greater patient comfort.[4,5] The decision of tracheostomy in ICU patients should be made on an individual basis and should depend on prognostic evaluations and not on "calendar watching".[6]

Seldinger described needle replacement over a guidewire for arterial catheterization in 1953. Later in 1955, Shelden et al. tried PCDT[7] with a slotted needle but unfortunately, have caused multiple complications, and fatalities. In 1969, Toye et al. described a tracheotomy technique using a single tapered dilator with a recessed cutting blade.[2] Many PCDT techniques have been evolved later. The differences between the various methods essentially relate to differences in identifying the trachea, insertion of guidewire and formation of the tracheal stoma by dilatation. PCDT technique can be broadly classified into two, based on the guidewire insertion.

 I Seldinger's technique (Anterograde)
 II Translaryngeal technique (Retrograde)

Percutaneous Dilatational Tracheostomy Methods using Seldinger's Technique (Anterograde)

These percutaneous techniques are based on the technique of needle replacement over a guidewire, initially described by Seldinger.[8] Under the bronchoscopic control, the trachea is identified by aspirating air through catheter introducer needle attached with syringe, between first and second or second and third tracheal rings. The J-wire is inserted through it into the trachea (Fig. 2). Subsequently different dilators have been used to form tracheal stoma guided over J-wire to facilitate placement of tracheostomy. This can be further divided on the basis of different methods of tracheal stoma dilatation:

Classification of Percutaneous Tracheostomy Methods using Seldinger's Technique

A. *Multiple (serial) dilatation method*
   (Multiple-dilator technique by Ciaglia)
B. *Single dilatation method*
   a. Single tapered dilator technique
      1. Blue Rhino
      2. Frova's PercuTwist
      3. Ambesh T-Trach technique
   b. Griggs' technique
   c. Balloon facilitation technique

A. Multiple-dilator Technique by Ciaglia

In 1985, Ciaglia et al. coined the term the PCDT, a method based on needle guidewire airway access by Seldinger's method followed by serial dilations with sequentially larger dilators.[9] Originally, Ciaglia et al. described the point of entry to be higher at the level of subcricoidal; which was associated with a risk of subglottic stenosis.[10,11] Therefore, the preferred site of entry is now between the first and the second or the second and third tracheal rings.[12,13] The serial dilational technique involves the insertion of prelubricated dilators that gradually enlarge the diameter of a tract made by a guidewire and guiding catheter, facilitating placement of a standard tracheostomy tube (Figs 2 and 3).

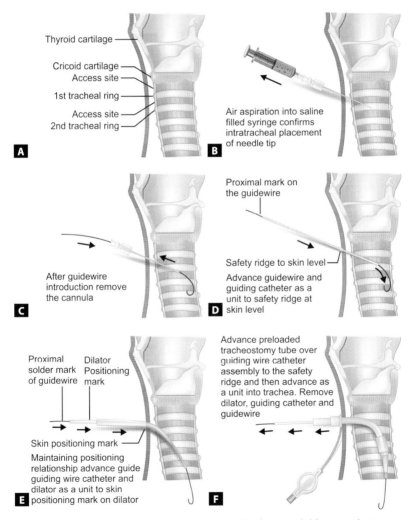

Figs 2A to F Multiple-dilator technique by Ciaglia using Seldinger technique

Source: Adapted from Figures 6.2A to D, and 6.3A and B Ciaglia's techniques of percutaneous dilational tracheostomy. Principles and Practice of Percutaneous Tracheostomy, SP Ambesh, Jaypee Brothers Medical Publishers (P) Ltd.

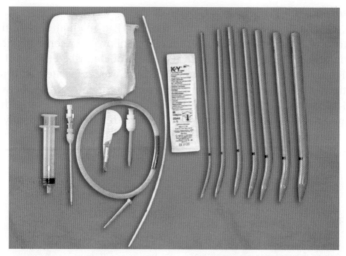

Fig. 3 Ciaglia's multiple dilator percutaneous tracheostomy kit

Source: Adapted from Figure 6.1 Ciaglia's techniques of percutaneous dilational tracheostomy, Principles and Practice of Percutaneous Tracheostomy, SP Ambesh, Jaypee Brothers Medical Publishers (P) Ltd.

B. *Single Dilatation Method*
a. *Single tapered dilator technique:*
   1. *Blue Rhino:* In 2000, Byhahn et al. introduced the Ciaglia Blue Rhino.[14] In this technique, a hydrophilically coated curved dilator (Blue Rhino, Portex single tapered dilator) is used for dilation of the tracheal stoma in a single step (Figs 4 and 5). Consequently, the risk of posterior tracheal wall injury and intraoperative bleeding is reduced. In addition, the adverse effect on oxygenation during repeated airway obstruction by the dilators is also reduced. The advantage with single dilatation is reduced loss of airway which happened repeatedly with serial dilatation and reduced blood loss. There is less chances of trauma and bleeding reported with single dilatation technique. Therefore, compared to serial multiple dilatation method, single-dilator PCDT technique is a safe, cost-effective, and more rapidly performed method of PCDT in the ICU.
   2. *Frova's PercuTwist:* In 2002 Frova introduced a controlled rotating dilation using a single step dilator with a self-tapping screw termed as PercuTwist technique.[15] The PercuTwist screw is commercially available for 7, 8, 9 mm ID cannula insertion (corresponding to 11.6, 13, and 14.3 mm outer screw diameter respectively) (Fig. 6). These are coated with hydrophilic film with lubricating property which is activated once screw is immersed in water for more than 15–20 seconds. There are more incidences of difficulty in tracheostomy tube insertion following the Forva PercuTwist method compared to Blue Rhino.[16] Many times during the process of rotation of Forva PercuTwist dilator, loose subcutaneous tissues are rolled up with screw of dilator.
   3. *Ambesh T-Trach technique:* SP Ambesh has introduced a new PCDT device using the "T-Dagger" (Criticure Invasives, India) for rapid bedside percutaneous tracheostomy[17] which is now available as Ambesh T-Trach

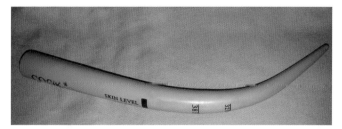

Fig. 4 Ciaglia blue rhino percutaneous tracheostomy single taped dilator

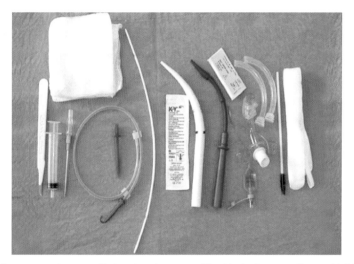

Fig. 5 Portex percutaneous dilational tracheostomy kit with single stage dilator with blue line ultra tracheostomy tube and introducer

Source: Adapted from Figure 6.4B, Ciaglia's techniques of percutaneous dilational tracheostomy, Principles and Practice of Percutaneous Tracheostomy, SP Ambesh, Jaypee Brothers Medical Publishers (P) Ltd.

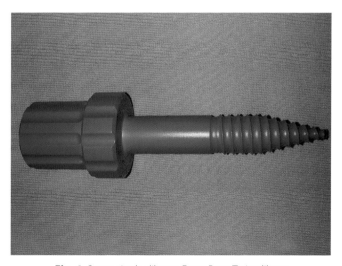

Fig. 6 Screw single dilators. Frova PercuTwist dilator

(Eastern Medikit Limited, India) (Fig. 7). The T-Trach is T-shaped tapered semi-rigid device. The T-Trach is smooth curved at middle part about 30°, ellipsoid in cross-section. It has numbers of hole in its shaft for the purpose of ventilation at the time of dilatation of trachea. At its proximal end it has 5 cm long soft guide catheter. The distal end has T-shaped shoulder for better grip (Fig. 8). Whole device has a central tunnel for guidewire passage. The T-Dagger™ forms the appropriate size of tracheal stoma for the corresponding size of tracheostomy tube with no under or over dilation. The elliptical shape of the shaft forms the tracheal stoma by splitting the inter-tracheal ring membrane and does not distort the tracheal rings as such. The oval holes in the shaft in T-Dagger™ provide access to the to-and-fro airflow during ventilation. Moreover, the elliptical shape of

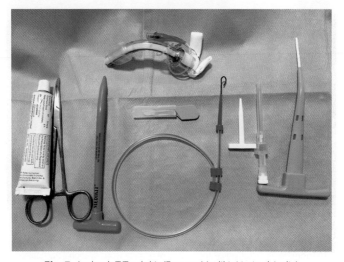

Fig. 7 Ambesh T-Trach kit (Eastern Medikit Limited, India)

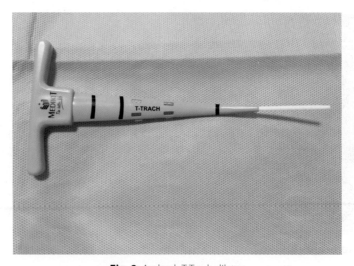

Fig. 8 Ambesh T-Trach dilator

the shaft leaves plentiful space in the tracheal lumen to accommodate the fiberoptic bronchoscope with no compromise in the ventilation.[17]

b. *Griggs' technique:* In 1990, Griggs and colleagues described a method based on a forceps, the guidewire dilating forceps (GWDF) method.[18] Unique forceps design allows passing guidewire between two blades of Griggs forceps (Figs 9 and 10). In the Griggs technique dilatation of the tracheal aperture is achieved by passing a dilating forceps (GWDF) over the guidewire, into the trachea. Opening these forceps forcibly dilates the tracheal aperture and any intervening tissue. Fikkers et al. showed that the greater number of difficult dilatations and minor bleeding were higher with the Ciaglia Blue Rhino dilation technique compared to Griggs' GWDF technique).[19] Voice problems and/or persistent hoarseness were also reported more frequently after colonic

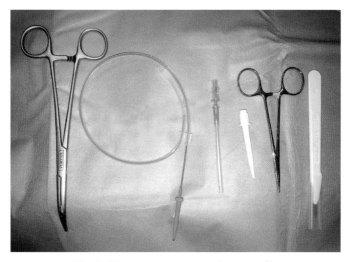

Fig. 9 Griggs percutaneous tracheostomy kit

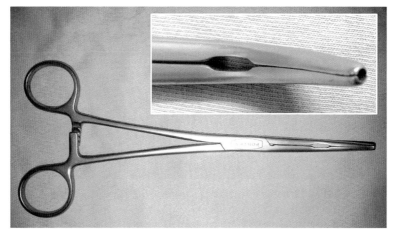

Fig. 10 Griggs' guidewire dilating forceps (GWDF), insect diagram showing channel in the GWDF for the passage of guidewire

dilatation. Contrary to common belief of higher complication rate with the use of sharp instruments (e.g., Griggs' GWDF technique), complications of percutaneous tracheostomy appear most likely to occur during the process of learning the technique—the "learning curve". There is increased risk of bleeding on opening the dilating forceps at the level tracheostomy site between first and second or between second and third tracheal rings because of presence of thyroid isthmus. Moreover, cosmetic problems were more associated with the GWDF technique than with single tapped dilator.[19]

c. *Balloon facilitation technique:* Combined balloon dilatation (CBD) is a new technique for PCDT using radial balloon dilation, offers a one-step solution for elective tracheostomies (Fig. 11). The balloon is made up of nylon and 5.4 cm long. It has an outer diameter of 16 mm when fully inflated. The maximum inflation pressure of the balloon is 11 atmospheres (ATM). PCDT is performed in an antegrade approach using the Seldinger guidewire technique with a tracheostomy tube preloaded onto a dilation balloon catheter.[20] The distal portion of CBD assembly holds a deflated balloon, while the proximal portion is armed with tracheostomy cannula (Fig. 11). The new balloon-facilitated Ciaglia Blue Dolphin dilatational tracheostomy technique uses mainly radial force to widen the tracheostoma thereby eliminating downward pressure during insertion and dilation. Because in most cases no soft tissue dissection is needed beyond a simple skin incision and no dilator is repeatedly advanced back and forth into the trachea, it reduces the patient risk associated with bleeding, ring fracture, posterior wall perforations and achieves good cosmetic results after decannulation. Many times temporary occlusion at the time of inflation of balloon for 15 seconds causes apnea or sometime life threatening hypoxemia.[20]

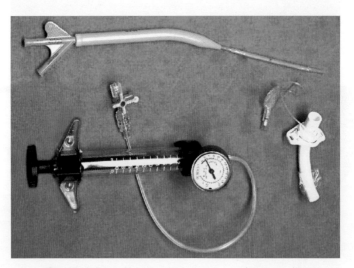

Fig. 11 Balloon dilatation percutaneous tracheostomy kit

Source: Adapted from Fig. 10.1, Balloon facilitated percutaneous tracheostomy, Principles and Practice of Percutaneous Tracheostomy, SP Ambesh, Jaypee Brothers Medical Publishers (P) Ltd.

Translaryngeal Technique (Retrograde)

In 1997 Fantoni devised translaryngeal tracheostomy (TLT) using a specially designed cannula to dilate the trachea in a retrograde manner.[21] This bronchoscopic guided PCDT was claimed to be a safe procedure when performed by experienced medical intensive care personnel in tertiary care institutions.[22] Bronchoscopy helps to reduce the risk of major complications and aids in the management of minor complications.

All TLT maneuvers took place under bronchoscopic visualization, and the TLT Kit (Mallinckrodt, Mirandola, Italy) was used. This technique of tracheostomy through translaryngeal approach comprises of passage of a dilator and tracheostomy tube from inside of trachea to outside of the neck. Unlike the other techniques, the initial puncture of the trachea is carried out with the needle directed cranially and the tracheal cannula inserted with a pull-through technique along the orotracheal route in a retrograde fashion. The cannula is then rotated downward using a plastic obturator. It should be noted that the procedure can only be carried out under endoscopic guidance, and rotating the tracheal cannula downward may pose a problem demanding that the surgeon have more experience (Figs 12A to G).

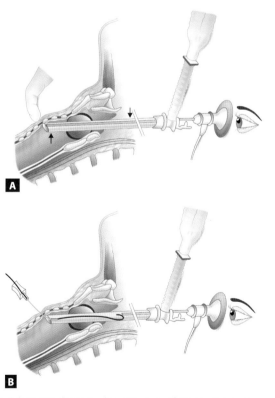

Figs 12A and B Schematic diagram showing step of Fantoni's translaryngeal tracheostomy technique. (A) The leverage of RTS enhances the transillumination and ensures palpation of the end of RTS from the outside. (B) Needle and wire insertion

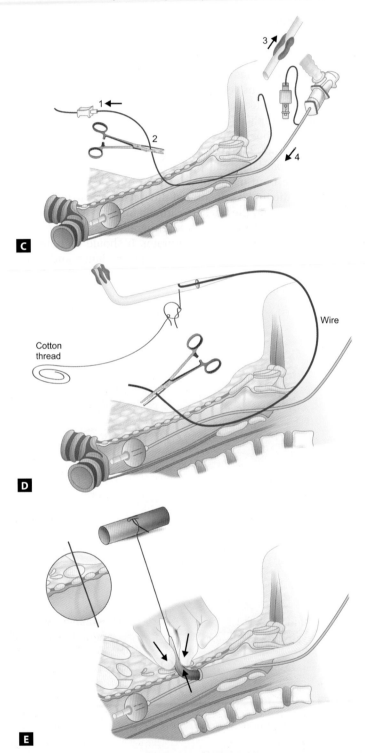

Figs 12C to E (C) Placement of ventilation catheter. (D) Wire and safety thread connection to the cone-cannula. (E) Cone-cannula extraction

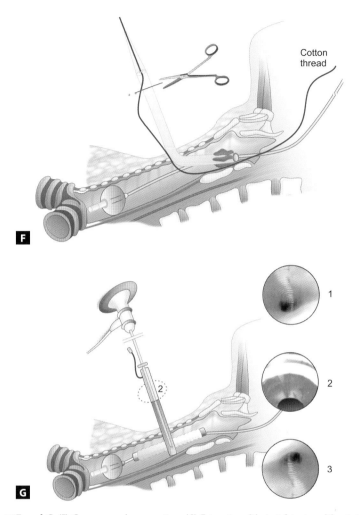

Figs 12F and G (F) Cone-cannula separation. (G) Extraction, (1) straightening, (2) rotation and (3) final positioning

Source: Adapted from A photo plate with combined diagram 9.11B, 9.12, 9.13B, 9.14B, 9.15B, 9.17, and 9.21 Fantoni's translaryngeal tracheostomy technique, Principles and Practice of Percutaneous Tracheostomy, SP Ambesh, Jaypee Brothers Medical Publishers (P) Ltd.

The biggest advantage of TLT is inside-outside dilation maneuver that avoid posterior tracheal wall injury and there is the minimal amount of skin incision required, with practically no bleeding observed. It has also been successfully carried out on infants and children.[23] It may be particularly useful in patients with bleeding diathesis and goiter. Disadvantage includes the rotating the tracheal cannula downward may pose a problem, thus demanding more experience. There is also an apnea phase of about 60–90 seconds during the procedure.[24] This technique should therefore be contraindicated in patients with severe respiratory insufficiency requiring extreme forms of mechanical ventilation (high positive end-expiratory pressure, high inspiratory oxygen concentration). Additionally, there is a significant amount of contamination since the tracheal cannula is pulled through the oropharynx.

Use of Bronchoscopy during Procedure

The PCDT should be performed under continuous bronchoscopic guidance.[25] Advantages of the continuous bronchoscopy during percutaneous tracheostomy are:

- Transillumination of tracheal region help in identification of anterior blood vessel
- Identification of tracheal ring and cricoids cartilage
- Reduction of risk of accidental loss of airway
- Helping in cannula placement in trachea under vision
- Protection of posterior tracheal wall injury
- Prevention of false tract formation
- Tracheal exploration during tracheal dilatation by different methods
- Early detection of complication, e.g. bleeding
- Facilitation of training and teaching

There are some potential risks of using bronchoscope during PDT that are partial occlusion of endotracheal tube and airway leading to carbon dioxide retention, hypoxia; and pneumothorax secondary to air trapping, and damage to the bronchoscope by needle puncture.

Recent studies showed the use of real-time ultrasonography, with actual visualization of the needle path up to the anterior tracheal wall further decreases the risk of puncture above the first tracheal ring as well as the risk of injury to surrounding structures and the posterior tracheal wall. Ultrasound imaging also outline the exact position of the tracheal rings prior to puncture in these patients even in the absence of clearly palpable tracheal anatomy (e.g., in patients with morbid obesity) and without extending the neck (in patients with cervical spine precautions).[26]

Ultrasound also helps in identification of blood vessels adjacent to the PCDT insertion site reducing risk of bleeding, estimating tracheal depth from the skin surface and tracheal diameter and ensuring accurate placement of the needle into the trachea.[27]

PREPARATION

Percutaneous dilatational tracheostomy is an elective procedure done on intubated adult patients with normal neck anatomy. The procedure should be performed during regular working hour when supporting staff is most readily available. Following are the common steps of preparation of the PDT which should be followed before percutaneous tracheostomy.

- *Risk assessment and consent:* Informed consent should be taken from family member of the patient following explaining the risk or benefit of the procedure including a review of absolute and relative contraindications. A detailed airway and clinical examination of the anterior neck anatomy must be performed with additional imaging as indicated (e.g., ultrasound or radiological) to identify potential difficulty.[27]
- *Fasting:* A minimum 4 hours of fasting is recommended. Residual gastric contents should be aspirated with wide bore nasogastric tube prior to the procedure.

- *Equipment:* All equipment of PDT should be ready like PCDT kit, crash cart, suction, monitor sterile sheet, gown, gloves, dressing trolley and fiberoptic video bronchoscope. Equipment related to emergency airway management should be available. The open surgical tracheostomy set should also be ready and person experienced of doing open tracheostomy should be kept as a backup.
- *Ventilation:* Preoxygenation and ventilation with 100% oxygen is recommended following proper suctioning of endotracheal tube. Ventilator setting should be changed pertinent to general anesthesia and ventilator requirement of the patient.
- *Monitoring:* Patient should be attached to the monitor and monitored for SpO_2, ECG, heart rate (HR), blood pressure (BP), end tidal CO_2.

PROCEDURE

The PCDT should be performed in an area with adequate light and sufficient space for performing the procedure and airway management at head end.
- *Medication:* Patient should have intravenous cannula and intravenous fluid should be started. Patients should be given hypnotics (midazolam and/or propofol), opioids (remifentanil or fentanyl) and muscle relaxant (vecuronium or atracurium).
- *Positioning:* Supine position with hyperextension of the neck should be made by putting a roll under the shoulder.
- *Skin preparation:* Operator should disinfect the skin and apply sterile full body drapes and identify the landmarks and mark the possible insertion site.
- *Fiberoptic bronchoscopy:* A trained person in airway management should be present at head end for the manipulation of endotracheal tube under direct laryngoscopy or under fiberoptic bronchoscope. At this stage oropharynx and endotracheal suctioning should be done.
- *Landmark identification:* The trachea is palpated for identification of cricoids and first, second and third tracheal ring. Operator should identify thyroid cartilage (most prominent cartilage in midline of the neck), followed by the cricothyroid membrane and cricoids cartilage and the tracheal rings.
- *Local anesthetic:* Local anesthetics 5–10 mL of 1% lignocaine with 1:200,000 adrenaline is infiltrated subcutaneously for local vasoconstriction once area of incision is defined.
- *Skin incision and dissection:* A midline, vertical, 2-cm incision is given just above the suprasternal notch. The subcutaneous tissues are dissected bluntly down up to the pretracheal fascia. The trachea is then manually palpated. It is essential that the tracheal puncture be made inferior to the cricoids cartilage landmark. Initial skin incision and blunt preparation of the pretracheal tissue may be helpful to identify the tracheal rings, thus avoiding either too high or too low tracheal puncture.
- *Airway manipulation:* The endotracheal tube cuff is deflated and endotracheal tube is retracted under guidance of the finger palpating the trachea and then the cuff is reinflated after final repositioning.
- *J-wire insertion:* The cannula included in the kit is introduced into the trachea, between the second and third tracheal rings after palpating tracheal space by little finger. Airflow in the syringe confirms the right position of the cannula tip (Fig. 1). Utmost care is done that needle is not injured posterior wall of

trachea. The cannula is advanced into trachea and needle is withdrawn. The J-tip Seldinger wire is introduced through the cannula. Free movement of guidewire in and out confirms its correct position. Many reports have been published regarding the lower rates of acute complications under endoscopic guidance.[28]

- *Tracheal dilatation:* Once guidewire is in place, trachea has been dilated with help of different methods of dilatation. Further the trachea has been dilated with different methods mentioned below:

Ciaglia Blue Rhino (Figs 13 and 14)

A small, firm introducing dilator is slide over the wire, through the soft tissues into the trachea. The dilator is then removed, keeping the wire in place. The stoma is then dilated, using a single curved tapered dilator "Blue Rhino" (COOK Critical Care, Bloomington) or White Dilator (Portex Ltd., UK). The dilator is slided over the "guiding catheter" until the blunt end of the dilator aligns with the "dilator-positioning" mark on the catheter (Figs 13 and 14).

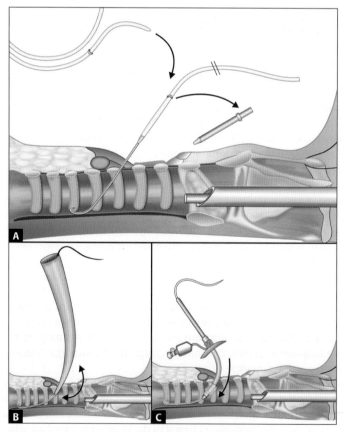

Figs 13A to C (A) Passage of guiding catheter following dilation with small dilator. (B) Dilatation of tracheal stoma with single tapered dilator. (C) Advancement of tracheostomy tube

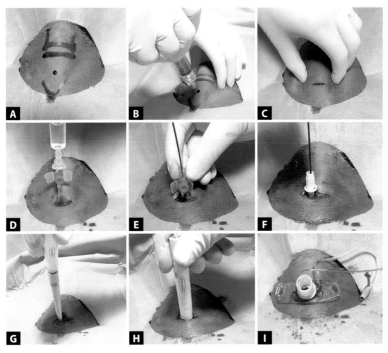

Figs 14A to I Step of percutaneous dilation tracheostomy by single taped dilation technique. (A) Landmark of percutaneous tracheostomy, (B) Infiltration of local anesthetics, (C) Skin incision, (D) Intratracheal cannula insertion. (E) Insertion of J-tip guidewire through cannula. (F) Tracheal stoma dilation with introducing dilator. (G) Passage of single tapered dilator with it guiding sheath over guidewire. (H) Full dilatation of trachea stoma with single tapered dilator. (I) Placement of tracheostomy tube

Lubricant with sterile aqueous jelly should be applied at the tip of the dilator. The dilator should be pushed in and out several times with firm pressure into the tracheal stoma. Once dilatation process is completed, the tracheostomy tube mounted on the corresponding size dilator is then threaded over the guidewire catheter assembly and inserted into dilated tracheal stoma.

Griggs' Technique (Figs 15A to I)

A 14G well-lubricated initial dilator is threaded over guidewire to make a small stoma in anterior tracheal wall. Following initial stoma formation, GWDF in closed state is advanced over guidewire into the tracheal stoma (Fig. 15). Once the tip of the GWDF is passed into the trachea, direction of the handle is now changed towards chin of the patient (Fig. 15). Once position of the GWDF is confirmed by fiberoptic bronchoscope, GWDF is opened. A great precaution is required to apply force to open the GWDF for tracheal dilatation. A rough assessment of degree of opening of GWDF can be made by checking, how much handle of GWDF get apart while holding the tracheostomy tube between GWDF flanges. GWDF is removed, keeping guidewire in trachea, in slight open state. Appropriate size tracheostomy tube with it obturator mounted on guidewire and inserted into dilated tracheal stoma.

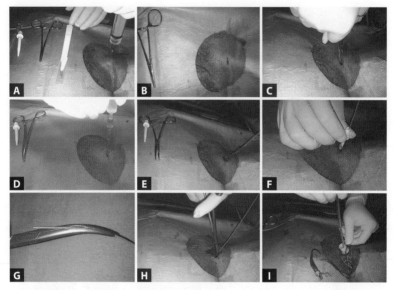

Figs 15A to I Step of percutaneous dilation tracheostomy by Griggs forceps (GWDF). (A) Infiltration of local anesthetics. (B) Skin incision. (C) Dissection of subcutaneous tissue. (D) Intratracheal cannula insertion. (E) Insertion of J-tip guidewire through cannula. (F) Tracheal stoma dilation with introducing dilator. (G) Loading of the Griggs forceps over guidewire. (H) Full dilatation of trachea stoma with Griggs forceps. (I) Placement of tracheostomy tube

Frova PercuTwist (Figs 16A to I)

Appropriate size PercuTwist screw after lubricated with saline is advanced over the guidewire. The PercuTwist is hold with its upper broad part (head) with index finger and thumb. A moderate downward pressure is needed to apply in first two to three twist (clockwise) of the screw in order to allow the screw to hold the tissue. Thereafter with the twisted movement, the PercuTwist is advanced into trachea without any downward force rather a PercuTwist is held slightly up with the help of fingers of non-dominating hand in order to prevent any injury to posterior tracheal wall (Fig. 16). Every complete screw turn corresponds to 2.5 mm advancement. During the entire procedure, guidewire should regularly be checked by to and fro movement of guidewire through PercuTwist. This confirms the position and correct progression of PercuTwist dilator. Once tip of PercuTwist is seen in trachea through bronchoscope, its head should be bent towards the chin of the patient. Screwing movement should be continued till full conic part of the PercuTwist is inside the trachea (6–7 twists). The PercuTwist then removed by making anticlockwise rotation without any traction force. Thereafter, tracheostomy tube with its semi-rigid round tipped introducer is inserted over guidewire and placed into trachea under bronchoscopic guidance. Thereafter, tracheostomy tube with its round tipped introducer is inserted over guidewire and placed into trachea under bronchoscopic guidance.

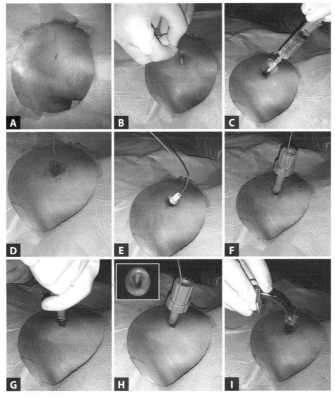

Figs 16A to I Step of percutaneous dilation tracheostomy by Frova PercuTwist. (A) Infiltration of local anesthetics. (B) Skin incision. (C) Intratracheal cannula insertion. (D) Insertion of J-tip guidewire through cannula. (E) Tracheal stoma dilation with introducing dilator. (F) Loading of the Frova PercuTwist dilator. (G) Insertion of Frova PercuTwist dilator by screw movement. (H) Full dilatation of trachea stoma with Frova PercuTwist (inset showed Frova PercuTwist dilator through bronchoscope). (I) Placement of tracheostomy tube

Ambesh T-Dagger (Figs 17A to L)

Once guidewire has been passed into trachea as described in Seldinger technique, a well lubricated 14-French initial dilator is advanced over guide to make tracheal stoma formation. The T-Trach then loaded over guidewire and tries to negotiate it proximal soft guide catheter into tracheal stoma. Once guide catheter is passed into trachea and its position is confirmed by fiberoptic bronchoscope, the T-Trach is then advanced slowly into trachea over guidewire. The direction of T-Trach dilator is then changed to about 60° and slowly it is advanced to its desire length (Fig. 17). The length of the T-Trach inserted into trachea depends on the size of the tracheosotmy tube to be inserted. After full dilatation of tracheal stoma, the T-Tract is removed. Thereafter, appropriate size tracheostomy tube will be loaded on introducer or obturator over guidewire and placed into trachea.

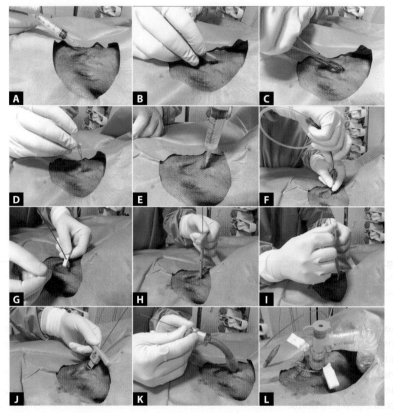

Figs 17A to L Step of percutaneous dilation tracheostomy by Ambesh T-Trach. (A) Infiltration of local anesthetics. (B) Skin incision. (C) Dissection of percutaneous tissue. (D) Intratracheal cannula insertion. (E) Confirmation of cannula position into trachea. (F) Insertion of J-tip guidewire through cannula. (G) Tracheal stoma dilation with introducing dilator. (H) Loading of the Ambesh T-Trach over guidewire. (I) Position of hand while advancing Ambesh T-Trach into trachea. (J) Full dilatation of trachea stoma with Ambesh T-Trach. (K) Placement of tracheostomy tube with tracheostomy tube introducer. (L) Tracheostomy tube attached with ventilator

Balloon Facilitation Technique

In manner to prepare the CBD, all the air should be purge out of inflation device, balloon and tubing. The inflation device should be filled with at least 20 mL of sterile saline. After generously lubricating the loading dilator, appropriate size of tracheostomy is loaded on to the loading dilator. Then prepared inflation device is attached to the balloon port on the balloon catheter assembly. There should be no air in the inflation device before connecting to balloon port. A 14 French short introducing dilator is advanced over guidewire. Using the twisting movement and controlled force dilator is pushed into the trachea to make an initial stoma. Dilator is removed while maintaining guidewire in position. Now with the balloon in fully deflated condition, whole balloon catheter and tracheostomy assembly is advanced over guidewire. The proximal end of balloon catheter is aligned at the mark on the proximal portion of guidewire. This will ensure

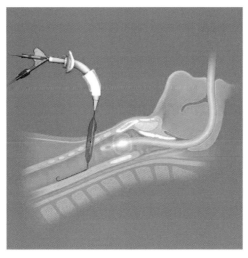

Fig. 18 Percutaneous dilation tracheostomy by balloon facilitating technique. Prepared inflation device is attached to the balloon port on the balloon catheter assembly and positioned into trachea and tracheal stoma dilatation by balloon inflation

the distal of the balloon catheter is correctly aligned on the guidewire, preventing possible trauma to the posterior tracheal wall during subsequent maneuver. Balloon catheter assembly along with guidewire is advanced into the trachea until balloon is halfway into trachea. The correct position of the balloon inside the trachea is confirmed by visualizing black mark on anterior tracheal wall on bronchoscopy. Balloon is now inflated while maintaining the visual reference point and positioning relation of guidewire and balloon catheter assembly (Fig. 18). Digital stabilization of balloon catheter is maintained during initial inflation of the balloon. Lock lever on the inflation device is disengaged (slide to left) to allow free movement of the plunger. After full inflation of the balloon the lever is engaged. Balloon is kept inflated for 10–20 seconds, lubricated with saline solution. Now lever is disengaged and balloon is deflated until all infused saline is withdrawn. Thereafter the proximal portion of balloon facilitated percutaneous tracheostomy (BFPT) device that carry tracheostomy tube is advanced into the trachea. The whole BFPT assembly should be directed perpendicular to the axis of the trachea during insertion for uniform dilatation between tracheal cartilages. Once the tracheostomy is in place, the balloon catheter, loading dilator and guidewire should be slowly removed. Position of tracheostomy is confirmed and connected to the ventilator.

Post-tracheostomy Tube Placement

Tracheostomy tube cuff is inflated once the appropriate size tracheostomy tube is placed into the trachea. Before connecting to the breathing circuit, suction catheter is passed into trachea through tracheostomy tube to ensure position of the tracheostomy tube and rule out any bleeding. The tracheostomy tube is now connected with ventilator circuit and confirm tube placement by seeing tidal volume or minute ventilation, chest inflation, chest auscultation, end-tidal CO_2 ($EtCO_2$).

Tracheostomy tube is secured in its position with suture and tie around the neck. A slit gauze piece is placed between the tracheostomy wings and the skin. A chest radiograph is mandatory after the procedure. Patient should be observer for any bleeding, high airway pressure or desaturation. Arterial blood gas should be done after half an hour thereafter ventilator settings should be readjusted.

POST-TRACHEOSTOMY CARE

- *Securing the tracheostomy tube:* Ties or cloth tapes should be checked for adequate grip and must be changed daily or when soiled or wet.[29] In case of neck surgery the tracheostomy tube should be stitched to the skin or else a breastplate can be used to secure if indicated. Tapes should be neither too tight nor very loose. This should be tested by putting two fingers between the tape and the patient's neck. If more than two fingers can be inserted then the tape is too loose.
- *Cuff pressure:* The cuff seals the space around the tracheostomy tube which prevent leak of the gas and prevent aspiration of oral or gastric secretions.[30] Cuff pressures should regularly be monitored to prevent tracheal injury and air leaks. Modern tracheostomy cuffs are high-volume, low-pressure to minimize tracheal wall ischemic necrosis. Cuff pressure must be checked a minimum of once per shift and maintained between 14 cm H_2O and 24 cm H_2O (10.36–17.76 mm Hg) using the tracheostomy cuff pressure gauge. As cuff leakage places the patient at an increased risk of aspiration, observe for clinical signs and symptoms of aspiration.[30]
- *Humidification*:
  - Heat moisture exchanger (HME) has limited ability of humidifying gas. Sometime copious, thick or bloody secretions block it easily thus increasing the risk of tube occlusion. Therefore, it should be observe for potential obstruction and possibly must be changed when soiled or every 24 hours.[31]
  - Hot water humidifier should be used when thick and copious secretions are present. In this, gas passes over the water bath, which is heated to body temperature and is then inhaled by the patient.[31] Water in the circuit is a good culture medium thus must be avoided.
  - Nebulization with bronchodilator mixed with saline must be administered 2–4 hourly and as required to provide fully saturated air with a fine mist of moisture.[31]
- *Stoma care:* The tracheal stoma site should be clean at least daily or more frequently if indicated. The choice of dressing is determined by condition of the stoma wound, amount of secretion and presence of granulation. Common problem which occur with tracheostomy stoma are: peri-stomal skin rashes, soft-tissue infection, excessive stomal granulation tissue, prolonged or renewed contraction, intratracheal erosions from irritation by the tube itself.
- *Abnormal bleeding:* Slight blood smears from the tracheostomy stoma are not unusual after percutaneous dilatation tracheostomy and usually subside within 24 hours.[32] Constant oozing may signal a bleeding vessel requiring intervention. Massive bleeding is life-threatening emergency and may warrants rupture of the any big vessel like innominate artery.[32] Overinflating the tracheostomy cuff is first line management. Translaryngeal intubation with digital compression may immediately be required to control bleeding.[33]

- *Suctioning:* Suctioning of the tracheostomy tube is necessary to remove mucus, maintain a patent airway, and avoid tracheostomy tube blockages. Acute care patients need to be assessed every 2 hours for the need for suctioning. However the frequency varies between patients and is based on individual assessment. Indications for suctioning include audible or visual signs of secretions in the tube, signs of respiratory distress or suspicion of a blocked or partially blocked tube, changes in ventilation pressure. Selection of the appropriate size suction catheter is vital in reducing the risk of trauma during suctioning. Correct size suction catheter in French gauge can be obtain by multiply the internal diameter (in mm) of the tracheostomy by three fourth.[34]

  The pressure setting for tracheal suctioning is 80–120 mm Hg (10–16 kpa) to avoid tracheal damage. The suction pressure setting should not exceed 120 mm Hg/16 kpa.[35] The episode of suctioning (including passing the catheter and suctioning the tracheostomy tube) should be completed within 5–10 seconds. Suctioning should be discontinued if heart rate drops by 20, increases by 40, drop in oxygen saturation by less than 90% or presence of arrhythmias. Routine use of 0.9% sodium chloride is not recommended however, in situations where this may be of benefit, e.g., thick secretions and to stimulate a cough 0.2–0.5 mL of 0.9% sodium chloride can be used.[36]

- *Changing tracheostomy tube:* Tracheostomy tube change in intensive care is very critical. Postoperative tracheostomy tube changes should be considered as a major procedure and not a part of routine care as it is associated complication leading to morbidity and even mortality.

  The most common accepted indications for tracheostomy change include the need for a size change (either decreased as part of weaning from mechanical ventilation and to facilitate vocalization and swallowing, or increased to allow passage of a bronchoscope into the airway); tube malfunction (e.g., fractured flange or nonfunctional cuff); need for a different type of tube (e.g., the need for a tube with an inner cannula); and routine changing as part of ongoing airway management. Conventional practice recommends changing the tube 7–14 days following placement;[37] however, there are no data to support that time frame, which was suggested to allow time for a stable endotracheal-cutaneous tract to form. A tract between the skin and the trachea develops after 1 week of tracheostomy tube placement. A mature stoma at the time of the tracheostomy tube change reduces the risk of establishing a false tract leading to subcutaneous emphysema, loss of the airway, mediastinitis and even death.

  In general, it is advisable to have two people present for any tracheostomy tube change and one must be experience of airway management. It is advisable that all the necessary instrument and percutaneous tracheostomy kit along with emergency endotracheal intubation equipment should be ready at the time of procedure. Nasogastric feed should be suspended for 4–6 hours to prevent inhalation of gastric contents. Important aspects to be considered when preparing to change the tracheostomy tube are, the timing, the type of tube being used, setting, frequency of previous tube changes, and individual patient characteristics such as age, weight, and general health factors.

  Prior to removing the old tube, all components of the new tracheostomy tube should be checked for integrity. The patient is placed either supine or semirecumbent, with the neck extended. The retaining sutures or ties are removed, the tracheostomy tube gently withdrawn, the new tracheostomy tube inserted, and the obturator removed. Removal of a tube through a tight stoma with a bulky cuff can be facilitated using 0.5–1 mL of lidocaine jelly (1%) inserted around the stoma or tube interface. It is important to remember that the first tracheostomy tube change can be associated with some risk. In a recent survey, surgical residents reported loss of airway in 42% and death in up to 15% of first tube changes.[38]

Patients with increased neck circumference, unusual airway anatomy, or with an elevated body mass index are at increased risk of having the tube placed into a false passage in the anterior mediastinum, especially during insertion of tracheostomy tube if the caudal turn is made prematurely before the distal end of tracheostomy tube reaches to tracheal lumen. If a difficult change is anticipated, tracheostomy tube change should be done by a skilled person trained in percutaneous tracheostomy. The use of a tube changer can help reduce the risk of airway loss. The "railroad" technique using an exchange device or "guiding" obturator, is recommended for difficult changes, e.g., immature tract, presence of factors contributing to tube change difficulties. The tube changer is passed through the existing tracheostomy tube into the trachea. The tracheostomy tube is then withdrawn while keeping the tube changer in place, and the new tube is then passed over the tube changer into the trachea. A fiberoptic tracheoscope can be very helpful to ensure correct placement of a tracheostomy tube and in addition allows for visual inspection of the airway anatomy, including the subglottic space.[39]

COMPLICATION/PROBLEM

There are risks and complications with this procedure. They include but are not limited to the following:

Perioperative

- Hemorrhage
- False passage
- Pneumothorax
- Lesion or laceration of the posterior tracheal wall
- Insertion failure
- Misplacement of insertion needle, J-tip wire or dilators
- Tracheal tube misplacement
- Hypoxia
- Hypotension
- Loss of airway
- Subcutaneous emphysema
- Death

Postoperative

- Hemorrhage
- Stomal infection
- Stomal granulation
- Tube displacement

Late Complication

- Stomal erosion or infection
- Laryngotracheal stenosis
- Tracheoinnominate artery fistula
- Tracheoesophageal fistula
- Ugly scar
- Voice change

Early Complications (Within the First 24 Hours)

Technical Problems

Accidental misplacement of the needle, guidewire or dilators into carotid artery, jugular vein, tracheal ring, esophagus, paratracheal tissues, endotracheal tube, cuff or Murphy's eye have all been reported.[40-42] Use of fiber optic during PCDT reduces the risk of misplacements. Failure to insert the tracheostomy tube appears to be greater when dilatation is insufficient or partial. The presence of tissue band around the stoma is common cause and pre-dilation dissection of the fascia and tissue can prevent it. Tracheal tube misplacement into the paratracheal tissues, posterior tracheal wall, esophagus and intrapleural space have all been reported.[43,44]

Hemorrhage

Controlled hemostasis is not possible in PCDT and therefore sometime leads hemorrhage. Minor bleeding usually stops with lateral pressure applied by the tracheostomy tube or with direct pressure applied to the wall of tracheal stoma. However, mortalities have been reported if a large vessel has been perforated (e.g., anterior jugular or thyroid veins) or presence of bleeding diathesis. In many cases a large bleed during tracheostomy necessitate reinsertion of the endotracheal tube, placement of the cuff over the tracheostomy stoma, and apply direct pressure over the stoma. If this does not control the bleeding, surgery is required.[45]

Barotrauma

There have been many published reports on incidence of barotrauma (e.g., subcutaneous emphysema, mediastinal emphysema, pneumothorax) after the PCDT.[44,46] After the percutaneous tracheostomy, airway pressure should be checked, bilateral air entry into the lungs should be confirmed and X-ray chest should always be done to rule any pneumothorax. Subcutaneous emphysema should be confirmed by palpation of supraclavicular space.

Tracheal Injury

The most feared complication associated percutaneous tracheostomy is tear or perforation of posterior tracheal wall incidence being 2–4%.[47,48] Serial dilatational technique required dilatation with multiple dilators and hence more chances of tracheal wall injury, this could be minimized with the use of single taped technique. Use of fiber optic cut down the incidences of posterior tracheal wall injury remarkably.[49]

Death

Though it is safe however, deaths been recorded which is usually due to misplaced tracheostomy tube insertion, premature decannulation or hemorrhage, with associated hypoxia and cardiac arrhythmia.[50-54]

Late Complications (After the First 24 Hours)

Late complications include wound infection or breakdown, skin tethering or scar and tracheal stenosis are usually less with PCDT.[55] Tracheal stenosis, tracheomalacia, tracheoinnominate fistula and tracheoesophageal fistula are usually infrequent complications. [56,57]

Delayed hemorrhage may also occur particularly in patients with secondary coagulopathies (e.g., in patients with multiple organ failure, renal failure, hepatic failure or trauma) and can lead to a life threatening complication of airway obstruction.[58] Bronchoscopy is helpful in diagnosing the cause of tracheal obstruction.

However, in case of acute obstruction tracheostomy must be taken out immediately and the patient intubated with an endotracheal tube. The ball valve clot usually "pops" out the tracheal stoma with removal of the tracheostomy tube. Rigid bronchoscopy is sometime needed to remove the clot from the trachea.

REFERENCES

1. Esteban A, Anzueto A, Alía I, Gordo F, Apezteguía C, Pálizas F, et al. How is mechanical ventilation employed in the intensive care unit? An international utilization review. Am J Respir Crit Care Med. 2000;161(5):1450-8.
2. Kumar M, Trikha A, Chandralekha. Percutaneous dilatational tracheostomy: Griggs guide wire dilating forceps technique versus ULTRA-perc single-stage dilator - A prospective randomized study. Indian J Crit Care Med. 2012;16(2):87-92.
3. Toye FJ, Weinstein JD. A percutaneous tracheostomy device. Surgery. 1969;65(2):384-9.
4. Astrachan DI, Kirchner JC, Goodwin WJ Jr. Prolonged intubation vs. tracheotomy: complications, practical and psychological considerations. Laryngoscope. 1988; 98(11):1165-9.
5. Diehl JL, El Atrous S, Touchard D, Lemaire F, Brochard L. Changes in the work of breathing induced by tracheotomy in ventilator-dependent patients. Am J Respir Crit Care Med. 1999;159(2):383-8.
6. Heffner JE. Timing tracheotomy: calendar watching or individualization of care? Chest. 1998;114(2):361-3.
7. Shelden CH, Pudenz RH, Freshwater DB, Crue BL. A new method for tracheostomy. J Neurosurg. 1955;12(4):428-31.
8. Seldinger SI. Catheter replacement of the needle in percutaneous arteriography; a new technique. Acta radiol. 1953;39(5):368-76.
9. Ciaglia P, Firsching R, Syniec C. Elective percutaneous dilatational tracheostomy. A new simple bedside procedure; preliminary report. Chest. 1985;87(6):715-9.
10. McFarlane C, Denholm SW, Sudlow CLM, Moralee SJ, Grant IS, Lee A. Laryngotracheal stenosis: a serious complication of percutaneous tracheostomy. Anaesthesia. 1994; 49(1):38-40.
11. van Heurn LW, Goei R, de Ploeg I, Ramsay G, Brink PRG. Late complications of percutaneous dilatational tracheotomy. Chest. 1996;110(6):1572-6.
12. Petros S, Engelmann L. Percutaneous dilatational tracheostomy in a medical ICU. Intensive Care Med. 1997;23(6):630-4.

13. Walz MK, Peitgen K, Thürauf N, Trost HA, Wolfhard U, Sander A, et al. Percutaneous dilatational tracheostomy--early results and long-term outcome of 326 critically ill patients. Intensive Care Med. 1998;24(7):685-90.
14. Byhahn C, Lischke V, Halbig S, Scheifler G, Westphal K. Ciaglia blue rhino: a modified technique for percutaneous dilatation tracheostomy. Technique and early clinical results. Anaesthetist. 2000;49(3):202-6.
15. Frova G, Quintel M. A new simple method of percutaneous tracheostomy: controlled rotating dilatation. A preliminary report. Intensive Care Med. 2002;28(3):299-303.
16. Byhahn C, Westphal K, Meininger D, Gürke B, Kessler P, Lischke V. Single-dilator percutaneous tracheostomy: a comparison of PercuTwist and Ciaglia Blue Rhino techniques. Intensive Care Med. 2002;28(9):1262-6.
17. Ambesh SP, Tripathi M, Pandey CK, Pant KC, Singh PK. Clinical evaluation of the 'T-Dragger': a new bedside percutaneous dilational tracheostomy device. Anaesthesia. 2005;60(7):708-11.
18. Griggs WM, Worthley LI, Gilligan JE, Thomas PD, Myburg JA. A simple percutaneous tracheostomy technique. Surg Gynecol Obstet. 1990;170(6):543-5.
19. Fikkers BG, Staatsen M, Lardenoije SGGF, van den Hoogen FJ, van der Hoeven JG. Comparison of two percutaneous tracheostomy techniques, guide wire dilating forceps and Ciaglia Blue Rhino: a sequential cohort study. Crit Care. 2004;8(5):R299-305.
20. Zgoda M, Berger R. Balloon-facilitated percutaneous dilational tracheostomy tube placement: preliminary report of a novel technique. Chest. 2005;128(5):3688-90.
21. Konopke R, Zimmermann T, Volk A, Pyrc J, Bergert H, Blomenthal A, Gastmeier J, Kersting S. Prospective evaluation of retrograde percutaneous translaryngeal tracheo- stomy (Fantoni procedure) in a surgical intensive care unit: Technique and results of the Fantoni tracheostomy. Head and Neck. 2006;28(4):355-9.
22. Byhahn C, Wilke HJ, Lischke V, Rinne T, Westphal K. Bedside percutaneous tracheo- stomy: clinical comparison of Griggs and Fantoni technique. World J Surg. 2001;25(3): 296-301.
23. Fantoni A, Ripamonti D. A non-derivative, non-surgical tracheostomy: the translaryn- geal method. Intensive Care Med. 1997,23(4):386-92.
24. Walz MK, Hellinger A, Walz MV, Nimtz K, Peitgen K. Translaryngeal tracheostomy. Technique and initial results. Chirurg. 1997;68(5):531-5.
25. Fernandez L, Norwood S, Roettger R, Gass D, Wilkins H 3rd. Bedside percutaneous tracheostomy with bronchoscopic guidance in critically ill patients. Arch Surg. 1996;131(2):129-32.
26. Rajajee V, Fletcher JJ, Rochlen LR, Jacobs TL. Real-time ultrasound-guided percuta- neous dilatational tracheostomy: a feasibility study. Crit Care. 2011;15(1):R67.
27. Hatfield A, Bodenham A. Portable ultrasonic scanning of the anterior neck before percutaneous dilatational tracheostomy. Anaesthesia. 1999;54(7):660-3.
28. Barba CA, Angood PB, Kauder DR, Latenser B, Martin K, McGonigal MD, et al. Bronchoscopic guidance makes percutaneous tracheostomy a safe, cost-effective, and easy-to-teach procedure. Surgery. 1995;118(5):879-83.
29. Dixon L, Wasson D. Comparing use and cost effectiveness of trachesostomy tube securing devices. Medsurg Nurs. 1998;7(5):270-4.
30. Crimlinsk JT, Horn MH, Wilson DJ, Marino B. Artificial airways: A survey of cuff management practices. Heart Lung. 1996;25(3):225-35.
31. Buglass E. Tracheostomy care: tracheal suctioning and humidification. Br J Nurs. 1999; 8(8):500-4.
32. Kapural L, Sprung J, Gluncic I, Kapural M, Andelinovic S, Primorac D, et al. Tracheo- innominate artery fistula after tracheostomy. Anesth Analg. 1999;88(4):777-800.
33. Solanki SL, Gupta D, Patil VP, Jain M. Tracheo-innominate artery fistula: report of two fatal cases and preventive measures. Anaesth Intensive Care. 2013;41(6):807-8.
34. Griggs A. Tracheostomy: suctioning and humidification. Nurs Stand. 1998;13(2):49-53.
35. Carroll P. Safe suctioning prn. RN. 1994;57(5):32-6; quiz 37.

36. Raymond SJ. Normal saline instillation before suctioning: helpful or harmful? A review of the Literature. Am J Crit Care. 1995;4(4):267-71.
37. De Leyn P, Bedert L, Delcroix M, Depuydt P, Lauwers G, Sokolov Y, et al. Tracheotomy: clinical review and guidelines. Eur J Cardiothorac Surg. 2007;32(3):412-21.
38. Tabaee A, Lando T, Rickert S, Stewart MG, Kuhel WI, et al. Practice patterns, safety, and rationale for tracheostomy tube changes: a survey of otolaryngology training programs. Laryngoscope. 2007;117(4):573-6.
39. White AC, Kher S, O'Connor HH. When to to change a tracheostomy tube. Respir Care. 2010;55(8):1069-75.
40. Hill SA. An unusual complication of percutaneous tracheostomy. Anaesthesia. 1995; 50(5):469-70.
41. Masterton GR, Smurthwaite GJ. A complication of percutaneous tracheostomy. Anaesthesia. 1994;49(5):452-3.
42. Kumar BN, Walsh RM, Courteney-Harris RG. Laryngeal foreign body: an unusual complication of percutaneous tracheostomy. J Laryngol Otol. 1997;111(7):652-3.
43. Noden JB, Kirkpatrick T. Intrapleural percutaneous tracheostomy. Anaesthesia. 1995; 50(1):91.
44. Schachner A, Ovil Y, Sidi J, Rogev M, Heilbronn Y, Levy MJ. Percutaneous tracheostomy—a new method. Crit Care Med. 1989;17(10):1052-6.
45. Griggs WM, Myburgh JA, Worthley LI. A prospective comparison of a percutaneous tracheostomy technique with standard surgical tracheostomy. Intensive Care Med. 1991;17(5):261-3.
46. Hutchinson RC, Mitchell RD. Life-threatening complications from percutaneous dilational tracheostomy. Crit Care Med. 1991;19(1):118-20.
47. Gardiner Q, White PS, Carson D, Shearer A, Frizelle F, Dunkley P. Technique training: endoscopic percutaneous tracheostomy. Br J Anaesth. 1998;81(3):401-3.
48. Trottier SJ, Hazard PB, Sakabu SA, Levine JH, Troop BR, Thompson JA, et al. Posterior tracheal wall, perforation during percutaneous dilational tracheostomy: an investigation into its mechanism and prevention. Chest. 1999;115(5):1383-9.
49. Polderman KH, Spijkstra JJ, de Bree R, Christiaans HM, Gelissen HP, Wester JP, et al. Percutaneous dilatational tracheostomy in the ICU: optimal organization, low complication rates, and description of a new complication. Chest. 2003;123(5): 1595-602.
50. Toye FJ, Weinstein JD. Clinical experience with percutaneous tracheostomy and cricothyroidotomy in 100 patients. J Trauma. 1986;26(11):1034-40.
51. Ivatury R, Siegel JH, Stahl WM, Simon R, Scorpio R, Gens DR. Percutaneous tracheostomy after trauma and critical illness. J Trauma. 1992;32(2):133-40.
52. Walz MK, Peitgen K, Thürauf N, Trost HA, Wolfhard U, Sander A, et al. Percutaneous dilatational tracheostomy—early results and long-term outcome of 326 critically ill patients. Intensive Care Med. 1998;24(7):685-90.
53. Hill BB, Zweng TN, Maley RH, Charash WE, Toursarkissian B, Kearney PA. Percutaneous dilational tracheostomy: report of 356 cases. J Trauma. 1996;41(2):238-43.
54. Cobean R, Beals M, Moss C, Bredenberg CE. Percutaneous dilatational tracheostomy. A safe, cost-effective bedside procedure. Arch Surg. 1996;131(3):265-71.
55. Whittet HB, Commins DJ, Waldmann CS. Skin tethering after dilatational percutaneous tracheostomy. Anaesthesia. 1995;50(10):892-4.
56. Callanan V, Gillmore K, Field S, Beaumont A. The use of magnetic resonance imaging to assess tracheal stenosis following percutaneous dilatational tracheostomy. J Laryngol Otol. 1997;111(10):953-7.
57. Charters P, Mannar R, Jones AS. Laryngotracheal stenosis after percutaneous tracheostomy. Anaesthesia. 1994;49(9):825-6.
58. Bernard SA, Jones BM, Shearer WA. Percutaneous dilatational tracheostomy complicated by delayed life-threatening haemorrhage. Aust NZ J Surg. 1992;62(2):152-3.

9
Surgical Tracheostomy

Kranti Bhavana, Amit Keshri

INTRODUCTION

Tracheostomy refers to creation of permanent opening or stoma between the trachea and skin of the neck. It is a commonly performed surgical procedure especially in emergency and ICU set up. It is an age old procedure finding its mention in the Hindu text of Rig Veda way back in 2000 BC. The first book of tracheostomy was written by Habicot and published in 1620.

The term tracheotomy refers to the formation of a surgical opening in the trachea. It refers strictly to a temporary procedure. Tracheostomy on the other hand refers to the creation of a permanent stoma between the trachea and the cervical skin.[1,2]

FUNCTIONS AND INDICATIONS OF TRACHEOSTOMY[3,4]

- Alternate pathway for breathing in cases of mechanical upper airway obstruction.
- Improves alveolar ventilation by reducing dead space and reducing the resistance to airflow.
- Protects the airway from pharyngeal secretions and blood aspirations in high risk patients.
- Permits removal of tracheobronchial secretions in patients who are unable to expectorate.
- To assist in intermittent positive-pressure ventilation where the endotracheal tube has to be kept for more than 3 days.
- To administer anesthesia in cases where intubation is difficult.
- Elective tracheostomy for major head and neck operations.

Mechanical Upper Airway Obstruction

Cause	Examples
Congenital	Subglottic or upper tracheal stenosis, laryngeal web, laryngeal and vallecular cysts, tracheoesophageal anomalies, hemangioma of larynx, bilateral choanal atresia
Infective	Acute laryngotracheobronchitis, acute epiglottitis, diphtheria, Ludwig's angina, peritonsillar, retropharyngeal or parapharyngeal abscess, tongue abscess

Cause	Examples
Trauma	External injury of larynx and trachea (e.g. gunshot and knife wounds), fractures of mandible or maxillofacial injuries, trauma due to endoscopies especially in infants and children
Tumor	Advanced tumor of larynx, tongue, pharynx , upper trachea or thyroid presenting with stridor
Foreign body larynx	Swallowed or inhaled object obstructing the upper airway and causing stridor
Vocal cord paralysis	Postoperative complication of thyroidectomy, cardiac or esophageal surgery, bulbar palsy
Edema	Edema of larynx due to steam, irritant fumes or gases, allergy (angioneurotic or drug sensitivity), radiation

Protection from Aspiration in High Risk Patients

Neurological diseases	Polyneuritis as in Guillain-Barré syndrome, motor neuron disease, multiple sclerosis, bulbar poliomyelitis, myasthenia gravis, tetanus, stroke, bulbar palsy
Coma	Situations where Glasgow Coma Scale is less than 8, e.g. head injury, poisoning, overdose, stroke and brain tumor
Trauma	Severe maxillofacial injuries leading to risk of aspiration of blood in upper airway.

Respiratory Failure

Tracheostomy reduces the respiratory dead space by 50% and hence results in less effort for respiration and improved alveolar ventilation. It also aids in better suctioning of bronchial secretions.

Pulmonary diseases	Chronic lung conditions like bronchitis, asthma, bronchiectasis, emphysema, atelectasis, severe pneumonia
Neurological diseases	Multiple sclerosis, motor neuron disease
Severe chest injury	Flail chest

Retained Bronchial Secretions

Inability to cough	• Coma of any cause, e.g. head injuries, cerebrovascular accidents, narcotic overdose • Paralysis of respiratory muscles-spinal injuries, polio, Guillain-Barré syndrome, myasthenia gravis • Spasm of respiratory muscles, tetanus, eclampsia, strychnine poisoning
Painful cough	Chest injuries, multiple rib fractures, pneumonia
Aspiration of pharyngeal secretions	Bulbar polio, polyneuritis, bilateral laryngeal paralysis

Elective Tracheostomy

- In major head and neck operations where there often are multiple comorbidities and one anticipates swallowing and breathing problem beforehand
- In ICU settings where the patient is already intubated

CONTRAINDICATION[4]

There are no absolute contraindications to surgical tracheostomy but certain factors have to be kept in mind before this procedure is attempted:
- If breathing difficulty is due to problems of the lower airway then a tracheostomy would not relieve the problem completely.
- Coagulation disorder should be corrected if elective tracheostomy is planned. It is not a contraindication for emergency tracheostomy.
- Any anatomical aberrations especially vascular anomalies in the neck renders this procedure is risky and adequate preparation should be done beforehand to deal with this.

APPLIED ANATOMY (FIG. 1)

The ideal tracheostomy site is at the second to fourth tracheal ring level, hence surface landmarks are important. The superior thyroid notch, cricoid and suprasternal notch usually can be easily palpated through the skin. The cricothyroid space can be identified by palpating a slight indentation immediately below the inferior edge of the thyroid cartilage. The anterior jugular veins lying in the superficial plane has to be dealt with in order to make the field bloodless. Cricothyroid arteries traverse the superior aspect of this space on each side and anastomose near the midline.

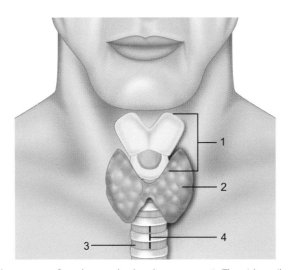

Fig. 1 Surgical anatomy of trachea and related structures: 1. Thyroid cartilage with cricoid cartilage. 2. Thyroid gland with isthmus. 3. Tracheal rings. 4. Site of tracheostomy incision (second to fourth tracheal ring)

The innominate artery crosses from left to right anterior to the trachea at the superior thoracic inlet. Its pulsations can be palpated and occasionally seen in the suprasternal notch especially in case of a high riding vessel, representing a contraindication for a bedside percutaneous or open tracheostomy. The knowledge of these vessels is of utmost importance as an anomalous course lead to devastating consequences if injured during surgery. One of the complications of tracheostomy is tracheoarterial fistula which can be fatal if left unattended.

The isthmus of the thyroid gland lies across the second to fourth tracheal rings and must be dealt with in any procedure at or around the upper trachea.

TECHNIQUE AND EQUIPMENT

Types of Tracheostomy[3,4]

1. *Emergency Tracheostomy*
   - Complete or near complete airway obstruction where intubation is not possible and there is urgent need to establish airway
2. *Elective or Tranquil Tracheostomy*
   - Planned procedure (commonly done now days in ICU where patients are already intubated)
   - Therapeutic to relieve obstruction, remove secretions, aid in positive pressure ventilation
   - Prophylactic in cases where there is risk of aspiration of blood or secretions as in extensive head and neck surgeries.
3. *Permanent Tracheostomy*
   - Total laryngectomy
   - Bilateral abductor paralysis of vocal cords
   - Laryngeal stenosis
4. *Percutaneous Dilatational Tracheostomy*
   - Common ICU intervention where patient is already intubated
5. *Mini Tracheostomy (Cricothyroidotomy)*
   - Emergency procedure
6. *High, Mid and Low Tracheostomy*
   - *High:* Done above the level thyroid isthmus
   - *Mid:* Second and third tracheal ring level (preferred)
   - *Low:* Done below the level of thyroid isthmus

Instruments Required

- Surgical handle
- Blade no. 15
- Retractor, sharp, 1 prong
- Retractor, sharp, 2 prongs
- Thymus retractor
- Langenbeck retractor
- Freer elevator, double-ended, semi-sharp and blunt
- Scissors, curved
- Tissue forceps
- Tracheal dilator
- Needle holder

- Mosquito forceps
- Allis forceps
- Sponge forceps
- Yankauer suction tube
- Catheter mount

Type of Tracheostomy Tubes[5]

There are various types of tracheostomy tubes available and the choice of tube is individualized:

- *Single lumen tubes:* It is for short-term use. It maximizes inner lumen diameter and reduces airway resistance.
- *Double lumen tubes:* It has an inner tube which can be removed and cleaned. The outer tube remains in situ. It can be used for longer duration. Double lumen metallic tubes are also available and they are easy to maintain at home.
- *Uncuffed tubes:* An uncuffed tube is suitable for a patient in the recovery phase of critical illness who has returned from intensive care and may still require chest physiotherapy, suction via the trachea and airway support. It also can be kept for longer period and is easy to insert and maneuver.
- *Cuffed tubes:* These tubes have cuff which can be inflated inside the trachea to form a seal and then it can be used for the purpose of positive pressure ventilation. Cuffed tube also prevents aspirations. Prolonged use and inflation of cuff can result in tracheal mucosal damage and sometimes result in tracheo-esophageal fistula. High volume low pressure cuffs can be used to avoid this complication.
- *Fenestrated tubes:* Commonly used to wean patients from tracheostomy. Airway can be established through the fenestra which can then pass through oropharynx. It also helps in making vocalization better. It also reduces work of breathing.
- *Adjustable flange tubes:* These are handy in patients who have low set trachea or very obese short neck or in patients with swelling or tumor in the neck.
- *Metallic tracheostomy tube:* Now not used commonly but is easier to maintain for long-term. These double lumen tubes are still in use in our country on routine basis when we discharge the patients with a tracheostomy.
- *Tracheostomy with speaking valve:* The Passy-Muir speaking valve is commonly used to help patients speak more normally. This one-way valve attaches to the outside opening of the tracheostomy tube and allows air to pass into the tracheostomy, but not out through it. The valve opens when the patient breathes in. When the patient breathes out, the valve closes and air flows around the tracheostomy tube, up through the vocal cords allowing sounds to be made. The patient breathes out through the mouth and nose instead of the tracheostomy.

Selection of Tracheostomy Tube Size

- There lies no definite formula for selection of tracheostomy tube size though some researchers have been able to derive some correlation between the age and the size of the tracheostomy tube to be used in them. This formula described by Behl and Watt in 2004 in the British Journal of Anaesthesia states that the size of the tracheostomy can be assessed by the following formula:[6]

ID (Internal diameter) = (age/3) + 3.5
OD (External diameter) = (age/3) + 5.5
   This formula is analogous to the one used to calculate the size of endotracheal tube also known as Cole's formula.[7]
- Further studies are required to establish a definite formula for tracheostomy tube size calculation.

PREPARATION

- Consent for tracheostomy is essential as it entails a major drift in lifestyle of the patient. Temporary loss of speech is to be explained beforehand. Patient can communicate initially by writing on a pad or have a bell by their bedside. A speaking valve can later be used with a fenestrated tracheostomy tube when mechanical ventilation is no longer required.
- Normal clotting parameters should be ascertained beforehand and any anti-coagulant should be stopped before surgery.
- Assessment of patient's neck is also important as an enlarged thyroid gland and a short neck poses additional challenge to the operating surgeon.

PROCEDURE

In major head and neck procedures and in ICU settings tracheostomy is often done electively. Whenever possible, endotracheal intubation should be done before elective cases. This is important in pediatric cases where tracheostomy becomes a safer surgery if the tube is in place.

- *Position:* Patient lies supine with a shoulder pad under the shoulders and a head ring to support the head. This position extends the neck and brings the laryngeal structure superficial which makes the surgery safer to perform. If this position is not maintained then there are chances that the surgeon may stray to either side with dire consequences. Over extension of head is to be avoided in elderly and pediatric age group. In the elderly there are chances of subluxation of cervical vertebra whereas in pediatric age group there are chances of injury to great vessels and pleura which can come above if neck is over extended.
- *Local anesthesia:* After palpation of laryngeal structures and ascertaining anatomical landmarks, the surgical site is infiltrated with 2% lidocaine with adrenaline. This gives a drier field during operation and is instrumental in providing postoperative pain relief.
- *Incision (Fig. 2):* Incision could be both vertical and horizontal with each having its advantages. A vertical incision is made in the midline of neck extending from cricoid cartilage to just above sternal notch. This incision is favored during emergency as it gives rapid access to trachea with minimal bleeding and tissue loss. A transverse incision is usually around 5 cm long and is given about two finger breaths above the sternal notch. This gives minimal scar and is preferred during elective tracheostomy.
- *Dissection (Figs 3 to 5):* Before we proceed further, one should make sure that correct size tube along with a catheter mount is available on the trolley with the scrub nurse. If patient is intubated then anesthetist should ensure that the tube is at the head end and tapes around the tube are released beforehand.

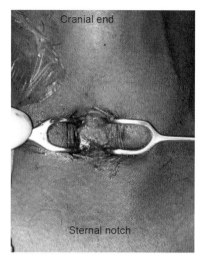

Fig. 2 Surgical step showing incision and initial plane of dissection showing the strap muscles underneath

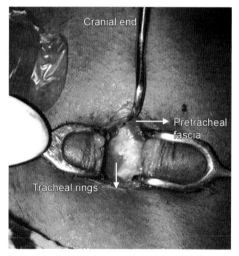

Fig. 3 The pretracheal fascia above the trachea is cleared and the white rings of trachea are clearly visible

This ensures that the tube can be easily manipulated once trachea is approached during dissection.

- Incision is then made through the skin, superficial fascia and platysma to reach up to the deep cervical fascia.
- Anterior jugular vein may need to be ligated or retracted laterally if they are in midline.
- Strap muscles are then exposed. It is retracted after blunt dissection and retracted on either side with the help of Langenbeck, double hook or a self-retaining retractor.

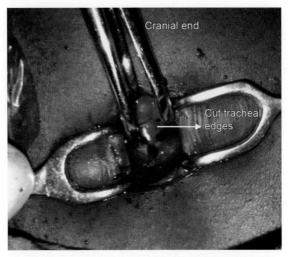

Fig. 4 The tracheal walls are cut and the endotracheal tube placed inside the trachea is visible

- After strap muscles the next important structure encountered is the thyroid isthmus which needs to be divided between two hemostats or can be retracted upwards to expose trachea.
- The trachea is approached after division of the thyroid isthmus. If the trachea is deep down then a cricoid hook is applied and the trachea is gently pull upward.
- It is important to avoid dissection on lateral aspect in order to prevent any injury to recurrent laryngeal nerves on either side.
- After division or retraction of thyroid isthmus the pretracheal fascia is exposed. It is important to achieve hemostasis at this stage with the use of bipolar cautery.
- Pretracheal fascia is incised and tracheal rings are well delineated.
- Tracheostomy should be done preferably between second and fourth tracheal rings. If the first tracheal ring is violated then there are chances of tracheal stenosis.
- When the endotracheal tube is in situ, anesthetist can either push the tube down to the carina or withdraw it upwards before tracheal wall incision is made. This ensures that the cuff of the endotracheal tube is not punctured during this step.
- Once the rings are well delineated, trachea is incised vertically and the opening is dilated with the help of a tracheal dilator. In pediatric cases it is advisable to place a stay suture in the trachea before placing the incision as it aids both in traction and tracheostomy tube change. In these cases a slit opening is made in the trachea and rings are not excised. This prevents laryngeal stenosis in near future.
- In cases of calcified cartilages in adults a window may need to be created by cutting a piece of tracheal ring anteriorly.
- Bleeding from cut tracheal edges is often controlled by tamponade effect of tracheostomy tube. Assistant holds the tube in its correct position and suction is done through the tube to remove secretions and blood from the airway.

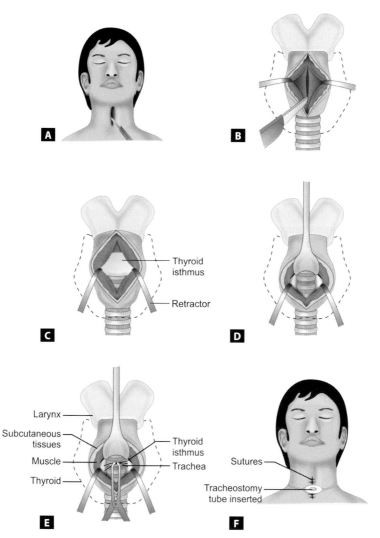

Figs 5A to F A schematic diagram showing the steps of surgical tracheostomy. (A) Vertical skin incision, (B) Splitting the strap muscles, (C) Isthmus of the thyroid over 1st and 2nd tracheal ring, (D) Pretracheal fascia over trachea is visible after retracting isthmus of the thyroid, (E) After removal of pretracheal fascia, tracheal rings are visible, (F) Tracheostomy tube in situ

- Correct size tube is then placed through the tracheal opening and secured both with straps and sutures. This prevents accidental de-cannulation in the immediate postoperative period.

POST-PROCEDURE CARE

- Care of a newly formed tracheostomy stoma should include frequent wound cleaning; two or three times a day with saline.[2,3]
- Tube can be changed after 3 days and then on alternate days.
- Humidified surrounding is very necessary to avoid formation of dry crusts.

- Dressing around the stoma should not be very tight as it may result in subcutaneous emphysema.
- If the patient is mechanically ventilated via the tracheostomy tube, the ventilator tubing must be supported to prevent tube displacement or trauma to the stoma site. A recognized cause of tracheal stenosis of the stoma site is excessive traction on the tracheostomy tube from the ventilator tubing.[1]
- Regular assessment of tracheostomy wound is essential as peristomal granulations are responsible for bleeding and later stenosis.

COMPLICATION/PROBLEM[3,4]

The complications can be intraoperative (including the first 24 hours), early postoperative (1–14 days) or late (>14 days). The incidence of overall complications depends on individual departments and ranges from 5% to 40%.[1,2] The most commonly occurring complications are hemorrhage, tube obstruction and tube displacement.

Intraoperative Complications

- *Primary Hemorrhage*
  - *Disturbed coagulation profile:* Try correcting the profile before surgery.
  - *Anterior jugular vein injury:* Ligation should be meticulous.
  - *Injury to thyroid isthmus:* Divided ends should be ligated properly.
  - *Injury to internal jugular veins and carotid artery:* Avoid dissecting lateral to the trachea.
- *Injury to Laryngeal Framework and Paratracheal Structures*
  - Injury to first tracheal ring and posterior tracheal wall is to be avoided as it can result in tracheal stenosis and tracheoesophageal fistula.
  - Injury to recurrent laryngeal nerves can result if dissection plane steers laterally. This leads to laryngeal paralysis and is to be avoided during tracheostomy.
- *Apnea*
  - This happens in patients who have had prolonged respiratory obstruction. Sudden wash out of CO_2 after tracheostomy results in this complication as CO_2 is a respiratory stimulant. Treatment is to administer 5% CO_2 in oxygen or assisted ventilation.
- *Cardiac Arrest and Arrhythmias*
  - The sudden swing in $PaCO_2$ level during procedure may results in extreme change in pH and/or potassium level, which may lead to this complication.[1]

Early Postprocedure Complications

- *Secondary Hemorrhage*
  - From incision edges after the effect of local anesthesia weans off. Controlled by pressure dressing.
  - Bleeding form granulation around the stoma—ensure adequate humidification and control of infection.

- *Surgical Emphysema*
  - Often results from tight dressing around the stoma which prevents air from the trachea to leak outside.
  - Usually resolves spontaneously but antibiotics may be needed to prevent cellulitis.
- Pneumothorax due to injury to apical pleura which may come in the surgical field especially in cases of prolonged respiratory distress.
- *Tube Displacement and Blockage*
  - This is a serious complication and may have disastrous consequences.
  - In order to prevent tube displacement, insertion of correct sized tube is recommended and securing it with ties and sutures is advisable. Stay sutures in the tracheal wall in pediatric cases prevents this complication.
  - Blockage of the tube due to crusting which in turn is the result of inadequate humidification.
- *Wound Infection*
  - Prolonged packing of the wound is to be discouraged as it becomes a breeding ground for microorganism to grow.
  - Tracheitis often results due to dry trachea which in turn results in perichondritis and then to tracheal necrosis.
- *Tracheal Necrosis*
  - Usually due to in appropriate tube size or excessive cuff pressure causing pressure necrosis of the posterior tracheal wall and eventually tracheal stenosis.
  - Tracheoesophageal fistula and tracheoarterial fistula may also result due to tracheal necrosis.

Late Postoperative Complications

- *Tracheal Stenosis*
  - Common if tracheostomy done at a higher level at first tracheal ring. Injury to cricoid ring is a major contributor to this complication.
  - Granulations also a causative factor
  - Tracheal necrosis can lead to tracheal stenosis
- *Tracheoesophageal Fistula*
  - Can result primarily during surgery when the posterior wall of trachea and anterior wall of esophagus, which are in contact, are injured during incision.
  - May result from pressure necrosis due to pressure from cuff of the tracheostomy tube on the posterior wall of trachea. This complication is compounded by presence of bigger size Ryles tube.
  - Cuff pressure should be regularly monitored and fine Ryles tube should be inserted in the esophagus.
- *Difficult Decannulation*
  - Often challenging in pediatric cases when they get dependent on tracheostomy tube breathing.
  - Granulations around the stoma may lead to this difficulty.
  - Always plan a slow decannulation and assessment of airway is necessary before planning decannulation. X-ray soft tissue neck to rule out any narrowing of airway is prudent before we plan decannulation.

- *Tracheocutaneous Fistula*
  - Usually seen in long-term tracheostomies where spontaneous closure of tracheal wound does not occur.
  - Epithelization of whole tract occurs and trachea cutaneous fistula results
  - Surgical closure is then indicated
- *Tracheoinnominate Fistula*
  - A disastrous complication with high morbidity and mortality

REFERENCES

1. Bradley PJ. Management of the obstructed airway and tracheostomy. In: Kerr AG, Booth JB (Eds). Scott-Brown's Otolaryngology, 6th edition. London: Butterworth-Heinemann. 1997. pp. 1-19.
2. Howard DJ. Emergency and elective airway procedures: Tracheostomy, cricothyroido-tomy and their variants. In: McGregor I, Howard D (Eds). Rob & Smith's Operative Surgery Head and Neck, 4th edition. Oxford: Butterworth-Heinemann. 1992. pp. 27-44.
3. Price T. Surgical tracheostomy. In: Russell C, Matta B (Eds). Tracheostomy: A Multi-Professional Handbook. Cambridge University Press. 2004. pp. 35-58.
4. Dhingra PL. Tracheostomy and other procedures for airway management. In: PL Dhingra (Ed). Diseases of Ear, Nose and Throat, 4th Edition. Elsevier. 2007. pp. 291-5.
5. NHS Greater Glasgow and Clyde. Types of Tracheostomy Tubes. [online] Available from www.nhsggc.org.uk/content/default.asp?page=s1214_8. [March, 2015]
6. Behl S, Watt JW. Prediction of tracheostomy tube size for paediatric long-term ventilation: an audit of children with spinal cord injury. Br J Anaesth. 2005;94(1):88-91.
7. Penlington GN. Letter: Endotracheal tube sizes for children. Anaesthesia. 1974;29(4): 494-5.

10

Bronchoscopy

Ravindra M Mehta, Rohan Aurangabadwalla

INTRODUCTION

In the last two decades, the application of bronchoscopy in the fields of pulmonology, intensive care unit (ICU) and thoracic surgery has widened tremendously. In the ICU specifically, the use of flexible bronchoscopy is increasing due to expanding indications. Although, critically ill patients in the ICU are considered to have higher risk of complications,[1] careful monitoring during and after the procedure[1] make it a relatively safe and useful procedure in trained hands.[2] This chapter comprehensively discusses the details of bronchoscopy in the ICU setting, from indications to technique and complications. A systematic approach helps to standardize the procedure, increase safety, maximize yield and reduce complications.

INDICATION

The indications for performing a bronchoscopy in the ICU can be diagnostic, therapeutic or often both together.[3,4]

Diagnostic

- *Infections*
    - Ventilator-associated pneumonia/hospital-acquired pneumonia [broncho-alveolar lavage (BAL)]
    - Immunocompromised hosts with infiltrates
    - Suspected viral and fungal infections
    - Community-acquired pneumonia—rarely
- Focal or diffuse lung lesions (infiltrates/mass)
- Interstitial lung disease with certain patterns
- *Airway trauma*
    - Blunt injury
    - Intubation injury
    - Post-operative including bronchial stump dehiscence.
- Stridor/localized wheeze to rule out airway stenosis or obstruction (Figs 1 to 3).
- Confirmation of endotracheal tube (ETT) placement
- Suspected laryngeal edema in intubated patients prior to extubation
- Acute inhalation injury/thermal or chemical burns

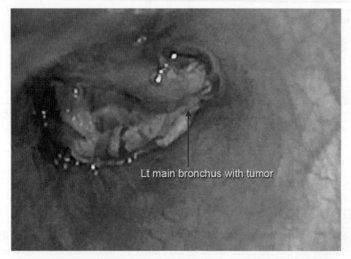

Fig. 1 Tumor mass occluding the left main bronchus

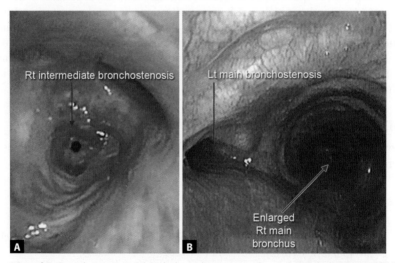

Figs 2A and B Bronchostenosis. (A) Right bronchus intermedius tight pin-hole stenosis; (B) Left main bronchus tight stenosis. Note the compensatory enlargement of the right main bronchus

- *Fistula*
    - Tracheo-esophageal fistula (TEF) (Fig. 4A)
    - Bronchopleural fistula.

Therapeutic

- *Difficult airway management*
    - Placement of single/double lumen tubes
    - Change of ETTs.
- Atelectasis—Lobar or complete lung collapse
- Tracheobronchial toilet with excessive airway secretions causing airway compromise (Figs 5A and B)

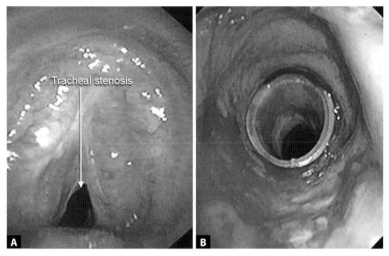

Figs 3A and B Role of bronchoscopy for diagnosis and treatment of tracheal stenosis. (A) Critical tracheal stenosis; (B) Tracheal stenosis-post silicone stenting

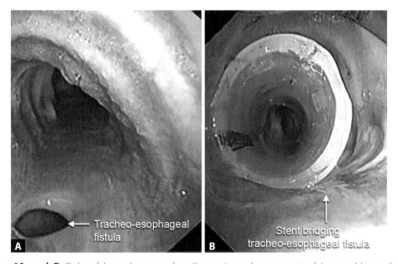

Figs 4A and B Role of bronchoscopy for diagnosis and treatment of inoperable tracheo-esophageal fistula. (A) Large tracheo-esophageal fistula; (B) Silicone stent placed across the tracheo-esophageal fistula

- Aspiration pneumonia, to remove aspirated material
- Massive hemoptysis (Figs 6A and B)
- Foreign body removal
- Pneumothorax with bronchopleural fistula to localize the leak and plan therapeutic options
- Stent placement for tracheo-esophageal fistula (Fig. 4B)
- Dilatation and stent placement for tracheobronchial stenosis (Figs 3A and B)
- Endobronchial thermal ablation for endobronchial tumors
- As a visual tool to guide percutaneous tracheostomy
- Lung abscess/bronchogenic cyst drainage.

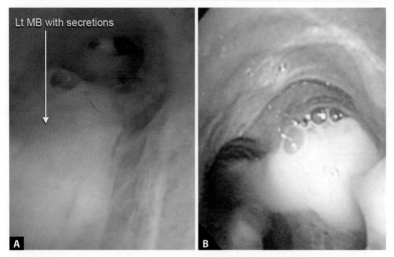

Figs 5A and B Secretions in the tracheobronchial tree. (A) Copious secretions in the left main bronchus; (B) Thick secretions in the trachea occluding the right main bronchus overflowing into the left main bronchus

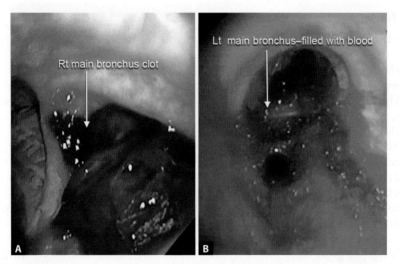

Figs 6A and B Massive hemoptysis. (A) Carina with massive clot occluding the right main bronchus; (B) Left main bronchus filled with fresh blood

CONTRAINDICATION[3,5,6]

There are very few absolute contraindications for performing ICU bronchoscopy with adequate training and in experienced hands.

Absolute

- Inability to maintain adequate oxygenation and ventilation
- Lack of adequate training and experience
- Lack of adequate infrastructure and equipment, especially complication management.

Relative

- *Acute myocardial infarction:* Avoid for 6 weeks unless imperative
- Unstable angina
- Status asthmaticus/active bronchospasm
- Oxygen saturation (SpO_2) less than 90% despite 100% fraction of inspired oxygen (FiO_2)
- Patients on mechanical ventilator with high positive-end expiratory pressure (PEEP)
- Chest radiograph showing presence of pneumothorax
- Severe pulmonary arterial hypertension
- Coagulation disorders, bleeding diathesis and thrombocytopenia (<50,000/ mm^3)—more true for transbronchial biopsy
- Severe uremia
- Increased intracranial pressure (ICP)
- Severe hemodynamic instability
- Unstable arrhythmias
- Acidosis (pH <7.2).

ANATOMICAL DETAILS AND PHYSIOLOGICAL CONSIDERATIONS

The knowledge of basic anatomy of the tracheobronchial tree is extremely important for performing ICU bronchoscopy. The trachea divides into the right and left main bronchus. The right main bronchus further divides into the right upper lobe and right intermediate bronchus, which further divides into the middle and lower lobe bronchi. The left main bronchus divides into the left upper lobe, lingular bronchus and lower lobe bronchus. The lobar bronchi further divide into segmental bronchi on each side (Figs 7A to F).

The presence of the bronchoscope in the airway can itself narrow the available space. In spontaneously breathing non-intubated patients in the ICU, the bronchoscope occupies only 10–15% of the cross-sectional area of the trachea. This does not result in any significant change in the tracheal pressures. However, in patients on mechanical ventilation and with an ETT in situ, an average adult bronchoscope with outer diameter of 5.7 mm occupies about 40% of the lumen of a size 9 ETT and about 66% of the lumen of size 7 ETT. This results in various pathophysiological changes, which can lead to significant alterations in the ventilatory parameters, gas exchange and hemodynamics as described below.

Increase in Airway Resistance

Insertion of a bronchoscope into the tracheobronchial tree leads to dramatic increase in the airway resistance. In intubated patients, this leads to increased peak inspiratory pressures and impedance to expiratory flow with incomplete emptying of the lungs during expiration causing a high intrinsic PEEP. These changes in peak inspiratory pressure, PEEP and the delivered tidal volume are closely linked to the size of the ETT as mentioned above and are also affected by the ventilator settings including the mode, flow and the respiratory rate. With the volume-controlled mode of ventilation the peak inspiratory pressures may be as high as 80–90 cm of H_2O.[7] These pressures represent the ventilator back

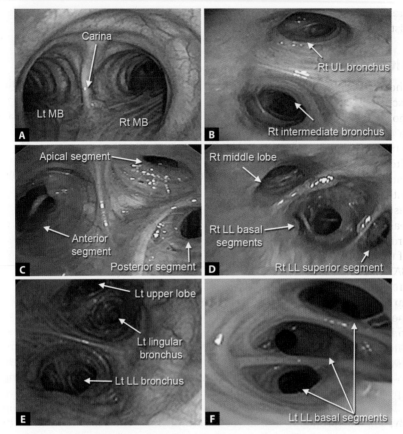

Figs 7A to F Anatomy of the tracheobronchial tree. (A) Carina; (B) Right main bronchus (MB) with divisions; (C) Right upper lobe with segments; (D) Right bronchus intermedius leading to middle and lower lobes; (E) Left main bronchus with divisions—Left upper lobe, lingular and lower lobe; (F) Left lower lobe basal segments

pressure, while the true intratracheal pressures are much lower. However, average pressures of up to 34 cm of H_2O have been recorded intratracheally. The average end-expiratory pressures are about 10–15 cm of H_2O, although pressures as high as 30 cm of H_2O have been recorded.[7] The pressure-controlled mode delivers more tidal volume as compared to the volume-control mode. High flow rates coupled with a lower respiratory rate are associated with lower auto-PEEP.[8] To ensure that an adequate tidal volume is delivered, the internal diameter of the ETT should be greater than or equal to 2 mm larger than the external diameter of the bronchoscope.

Decrease in Lung Compliance

Application of suction and instillation of saline for BAL can lead to changes in the static and dynamic lung compliance. Instillation of saline leads to wash-out of surfactant. These changes can have a significant effect in patients with pre-existing reduced lung compliance such as in atelectasis, acute respiratory distress syndrome (ARDS) and consolidation.

Alterations in Gas Exchange

The presence of a bronchoscope in the airway leads to alterations in gas exchange leading to hypoxemia and hypercapnia. Transient hypoxemia is the most common gas exchange abnormality encountered during bronchoscopy in the ICU, secondary to reductions in the delivered tidal volume, PEEP and intra-alveolar oxygen depletion due to suctioning and alveolar collapse. These alterations in gas exchange are magnified during suctioning, which removes about 200–300 mL of tidal volume. These reductions in lung volumes, coupled with reduction in the functional residual capacity can lead to alveolar closure, resulting in hypoxemia which can last for a few hours after the procedure. Air leaks in the ventilator circuit including the swivel adaptor of the ETT, reflex bronchospasm due to sub-epithelial vagal receptor stimulation, and flooding of the alveoli with BAL fluid are additional factors which can cause hypoxemia. BAL-induced hypoxemia occurs as result of reduction in the gas exchange surface area and release of inflammatory mediators. Suctioning for shorter periods of up to 3 seconds and utilization of adequate topical anesthesia are some of the measures to minimize the extent of hypoxemia. Hypercapnia occurs secondary to hypoventilation due to airway obstruction, due to factors mentioned earlier. These gas exchange abnormalities usually return back to the baseline in about a few minutes to few hours, depending upon the condition of the underlying lung.

Hemodynamic Effects

Hypoxemia and hypercapnia changes in the intrathoracic pressure and reflex sympathetic stimulation due to mechanical airway irritation cause a significant change in the hemodynamics, by altering the vascular tone. Thus, the cardiovascular system is indirectly affected by the presence of a bronchoscope in the airway. Sympathetic stimulation can result in tachycardia, elevation of the arterial pressure and pulmonary arterial pressure. In addition, changes in the intrathoracic pressure bring about alterations in the venous return and the cardiac afterload, significantly affecting the hemodynamics.

TECHNIQUE AND EQUIPMENT

There are two categories of patients in the ICU who require bronchoscopy—the spontaneously breathing patient, and the patient on mechanical ventilation.

In spontaneously breathing patients, bronchoscopy can be performed by the transnasal or the transoral route with the help of local anesthesia and conscious sedation as appropriate. In patients with hypoxemia, the use of non-invasive positive pressure ventilation (NIPPV) with titrated oxygen helps to prevent desaturation and reduces the need for postprocedure ventilatory support, as detailed below.[1,9] In patients on mechanical ventilation, bronchoscopy is performed via the endotracheal tube or tracheostomy, with a swivel adapter and rubber diaphragm with a central orifice (Fig. 8). Appropriate alterations in

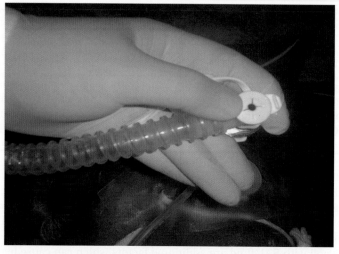

Fig. 8 Swivel adapter with central orifice to admit scope

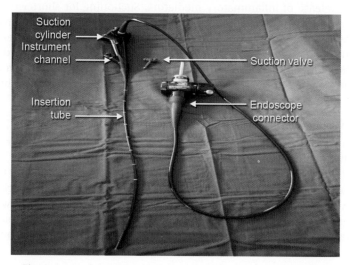

Fig. 9 A typical diagnostic bronchoscope (Olympus BF-Q180 SCOPE)

the ventilatory settings, with careful monitoring can help minimize the risk of bronchoscopy, described in detail in the procedure section below.

Bronchoscope

The major discussion in this chapter is on flexible bronchoscopy. The Figure 9 depicts a typical flexible video bronchoscope, with its parts. The diagnostic scope has an insertion tube outer diameter of 5.1 mm, with a working channel diameter of 2.0 mm and can move unidirectionally with an upward bending of 180° and downward bending of 130°. The latest generation therapeutic scope has an insertion tube outer diameter of 6.0 mm, with a working channel diameter of 2.8 mm and moves bidirectionally with an upward bending of 210°, downward

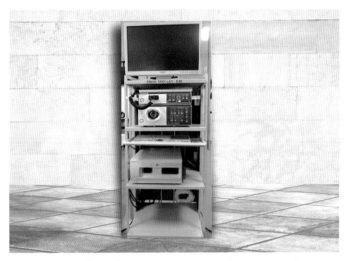

Fig. 10 A typical bronchoscopy cart: processor, light source and monitor

bending of 130° and 120° to the right and left. It can be used for therapeutic bronchoscopies in the ICU including superior suctioning capability for thick secretions. The video bronchoscopes typically need a light source, a processor and a monitor, usually mounted in a single tower (Fig. 10). Currently, portable scopes with an inbuilt light source for rapid transport and disposable bronchoscopes are available internationally.

PREPARATION

Consent
- The indication for bronchoscopy and the relevant imaging (chest radiograph, computed tomography of the chest if done) should be reviewed prior to the procedure.
- A written informed consent has to be taken, as per standard guidelines.

Patient Preparation
- Discontinue enteral feeding at least 4–6 hours prior to the procedure or empty the stomach contents prior to the procedure, if the procedure is emergent
- Ensure the presence and patency of adequate intravenous access.

Medications Needed
- Topical anesthetics like lidocaine (concentration 10 mg/mL)
- Sedatives like midazolam, fentanyl, propofol or dexmedetomidine in appropriate amounts
- Short acting neuromuscular blocking agents like atracurium or vecuronium can be used as needed
- Hemostatic agents like ice-cold saline, diluted epinephrine (1:10,000)
- Atropine or glycopyrrolate to reduce secretions are not recommended.

Monitoring

Multimodal physiologic monitoring during and after the procedure is very important considering the alterations in gas exchange and hemodynamics as described above.[1]

- Electrocardiogram (ECG) to monitor the heart rate and rhythm
- Blood pressure monitoring (intermittent cuff or continuous intra-arterial blood pressure monitoring, if in place)
- Pulse oximetry
- Monitoring of the ventilator parameters including tidal volume, peak inspiratory pressures, PEEP and end-tidal carbon dioxide ($EtCO_2$) enhances the safety during the procedure. Monitoring the $EtCO_2$ is especially important in patients with head injury, where sudden rise in ICP is to be avoided. Adequate sedation and neuromuscular blockade is required in patients with head injuries undergoing bronchoscopy.

Equipment

- The equipment essential for bronchoscopy in the ICU are as follows (Fig. 11):
  - *Appropriate bronchoscope(s):* Diagnostic/therapeutic, as discussed above
  - Suction
  - Bite block/mouthguard
  - Swivel adapter
  - Lubricating jelly
  - *Local anesthesia:* Lignocaine 1–2%
  - *Hemostatic agents:* Ice-cold saline/epinephrine
  - *Accessories:* Traps/forceps/brush/transbronchial needle aspiration (TBNA) needle
  - *Documentation:* Pictures/videos

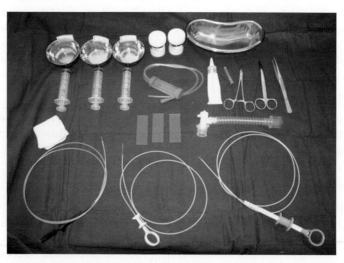

Fig. 11 *Preparation table:* Saline, local anesthesia, hemostatic agents (diluted epinephrine), accessories (forceps, brush, needle), catheter mount and mucus trap

PROCEDURE

Bronchoscopy in the Intubated Patient

- The size of the ETT should be at least greater than or equal to 2 mm larger than the outer diameter of the bronchoscope, as discussed earlier. The ETT should be of size 8 mm or larger to pass an adult scope of size 5.7 mm. If the tube diameter is smaller, the ETT has to be replaced by a tube of larger diameter. If replacement of tube is not possible, then a smaller diameter scope or a pediatric or an ultrathin bronchoscope (2.8 mm outer diameter) can be used.
- The ETT should not be too long. It should be shortened as much as possible by cutting the proximal end to facilitate the rapid passage and withdrawal of the scope.
- Use a swivel adapter with an attached rubber diaphragm and adequate central orifice (see Fig. 8) which admits the bronchoscope and maintains a seal to minimize air leak and loss of tidal volume.
- A mouthguard or an oral airway should be used to prevent the patient from biting and preventing scope damage.
- Increase the FiO_2 to 100% prior to, during and for an hour after the procedure to maintain the SpO_2 more than 90% at all times.
- If the SpO_2 is less than 90% despite a FiO_2 of 100%, the procedure indication and risk-benefit ratio should be carefully reviewed, and the most experienced operator should do the procedure. In certain conditions like hemoptysis, retained secretions and lobar or lung collapse, clearance of the blood or secretions can result in improvement of oxygenation and can be life saving.
- Adequate sedation and if required, neuromuscular blockage should be given.
- Bronchodilators prior to the procedure can be considered in patients with a propensity for bronchospasm after the procedure, such as in asthmatics.
- Make appropriate alterations in the ventilatory settings to maintain adequate tidal volume, minute ventilation and gas exchange. In case of volume-control mode, the peak airway pressure alarm needs to be increased appropriately, while in case of pressure-control mode, the pressure control setting is increased to compensate for loss of tidal volume caused by increased airway resistance. The peak airway pressure should be documented prior and after the procedure.
- Positive end-expiratory pressure is discontinued or if not possible or safe, reduced by 50%.
- The operator has to be preferably at the head end of the patient to facilitate understanding of the anatomy, especially in the early part of the learning curve of bronchoscopy (Fig. 12).
- Ensure adequate lubrication of the bronchoscope using a thin layer of viscous jelly, prior to insertion of the scope.
- Use of small amounts of topical lignocaine (1–2%) for instillation in the trachea, at the carina and in both main bronchi, to facilitate airway anesthesia.
- Suction to be used for short periods of 3 seconds or less.
- Monitoring of parameters as mentioned above, and the exhaled tidal volume/minute ventilation as there is a potential for loss of tidal volume due to leaks in the ventilator circuit, around the swivel adapter orifice, and during suctioning.

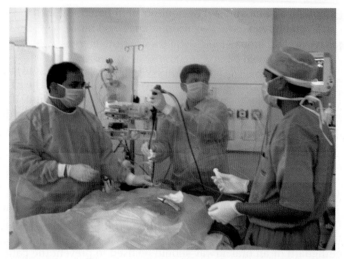

Fig. 12 *Position during ICU bronchoscopy:* Operator at the head end of the patient with assistant and technician

- Discontinue the procedure temporarily in case of desaturation, arrhythmias or hemodynamic instability. The procedure can be restarted after careful consideration, when the vital parameters return to normal.
- If a BAL is done, careful consideration for the amount of fluid used. If a transbronchial biopsy is done, the ventilator should be disconnected briefly for a few seconds at actual biopsy time, to avoid positive pressure and reduce the risk of pneumothorax.
- Reconfirm the position of the ETT bronchoscopically under vision, at the end of the procedure.

Bronchoscopy for the Spontaneously Breathing Patient

- In the spontaneously breathing patient, the nose and the pharynx can be sprayed with topical lidocaine (1–2%) or nebulized with aerosolized lidocaine for local anesthesia
- The trans-nasal route should be avoided in individuals with coagulopathy, as it can lead to bleeding
- The trans-oral approach requires a mouthguard to prevent biting of the scope
- Oxygen supplementation can be done with the help of nasal cannulae, high flow mask, non-rebreather mask or NIPPV
- A small hole can be made in the high flow mask and the non-rebreathing mask opposite the nostril to facilitate the insertion of the bronchoscope
- Consideration for using NIPPV in these patients is discussed below.

Bronchoscopy Using NIPPV

- Non-invasive positive pressure ventilation has been described as an additional tool for bronchoscopy in the borderline patient, where there is a significant risk of worsening of the respiratory status requiring intubation following bronchoscopy.

- In a prospective study by Heunks et al.[9] 12 patients for bronchoscopy/BAL who were at high-risk for worsening hypoxemia and respiratory distress after procedure were included. In this study, 20 minutes before bronchoscopy, the patients were connected to NIPPV with the pressure support (PS) mode 10 cm H_2O, PEEP 6 cm H_2O and FiO_2 100%. Standard bronchoscopy with BAL was done. After bronchoscopy, PS and FiO_2 were tapered with target SpO_2 kept greater than 92%. Once the FiO_2 was less than 40% with maintained SpO_2 and without respiratory distress, NIPPV was discontinued, supplemental oxygen was continued and the patients were monitored in the ICU for 12–24 hours. The mean duration of NIPPV was 6 hours (range 2–24 hours), 10 of 12 patients were transferred out of the ICU within 24 hours, and only one patient required intubation after 28 hours. In terms of yield, in 8 of 12 patients a causative infectious agent was isolated.
- The most important features recommended are meticulous preparation, using the right interface and protocol, an experienced bronchoscopist and adequate monitoring post-procedure in case emergent endotracheal intubation is needed. A sample NIPPV mask and set-up are shown in Figures 13 and 14.

Clinical Pearls in High-risk Patients

Bronchoscopy in certain critical or borderline situations can be challenging. The precautions recommended while performing bronchoscopy in these special groups are:

The hypoxemic non-intubated patient:
- Non-rebreather mask to give maximum possible FiO_2
- Non-invasive positive pressure ventilation with titrated O_2
- Intubate electively for procedure
- Rapid procedure
- Limited washings to minimize desaturation
- Close prolonged observation for post-procedure complications and rapid intervention

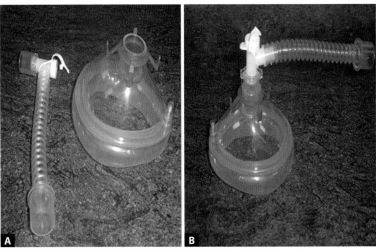

Figs 13A and B Non-invasive positive pressure ventilation mask which can be used with a swivel adapter (Please note that this needs an inspiratory and expiratory circuit)

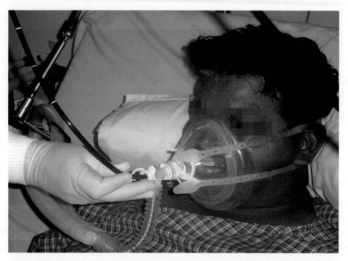

Fig. 14 Bronchoscopy using non-invasive positive pressure ventilation

High FiO$_2$/PEEP patient on ventilator:
- Experienced operator to do procedure to minimize procedure time
- Careful obsessive preparation to minimize procedure time
- Consider paralysis with sedation to avoid desynchrony
- May go in with trap attached to reduce procedure time
- Rapid procedure
- Limited washings/suctioning to minimize desaturation
- Recruitment after procedure as needed

Immunosuppressed patients:
- Heightened sterility precautions, to prevent infection
- Avoid intubation (mortality high after intubation)
- Use NIPPV, if possible to avoid intubation
- Consider transbronchial biopsy for accurate diagnosis

POST-PROCEDURE CARE

Clinical Aspects
- Monitor the vital parameters including heart rate, blood pressure and saturation
- Careful monitoring of patients for worsening respiratory distress or desaturation
- Assess for bronchospasm by auscultation, monitoring of peak airway pressure for mechanically ventilated patients
- Check peak airway and plateau pressures at the end of the procedure. These may rise after procedure and should reduce over time
- If a transbronchial biopsy is done, a chest radiograph is recommended after procedure to rule out any complications
- Repeat arterial blood gas analysis, if clinically indicated
- Ensure prompt labeling and early dispatch of collected samples for processing appropriate investigations.

Documentation

This includes a comprehensive report incorporating all relevant aspects mentioned below and follow-up advice to the patient/family and ICU team:
- Pre-medications used
- Details of the procedures done
- Photos and videos (as needed) of the procedure
- Note complications if any during the procedure
- Post-procedure advice, including expected complications in the next 24 hours.

Cleaning and Disinfection of Bronchoscope

This is done by the technician responsible for scope disinfection and maintenance.

Cleaning

- The insertion tube has to be wiped with a detergent soaked cloth
- Aspirate detergent, then air, through the suction channel using the suction valve
- Detach the suction and biopsy valve, which are intended for single use only
- Perform the leak test to check for damage to the scope
- Immerse the scope in freshly prepared detergent solution and clean all external surfaces and the distal tip
- Clean the suction and instrument channels with the recommended brush until all the debris is removed
- Aspirate detergent solution through the bronchoscope with the help of the suction cleaning adapter
- Rinse the equipment with water and subsequently aspirate water through the scope
- Remove the scope from water and aspirate air
- Wipe the equipment with cloth to remove excess moisture prior to disinfection.

Disinfection

- Disinfection should be carried out before the procedure and also after each patient use
- Disinfectants like cidex OPA (ortho-phthalaldehyde) (0.55% benzene dicarboxaldehyde) can be used
- The equipment should be soaked in the disinfectant at temperature and duration as recommended by the disinfectant manufacturer
- Distal end of the scope is immersed in 70% alcohol, followed by aspiration of alcohol for 5 seconds
- Distal end is removed from alcohol and air is aspirated
- Bronchoscope and adapter is dried with the help of alcohol moistened cloth
- Ensure that the equipment is completely dried prior to storage.

Washing and disinfection can also be done with commercially available machines.

COMPLICATION/PROBLEM

The incidence of complications during flexible bronchoscopy is very low, making it an extremely safe procedure in experienced hands. The overall complication rate for ICU flexible bronchoscopy is less than 10%.[4-6,10] The mortality rate in various series ranges from 0.01% to 0.02% and rate of major complications ranging from 0.08% to 0.3%.[5,6,11] The potential complications are mentioned below:

- *Sedation and premedication related:* Hypotension, respiratory depression and hypoventilation, more relevant for non-intubated patients
- *Topical anesthesia related:* Cardiovascular collapse, respiratory arrest, convulsions
- *Bronchoscopy related:* Bleeding, laryngospasm, bronchospasm, hypoxemia, hypotension, cardiac arrhythmias, myocardial ischemia, vasovagal reaction, infection, fever
- *Biopsy related:* Bleeding, pneumothorax [more with transbronchial biopsy (TBB)].

A few of the important complications are described below:

- *Bleeding:* Patients undergoing TBB, endobronchial biopsy and brushings are at a higher risk of bleeding, with the highest risk for TBB. The mortality rates related to bleeding during bronchoscopy range from 0.03% to 0.05%. Blood loss of greater than 50 mL is defined as significant bleeding. Most of the bleeding is self-limiting and resolves spontaneously or can be controlled by segmental tamponade, instillation of ice-cold saline, dilute epinephrine or a combination of both. The risk of bleeding is higher in individuals with liver disease, renal disease, pulmonary arterial hypertension, platelet counts below 50,000/mm³, platelet dysfunction, coagulopathy, and malnutrition. Administration of fresh frozen plasma is recommended before doing brushings or biopsy in patients with an international normalized ratio (INR) greater than 1.5. Cryoprecipitate may be helpful in patients with dysfunctional platelets. It is recommended to stop unfractionated heparin at least 6 hours prior and low molecular weight heparin at least 1 day prior to the procedure. The procedure and biopsy can be done with aspirin, but clopidogrel should be ideally stopped only for TBB at least 5 days prior to the procedure. However, the indications for performing a TBB need to be clearly defined before stopping a beneficial drug for patients with cardiovascular disease.
- *Pneumothorax:* The overall risk of pneumothorax during bronchoscopy is very low, happening predominantly with TBB. The risk of pneumothorax in spontaneously breathing patients undergoing TBB is much lower (2%) as compared to patients on mechanical ventilator (7–15%). The signs and symptoms of pneumothorax after TBB can be delayed, but it is rare for a pneumothorax to develop an hour after the TBB, especially on positive pressure ventilation. The use of fluoroscopy for performing TBB in mechanically ventilated patients not only increases the diagnostic yield but also enhances the safety of the procedure.
- *Cardiac arrhythmias:* Patients with cardiovascular disease, unstable angina and severe hypoxemia are at a higher risk of developing cardiac arrhythmias.
- *Hypoxemia:* It is one of the most common complications associated with bronchoscopy. It is especially common in ARDS patients. The drop in partial pressure of oxygen (PaO_2) in critically ill patients can be as high as 30–60 mm Hg and can persist for several hours post-procedure.

- *Laryngospasm and bronchospasm:* These are common airway complications seen in about 0.1–0.4% of nonintubated patients undergoing bronchoscopy. It is common in patients with underlying bronchospastic conditions. Nebulization with beta-agonists reduces the incidence of laryngospasm and bronchospasm. It rarely occurs in patients on mechanical ventilation.
- *Lignocaine toxicity:* Lignocaine is commonly used as a topical anesthetic agent during bronchoscopy, as outlined earlier. The maximum recommended safe dose is 4–5 mg/kg ideal body weight. Lignocaine toxicity can cause tremors, convulsions, respiratory arrest, arrhythmias and cardiovascular collapse.
- *Postbronchoscopy fever:* It is a self-limiting fever occurring in about 5–16% of the patients undergoing bronchoscopy. It can be associated with leukocytosis and neutrophilia. The presence of fever and leukocytosis in association with a negative culture suggests a systemic inflammatory response. It usually occurs as a result of release of inflammatory mediators, transient bacteremia and release of endotoxins.

REFERENCES

1. Du Rand IA, Blaikley J, Booton R. British Thoracic Society Guideline for diagnostic flexible bronchoscopy in adults: accredited by NICE. Thorax. 2013;68(Suppl 1):i1-44.
2. De Castro FR, Violan JS. Flexible bronchoscopy in mechanically ventilated patients. J Bronchol. 1996;3:64-8.
3. Silver MR, Balk RA. Bronchoscopic procedures in the intensive care unit. Crit Care Clin. 1995;11(1):97-109.
4. Turner JS, Willcox PA, Hayhurst MD, Potgieter PD. Fiberoptic bronchoscopy in the intensive care unit—a prospective study of 147 procedures in 107 patients. Crit Care Med. 1994;22(2):259-64.
5. Mehta AC, Tai DYH, Khan SU. Bronchoscopy: Common problems and solutions. Mediguide to Pulmonary Medicine. 1996;3:1-7.
6. Olopade CO, Prakash UB. Bronchoscopy in the critical care unit. Mayo Clin Proc. 1989; 64(10):1255-63.
7. Lindholm C, Ollmann B, Snyder JV, Millen EG, Grenvik A. Cardiorespiratory effects of flexible fiberoptic bronchoscopy in critically ill patients. Chest. 1978;74(4):362-8.
8. Lawson RW, Peters JI, Shelledy DC. Effects of fiberoptic bronchoscopy during mechanical ventilation in a lung model. Chest. 2000;118(3):824-31.
9. Heunks LM, deBruin CJ, van der Hoeven JG, van der Heijden HF. Non-invasive mechanical ventilation for diagnostic bronchoscopy using a new face mask: an observational feasibility study. Intensive Care Med. 2010;36(1):143-7.
10. Jolliet P, Chevrolet JC. Bronchoscopy in the intensive care unit. Intensive Care Med. 1992;18(3):160-9.
11. Pue C, Pacht E. Complications of fiberoptic bronchoscopy at a university hospital. Chest. 1995;107(2):430-2.

11

Bronchoalveolar Lavage (BAL) and Mini-BAL

Sanjay Singhal

INTRODUCTION

Flexible bronchoscopy has become one of the most frequently performed invasive procedures in respiratory medicine. Since its introduction, flexible fiberoptic bronchoscope (FOB) has become the instrument of choice because of its ability to safely visualize and biopsy bronchial lesions. It visualizes the trachea, proximal airways and segmental airways up to the third generation of branching, and can be used to sample and treat lesions in those airways. However, we could not visualize the orifices of subsegmental bronchi, hence, bronchoalveolar lavage (BAL) is used for sampling the contents of lower respiratory tract. BAL is a technique to samples the cellular and acellular components of distal bronchiole unit and gas exchange units through the channel of a wedged bronchoscope after saline has been injected. BAL differs from bronchial washing, which samples the secretions or small amounts of instilled saline from the large airways. BAL is a standard diagnostic procedure in all patients with diffuse lung diseases of unknown cause whether an infectious, noninfectious, immunologic or malignant cytology is suspected.

INDICATION

Bronchoalveolar lavage is an important tool for evaluation of pulmonary diseases. In some of the pulmonary diseases, the findings of BAL are diagnostic whereas in other diseases, they may contribute to the diagnosis and management (Table 1).

- *Infectious disease:* BAL helps in diagnosis of several lung infections. But, the recovery of a potentially pathogenic organism should be considered diagnostic only if colonization of the respiratory tract with that organism is not known. However, it is considered diagnostic only if colonization of that particular organism is not known and if colonization is known, semi-quantitative culture should be positive (10^5 colony forming unit/mL).[1] Measurement of $(1,3)$-β-D-glucan content in BAL fluid is also studied with reasonable accuracy in diagnosis of pulmonary fungal infections.[2,3]
- *Noninfectious disease:* BAL analysis when used in conjunction with clinical and radiological information is very useful for the diagnostic evaluation of

Table 1 Uses of bronchoalveolar lavage

Infectious diseases	
Diagnostic (colonization not known)	*Pneumocystis jirovecii*
	Legionella
	Mycoplasma
	Toxoplasma gondii
	Histoplasma
	Strongyloides
	Paragonimus westermani
	Mycobacterium tuberculosis
Non-diagnostic (colonization known)	Herpes simplex
	Cytomegalovirus
	Bacteria
	Aspergillus
	Candida
	Cryptococcus
	Atypical mycobacteria
Non-infectious diseases	
Diagnostic	Alveolar proteinosis (milky BAL)
	Histiocytosis-X
	Malignancies
	Eosinophilic pneumonia
Non-diagnostic	Pulmonary hemorrhage
	Hypersensitivity pneumonitis
	Interstitial lung disease
	Asbestosis, berylliosis, silicosis

patients with suspected interstitial lung disease (ILD).[1,4] However, lung cancer and some rare ILD can be diagnosed by BAL alone.

CONTRAINDICATION

There is no definitive contraindication for BAL. The relative contraindications are uncooperative patient, hypercapnia, hypoxemia (oxygen saturation <90% or PaO_2 <75% on supplemental oxygen), serious cardiac instability (arrhythmias and myocardial infarction within 6 weeks) and severe hemorrhagic diathesis.[1]

TECHNIQUE

Irrigation of bronchial tree with saline via catheter passed through rigid broncho-scope was first reported in 1927. Subsequently, the term "bronchial lavage" was coined by Stitt in 1932. Initially, it was used as a therapy for septic lung disease or pulmonary alveolar proteinosis. Reynolds and Newball introduced saline lavage of a portion of lung via flexible bronchoscope, which was now known as bronchoalveolar lavage (BAL). BAL is a part of routine bronchoscopy. When bronchoscopy is carried out, it is very important to inspect the airway lumen, surface of the bronchial mucosa and movement. BAL is performed before brushing or biopsy in order to avoid alteration of recovered fluid.

- Fluid recovery is optimum when bronchoscope occludes the bronchial lumen completely (bronchoscope of 5.2 mm in diameter permits easy wedging of bronchial subsegments).
- To perform BAL in intubated patient, bronchoscope is inserted through the endotracheal tube (ETT) with the use of swivel Y connector. ETT should be of at least 8 mm in size, If not possible, pediatric FOB is used.
- BAL target site should be selected on the basis of high resolution computed tomography (HRCT) performed before the procedure, rather than traditional BAL site (middle lobe or lingula).[4]

Non-bronchoscopic Bronchoalveolar Lavage

Non-bronchoscopic BAL, also known as mini or blind BAL is collected by double catheter technique (Figs 1 to 4).[5] For this method, we need two different size suction catheters, where smaller one could pass easily through the larger one, e.g. 16 Fr and 8 Fr catheters. Mini-BAL is an inexpensive, simple and useful technique for the diagnosis of lower respiratory tract infection and also can be used for diagnosis, prognosis and severity of acute respiratory distress syndrome (ARDS).[5,6]

PREPARATION

Equipment: Flexible bronchoscope, sterile collection trap, suction tubing, sterile saline, vacuum source, syringe.

Fiberoptic bronchoscopy can be performed under either general (children) or local anesthesia (adults).

- Patients must not take any food or drink for at least 4 hours before the procedure.
- Appropriate monitoring (continuous cardiac monitor and pulse oximetry) and resuscitative equipment with an intravenous line must be available.

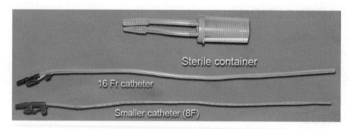

Fig. 1 Sterile container with suction catheter of two different sizes (where small catheter can pass easily through the larger catheter)

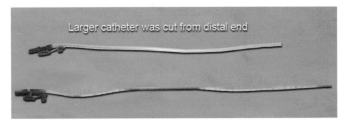

Fig. 2 Distal end of large catheter has been cut so that tip of small catheter can cross its tip during suctioning

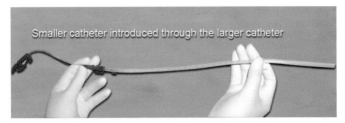

Fig. 3 Tip of inner smaller catheter coming out through larger catheter

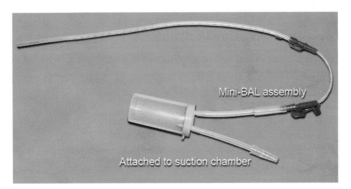

Fig. 4 Assembly of sterile container with catheter in catheter during sample collection

- Patients with history of bronchial asthma or chronic obstructive pulmonary disease (COPD) should be nebulized with bronchodilator before procedure.
- Sedation with a benzodiazepine (adult dose midazolam 2.0 mg IV bolus) with a narcotic (fentanyl 25–100 µg IV adult dose) or propofol (adult dose 20 mg IV bolus) will make patient comfortable and minimize cough reflex.[7]

Spontaneously Breathing Patients

- The patient should be explained about the procedure to alleviate any anxiety and facilitate cooperation.
- Lignocaine is the most common used local anesthetic agent (maximum safe dose 4–5 mg/kg). Usually, we start with 3 mL of 2% lignocaine given via nebulizer with the patient in sitting position. Then the oral lumen and pharynx are sprayed using the lignocaine spray. After this, the patient pulls out the

tongue; puffs of lignocaine are sprayed over the vocal cord at the beginning of inspiration. Instruct the patient not to swallow the lignocaine mixed with sputum. He should be provided with a cup for spitting.

Mechanically Ventilated Patients[8]

- ETT is shortened as much as possible to allow tip of flexible fiberoptic bronchoscopy (FOB) to reach the periphery of bronchial tree.
- Portex adapter with a fitted rubber cap may be used to minimize loss of tidal volume (TV).
- A mouth guard must be used to prevent patient biting the scope.
- Increase FiO_2 to 100%, 5–15 minutes before, during and up to an hour after the procedure with the aim of maintaining the SpO_2 close to 100%.
- Check arterial blood gas (ABG) before and 10 minutes postbronchoscopy. Postpone FOB if $SaO_2 < 90\%$ on FiO_2 100% (except gross hemoptysis).
- Positive end-expiratory pressure (PEEP) is taken off during FOB. If the discontinuation of PEEP is not feasible, reduce PEEP by 50%.
- Volume mode is preferred so that increased airway resistance secondary to FOB would not result in reduced TV. If pressure-controlled mode is used, peak pressure setting is increased to compensate for the loss of TV consequent to increased resistance.

Patients on Non-invasive Ventilation[9]

- The patient is connected to the ventilator via a full face mask and secured to the patient's face with elastic straps.
- In patients on noninvasive ventilation (NIV), full face mask with dual axis swivel adapter is used.
- Lubricant jelly is applied to the bronchoscope to facilitate its advancement through the swivel adaptor.
- NIV setting depends on clinical condition for example in COPD patients, inspiratory positive airway pressure (IPAP) is set at 15–17 cm H_2O and expiratory positive airway pressure (EPAP) is set at 5 cm H_2O with FiO_2 of 1.0.

PROCEDURE

- During standard flexible bronchoscopy, the bronchoscope is wedged in the selected bronchopulmonary segment. Good wedge position means that the bronchoscope is advanced as far as possible without losing the view.
- 20–50 mL of normal saline (at room temperature) is instilled and recovered by negative pressure through the bronchoscope three to six times.
- The recommended negative suction pressure is less than 100 mm Hg.
- The minimal retrieved volume should be more than 5% of the instilled volume (optimal retrieves ≥30%).
- The first BAL sample represents a disproportionate amount of bronchial airway material rather than alveolar return. There is no consensus whether or not to pool this sample with fluid recovered subsequently. The first sample may be of interest in diseases with primary bronchial component (e.g. asthma and bronchitis) and for microbiological cultures.[1,10]

- Subsequently, all the aliquots of retrieved BAL fluid are pooled for routine analysis.
- BAL sample should be transported immediately to the laboratory for analysis.[4] If the delay between BAL fluid retrieval and delivery to the laboratory is 30–60 minutes, specimen should be transported at 4ºC (on ice) and if anticipated delay is more than 1 hour, nutrient-supplement medium could be added to the pooled sample with subsequent storage at 4ºC for up to 12 hours.[4] BAL fluid should not be frozen.[4]

Non-bronchoscopic Bronchoalveolar Lavage Sampling in Patient Having Artificial Airway (Figs 1 to 4)

- A sterile suction catheter of larger size is cut about 2–5 cm from the distal end and advanced through the endotracheal tube into the distal airway till resistance is felt.
- The catheter is wedged in this position and another catheter of smaller size is passed through the first catheter as far as possible.
- 20 mL of sterile normal saline is instilled through the inner catheter and aspirated fluid is collected in a sterile container.
- Repeat procedure if aspirate fluid is less than 5 mL.

POST-PROCEDURE CARE

Oxygen saturation should be measured as transient decrease in oxygen saturation is anticipated after BAL. In patients with already compromised respiratory status and on invasive or noninvasive ventilation, FiO_2 is kept at 1.0 up to an hour after the procedure with the aim of maintaining the SpO_2 close to 100% and decreased to prebronchoscopy level if the patient is able to maintain oxygen saturation more than 92%.[8-9]

Bronchoalveolar Lavage Analysis and Interpretation

A variety of diagnostic studies may be performed on BAL fluid. Typical diagnostic studies are gross observation, differential cell count, microbiological studies and cytopathology.[1,4]

- *Gross observation:* Lavage fluid is opaque and/or milky establish diagnosis of pulmonary alveolar proteinosis and sequentially more hemorrhagic with each aliquot suggests alveolar hemorrhage.
- *Interpretation of differential cell count:* In normal, non-smoker adult, BAL differential cell counts are alveolar macrophage more than 85%, lymphocyte 10–15% (CD4+/CD8+ = 0.9–2.5), neutrophil less than or equal to 3%, eosinophils less than or equal to 1%, epithelial cell less than or equal to 5% (>5% suggests suboptimal sample).
- *Lymphocyte differential count more than or equal to 25%* suggests granulomatous disease [sarcoidosis (CD4+/CD8+ > 4 is highly specific), hypersensitivity disease and chronic beryllium disease], cellular nonspecific interstitial pneumonitis, lymphoid interstitial pneumonitis, cryptogenic organizing pneumonia, drug reaction and lymphoma.

- *Lymphocyte differential count more than 50%* suggests hypersensitivity pneumonitis or cellular nonspecific interstitial pneumonitis.
- *Eosinophils differential count more than 25%:* Virtually diagnostic of acute or chronic eosinophilic pneumonia.
- *Microbiological studies:* Infectious organisms suggest lower respiratory tract infection.
- *Cytopathology:* Malignant cell suggest malignancy.

COMPLICATION/PROBLEM

Fiberoptic bronchoscopy with BAL is a safe procedure in majority of patients. Only less than 5% of the BAL procedures were associated with minor complications including postbronchoscopy fever (2.5%), pneumonitis (0.4%), bleeding (0.7%). None of these complications required therapy.

REFERENCES

1. Goldstein RA, Rohatgi PK, Bergofsky EH, Block ER, Daniele RP, Dantzker DR, et al. Clinical role of bronchoalveolar lavage in adults with pulmonary disease. Am Rev Respir Dis. 1990;142:481-6.
2. Yang WL, Cao J, Chen BY, Xie W, Dong LX, Wu YQ, et al. A preliminary study on the measurement of (1, 3)-β-D-glucan in bronchoalveolar lavage for the diagnosis of pulmonary fungal infections. Zhonghua Jie He He Hu Xi Za Zhi. 2012;35:897-900.
3. Limper AH, Knox KS, Sarosi GA, Ampel NM, Bennett JE, Catanzaro A, et al. An official American Thoracic Society statement: Treatment of fungal infections in adult pulmonary and critical care patients. Am J Respir Crit Care Med. 2011;183:96-128.
4. Meyer KC, Raghu G, Baughman RP, Brown KK, Costabel U, du Bois RM, et al. An official American Thoracic Society clinical practice guideline: the clinical utility of bronchoalveolar lavage cellular analysis in interstitial lung disease. Am J Respir Crit Care Med. 2012;185:1004-14.
5. Khilnani GC, Arafath TK, Hadda V, Kapil A, Sood S, Sharma SK. Comparison of bronchoscopic and non-bronchoscopic techniques for diagnosis of ventilator associated pneumonia. Indian J Crit Care Med. 2011;15:16-23.
6. Singh C, Rai RK, Azim A, Sinha N, Baronia AK. Mini-bronchoalveolar lavage fluid can be used for biomarker identification in patients with lung injury by employing 1H NMR spectroscopy. Crit Care. 2013;17:430.
7. Wahidi MM, Jain P, Jantz M, Lee P, Mackensen GB, Barbour SY, et al. American College of Chest Physicians consensus statement on the use of topical anesthesia, analgesia, and sedation during flexible bronchoscopy in adult patients. Chest. 2011;140:1342-50.
8. Tai DYH. Bronchoscopy in the intensive care unit (ICU). Ann Acad Med Singapore. 1998;27:552-9.
9. Murgu SD, Pecson J, Colt HG. Bronchoscopy during noninvasive ventilation: indications and technique. Respir Care. 2010;55:595-600.
10. Blic Jd, Midulla F, Barbato A, Clement A, Dab I, Eber E, et al. Bronchoalveolar lavage in children. ERS Task Force on bronchoalveolar lavage in children. European Respiratory Society. Eur Respir J. 2000;15:217-31.

12

Thoracentesis

Pralay K Sarkar

INTRODUCTION

Thoracentesis is a commonly performed bedside procedure in clinical practice. If performed correctly, it has low risk of complications. Knowledge of the anatomy of the intercostal space, a familiarity with the equipment and use of ultrasound improve the safety and success rate of this procedure.

INDICATION

- *Diagnostic thoracentesis:* To find cause of a pleural effusion when etiology is not clear from history, physical examination and other laboratory and radiological studies.
- *Therapeutic:* If a patient has symptoms attributable to a large pleural effusion, e.g. dyspnea, chest discomfort, hypoxemia.

CONTRAINDICATION

There is no absolute contraindication for thoracentesis.
- The procedure cannot be performed in an uncooperative patient.
- In case of thrombocytopenia and coagulopathy, the risks and benefits should be carefully balanced. Thrombocytopenia and coagulopathy need not be corrected to normal levels for safe performance of thoracentesis. In any patient with significant thrombocytopenia and coagulopathy, smaller size needles/catheters should be used and careful attention should be paid to anatomy and technique to avoid injury to the intercostal artery.
- If under ultrasound, the effusion is small and there is no safe window, the procedure should not be attempted.

APPLIED ANATOMY

Relevant anatomy of the intercostal space has been described elsewhere in this manual. It is important to be aware of the position of the neurovascular bundle to avoid injury to it.

The intercostal artery runs along a groove at the lower margin of the upper rib forming an intercostal space. The needle entry point should be at the upper border of the lower rib forming the space.

TECHNIQUE AND EQUIPMENT

The procedure can be performed with or without using ultrasound for localization of fluid. A real-time guidance of the needle is not necessary. If real-time ultrasound is not used, both hands of the clinician are free for operating needle-syringe assembly, giving better control over the movement of needle.

Equipment

One can use commercially available thoracentesis kits, e.g. Arrow-Clarke™ Pleura-Seal® thoracentesis kit (Fig. 1) containing a needle catheter assembly

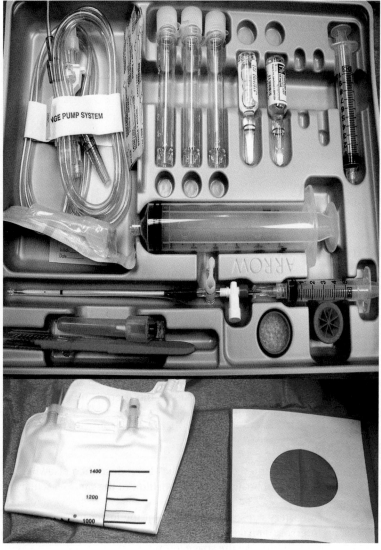

Fig. 1 Arrow-Clarke™ Pleura-Seal® thoracentesis kit. The catheter is 8 Fr over a 19 cm long 18 G needle. A three-way stopcock and a self-sealing valve system are parts of the catheter

(8 Fr catheter over 18 Ga needle) or other specialized needles, e.g. Argyle-Turkel safety needle, as may be available in a given institution. Alternatively, a simple inexpensive system can be assembled using an intravenous cannula, an intravenous infusion set and a three-way stopcock.

PREPARATION

- *To gather necessary adjunct equipment:*
  - Local anesthetics: 1% or 2% lidocaine
  - Skin disinfectant: Chlorhexidine solution or povidone-iodine solution
  - Sterile gloves
  - Sterile drape
  - Drainage bottles
  - Sterile cups/tubes for collection of specimen
  - Syringes: 10 cc and 50 cc
  - Three-way stopcock.
  Commercial kits come complete with all the above supplies.
- *Informed consent:* Prior to starting the procedure, the patient or if the patient is medically incompetent to make an informed decision, his/her relatives should be informed about the indication for thoracentesis, the procedure itself, associated risks and benefits, any alternative management option and a written informed consent should be obtained.
- The indication for thoracentesis should be reviewed and any contraindication should be ruled out.
- *Localization of fluid and identification of site:* It is important that fluid is localized and the site identified after the patient has been placed in the position in which the procedure will be performed (see below).
  - Review of all relevant chest radiology should be performed to identify the best site for thoracentesis.
  - If ultrasound guidance is not available, clinical examination should be used as a guide. Percussion should be performed to identify an area of definitive dullness. Auscultation should be performed to identify the level where diminution of breath sounds starts and the intercostal space below is usually a good site. Often, the site such identified is 2–3 finger-breadths below the tip of scapula, slightly medial or lateral to the midscapular line.
  - *Use of ultrasound for localization of site:*
    - The purpose of ultrasonography for procedural guidance of thoracentesis is to identify a safe site, angle, and depth for needle penetration that avoids injury to lung, subdiaphragmatic organs and the heart.
    - The three cardinal features of ultrasonographic identification of pleural effusion are:
      1. Presence of a relatively echo-free space.
      2. *Typical anatomic boundaries that surround this space:* The chest wall, the diaphragm and the visceral pleural surface of the lung (Fig. 2).
      3. Typical dynamic findings: Movement of compressed lung during respiration.
    - The transducer is angled and/or moved to find an anechoic space that is subtended by typical anatomical boundaries and that has typical dynamic findings, consistent with a pleural effusion.

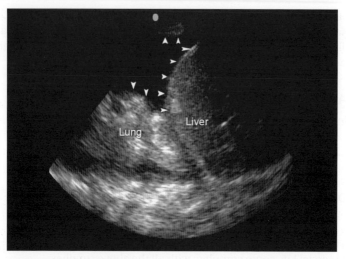

Fig. 2 Identification of pleural effusion by ultrasonography. A pleural effusion is identified by locating the typical anatomic boundaries (Arrowheads)

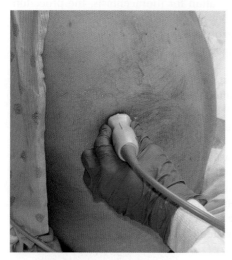

Fig. 3 In the photograph, ultrasound beam is directed slightly medially to visualize the effusion. The needle-syringe assembly should be inserted maintaining the same angle and direction

- Once a suitable site is identified and marked, the depth of the penetration is measured from a frozen ultrasound image. Thoracentesis should be performed promptly after ultrasound marking without any patient movement to avoid shifting of fluid from the intended aspiration site.
- Before any consideration of needle insertion, the examiner must make unequivocal identification of the diaphragm.
- There should be at least 10 mm of space between the inside of chest wall and the visceral pleural surface for safe performance of thoracentesis.
- The syringe and the needle assembly should be introduced in the same angle in which the transducer was held while determining the best access site (Fig. 3). This is best accomplished when the operator performs the procedure immediately following the examination.

- It is important that the patient is instructed not to move after localization and the procedure is performed immediately after ultrasound localization.
- Routine monitoring is not indicated. However, if the patient is very symptomatic or hypoxic, monitoring of vital signs is important.
- *Premedication:* Not indicated. There is no evidence that premedication with atropine decreases the risk of vasovagal syncope.
- If the patient's medical history does not suggest any bleeding diathesis, routine checking of platelets and coagulation parameters is not necessary.

PROCEDURE

- Patient is positioned and fluid is localized. It is most convenient to perform thoracentesis if the patient can sit upright. The patient can sit at the side of the bed or on a chair with feet supported on ground or on a stool (Fig. 4). In case of a large effusion, if patient is unable to sit upright, a supine recumbent position can be chosen. If there is an accessible pocket of fluid, the procedure can be performed with the patient lying supine with the arm on the side of the effusion behind the patient's head. If the procedure is being performed in an ICU patient and the effusion is small, being localized mainly posteriorly, the patient may have to be positioned carefully in a lateral position and stabilized in that position.
- *Marking the identified site:* Either with nonerasable ink or by creating a skin dimple with a needle cap or other suitable blunt object.
- Skin disinfection performed at the site of proposed puncture and around it.
- Sterile drape is placed.
- Administration of local anesthesia: Adequate and effective local analgesia should be ensured to minimize patient discomfort and maximize patient co-operation.
  - Intradermal injection of small amount of local anesthetics with a 25 G needle to raise a wheal (Fig. 5A).
  - A larger needle (20–22 G) is advanced through the wheal for additional administration of local anesthetics to intercostal tissue (Fig. 5B).

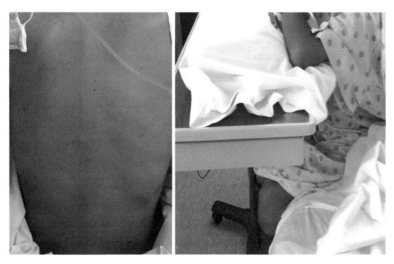

Fig. 4 Positioning of patient for thoracentesis

- With each small advance of the needle, a small amount of local anesthetics should be injected after confirming at each step by negative suction that the needle has not punctured any blood vessel.
- Pleural entry is confirmed by free aspiration of pleural fluid.
- Once pleural fluid is aspirated, the needle is then slightly withdrawn till fluid can no longer be aspirated; at this point, which marks the parietal pleura and surrounding tissue, sufficient amount of local anesthetics should be injected.

- *Placement of small skin incision:* If a larger bore catheter is being used, a small incision is placed to facilitate the entry of the needle. The depth of the incision should involve only skin and subcutaneous tissue (Fig. 5C).
- The catheter/needle is introduced placing a finger guard at the level where fluid aspiration is anticipated (Fig. 5D). This is important particularly in case of small pleural effusion to avoid accidental injury of the visceral pleura and lung.
- From the point first fluid is aspirated, the needle-catheter assembly is advanced slowly for a few millimeters (Fig. 5E). Then the needle is held steady and the catheter is advanced into the pleural cavity over the needle. The needle is withdrawn (Fig. 5F).
- If only a diagnostic thoracentesis is being performed, the needle that is being used to infiltrate local anesthetics is withdrawn into the rib space until fluid return stops; the syringe containing the local anesthetics can then be exchanged for a larger clean syringe and the needle is reinserted to the same depth at which pleural fluid was obtained initially.
- For therapeutic drainage, the catheter is connected to the drainage system through a 3-way stopcock to facilitate aspiration and drainage of pleural fluid without risk of introducing air into the pleural space (Figs 5G and H).

The color, character and odor (if any) of the pleural fluid and the amount of fluid removed should be documented in procedure note.

Pearls and Pitfalls

- If a kit is being used, the operator should familiarize himself/herself with all the components and their proposed functioning.
- If ultrasound is being used, a serious error is wrongly identifying the hepatorenal or splenorenal space, which is curvilinear, as the diaphragm. This error, if happens, can lead to laceration of these organs (Fig. 6).
- If ultrasound is used for localization of fluid and determining the depth of needle penetration, an important pitfall is that firm pressure by the probe on the skin, particularly in an edematous patient, may indent the skin at the site of examination. This leads to the underestimation of the depth at which fluid will be reached when aspiration is attempted. The operator should be able to recognize this problem and needs to insert the needle more than the measured distance.
- It is important to remember that fluid return can be expected approximately within 5 mm after crossing the upper margin of the lower rib. Blind plunging of the needle till the hub should be avoided.
- The needle should always be kept horizontal while advancing through the intercostal space; angling the needle cephalad increases the risk of intercostal artery damage.

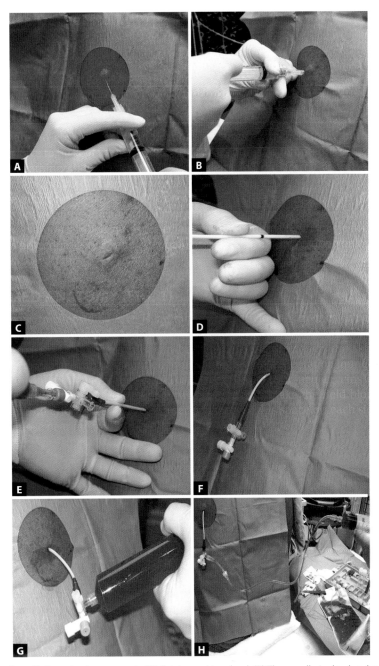

Figs 5A to H Steps in thoracentesis. (A) Raising a skin wheal; (B) The needle is slowly advanced, aspirating and injecting local anesthetics in steps, till pleural space is entered; (C) A small skin incision is placed to facilitate entry of the catheter; (D) A finger guard is placed to protect against accidental needle entry beyond the desired distance; (E) After first fluid aspiration, the catheter is advanced few millimeters; (F) Keeping the inner needle steady, the catheter is advanced and then the needle removed; (G and H) Using the three-way stopcock, the desired amount of fluid is aspirated/drained

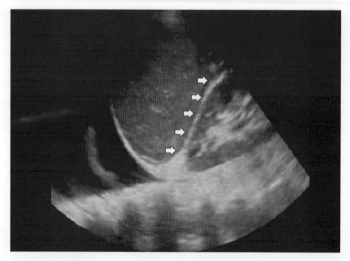

Fig. 6 Inexperienced operator can mistakenly identify the hepatorenal space (Arrows) or splenorenal space as the diaphragm

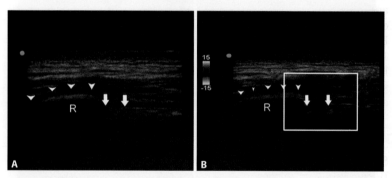

Figs 7A and B Longitudinal scan through an intercostal space showing intercostal vessels exposed in the intercostal space. R = acoustic shadow of the rib at the upper margin of the intercostal space (Arrowheads point to the anterior surface of the rib). Note the intercostal vessels are exposed in the space (Arrows)

- The immediate paraspinal area should be avoided as radiological studies have shown that the intercostal artery can become exposed within the intercostal space in the first ~ 6 cm lateral to the spine (Figs 7A and B). The identified site can be carefully examined with ultrasonography for presence of intercostal vessels.
- If removal of pleural fluid is done slowly, the patient is less likely to have chest discomfort and/or cough, which are usually due to rapid re-expansion of lung.
- If a therapeutic drainage is being performed, the amount of fluid removal should be limited to less than 1.5 L in one sitting unless pleural pressure is also being simultaneously monitored.
- If the patient starts to have violent or frequent cough, the procedure should be terminated.

Drained Fluid for Laboratory Testing

- Usually, 50–100 mL of pleural fluid is enough for complete analysis including cytology.
- Ideally, all pleural fluid samples should be analyzed/processed promptly. If prompt processing is logistically not possible, the sample should be refrigerated.
- If a diagnostic thoracentesis is being performed, initial analysis should include total and differential leukocyte count; initial biochemical analysis should include estimation of glucose, protein and lactate dehydrogenase (LDH). These initial tests help differentiate between an exudate and a transudate and suggest possible etiologies.
- The sample for cell count should be collected in an ethylenediamine tetra-acetic acid (EDTA)-coated tube/vial. The pleural fluid WBC count has been reported to be lower if the pleural fluid has been collected in tubes without an anticoagulant. Refrigerated storage for up to 24 hours has no significant effect on the total WBC count or on the WBC count differential.
- Temperature and storage time can introduce potential errors in estimation of pleural fluid glucose and LDH, falsely showing lower values.
- If cultures need to be sent, the fluid needs to be collected in a sterile container and should promptly be transported to the laboratory. Blood culture bottles can be inoculated at bedside for bacterial culture.
- For cytological analysis, the pleural fluid should be delivered promptly (within 1 hour) to the laboratory.
- For estimation of pleural fluid pH, the fluid should be collected in a blood gas syringe avoiding prolonged contact with air, and pH should be measured with a blood gas analyzer.

POST-PROCEDURE CARE

- Skin is cleaned of blood and antiseptic stain and a small sterile dressing or a BAND-AID® can be placed.
- Patient should be watched for any sign of respiratory distress or development of chest pain.
- A routine chest X-ray (CXR) is not necessary to rule out pneumothorax, though it is a common practice in most institutions. CXR should definitely be performed if the patient develops chest pain or worsening shortness of breath after thoracentesis. A CXR may also be indicated if the therapeutic effect of the thoracentesis needs to be judged or the underlying lung parenchyma needs to be examined with re-expansion of lung after drainage of fluid.
- If ultrasound has been used to localize fluid, it can also be used to rule out pneumothorax after completion of the procedure.

COMPLICATION/PROBLEM

- *Pneumothorax:* It happens if there is accidental puncture of visceral pleura or if there is accidental entry of atmospheric air into pleural cavity. This complication can be avoided by careful control of needle movement, prevention of patient movement, and maintenance of a closed drainage system

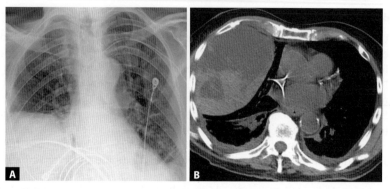

Figs 8A and B Large hemothorax after thoracentesis. (A) CXR showed increased right pleural effusion after thoracentesis; (B) CT scan showed large intrapleural fluid collection. Note that the fluid in pleural space is hyperdense in this non-contrast scan, suggesting presence of blood

at all time while performing the procedure. If ultrasound is available, it can be used immediately at the end of thoracentesis to rule out pneumothorax.

- *Re-expansion pulmonary edema:* Risk can be minimized by slow withdrawal of fluid.
- *Infection:* Unusual, if appropriate aseptic technique is used.
- *Intercostal artery laceration and hemothorax:* It is the most dreaded complication and largely reported in the elderly patients. It should be suspected if the patient develops new chest pain and shortness of breath after thoracentesis and CXR shows substantial increase in the pleural effusion (Figs 8A and B).
- *Dry tap:* It is usually due to one of the following reasons:
  - Failure to correctly localize pleural fluid.
  - The needle length is not adequate to traverse the whole thickness of chest wall, particularly in an obese patient.
  - The fluid is too thick, particularly if a smaller gauge needle is being used.
  - The needle is blocked by clot or fibrinous material. If needle occlusion is suspected, the lumen can be cleared by injecting small amount of local anesthetics.
- *Vasovagal syncope:* If it happens, the procedure should be immediately halted and the patient should be placed in the Trendelenburg position.

SUGGESTED READING

1. Helm EJ, Rahman NM, Talakoub O, Fox DL, Gleeson FV. Course and variation of the intercostal artery by CT scan. Chest. 2013;143:634-9.
2. Mayo PH, Goltz HR, Tafreshi M, Doelken P. Safety of ultrasound-guided thoracentesis in patients receiving mechanical ventilation. Chest. 2004;125:1059-62.
3. Petersen WG, Zimmerman R. Limited utility of chest radiograph after thoracentesis. Chest. 2000;117:1038-42.

13
Tube Thoracostomy

VN Maturu, Ritesh Agarwal

INTRODUCTION

Intercostal chest tube placement (tube thoracostomy) is a procedure that is commonly performed in the emergency department, intensive care setting, and even the general wards. The aim of chest tube placement is drainage of abnormal collection of air or fluid from the pleural space. First described by Hippocrates in the fifth century, there have been several modifications of the intercostal tubes and the drainage systems used. Although a very simple procedure, an improperly placed tube can lead to life-threatening complications.[1,2] In this chapter, we review in detail the technique for placement of an intercostal tube.

INDICATION

- *Pneumothorax:* A pneumothorax is defined as the presence of air in the pleural cavity. Pneumothoraces can be classified as traumatic, spontaneous (primary or secondary) or iatrogenic. All pneumothoraces do not need placement of a chest drain.
  - *Primary spontaneous pneumothorax:* The British Thoracic Society (BTS) guidelines[3] recommend single time manual aspiration of pneumothorax if the size is greater than 2 cm or the patient is breathless, and recommend insertion of a small bore chest drain only if manual aspiration fails (pneumothorax >2 cm or persistent symptoms despite aspiration). The American College of Chest Physicians (ACCP) Delphi statement also recommends insertion of chest drain only if the pneumothorax is large (apex to cupola distance ≥3 cm) or if the patient is clinically unstable (defined as any one of the following: respiratory rate >24/min, heart rate >120/min, room air oxygen saturation <90% or unable to speak whole sentences in a single breath).
  - *Secondary spontaneous pneumothorax:* Most authorities recommend performance of tube thoracostomy in all symptomatic patients with secondary spontaneous pneumothorax.[3-5] Even patients with smaller pneumothoraces need to be closely monitored for progression of size or symptoms. Manual aspiration is usually not recommended for secondary spontaneous pneumothoraces as it is unlikely to be successful. Moreover, all patients require chemical pleurodesis, which can only be performed with chest tube in the pleural cavity.

- *Iatrogenic pneumothorax:* The incidence of iatrogenic pneumothoraces is increasing due to the explosion of invasive diagnostic and therapeutic modalities. As recurrence is not an issue in the management of iatrogenic pneumothorax, the management mainly focuses on relieving the patient's symptoms with the least invasive approach possible. The common causes of an iatrogenic pneumothorax include transthoracic needle aspiration, transbronchial lung biopsy, placement of subclavian catheters and diagnostic thoracentesis. The factors deciding the treatment strategy include the presence or absence of underlying lung disease, clinical status of the patient and size of the pneumothorax. Most cases can be successfully management by close observation, oxygen supplementation and single time aspiration. A chest drain is indicated only if the underlying lung is diseased, the patient is clinically unstable or deteriorating, or if the conservative approach fails.
- *Traumatic pneumothorax:* Pneumothorax is the second most common complication of chest trauma after rib fracture and is seen to occur in up to 50% of chest trauma patients. All overt traumatic pneumothoraces are managed with a chest drain insertion. An occult pneumothorax (defined as that not obvious on initial chest radiograph but is detected on subsequent imaging like a computed tomography scan or a subsequent chest radiograph) is also common. Although some recommend placing a chest drain even in occult pneumothoraces, a more conservative approach may also be considered. However, if mechanical ventilation is anticipated, even an occult pneumothorax may be treated with a chest drain.

  It is also important to remember that most pneumothoraces in a mechanically ventilated patient or any pneumothorax that causes hemodynamic instability (tension pneumothorax), should be drained with a chest tube.
- *Pleural effusion:* A chest drain in pleural effusion is placed with the aim of relieving patient's symptoms or drainage of pleural contents (pus, blood). The indications of chest drain include rapidly reaccumulating pleural effusion (usually in cases of malignancy and occasionally in those with benign diseases like uremia), empyema or a complicated parapneumonic effusion (pleural fluid glucose <60 mg/dL, pH <7.2, Gram stain or culture positivity) and hemothorax (spontaneous or traumatic).
- *Post-surgery:* Chest drains are also routinely placed following thoracic or cardiothoracic surgeries.

CONTRAINDICATION

There is no absolute contraindication for the placement of a chest drain. The relative contraindications include:

- *Bleeding diathesis:* Deranged clotting profile or thrombocytopenia needs to be corrected before the procedure provided the indication is not an emergency.
- *Trapped lung:* A trapped lung is identified by the presence of a thick fibrous pleural peel resulting from a remote pleural space infection, which prevents the lung from expanding on fluid removal. A chest tube should not be placed as the lung does not expand.

- *Endobronchial obstruction:* A complete endobronchial obstruction on the side of pleural effusion (which might coexist in malignant pleural effusions) is also a contraindication for chest tube placement as the lung will not expand even if the fluid is drained. It can be suspected by lack of contralateral mediastinal shift on chest radiograph, and lack of improvement in dyspnea following a therapeutic thoracentesis.
- *Loculated effusion:* This is a contraindication for blind placement of a chest drain. An image-guided chest drain or a pigtail should be placed.

APPLIED ANATOMY

It is essential to know the anatomy of lungs and pleura for comfortable performance of the procedure and prevention of complications. The usual site for the placement of chest drain is the triangle of safety, which is bounded anteriorly by the lateral border of pectoralis major, posteriorly by the anterior border of latissimus dorsi and inferiorly by an imaginary line drawn at the level of the nipple. The apex of the triangle is formed by the axilla. This usually corresponds to the fourth or fifth intercostal space in the midaxillary line. The safe triangle avoids damage to the internal mammary artery and also avoids dissection through the muscles and breast tissue (Fig. 1). The midaxillary line is chosen because the innermost layer of intercostal muscle is poorly developed at this point and also it is more comfortable to the patient and allows him/her to lie down supine. A more posterior approach though feasible makes lying down supine uncomfortable for the patient. Also there is chance of injury to the long thoracic nerve which lies on the surface of serratus anterior and segmentally supplies this muscle.

There are three layers of intercostal muscles (the external intercostal, internal intercostal and innermost intercostal) between the ribs (Fig. 2). As the intercostal neurovascular bundle lies in the groove on the inferior margin of the superior rib, the chest drain is typically inserted just superior to the lower rib so as to avoid injury to the same. However, as the collateral intercostal vessels run along the superior margin of the inferior rib, the ideal site for insertion should be 50–70% of

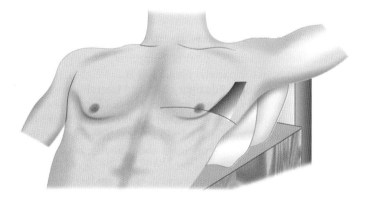

Fig. 1 Diagram to illustrate "safe triangle"
Source: Reproduced with permission from Reference 3

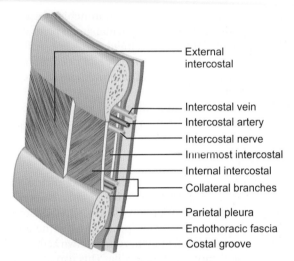

Fig. 2 Anatomy of the intercostal space

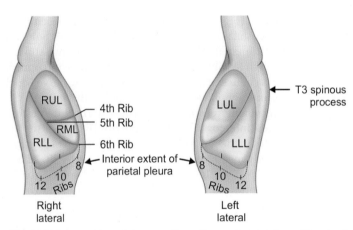

Fig. 3 Surface marking of pleura and lung fissures (Lateral view of the chest)

the way down the intercostal space.[6] Despite adequate precautions, injury to the neurovascular bundles remains a potential complication of the procedure.

The inferior margin of the parietal pleura lies at the eighth, tenth and twelfth ribs in the midclavicular line, midaxillary line and lateral border of the erector spinae respectively (Fig. 3).[7] However, the superior border of the diaphragm lies at much higher levels, especially in expiration (fourth space on right side and fifth on the left side). Hence, a drain placed too low can traverse the pleural space and injure the diaphragm and also the intra-abdominal organs, if undue force is used. The major fissure runs from the second spinous process posteriorly to the sixth costochondral junction anteriorly and cuts the midaxillary at the fifth rib. The minor fissure runs horizontally from the fourth costochondral junction to cut the oblique fissure at the fifth rib. Hence, there is a high chance of intrafissural placement of the tube if it is placed at the midaxillary line in the safety triangle and not angulated upward.

TECHNIQUE AND EQUIPMENT

There are three methods of insertion of chest tube: blunt dissection into pleura (operative tube thoracostomy), Seldinger guidewire technique (guidewire tube thoracostomy), and trocar tube thoracostomy.[8,9]

1. *Operative tube thoracostomy:* Blunt dissection into the pleura is the oldest and probably the safest technique for chest drain insertion. This is the most commonly used technique in resource-constrained settings and is typically used when larger bore tubes have to be placed. The advantages of this technique include the ability to perform digital exploration of the pleural space and therefore direct the tube into the most appropriate position in the thoracic cavity. However, this is also the most painful technique as it needs a larger incision and also leaves a larger scar.

2. *Guidewire tube thoracostomy (Seldinger technique):* With an increasing trend toward the use of smaller chest tubes and pigtail catheters, this Seldinger technique is more commonly being used now. This technique also causes less pain, is more patient-friendly and does not leave an unsightly scar. Commercial kits are available for guidewire tube thoracostomy. Chest tubes of varying sizes (8–36 Fr) can be inserted with this technique.

3. *Trocar tube thoracostomy:* This is similar to the guidewire technique except that there is no sequential dilation. Considerable force is used while inserting the metal trocar into the pleural space, thereby increasing the risk of damaging internal organs. This technique is not recommended for routine use.

Equipment

The equipment needed for operative tube thoracostomy include: (1) chest tube (of the desired size); (2) underwater seal bag of the desired type (described below); (3) normal saline (to be filled in the water seal bag); (4) chest tube insertion tray (scalpel, blunt-tipped artery forceps, scissors, nonabsorbable suture with a cutting needle, needle holding forceps, syringes, sterile drapes, sterile dressings, cotton and gauze); (5) local anesthetic agent (usually lignocaine); (6) sterile skin preparation solution (povidone iodine, chlorhexidine); (7) sterile gown, face mask and cap (Fig. 4). Commercial kits with sequential dilators are available for guidewire tube thoracostomy.

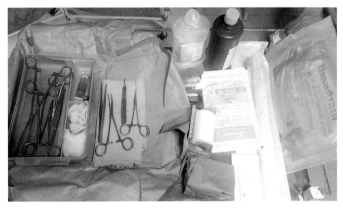

Fig. 4 Equipment needed for operative tube thoracostomy

Intercostal Drainage Tube

Intercostal tubes/drains are hollow cylindrical tubes made of polyvinyl chloride or silicone designed to be placed within the pleural cavity. They also have side holes designed to increase the surface area of absorption of fluid or air and to allow alternate path for drainage in case the tip of the tube gets blocked. A radiopaque strip is present on the side of the chest tube to assist visualization on chest radiographs. The most proximal hole on the chest tube, the sentinel eye, is usually situated on this strip and is visible on the chest radiograph as a defect in the line. The position of this sentinel eye helps us ensure that all the holes are inside the pleural cavity (Fig. 5). The length markings on the tube note the distance of the sentinel eye from the skin insertion site.

Chest tubes come in varying sizes ranging from 6 French (Fr) to 40 Fr (The Fr refers to the outer diameter of the cylindrical tube and is equivalent to 0.333 mm). The flow rate however is determined by the chest drain's internal but not external diameter. This varies even amongst tubes of the same external diameter due to differences in the wall thickness. Chest tubes are classified as small bore and large bore chest tubes. The ACCP Delphi consensus statement has classified tubes into three categories: small (≤14 Fr), medium (16–24 Fr) and large (24 Fr and above).[7] Others have used cutoffs ranging from 14 to 20 Fr to differentiate small from large bore chest tubes.[8,10]

There is an increasing trend to use small bore chest tubes for pleural drainage. The traditional concerns raised against the use of small bore chest tube are the low flow rates, and the increased tendency to get blocked, kinked or displaced.[11] However, several recent studies have disproved these concerns and have shown that even small bore chest drains can effectively drain fluid and air from the chest. Other advantages of small bore chest drains include less pain, more patient comfort and smaller scars. The only indications for placement of large bore chest drains are pneumothorax in a mechanically ventilated patient (to effectively drain larger

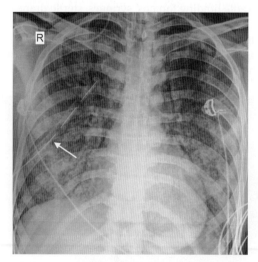

Fig. 5 Chest radiograph showing an intercostal tube placed in the right pleural cavity. Note the radiopaque line (arrow) on the chest tube with side drainage holes visualized as defects in this line. Also note the fully expanded lung

air leaks which are expected), hemothorax and empyema (as there is an increased chance of tube blockage when small bore tubes are used).[8,10] Recent studies have shown that even empyemas can be effectively drained using small bore chest tubes with periodic flushing and use of intrapleural fibrinolytic agents.[12,13]

Intercostal Drainage Bags

There are various types of drainage systems which can be connected to the chest tube. Conventionally, glass or plastic bottles were used for pleural drainage. However, these have been replaced by various types of ambulatory drainage systems. The collection bags are purely gravity-assisted drainage systems or gravity plus negative suction-assisted drainage systems. There are also waterless variants of these drainage systems. The basic principles of underwater seal drainage are best understood with the bottle system,[9,14] which shall be briefly described here. The various types of bottle systems are:

One-bottle system: The same chamber acts both as a water seal and a collection chamber (Fig. 6). The drainage tube extends into a sterile plastic or glass bottle such that it is submerged 2 cm under the level of sterile saline. Air escapes from this chamber to the atmosphere via an exit vent which should always be kept open. As the collection chamber fills with blood or fluid, the drainage tube becomes submerged to a greater depth and this results in an increased resistance to drainage. A regulated suction cannot be applied to this system.

Two-bottle system: There are two bottles, the one proximal to the patient acts as a collection chamber and the other one acts as a water seal chamber and has the air vent (Fig. 7). Blood or fluid drains into the proximal collection chamber and only the air flows into the underwater seal chamber and escapes through the air vent. This ensures that the underwater seal is always kept at a fixed level. Thus, there is no increase in resistance as the fluid gets drained and is ideal when large amount of fluid needs to be drained. A regulated suction cannot be applied to this type of drainage system also.

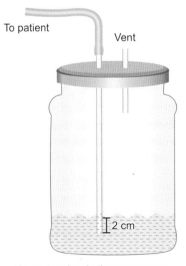

Fig. 6 One-bottle drainage system

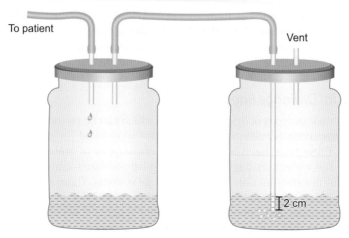

Fig. 7 Two-bottle drainage system

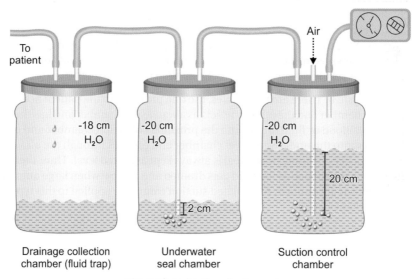

Fig. 8 Three-bottle collection system

Three-bottle system: This is designed for safe application of negative suction pressure and involves the addition of a suction control bottle between the underwater seal and the suction apparatus (Fig. 8). The suction control chamber is connected to the exit vent of the underwater seal on one end and the suction device on the other end. This chamber also has a control tube which is immersed approximately 20 cm in water and is open to the atmosphere. The depth to which the control tube is immersed determines the upper limit of negative pressure in the system. The major disadvantages of the three-bottle system are greater complexity, noise due to continuous bubbling in the third bottle, and lack of an exit vent if suction fails.

Four-bottle system: The four-bottle system consists of a fourth bottle, a safety underwater seal which is connected to the collection chamber (fluid trap) of the three-bottle system (Fig. 9). This will vent the entire system and relieve any pressure build-up in case of a failure of suction.

Ambulatory Drains

These are basically modifications of the traditional bottle systems with which the patient can ambulate.[15] The simplest of these, the Heimlich valve, needs special mention. Heimlich valve is a one-way flutter valve (Figs 10A and B), which is constructed such that the tubing gets occluded whenever the pressure inside the tubing (same as the intrapleural pressure) is less than the atmospheric pressure (inspiration) and is patent when the pressure inside the tube is above atmospheric pressure (expiration). As there is no collection chamber attached to this valve, this is most useful for patients with pneumothorax where there is no fluid which needs to be drained. It is also important to know that if attached in the wrong direction, it can lead to a tension pneumothorax.

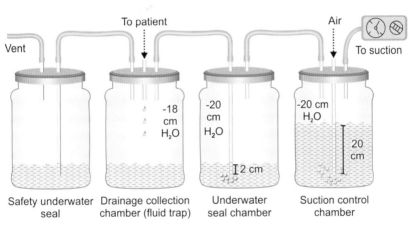

Fig. 9 Four-bottle collection system

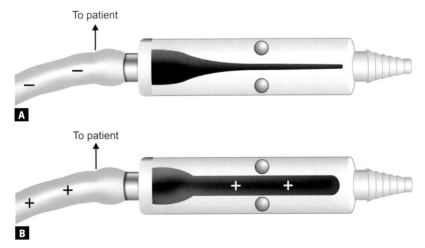

Figs 10A and B Heimlich's valve—schematic diagram. (A) During inspiration; (B) During expiration

PREPARATION

Informed Consent

Prior to starting the procedure, the patient (or his/her relatives) should be informed about the indication for chest tube placement, the procedure itself and its attendant complications, and a written informed consent should be obtained.

Patient Preparation

- The indication for chest tube insertion should be reconfirmed and any contraindications if present should be ruled out.
- The side of placement of intercostal drain should be reconfirmed by auscultation and chest radiograph.
- *Positioning the patient:* The preferred position for intercostal drain insertion is patient lying supine with the arm on the side of the lesion behind the patients head so as to expose the axillary region. Chest drains can also be inserted with the patient lying in lateral decubitus position with the affected side facing upward. Some authors have also described placing chest tube with the patient sitting and leaning forward with the arms resting over an adjacent table or a pillow. We do not recommend this position as there is a possibility of vasovagal syncope during the procedure.
- *Establishing an intravenous access:* It is important to have a functional intravenous access before starting the procedure so that no time is wasted in securing an access in the event of an emergency.
- It is advisable to monitor the pulse rate, blood pressure and arterial saturation throughout the procedure. Patients may need supplemental oxygen during the procedure.
- *Premedication:* As intercostal drain placement is a painful procedure, adequate analgesia needs to be given. BTS guidelines recommend the use of an anxiolytic/sedative, either a benzodiazepine or an opioid, before the procedure. However in patients who are prone to respiratory depression, e.g. patients with chronic obstructive pulmonary disease (COPD), deep sedation should be avoided.

PROCEDURE

Operative Tube Thoracostomy[3,16]

Identifying the Site of Insertion

The most common site for chest tube insertion is the safe triangle in the midaxillary line (Fig. 11A). Once identified, it is preferable to mark the site of insertion with a skin marker. We usually perform a chest ultrasonography in the presence of loculations. If there are extensive adhesions, an image-guided pigtail insertion is then performed. It was earlier thought that the chest drain should be placed more superiorly, in the second intercostal space in midclavicular line for draining a pneumothorax. However, it has been shown that lateral placement of chest tube through the midaxillary line drains pneumothoraces equally well.

Skin Sterilization

Chest tube insertion should be performed under strict aseptic precautions. The operator and the assistant should wear a sterile gown, face mask, cap and gloves. The patient's skin should be disinfected from the axilla to the iliac crest and from the nipple line to the midline posteriorly. Thereafter, the area should be draped with sterile towels on all sides, leaving only a few inches exposed on either side of the proposed site of insertion (Fig. 11B). It is necessary to prepare and drape a wide area so that asepsis is not breached during the procedure. Failure of asepsis may lead to iatrogenic wound site infection and may even turn an uncomplicated effusion into an empyema. The role of prophylactic antibiotics to prevent wound infection is controversial. In the setting of chest trauma (penetrating or blunt), a meta-analysis found the use of prophylactic antibiotics beneficial (decline in the absolute risk of empyema by 5.5-7.1% and all infectious complications by 12.1-13.4%).[17] However, we do not recommend the routine use of prophylactic antibiotics for preventing wound infection.

Local Anesthesia

A local anesthetic agent, usually lignocaine (up to a maximum dose of 3 mg/kg) is infiltrated at the site of insertion for adequate analgesia. The skin is infiltrated first followed by injection into the deeper layers. It is advisable to anesthetize a slightly wider area than the size of anticipated incision. The periosteum of the underlying ribs also needs to be anesthetized. The volume given is considered to be more important than the concentration to aid spread of the effectively anesthetized area. After infiltration of the anesthetic agent, adequate time (usually 3-5 minutes) must be given for the drug to act.

Incision and Dissection

The skin is incised parallel to and above the upper margin of the lower rib (Fig. 11C). The length of the incision is slightly larger than the diameter of the tube to be inserted and large enough to allow the operators finger to be inserted. Once the incision is made, blunt dissection of the underlying subcutaneous tissue and muscles should be done using a curved artery forceps till the pleura is reached (Fig. 11D). The pleura is punctured using the same blunt-tipped forceps. The feel of a pleural puncture is like that of a sudden give away of resistance. There will be a gush of air or of fluid the moment the pleural cavity is punctured. Next, the artery forceps should be gently opened in one direction and then again at right angles to dilate the tract, so that the chest tube can be inserted (Fig. 11E). It is important to keep the artery forceps in an open position for a few seconds to allow the tract to be adequately dilated. The creation of a patent adequately dilated track into the pleural cavity ensures that excessive force is not needed during drain insertion. The operator's finger may be used if required to explore the tract and to ensure proper placement (Fig. 11F).

Insertion of the Chest Drain

The chest tube is to be held by the artery forceps just proximal to its tip and inserted through the surgical tract (Fig. 11G). Undue force should not be used during insertion of the chest tube so as to avoid damage to the internal organs. If there is resistance during insertion, the chest tube should be removed and the tract explored and dilated using the curved artery forceps. The artery forceps should be used to ensure the entry of the tip of the chest tube into the pleural cavity and should be withdrawn thereafter (Figs 11H and I). An appropriate length of the chest tube can now be pushed inside in the desired direction. It was earlier postulated that the tip of the tube should be aimed apically to drain air and basally for fluid. However, successful drainage of air as well as fluid can be achieved with the drain in any position. The length of tube to be pushed inside will vary according to the patient's body habitus. Once the tube is inserted, the outer end of the chest tube should be cut and attached to the underwater seal bag (Fig. 11J). The proper positioning of the chest drain in the pleural cavity is confirmed by the movement of the water column in the water seal bag. The physician or assistant's left hand should press the site of insertion of the chest tube with a gauze piece so as to prevent peritubal leak of pleural fluid or air entering the pleural cavity till the tube is secured.

Securing the Chest Drain

The incision should be closed using one stay suture placed across at right angles to the incision (Fig. 11K). An inadvertently placed large incision may need two sutures placed across the incision. The chosen suture should be stout and nonabsorbable (silk) to prevent breakdown, and adequate depth of skin and subcutaneous tissue should be included in the suture to ensure that it is secure. The chest drain should be secured to the chest wall with the same suture which was used to close the incision using figure of 8 knots (Figs 11L and M). This is to prevent the tube from accidentally slipping out. Care should be taken to make the site of entry air tight so as to avoid any peritubal leak. Complicated "purse string" sutures must not be used to secure the chest drain as they convert a linear wound into a circular one that is painful for the patient and may leave an unsightly scar. The site of insertion of the chest tube is once again cleaned, covered with a sterile piece of gauze and an adhesive tape applied after drying the skin (Fig. 11N). Large amounts of tape and padding to dress the site are unnecessary and may restrict chest wall movement or increase moisture collection. An "omental" tag of tape may also be applied which allows the tube to lie a little away from the chest wall to prevent tube kinking and tension at the insertion site (Fig. 11O).

Guidewire Tube Thoracostomy

All the steps till infiltration of local anesthesia are same as that described for operative tube thoracostomy. However, premedication with a benzodiazepine or opioid is not always necessary as it is a less painful technique. The site of insertion is confirmed using an ultrasound.
- A needle attached to a syringe is introduced into the pleural cavity at the identified site. Fluid or air is aspirated to confirm the intrapleural location.
- The syringe is then removed and a 'J' tipped guidewire is introduced into the pleural cavity through the needle. This needle also is finally removed leaving the guidewire in position.

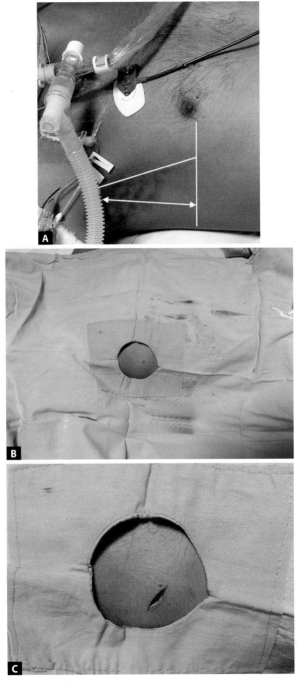

Figs 11A to C Stepwise demonstration of an intercostal drain placement by operative tube thoracostomy. (A) Identification of the site of insertion, the safe triangle; (B) Cleaning and draping. Note that a wide area is draped so as to ensure proper asepsis; (C) An incision is placed parallel to the rib margin

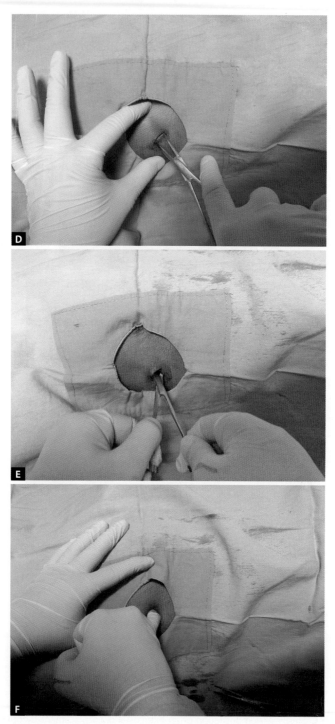

Figs 11D to F (D) Blunt dissection and creation of the tract being done with a blunt-tipped curved artery forceps; (E) Pleural puncture and dilation of the tract; (F) Exploration of the tract using operator's finger

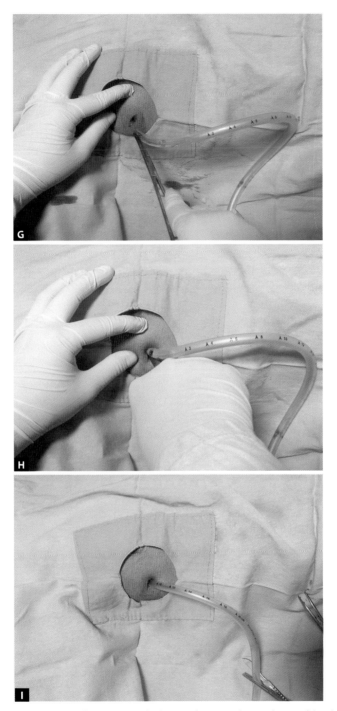

Figs 11G to I (G) Insertion of the intercostal tube into the created tract. The tip of the chest tube is held with the blunt-tipped forceps and is being inserted; (H) The chest drain is held with the forceps till it is in the pleural space; (I) The forceps is then withdrawn out leaving the chest tube in the pleural space. The free end of the chest tube is now cut and the tip blocked with an artery forceps

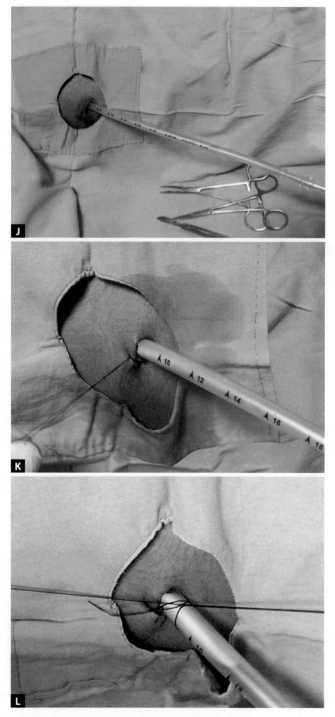

Figs 11J to L (J) The chest tube is now attached to the underwater seal bag; (K) Placement of a linear incision closing suture; (L) The chest tube being secured to the chest wall using the same incision closing suture thread

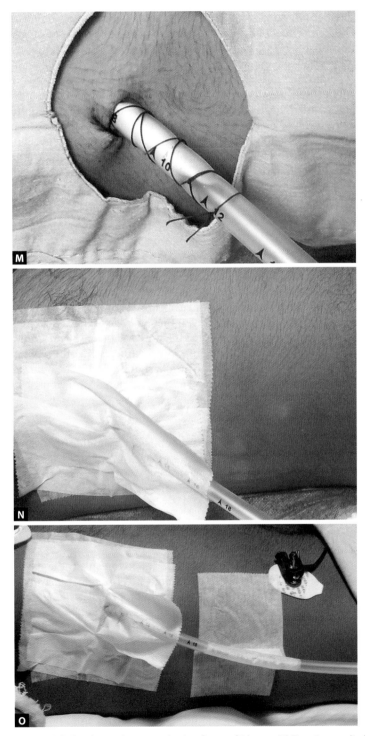

Figs 11M to O (M) The chest tube secured using figure of 8 knots; (N) Dressing applied at the chest drain insertion site; (O) The chest drain also secured using an omental tag of tape

- A small incision is made at the guidewire entry site and the guidewire tract is then dilated sequentially using dilators of progressively increasing size. The smallest dilator is inserted first with a rotating movement until a sensation of giveaway is felt upon entry into the pleural cavity. The dilator is then removed and the next size dilator is advanced similarly over the guidewire. The guidewire should always project beyond the end of the dilator. If large bore tubes are to be inserted, a small incision or nick may be required at the site of insertion to facilitate the entry of larger dilators and the chest tube.
- The chest tube is loaded onto a stylet and is then passed into the pleural cavity over the guidewire. Once inside the pleural space, the chest tube is advanced making sure that all the side holes are in the pleural space. The stylet along with the guidewire is then removed.
- The chest tube is attached to the underwater seal and is secured to the chest wall as described above.

Trocar Tube Thoracostomy

After identifying the site of insertion, an incision is made and the skin and subcutaneous tissue dissected as described in the operative thoracostomy section. A chest tube with the trocar positioned inside the tube is used. The trocar is then inserted into the pleural space with the flat edge of the stylet cephalad. As described earlier, there is no sequential dilation and hence a considerable force would be required to puncture the pleura with the trocar. Once the pleural space is entered, the trocar is removed, leaving the chest tube inside. The tube is attached to the underwater seal bag and secured as described in the previous sections.

POST-PROCEDURE CARE

- *Confirming tube position:* The tube position should be confirmed by observing the movement of the water column in the drainage system. In a normally breathing patient, the water level will move higher on inspiration indicating a more negative pleural pressure. However in a patient on mechanical ventilation, the water level will move down with inspiration because the pleural pressure becomes more positive. A chest radiograph (both posteroanterior and lateral) should be done to confirm the position of chest tube within the pleural cavity.
- *Patient instructions:* It is of utmost importance to explain the patient about proper chest tube care. The patient should be given clear instructions (and if possible provided with a patient information leaflet) as follows: (1) To keep the chest drain upright below the insertion site at all times; (2) to avoid compression of the tube; (3) to report to medical staff immediately in case of any distress; and (4) if being discharged, daily drain output monitoring and instructions for changing the fluid in the collection system should be taught.
- *Analgesia:* All patients should be given adequate analgesia following the procedure.
- *Monitoring:* A chest drain monitoring chart should be used for all patients. The frequency of monitoring can be variable ranging from hourly to at least once a day. The parameters which need to be monitored are: (1) functionality of the tube which is assessed by movement of the water column; (2) presence

and quantification of air leak, described later in the complications section; (3) volume of drain output; (4) type of drainage with regard to color and turbidity.

- *Changing the drain fluid:* The fluid in the water seal bag should be changed at least daily and even more frequently if the drainage is excessive. The amount of fluid and also the amount of sediment collected should be noted before emptying the bag. The tube should be clamped before emptying the fluid. The fluid collected in the drainage bag should be emptied and sterile fluid (normal saline) should be filled up to the mark provided. The tube should be unclamped after changing.
- *Applying suction:* A low pressure suction (20–40 cm H_2O) may be applied if either the lung does not expand on its own or if there is a persistent air leak.
- *Chest tube dressing:* The dressing applied should be changed daily or at least once every other day. The local site should be examined for any erythema, subcutaneous emphysema, peritubal leak and pus discharge.

COMPLICATION/PROBLEM

There are various complications of tube thoracostomy ranging from minor complications not requiring any intervention to life-threatening ones.[18] It is important to understand each of these complications, strategies to prevent them and prompt identification and management once they occur.

Tube Malposition

This is the most common complication of intercostal tube drainage. Most of these occur because of failure to identify the triangle of safety of if the tube is placed during an emergency setting. Hence, it is always essential to get a chest radiograph to confirm the proper positioning of the chest tube. In two different audits performed, up to 50% of the junior doctors would have placed the chest drain outside the triangle of safety.[19,20] Tube malposition can further be classified as: (1) intraparenchymal placement; (2) intrafissural placement; and (3) extrathoracic placement (subcutaneous, mediastinum, abdomen). Intraparenchymal malpositioning usually occurs when the lung is adherent to the chest wall at the site of insertion, when undue force is used to insert the chest tube or when trocars are used without blunt dissection. It generally cannot be detected on a chest radiograph. It is identified by poor drainage and is confirmed by a computed tomography scan. The chest tube requires only to be repositioned; surgical intervention is rarely required. Intrafissural placement, though classified as a malposition, does not affect the drainage of fluid and does not need repositioning if the drain is functional. Extrathoracic subcutaneous placement is common in patients with chest trauma and in obese patients. It is identified on chest radiograph and needs repositioning. Placement into mediastinum may cause injury to heart, pulmonary artery, esophagus and nerves. Similarly, a chest tube placed too low may cause injury to abdominal organs including liver, spleen and stomach. Extrathoracic placement can also be identified at the time of insertion itself by lack of column movement. Mediastinal or abdominal organ injury needs prompt surgical correction.

Re-expansion Pulmonary Edema

This is an uncommon (0–1%) but a serious complication of tube thoracostomy. It usually occurs when chest drain is inserted for a massive pleural effusion or a large pneumothorax. Risk factors include young age (<40 years), underlying lung collapse for >7 days, large effusion or pneumothorax, rapid lung re-expansion and use of negative pressure suction. The postulated mechanism for development of this edema is increased endothelial permeability leading to exudation of a protein-rich fluid. The reason for endothelial damage is: (1) ischemia reperfusion leading to oxygen free radicals and neutrophils influx; (2) damage to the vascular endothelium in the collapsed lung due to mechanical stress; and (3) stress injury to the vascular endothelium of the normal vessels due to sudden expansion. The clinical spectrum ranges from asymptomatic radiologic finding, symptoms of chest pain, breathlessness and dry cough, to frank cardiorespiratory failure requiring mechanical ventilation and inotropic support. Re-expansion pulmonary edema can be prevented by slowly draining the massive effusion, not draining more than 1.5 liters in one setting and clamping the tube if patient develops symptoms of chest pain or dry cough. Treatment is institution of supportive measures.

Bleeding

Intercostal arteries, if injured during dissection for insertion of the chest drain, may bleed profusely. The safest zone to perform tube thoracostomy should be between 50% and 70% of the way down an interspace to avoid the variably positioned superior intercostal neurovascular bundle and the inferior collateral vessels. Systemic arteriovenous fistula (SAVF) involving an intercostal artery and subcutaneous vein can result after tube thoracostomy. The clinical manifestations of a traumatic SAVF may be immediate or delayed, ranging from 1 week to 12 years.

Subcutaneous Emphysema

This presents as a soft tissue swelling with crepitus at the site of chest drain insertion. It is usually minor and self-limited but sometimes can spread widely leading to cosmetic disfigurement and even respiratory distress. Subcutaneous emphysema develops when a side hole of chest tube is lying in the subcutaneous space or if there is obstruction of chest tube drainage system or if the drainage system cannot cope up with the air leak (Fig. 12). When extensive and correction of the above factors fail to control the emphysema, insertion of a fenestrated angiocatheter into the subcutaneous tissue (Fig. 13) or subcutaneous pigtail insertion may be required.[21]

Infectious Complications

Breach in asepsis while inserting a chest tube or in managing a chest drain leads to infectious complications. The infectious complications include empyema, surgical site infection (ranging from cellulitis to necrotizing fasciitis) and pneumonia (uncommon). Prompt identification and treatment with antibiotics is required. It is more important to prevent the development of these infectious complications.

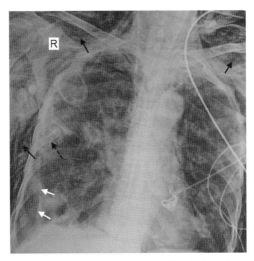

Fig. 12 Chest tube placed in the right pleural space (black dotted arrow) after the patient developed a spontaneous tension pneumothorax due to rupture of a peripheral cavity. Note the development of extensive subcutaneous emphysema (black arrows). Also note the presence of a loculated residual pneumothorax (white arrows)

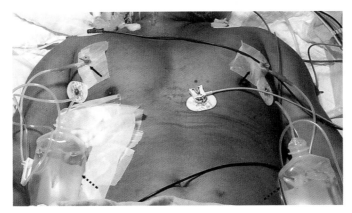

Fig. 13 The subcutaneous emphysema being drained using bilaterally placed fenestrated angiocatheters (black solid arrows) connected to underwater seals (black dotted arrows)

Blocked Chest Tube

Blockade of chest drain with fibrin deposits/clots is a commonly encountered complication with the increasing use of smaller bore chest drains. It is identified by lack of movement of the water column with respiration. Milking of the chest drain is not recommended as it increases the pressures inside the pleura. Flushing the chest drain with 50 mL normal saline under sterile conditions usually restores the patency. If the cause of blockage is kinking of the chest tube, the chest drain may need to be repositioned.

Prolonged Air Leak

An air leak is defined as the presence of air bubbling in the underwater seal bag. Causes of air leak include:

- *Bronchopleural fistula:* An air leak due to a communication between a large bronchus (mainstem, lobar or segmental) and the pleural space
- *Alveolopleural fistula:* An air leak due to a communication between the pulmonary parenchyma distal to a segmental bronchus and the pleural space.
- *Peritubal leak:* An air leak due to poorly applied skin incision closing suture, which leads to air being sucked into the pleural cavity with each inspiration. The most definite way to confirm a peritubal leak is to check the $PaCO_2$ of the air coming from the chest tube. If $PaCO_2$ is less than 10 mm Hg, then it confirms a peritubal leak as the air has not participated in gas exchange.
- *System leak:* An air leak due to loose connections in the chest drainage system.

The terms alveolo- and bronchopleural fistula should not be used interchangeably as the treatment strategies differ.[22] A bronchopleural fistula usually develops only after a major pulmonary resection surgery and its management usually requires surgery. An alveolopleural fistula is the more common form of air leak that develops spontaneously or following iatrogenic trauma. Most of these heal on their own and do not need any therapeutic intervention. They also occur more commonly in mechanically ventilated patients.

There are various ways to quantify an air leak. The earliest proposed semiquantitative and qualitative classification is the Robert David Cerfolio (RDC) classification system in which the air leak is classified as continuous (C), inspiratory (I), expiratory (E) or a forced expiratory (FE) air leak depending on the phase of respiration in which the bubbling is seen.[23] This is however highly subjective. Another semiquantitative method of classifying air leaks is by using Sahara S1100 a Pleur-evac drainage bag. The air leak is quantified on a scale from 1 to 7. A number 1 leak indicates a small leak and a number 7 leak indicates a large air leak.[24] The latest and more accurate quantitative estimation of air leaks is using digital air leak monitoring meters. The air leak is quantified in mL/min. The commercially available systems are the Thopaz and Atmos pleural drainage systems.[25]

An air leak is common after the insertion of chest drain. After a system leak and a peritubal leak are ruled out, a period of observation is all that is required in most cases. If the air leak does not heal by 5 days (ACCP Delphi statement), a thoracoscopic procedure or thoracotomy might be needed. Other techniques include blood patch pleurodesis or endobronchial management (valves or glue insertion). It has also been shown that chest drains can also be removed safely even in the presence of a persistent minor air leak as long as there is no symptomatic pneumothorax after provocative clamping.[26] If an air leak develops in a mechanically ventilated patient, the patient should be shifted to a pressure-controlled mode of ventilation and patient ventilated with the minimum possible pressures needed.

Failure of Lung Expansion

Failure of the lung to expand despite a functional and properly placed chest drain is a commonly encountered clinical scenario.[27,28] The common causes of a nonexpanding lung include:

- *Lung entrapment:* A lung is said to be entrapped when an inflammatory visceral pleural peel resulting from an active pleural process prevents the

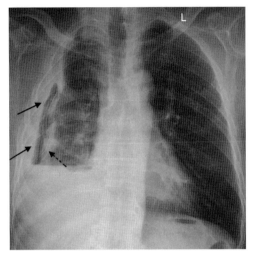

Fig. 14 Non-expanding lung after placing a chest tube (black dotted arrow) due to the presence of thick pleural peel (black solid arrows). This patient was later managed with surgical lung decortication

lung from expanding. The common causes include active pleural infection, malignancy and inflammatory diseases like rheumatoid arthritis. The pleural fluid is exudative in character and treatment of the underlying disease usually results in lung re-expansion.

- *Trapped lung:* Trapped lung is the development of a mature, fibrous pleural membrane as a sequel of remote pleural space inflammation that impedes lung expansion during fluid removal. The pleural fluid is usually a transudate and management requires decortication (Fig. 14).
- Endobronchial obstruction
- *Chronic atelectasis:* In patients with chronic atelectasis, the lung may take longer time than usual to expand unless a significant amount of parenchymal fibrosis has already set in.
- Persistent alveolopleural or bronchopleural fistula
- *Peritubal leak:* This leads to air being sucked into the pleural space with each inspiration.

Treatment depends on identification of the cause and institution of appropriate treatment.

REFERENCES

1. Harris A, O'Driscoll BR, Turkington PM. Survey of major complications of intercostal chest drain insertion in the UK. Postgrad Med J. 2010;86:68-72.
2. Maritz D, Wallis L, Hardcastle T. Complications of tube thoracostomy for chest trauma. S Afr Med J. 2009;99:114-7.
3. MacDuff A, Arnold A, Harvey J. Management of spontaneous pneumothorax: British Thoracic Society Pleural Disease Guideline 2010. Thorax. 2010;65(Suppl 2):ii18-31.
4. Baumann MH, Strange C, Heffner JE, Light R, Kirby TJ, Klein J, et al. Management of spontaneous pneumothorax: an American College of Chest Physicians Delphi consensus statement. Chest. 2001;119:590-602.

5. Laws D, Neville E, Duffy J. BTS guidelines for the insertion of a chest drain. Thorax. 2003; 58(Suppl 2):ii53-9.
6. Wraight WM, Tweedie DJ, Parkin IG. Neurovascular anatomy and variation in the fourth, fifth, and sixth intercostal spaces in the mid-axillary line: a cadaveric study in respect of chest drain insertion. Clin Anat. 2005;18:346-9.
7. Yalcin NG, Choong CK, Eizenberg N. Anatomy and pathophysiology of the pleura and pleural space. Thorac Surg Clin. 2013;23:1-10, v.
8. Mahmood K, Wahidi MM. Straightening out chest tubes: what size, what type, and when. Clin Chest Med. 2013;34:63-71.
9. Light RW. Chest tubes. In: Rhyner S (Ed). Pleural Diseases. Philadelphia, PA 19106 USA: Lippincott Williams & Wilkins. 2007. pp. 404-12.
10. Cooke DT, David EA. Large-bore and small-bore chest tubes: types, function, and placement. Thorac Surg Clin. 2013;23:17-24, v.
11. Fysh ET, Smith NA, Lee YC. Optimal chest drain size: the rise of the small-bore pleural catheter. Semin Respir Crit Care Med. 2010;31:760-8.
12. Rahman NM, Maskell NA, Davies CW, Hedley EL, Nunn AJ, Gleeson FV, et al. The relationship between chest tube size and clinical outcome in pleural infection. Chest. 2010;137:536-43.
13. Rahman NM, Maskell NA, West A, Teoh R, Arnold A, Mackinlay C, et al. Intrapleural use of tissue plasminogen activator and DNase in pleural infection. N Engl J Med. 2011;365:518-26.
14. Kam AC, O'Brien M, Kam PC. Pleural drainage systems. Anaesthesia. 1993;48:154-61.
15. Joshi JM. Ambulatory chest drainage. Indian J Chest Dis Allied Sci. 2009;51:225-31.
16. Kumar A, Dutta R, Jindal T, Biswas B, Dewan RK. Safe insertion of a chest tube. Natl Med J India. 2009;22:192-8.
17. Fallon WF Jr, Wears RL. Prophylactic antibiotics for the prevention of infectious complications including empyema following tube thoracostomy for trauma: results of meta-analysis. J Trauma. 1992;33:110-6; discussion 116-7.
18. Kesieme EB, Dongo A, Ezemba N, Irekpita E, Jebbin N, Kesieme C. Tube thoracostomy: complications and its management. Pulm Med. 2012;2012:256878.
19. Elsayed H, Roberts R, Emadi M, Whittle I, Shackcloth M. Chest drain insertion is not a harmless procedure—are we doing it safely? Interact Cardiovasc Thorac Surg. 2010;11:745-8.
20. Griffiths JR, Roberts N. Do junior doctors know where to insert chest drains safely? Postgrad Med J. 2005;81:456-8.
21. Srinivas R, Singh N, Agarwal R, Aggarwal AN. Management of extensive subcutaneous emphysema and pneumomediastinum by micro-drainage: time for a re-think? Singapore Med J. 2007;48:e323-6.
22. Singh N, Agarwal R. Bronchopleural fistula or alveolopleural fistula? Not just semantics. Chest. 2006;130:1948; author reply 1948-9.
23. Cerfolio RJ, Bass C, Katholi CR. Prospective randomized trial compares suction versus water seal for air leaks. Ann Thorac Surg. 2001;71:1613-7.
24. Cerfolio RJ, Bryant AS. The quantification of postoperative air leaks. Multimed Man Cardiothorac Surg. 2009;2009(409):mmcts.2007.003129.
25. Cerfolio RJ, Varela G, Brunelli A. Digital and smart chest drainage systems to monitor air leaks: the birth of a new era? Thorac Surg Clin. 2010;20:413-20.
26. Cerfolio RJ, Minnich DJ, Bryant AS. The removal of chest tubes despite an air leak or a pneumothorax. Ann Thorac Surg. 2009;87:1690-4; discussion 1694-6.
27. Huggins JT, Doelken P, Sahn SA. The unexpandable lung. F1000 Med Rep. 2010;2:77.
28. Huggins JT, Sahn SA, Heidecker J, Ravenel JG, Doelken P. Characteristics of trapped lung: pleural fluid analysis, manometry, and air-contrast chest CT. Chest. 2007;131: 206-13.

14

Non-invasive Ventilation for Acute Respiratory Failure

Raj Kumar Mani, Prashant Saxena

INTRODUCTION

Non-invasive ventilation (NIV) provides support to ventilation in appropriate settings with the help of a mask or similar interface. Its advantages is that tracheal conduit such as endotracheal or tracheostomy tube is not required to provide respiratory support. Thus, NIV-assisted patients are at a lesser risk of nosocomial pneumonia, have more comfort and can feed and speak.[1-3] One must always remember that NIV is appropriate only for intermittent partial respiratory support and one should not delay invasive mechanical ventilation when clearly indicated. Non-invasive positive pressure ventilation (NIPPV) can also be used as an abbreviation instead of NIV.

INDICATIONS OF NON-INVASIVE VENTILATION[1-22]

Well-evidenced Indications

- Exacerbations of chronic obstructive pulmonary diseases (COPD)
- Weaning from invasive ventilation in COPD
- Cardiogenic pulmonary edema
- Respiratory failure in immunocompromised patients.

Indications Based on Lesser Grades of Evidence

- Hypoxemic respiratory failure in early acute respiratory distress syndrome (ARDS)
- COPD patients with pneumonia and hypoxic respiratory failure
- Respiratory failure due to obesity hypoventilation syndrome
- Obstructive sleep apnea
- Acute bronchial asthma
- Post-extubation failure in COPD patients
- Respiratory failure in neuromuscular diseases or chest wall deformity
- Flail chest
- Patient for palliative or end-of-life care
- To assist bronchoscopy (Fig. 1).

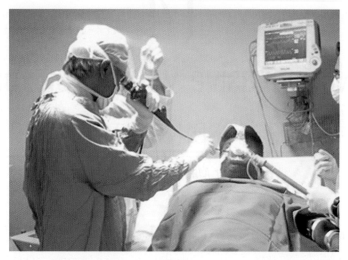

Fig. 1 Non-invasive ventilation-assisted bronchoscopy

CONTRAINDICATIONS OF NON-INVASIVE VENTILATION[1-4]

Absolute

- Respiratory arrest
- Cardiac arrest
- Hemodynamic instability or malignant arrhythmias
- Life-threatening hypoxemia

Relative

- Recent or ongoing myocardial ischemia
- Inability to protect upper airway
  - Coma with Glasgow Coma Scale (GCS) less than 8
  - Copious secretions
  - High-risk of aspiration
- Faciomaxillary injuries or surgery or deformity
- Gastric distension
- Claustrophobia or inability to accept mask interface
- Failure of a NIV trial after half to 1 hour of hypoxic failure and 4 hours after hypercarbic failure
- Upper gastrointestinal (GI) bleeding
- Recent upper GI surgery.

TECHNIQUE AND BASIC PRINCIPLES OF NON-INVASIVE VENTILATION

In the earlier days of development of mechanical ventilation, the concept of negative pressure ventilation emerged with the development of an iron lung by Woillez in 1876. Subsequently, in 1889, Alexander Graham Bell came up with an "iron lung" for use in newborns. The earlier NIV devices were external negative pressure ventilators, including the body ventilator and the iron lung. Negative pressure ventilators were widely used during the polio epidemics of the 1930s and 1960s, but these ventilators gradually went out of fashion as they were large, bulky and less easy to use.[1] The new generation cuirass ventilators in the form of a "shell" or "chest wrap" are more user-friendly but carry the risk of increased airway collapse in some patients.[5] With the invention of mask interface in 1981 for obstructive sleep apnea,[6] NIV was applied first for respiratory support in neuromuscular disease[7] in the mid-1980s and later in chronic obstructive airways disease in the 1990s.[8] With the evolution of new technologies for devices, interfaces and evidence basis for clinical use along with ease of use, comfort, low cost and portability, positive pressure ventilation via NIV became the first choice of physicians in appropriate settings.[1-3]

Mechanism of Action of Non-invasive Ventilation[1-3]

- *Improved oxygenation:* By increasing the functional residual capacity (FRC) oxygenation is improved and gas exchange is facilitated
- Partial unloading of respiratory muscles thereby reducing work of breathing
- Reduction of upper airway resistance overcomes obstructive sleep apnea and reduces work of breathing
- Augmented tidal volume when bilevel pressure is applied
- Improved cardiac function in the setting of LV dysfunction through reduction of preload (venous return) and afterload (decrease in left ventricular transmural pressure)
- In COPD patients reduced work of breathing and improved triggering by overcoming auto positive end-expiratory pressure (auto-PEEP).
- In the chronic setting, it helps in resetting the respiratory center by reducing the nocturnal peaks of hypercarbia.

Types of Non-invasive Ventilation Support[1-3,23]

Many types of ventilators are used nowadays for the purpose of NIV. Experience, training and familiarity with the ventilators impact on the criteria for choosing a particular ventilator. Most units prefer to use a single model for easy operability by the staff. Broadly, the ventilators can be grouped as follows:
- *Critical care ventilators (Fig. 2):* Some of the modern ventilators have an NIV module or any critical care ventilator can be used to provide NIV support. The main advantage of this form of support is that oxygen concentration can be better regulated and carbon dioxide rebreathing is minimized since a double limb circuit is employed. Respiratory monitoring and alarm systems are also available. The disadvantage is that the system can also be complex and sensitive with propensity for continual alarms resulting in patient disturbance.
- *Ventilators specifically designed for NIV (Fig. 3):* Bilevel pressure ventilators are lightweight portable devices with a single limb circuit attached to a mask or similar interface. It may be a simple pressure support device or a more sophisticated one with the capability of providing timed breaths of a variety of ventilatory modes. Usually, oxygen is not blended into the system but provided separately through a port located either in the mask or in the tubing.

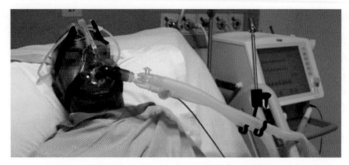

Fig. 2 Non-invasive ventilation using a full facemask through a critical care ventilator

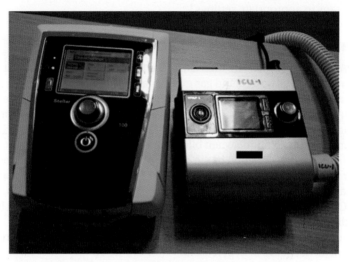

Fig. 3 A sample of portable bilevel pressure devices

Modes of Non-invasive Ventilation[1,2]

Usually, most of the modes used invasively in modern ventilators can be used for NIV. The commonly used modes are:

- *Bilevel positive airway pressure (BIPAP):* BIPAP is the most frequently utilized and understood mode. Here, two pressure levels, inspiratory positive airway pressure (IPAP) and expiratory positive airway pressure (EPAP) assist spontaneously triggered breaths (pressure support). This is also called S or spontaneous mode as opposed to timed breaths that can be delivered in the form of a back-up rate also called S/T or spontaneous-timed mode.[1-3]
- Continuous positive airway pressure (CPAP) delivers a fixed pressure through both inspiration and expiration. Used in obstructive sleep apnea (OSA)/obesity hypoventilation syndrome (OHS), pulmonary edema and bronchial asthma.[1-3]
- *Volume/assist control modes:* Aimed at delivery of a preset tidal volume (7–12 mL/kg) especially in chest wall deformities or neuromuscular diseases.

Inspiratory Time

Timed modes are primarily used to provide a backup breath rate, if the patient is liable to central apneas when asleep. Remember, pressure support ventilation is flow cycled, and thus inspiratory time can be adjusted only when there is no spontaneous breath and the back-up rate is activated.

Prediction of Non-invasive Ventilation Success[1-3,9,10]

- Relief of dyspnea and work of breathing within half to 1 hour in case of hypoxemic failure and 1–4 hours in case of hypercarbic failure.
- Improvement in the GCS within 2–4 hours in case of hypercarbic failure
- Improvement in arterial blood gas analysis (ABGA) (desired reduction in $PaCO_2$, an increase in PaO_2 and improvement in pH) within half to 1 hour in hypoxemic failure and 2–4 hours in case of hypercarbic failure.

Prediction of Non-invasive Ventilation Failure[1-3,8,9]

- No relief in dyspnea or work of breathing after half to 1 hour in case of hypo-xemic failure and after 4 hours in case of hypercarbic failure
- Worsening of sensorium at any time
- Worsening ABGA after half to 1 hour in case of hypoxemic failure and after 2–4 hours in case of hypercarbic failure.
- Hemodynamic instability at any time
- Intolerance to mask leading to anxiety or agitation
- Patient's subjective impression of worsening
- Physician assessment of increasing exhaustion.

Non-invasive Ventilation Machine

- Provision of NIV requires a machine capable of delivering pressurized gas to the patient through an interface. Modern intensive care ventilators may be used, if equipped with the appropriate software. An ideal NIV machine should have the following features:[2]
  - Provision of at least 30 cm H_2O pressure control
  - Flow rates of at least 60 L/min
  - Should have both pressure support and assist-control modes
  - Respiratory rate of 40 breath/min
  - Flow triggering and leak alarms.
- The machine is attached to the patient via a breathing circuit. The circuit can be single or double limb. Single limb circuits are typically used with portable NIV machines whereas double limb circuits are used with critical care ventilators.
- Humidification of air may be required in some patients on long-term venti-lation or those who develop dryness of mouth or nostrils. Usually, a water bath humidifier is used but a heated humidifier or an HME (Heat and moisture exchange) filter can also be used. HME filters can increase airway resistance and dead space and are not used routinely.[2]

Interfaces[1,2,4]

Many kinds of masks and interfaces of different sizes are available for provision of NIV, such as face (Figs 2, 4 and 5), nasal (Figs 6 and 7) or total facemasks (Fig. 8), helmets (Fig. 9) and nasal pillows. A full-facemask is preferred in the acute setting though it is less comfortable, has higher aspiration risk, and limits communication and oral intake as compared to a nasal mask. It could be replaced by a nasal mask in case of noncompliance or partial resolution of the acute process. Nasal masks are generally preferred in patients with chronic ventilatory insufficiency. They require a patent nasal passage and the mouth may need to be kept closed with a chin strap to minimize air leaks. There is no evidence to support the use of

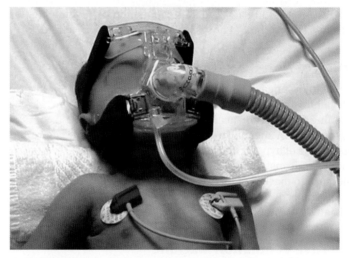

Fig. 4 Non-invasive ventilation with facemask in a child

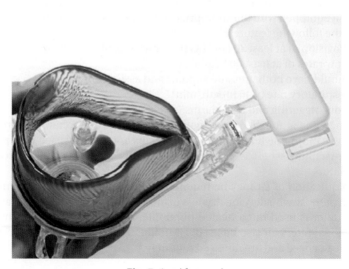

Fig. 5 A gel facemask

Source: Philips Respironics, India

one interface device over others. It is known that full-facemasks improve efficacy by reducing air leaks and may be the appropriate choice in the acute setting of severe hypoxemic respiratory failure.

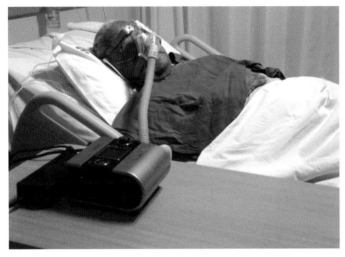

Fig. 6 Non-invasive ventilation using a nasal mask through a portable bilevel device

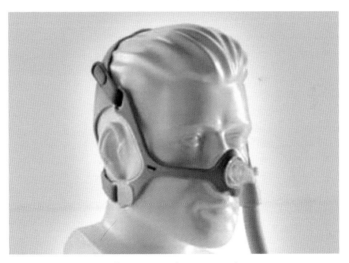

Fig. 7 Minimal contact mask
Source: Philips Respironics, India

Infection Control and Equipment Safety[1,2]

- Ideally single use masks and circuits should be used for every patient
- Automated washer may be used for disinfection of reusable masks, valves and circuits.
- Surface cleaning of the ventilator must be ensured on a daily basis with appropriate disinfectant.
- Regular maintenance and checks for electrical safety must be done.

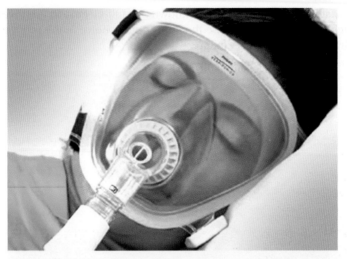

Fig. 8 Non-invasive ventilation using a total facemask
Source: Philips Respironics, India

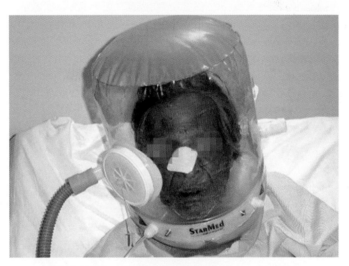

Fig. 9 Non-invasive ventilation using a helmet interface

PREPARATION FOR NON-INVASIVE VENTILATION

- *Clinical evaluation:* General examination of the patient including vital signs must be documented with special reference to GCS, chest wall movements, accessory muscle use and respiratory rate. A patient who is unable to protect the airway due to low GCS or secretions, etc. is not an appropriate candidate for NIV. A baseline and subsequent ABG analysis will help monitoring the response to therapy.[2]
- Carefully select the patient according to the inclusion and exclusion criteria
- Perform oral suctioning, if required.

- *Determination of mask type and size:* Nasal masks usually extend from the bridge of nose to the bottom of upper lip and should not touch the side of nose. An adequately sized full-facemask extends from the bridge of nose and between the chin and lower lip. Various manufacturing companies provide measuring scales along with the masks to help choose the size of the mask. Carefully select appropriate size of mask. Sizing scales (Figs 10 and 11), if available can be useful.
- Full-facemasks are preferable in an acute situation unless the patient is claustrophobic. If the patient is unable to tolerate an interface, try switching to a nasal mask or to a smaller size.

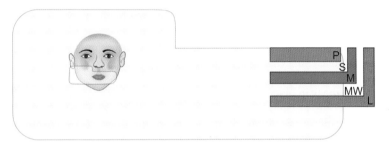

Fig. 10 Measuring scale for nasal mask
Source: Philips Respironics, India

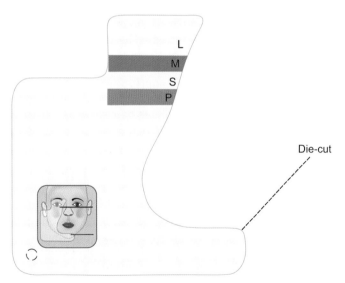

Fig. 11 Measuring scale for facemask
Source: Philips Respironics, India

STARTING, MONITORING AND WEANING OF NON-INVASIVE VENTILATION

Setting up of Non-invasive Ventilation[1,3,4,9,11]

Depending upon the severity of the illness, NIV can be applied in an emergency room (ER), intensive care unit (ICU), high dependency unit (HDU) or ward setting.

- Explain the procedure and benefits of NIV to the patient. Allay his apprehensions.
- Carefully position the patient in at least 30–45 degree supine
- Turn on the NIV machine
- Select the desired NIV mode: usually spontaneous mode is used with IPAP and EPAP settings.
- Oxygen supplementation may be required in some patients to target a saturation of at least 90% via nasal prongs or through ports in the mask. Flow rate is usually set at 2–4 L/min.
- Hold the mask in place first without the straps, so that the patient can adapt to the mask (Fig. 12, Step 1)
- After adaptation, apply the straps to secure the mask (Fig. 12, Step 2, 3, 4). Avoid excessive pressure over the face and nose.
- Check for major air leaks through the mask. Air leaks to the eye are to be strictly avoided while a degree of air leaks over or under the face is acceptable after adaptation (Nowadays, NIV devices have in-built leak compensation of up to 60 liter/min).
- First adjust the EPAP, starting EPAP level should be set at 2–3 cm H_2O
- In case of hypoxic failure, EPAP is increased in steps of 1–2 cm H_2O until SPO_2 is more than 89% or a maximum of 10 cm is achieved. Add supplemental oxygen, if SPO_2 targets are not achieved.
- In case of hypercarbic failure, EPAP should be set 4–6 cm H_2O in order to avoid CO_2 rebreathing
- IPAP is set at least 4 cm H_2O above the set EPAP. Thereafter, IPAP is increased in steps of 1–2 cm H_2O targeting reduction in sternomastoid activity.
- Subsequent adjustments are based on the nature of illness, target tidal volume (usually 5–7 mL/kg) and patient's clinical status.

Monitoring during Non-invasive Ventilation[1,3,4,9-11]

- Regularly assess patient comfort, conscious level, chest wall motion, accessory muscle recruitment, and coordination with the ventilator, air leaks, respiratory rate and heart rate. Regular assessment of comfort, GCS, chest wall movements, accessory muscle use and vital signs must be done along with checks for air leak.
- Stay at the beside of the patient in the initial half to 1 hour for reassurance, coaching, monitoring and final adjustments
- Regular arterial blood gas analyses to assess patient's clinical progress (baseline, 0.5–1 hourly and then as indicated)
- Monitor oxygen saturation continuously and maintain between 90–93% with or without supplementary oxygen.

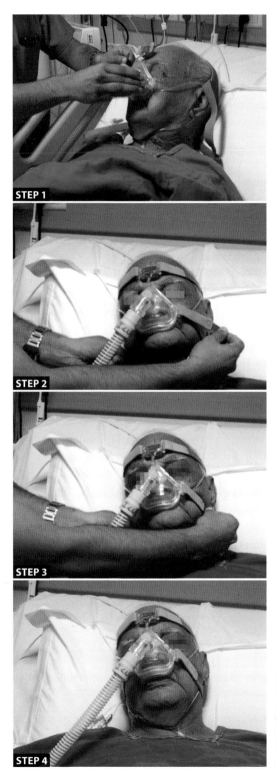

Fig. 12 Steps of application of mask interface. *Step 1:* Initially hold mask without the straps to allow for adaptation; *Step 2:* First secure the forehead straps; *Step 3:* Secure the cheek straps; *Step 4:* Nasal mask secured

Monitoring and Continuous Assessment[1,3,4,9,11]

- In case of hypoxemic failure, usually patients should show improvement within half to 1 hour of NIV initiation.
- In case of hypercarbic failure, clinical improvement in terms of sensorium and work of breathing should improve over 3–4 hours. Biochemical improvement in terms of $PaCO_2$ and pH sometimes takes longer.
- Patient need not receive NIV continuously. Discontinuation for feeding, drinking or toileting should be allowed any time.
- Setting may be changed to suit comfort at any time. Comfort takes precedence over PaO_2 or $PaCO_2$ targets.
- Bronchodilator aerosols can be administered via the NIV circuit.

Weaning from Non-invasive Ventilation[1,2]

- Assess for the achievement of clinical targets, e.g. target PaO_2, $PaCO_2$, relief of dyspnea and work of breathing, improvement in GCS
- Continue NIV support until the acute cause is resolved and the targets of therapy are maintained for at least 24–48 hours
- Plan intermittent NIV support with gradual increase in duration of NIV-free periods during the day, e.g. use NIV for 12–16 hours on day 3 followed by 8–10 hours on day 4 and then nocturnal NIV subsequently for 6–8 hours by day 5.
- Aim to consolidate NIV application to nocturnal use only.
- When patient is stable for 48 hours on nocturnal NIV support, gradually reduce NIV pressures in steps of 2 cm/day until an IPAP of 8 cm H_2O and EPAP 4 cm H_2O is achieved
- Remember, some patients can improve quickly during NIV and may require early weaning from NIV.
- Assess with overnight pulse oximetry and morning arterial blood gas analysis, for the need of long-term support prior to discharge.

COMPLICATIONS OF NON-INVASIVE VENTILATION[1-3,9]

- Risk of aspiration
- Gastric dilatation
- Interface injury—Facial and nasal ulcerations
- Air leaks
- Dryness of airway
- Pneumothorax
- Eye irritation.

REFERENCES

1. Keenan SP, Sinuff T, Burns KE, Muscedere J, Kutsogiannis J, Mehta S, et al. Clinical practice guidelines for the use of Noninvasive positive-pressure ventilation and noninvasive continuous positive airway pressure in the acute care setting. CMAJ. 2011; 183(3):e195-214.
2. British Thoracic Society Standards of Care Committee. Non-invasive ventilation in acute respiratory failure. Thorax. 2002;57:192-211.
3. ATS-International Consensus Conferences in Intensive Care Medicine: noninvasive positive pressure ventilation in acute respiratory failure. Am J Respir Crit Care Med. 2001;163:283-91.

4. Mehta S, Hill NS. Noninvasive ventilation. Am J Respir Crit Care Med. 2001;163:540-77.
5. Linton DM. Cuirass Ventilation: a review and update. Crit Care Resusc. 2005;7:22-8.
6. Sullivan CE, Issa FG, Berthon-Jones M, Eves L. Reversal of obstructive sleep apnoea by continuous positive airway pressure applied through the nares. Lancet. 1981;1(8225): 862-5.
7. Ellis ER, Bye PT, Bruderer JW, Sullivan CE. Treatment of respiratory failure during sleep in patients with neuromuscular disease. Positive-pressure ventilation through a nose mask. Am Rev Respir Dis. 1987;135:148-52.
8. Brochard L, Isabey D, Piquet J, Amaro P, Mancebo J, Messadi AA, et al. Reversal of acute exacerbations of chronic obstructive lung disease by inspiratory assistance with a facemask. N Engl J Med. 1990;323:1523-30.
9. Curtis JR, Cook DJ, Sinuff T, White DB, Hill N, Keenan SP, et al. Noninvasive positive pressure ventilation in critical and palliative care settings: understanding the goals of therapy. Crit Care Med. 2007;35:932-9.
10. Barreiro TJ, Gemmel DJ. Noninvasive ventilation. Crit Care Clin. 2007;23:201-22.
11. Sinuff T, Keenan SP. Department of Medicine, McMaster University. Clinical practice guideline for the use of non-invasive positive pressure ventilation in COPD patients with acute respiratory failure. Crit Care Med. 2004;19:82-91.
12. Confalonieri M, Potena A, Carbone G, Porta RD, Tolley EA, Umberto Meduri G. Acute respiratory failure in patients with severe community acquired pneumonia: a prospective randomized evaluation of noninvasive ventilation. Am J Res Crit Care Med. 1999;160:1585-91.
13. Mani RK. Noninvasive ventilation for hypercapnic respiratory failure in COPD: encephalopathy and initial post-support deterioration of pH and $PaCO_2$ may not predict failure. Indian J Crit Care Med. 2005;9:217-24.
14. Nava S, Gregoretti C, Fanfulla F, Squadrone E, Grassi M, Carlucci A, et al. Noninvasive ventilation to prevent respiratory failure after extubation in high-risk patients. Crit Care Med. 2005;33(11):2465-70.
15. Nava S, Ambrosino N, Clini E, Prato M, Orlando G, Vitacca M, et al. Noninvasive mechanical ventilation in the weaning of patients with respiratory failure due to chronic obstructive pulmonary disease. A randomized, controlled trial. Ann Intern Med. 1998;128(9):721-8.
16. Mehta S, Jay GD, Woolard RH, Hipona RA, Connolly EM, Cimini DM, et al. Randomized, prospective trial of bilevel versus continuous positive airway pressure in acute pulmonary edema. Crit Care Med. 1997;25(4):620-8.
17. Hilbert G, Gruson D, Vargas F, Valentino R, Gbikpi-Benissan G, Dupon M, et al. Noninvasive ventilation in immunosuppressed patients with pulmonary infiltrates, fever, and acute respiratory failure. N Engl J Med. 2001;344(7):481-7.
18. Caples SM, Gay PC. Noninvasive positive pressure ventilation in the intensive care unit: a concise review. Crit Care Med. 2005;33(11):2651-8.
19. Shneerson JM, Simonds AK. Noninvasive ventilation for chest wall and neuromuscular disorders. Eur Respir J. 2002;20(2):480-7.
20. Burns KE, Adhikari NK, Keenan SP, Meade M. Use of non-invasive ventilation to wean critically ill adults off invasive ventilation: meta-analysis and systematic review. BMJ. 2009;338:b1574.
21. Esteban A, Frutos-Vivar F, Ferguson ND, Arabi Y, Apezteguía C, González M, et al. Noninvasive positive-pressure ventilation for respiratory failure after extubation. N Engl J Med. 2004;350(24):2452-60.
22. Antonelli M, Conti G, Bufi M, Costa MG, Lappa A, Rocco M, et al. Noninvasive ventilation for treatment of acute respiratory failure in patients undergoing solid organ transplantation: a randomized trial. JAMA. 2000;283(2):235-41.
23. Ferreira JC, Chipman DW, Hill NS, Kacmarek RM. Bilevel vs ICU ventilators providing non-invasive ventilation: effect of system leaks, a COPD lung model comparison. Chest. 2009;136(2):448-56.

15

Aerosol Drug Delivery

Sanjay Singhal, Mohan Gurjar

INTRODUCTION

Aerosol therapy refers to the delivery of a drug to the lower airways in an aerosolized form for either local or systemic effect. Inhaled aerosol therapies are the mainstay of treatment of several respiratory diseases including obstructive lung disease. Because inhaled drug is directly delivered to the site of action, there is rapid onset of action. Moreover, a small dose of aerosolized drug is needed to produce an effect comparable to the effect obtained with large dose of same drug given systemically and hence limiting systemic toxicity.

Depending upon drug, aerosol can be categorized into bland (sterile water or hypotonic, normotonic and hypertonic saline delivered with or without oxygen) and pharmacologically active aerosols (delivers drugs). Aerosol delivery to lung depends on the characteristics of these drugs.

INDICATIONS FOR USES OF AEROSOL THERAPY

- Relief of bronchospasm with use of β-adrenergic or anticholinergic agents
- Relief of airway inflammation with use of inhaled corticosteroids
- Mobilization and hydration of bronchial secretions
- Aerosolized antimicrobial therapy (ventilator-associated pneumonia and cystic fibrosis)
- Pulmonary artery hypertension (prostacyclin, iloprost)

CONTRAINDICATION

- Hypersensitivity or allergy to drug
- Cardiac arrhythmias to propellants

PRINCIPLES OF AEROSOL THERAPY

The practice of delivering aerosolized medications has been used for thousands of years. Since long time, the smoke from burning compounds is used for enjoyment. Asthma cigarette containing *Datura stramonium*, an anticholinergic were available until 1970.[1] The modern era of aerosol therapy began in 1778. Metered dose inhaler (MDI) is invented by Charlie Thiel and colleagues, just 50 years back.[1] However, better understanding of factors that influences aerosol delivery to mechanically ventilated patients occurred over past 15 years.

Types of Devices

Presently, three major types of aerosol generation devices are available: MDI, dry powder inhaler (DPI), nebulizers.[1-5]

1. *Metered dose inhalers:* MDI contain a mixture of medication and propellant in a pressurize canister, depression of which actuates the aerosol into the mouthpiece. However, breathe actuated MDIs are also available, in which inhalation through the mouthpiece triggers aerosol release (Figs 1A to D).
2. *Dry powder inhalers:* In DPI, aerosol is created by the patient's inspiratory flow from the powdered medication within the device. DPI is available in two forms: multiple dose (aerosolized one at a time) or single dose (medication capsule need to be loaded every time) (Figs 1A to D).
3. *Nebulizers:* It creates an aerosol by agitating a medication solution held in a small reservoir (Fig. 2). The patient has to load the medication every time for use. Three types of nebulizers are available: traditional jet nebulizers use a stream of compressed air or oxygen, ultrasonic nebulizers use high frequency ultrasonic waves to generate aerosols and newer-generation vibrating-mesh nebulizers which uses a vibrating mesh or plate with multiple apertures to produce an aerosol.

Factors Affecting Delivery of Aerosols

An understanding of factors affecting delivery of aerosols is essential before using these devices. These factors can be categorized into aerosol factors and host factors.

Aerosol Factors

Aerosol is defined as a group of particles that remains suspended in air because of a low terminal settling velocity. The terminal velocity is a result of particle size and density. Size of the aerosol droplets is generally characterized by mass median aerodynamic diameter (MMAD). MMAD for spherical particle is the product of the diameter and square root of particle density. But aerosol particles are rarely spherical and have heterogeneous size distribution. The distribution of particle size is known as geometric standard deviation (GSD), which depends on

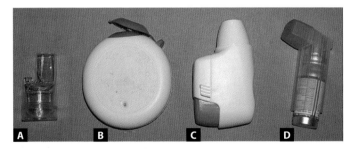

Figs 1A to D Examples of commercial available devices. (A) Single dose dry powder inhaler device (Rotahaler, Cipla Ltd.); (B) Multidose dry powder inhaler (Multihaler, Cipla Ltd); (C) Multidose dry powder inhaler (Novolizer, German Remedies); (D) Metered dose inhaler (MDI, Lupin Ltd.)

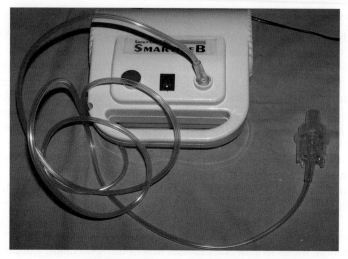

Fig. 2 A jet nebulizer and compressor

the uniformity of particle size. Aerosol with GSD less than 1.22 is considered as monodisperse aerosol. But most aerosols used in clinical practice are polydisperse (high GSD), thus, portion of aerosol particles of specific size range will be less.[1-5]

Aerosol particles (MMAD > 5 μm) can be filtered out in the upper airways and fails to reach even the larger airways, while extremely small particles (MMAD < 0.5 μm) may not settle in the airway after inhalation and thus are exhaled. Therefore, particles with MMAD of 0.5–5 μm are considered to be respirable and respirable mass is the volume of particles of respirable size range available for patient's inhalation.

Respirable mass is the primary factor for differences between different aerosol devices. Nebulizers, MDI and DPIs may have similar MMAD, but aerosol generated from nebulizer is having high GSD, hence, a small proportion of these particles are of respirable size and thus the respirable mass is smaller. Moreover, particles more than 5 μm MMAD can deposit on the oral pharynx leading to drug loss and systemic side effects (tachycardia, oral candidiasis or hoarseness).

Host Factors

Aerosol therapy should be given preferably in sitting position. Patients who are not able to erect during aerosol administration, a semi-recumbent position with head of bed elevated to 20–30° above horizontal is sufficient.

- *In ambulatory patients:* Host factors are related to the ventilatory and airway status of the patient.[5,6] Among ventilatory factors: inspired volume, inspired time, breath-hold duration and timing of aerosol delivery during inspiration are important. With increasing inhalation volume, particles are more likely to be carried into the peripheral airways. Hence, instructions are given to the patients to take a deep breath while actuation of aerosol delivery device. They are also instructed to exhale maximally to functional residual capacity (FRC) before initiating inspiration. However, forced exhalation to residual volume prior to inhalation is not recommended since this may lead to temporary collapse of some airways reducing drug delivery. Breath-holding increases the penetration as well as deposition of drugs into the lung. Finally, it is important to coordinate inspiration with the delivery of aerosol especially while using MDI. This is not a major problem while using the nebulizer or DPI. Airway status do not affect the total drug dose delivered to the airways but may play a major role in deciding the fraction of dose reaching the desired site. For example in smokers and patients with obstructive lung disease, aerosol particles may get deposited in the proximal airway depending upon the airway resistance.

- *Mechanically ventilated patients:* In intubated and mechanically ventilated patients, the presence of an artificial airway significantly reduces the efficiency of aerosol therapy.[7-9] The low efficiency of aerosol therapy means that high drug doses are required for ventilated patients than for ambulatory patients. Recently, with the advent of optimal aerosol delivery techniques, efficiency of aerosol delivery in mechanically ventilated patients has improved to the level of ambulatory patients. Optimal aerosol therapy in mechanically ventilated patients requires consideration of several factors.

  - Ventilator-related
    - Tidal volume more than or equal to 500 mL (in adult) ensures that dead space is cleared of aerosol, hence improving aerosol delivery to lower respiratory tract.
    - *Duty cycle and inspiratory flow:* Aerosol delivery increases with longer duty cycle (ratio of inspiratory time to total breathing cycle time). With same duty cycle, MDI drug delivery was significantly better with slow inspiratory flow (40 L/min) than faster inspiratory flow (80 L/min).
    - *Mode of ventilation and spontaneous breath:* With nebulizer, aerosol delivery is better during volume controlled mode whereas with MDI, aerosol delivery is better during pressured-controlled mode. MDI synchronized with spontaneous breath deliver drug more effectively as compared to controlled breath of similar tidal volume.

  - Circuit-related
    - *Humidity:* Heating and humidification of inspired gas in the ventilatory circuit prevents drying of airway mucosa, but it reduces aerosol delivery to lower respiratory tract by 40% from both MDIs and nebulizer. Although humidification reduces aerosol delivery, still bypassing or switching off the active humidifier is not recommended routinely, but its impact can be overcome by increasing the dose. Heat and moisture exchangers (HMEs) are passive humidification systems that capture the heat and moisture from breath and transfer part of it to next inspired breath. This filter is barrier to aerosol therapy and should be removed during aerosol therapy. With CircuVent HME/HCH Bypass, the HME removal can be avoided. A piece of tubing bypasses the HME by turning a dial on the device during aerosol delivery (Fig. 3). After aerosol delivery is completed, the dial is turned back to allow inspiratory airflow to pass through the HME.
    - *Gas density:* Inhalation of less dense gas such as helium-oxygen (Heliox) improves aerosol delivery by making airflow less turbulent and more laminar. To maximize efficiency of nebulizer aerosol in a patient on mechanical ventilation is to operate the nebulizer with

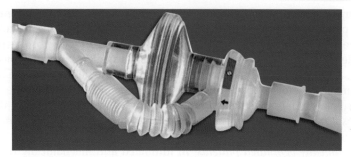

Fig. 3 Commercially available spacer and adapter (ACE® MDI holding chamber, Smiths Medical) that are used to connect a metered dose inhaler canister to a ventilatory circuit and CircuVent® (*Courtesy*: Smith Medical, India)

oxygen at 6–8 L/min and entrain the aerosol into a ventilator circuit containing Heliox further improves aerosol delivery.

- *Artificial airway:* Aerosol impaction in the endotracheal tube (ETT) reduces lower airway delivery in ETT of inner diameter 3–6 mm;[10] however, the efficacy of nebulizer aerosol delivery remains same when compared with ETT of inner diameter 7 mm versus inner diameter 9 mm.[11]
- *Device-related*
  In ambulatory patients, all types of aerosol generating devices can be used whereas in patients on mechanical ventilation, only MDI and nebulizers can be used.
  - *MDI:* Commercially available MDIs are designed for ambulatory patients. To use an MDI in ventilated patients, the canister must be removed from the actuator and connected to ventilator circuit with a different adaptor.
    - Adaptors are used to connect MDIs with the ventilator circuits, e.g., elbow adapters (connected directly to ETT), inline and chamber adapters (both are used to connect to the inspiratory limb of the ventilatory circuit). A chamber spacer with an MDI is having high aerosol delivery as compared to elbow or inline adapter.
    - An MDI with chamber spacer connected to ventilatory circuit at approximately 15 cm from the ETT provides efficient aerosol delivery to ventilated patients.
    - The actuation of MDI must be synchronized with the onset of inspiration (go with the flow).
  - Nebulizer
    - *Type:* Jet nebulizer is preferred in ventilated patients because of several problems associated with the ultrasonic nebulizer. Larger size of aerosol particle, bulky, relative inefficiency in nebulizing drug suspension, expensive and while operating for few minutes, drug solution becomes more concentrated and heated by 10–15°C resulting denaturation of some drugs are the major drawback of ultrasonic nebulizers. Recently, new generation vibrating mesh nebulizers having many advantages over jet nebulizers became available and is likely to find increasing use in future.

- Placing the jet nebulizer at a distance from the ETT (inspiratory limb of the ventilator circuit) offer better efficiency.
- Intermittent operation of nebulizer that is synchronized with inspiration is more effective than continuous nebulizer, because it minimizes the drug wastage during exhalation.

PREPARATION

Selecting Aerosol Device

- *Ambulatory patients:* It is well established that MDI and DPI are the most convenient and cost-effective delivery system and should be the first choice.[5,6] In patients with improper technique and when pharyngeal deposition is a concern such as with inhaled steroids, a valved spacer should be used with MDI. A nebulizer may also be indicated if the drug is available only in solution form or MDI or DPI is not effective. It is well established that nebulizers, DPIs and MDIs are equally effective, if used appropriately by the patients.[4] Moreover, in acute exacerbations of obstructive lung disease, β-agonists given via an MDI with spacer is as effective as nebulizer.[4] But some patient might prefer a nebulizer over an MDI or DPI because of better response, but mostly it is because of higher dose. In such case, increasing the dose of MDI or DPI might be useful.
- *Mechanically ventilated patients:* In patients on mechanical ventilation,[7,8] both MDI and nebulizers can be used as compared to ambulatory patients where all mode of aerosol delivery (MDI, DPI or nebulizers) can be used. But, nebulizers are most preferred mode of aerosol delivery in hospitalized patients which lead to an interpretation that nebulizers are more effective in comparison to MDI. Studies have shown that both MDI and nebulizers are equally effective in the treatment of ventilated patients of obstructive lung disease. However, nebulizers need to be employed for delivery of antibiotics, surfactant, prostaglandins and other formulations that are not available in MDIs.

PROCEDURES FOR DELIVERING AEROSOL THERAPY

- *Ambulatory Patients*
  - *Steps for use of MDI (Figs 4A to E)*
    - Shake the canister
    - Hold the canister upright
    - Gently exhale to FRC
    - Place the mouthpiece in mouth between teeth and close lips
    - With initiation of inhalation, press the canister to actuate
    - Slowly inhale up to the maximum capacity
    - Hold breath for 10 seconds or as long as possible
    - Wait for at least 1 minute before next actuation
    - Rinse the mouth after taking puff

    The commonest error in the usage of an MDI is the lack of coordination between actuation and inspiration. To overcome this problem, a valved spacer may be used. It should be explained to the patient that aerosol must be inhaled immediately after the MDI is actuated into the spacer and single puff should be actuated into the spacer for each inhalation (Figs 5A to C).

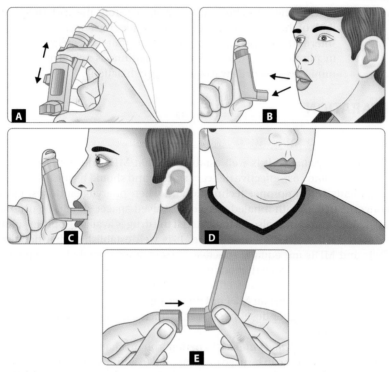

Figs 4A to E Demonstration of correct technique for use of metered-dose inhaler (MDI) (*Courtesy*: Cipla Ltd., Mumbai, India). (A) Remove mouthpiece and shake well before use; (B) Breathe out fully through the mouth; (C) Place the mouthpiece of the inhaler in the mouth. Start breathing in slowly through the mouth and press down the canister firmly and fully to release one spray while continuing to breathe in slowly and deeply; (D) Remove the inhaler from the mouth and hold the breath for 10 seconds; (E) Replace the mouthpiece cap firmly

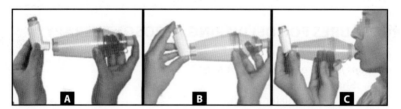

Figs 5A to C Demonstration of correct technique for use of metered-dose inhaler (MDI) with spacer (*Courtesy*: Cipla Ltd., Mumbai, India). (A) Insert the inhaler firmly into the opposite end of the spacer; (B) Holding the inhaler, press down on the canister to release a dose into the spacer; (C) Remove the mouthpiece cap from the spacer and inhale accordingly

- *Steps for use of DPI (Figs 6A to E)*
    - Check the device is clean and free from obstruction
    - Load a dose into the device
    - Hold the inhaler with mouthpiece facing down
    - Gently exhale to FRC without straining or breathing into the device
    - Place the mouthpiece in mouth between teeth and close lips
    - Breath in quickly and deeply through the mouthpiece

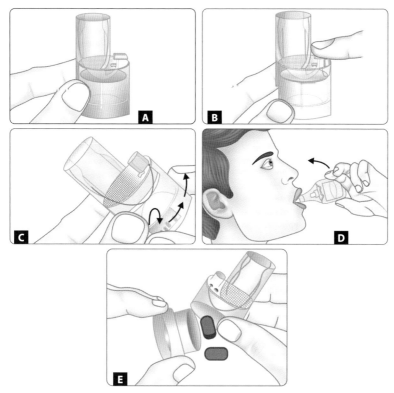

Figs 6A to E Demonstration of correct technique for use of Rotahaler® (*Courtesy*: Cipla Ltd., Mumbai, India). (A) Position the two halves of Rotahaler®; (B) Insert the capsule into the hole with the transparent end facing down. Press the capsule firmly so that the top end is level with the top of the hole; (C) Holding the mouthpiece firmly with one hand, rotate the base. This will separate the two halves of the capsule and now it is ready for use; (D) Place the mouthpiece between the teeth and close the lips tightly around it. Sit or stand upright, tilt the head as shown and breathe in through the mouth rapidly and deeply; (E) After use, separate the two halves of the Rotahaler® and discard the empty capsule. Rejoin the two halves of the Rotahaler®

- Remove the device and hold breath for 10 seconds and breathe out slowly against pursed lips.
- Rinse the mouth after taking puff
– *Steps for use of nebulizer*
  - Hand should be washed prior to preparing each nebulizer solution
  - If using multi-dose vial of medicine, put the correct amount of medicine into the nebulizer chamber along with saline solution.
  - The mouthpiece should be connected to the adaptor of nebulizer chamber
  - Connect the nebulizer tubing to the compressor port
  - Hold the nebulizer in an upright position to prevent spilling
  - Turn the compressor on and check for misting
  - As the mist starts, patient should inhale slowly and deeply through the mouth
  - Continue till the medicine is finished in the chamber (may last for 10 minutes).

- *Intubated Patients*
  - *Optimal Technique for Delivering MDI*
    - Suction endotracheal or tracheostomy tube and airway secretions
    - Shake the canister
    - Place MDI in spacer chamber adapter in inspiratory limb of the ventilatory circuit (Fig. 3)
    - *Use of humidifier during aerosol therapy:* If HME, then remove it; if active humidifier, then no need to remove it
    - Coordinate MDI actuation with the beginning of inspiration
    - Wait for at least 15 seconds between actuations and administer total dose
    - Reconnect HME
  - *Optimal Technique for Delivering Jet Nebulizer Aerosol*
    - Suction ETT and airway secretions
    - Place drug in nebulizer to fill volume of 4–6 mL
    - Place nebulizer in the inspiratory limb of ventilatory circuit 15 cm from the ventilator (if nebulizer is of jet type) and 15 cm from the Y-piece adapter if nebulizer is vibrating-mesh or ultrasonic.[12]
    - Remove HME and do not disconnect humidifier
    - Set gas flow to nebulizer at 6–8 L/min
    - Use a ventilator if it meets the nebulizer flow requirements and cycles on inspiration
    - Use continuous flow from an external source
    - Adjust ventilator volume limit or pressure limit to compensate for flow added by nebulizer.
    - Tap nebulizer periodically until nebulizer begins to sputter.
    - Remove nebulizer from the circuit, rinse with sterile water and run dry; store in dry place.
    - Reconnect humidifier or HME, return ventilator settings and alarm to previous values.

Patients on Non-invasive Ventilation

Patient with acute or acute on chronic respiratory failures who are receiving noninvasive ventilation (NIV) often requires inhaled bronchodilator for relief of airway obstruction. But to deliver aerosol therapy, NIV has to be removed intermittently. Aerosol with MDI takes less time for off NIV duration but inadequate delivery expected due to poor inspiratory effort, while nebulizers take long time for off NIV. However, both MDIs and nebulizers can be used during NIV, but further studies are needed to optimize drug delivery from these devices.

POST-PROCEDURE CARE

- Always documents the dose and clinical effects of aerosol therapy in hospitalized patients.
- *Handling of the device:* Clean the device or spacer regularly (at least once a week). For cleaning dismantle the device or spacer, rinse with clean water, then shake to remove excess water and leave it to air dry. Ensure that spacer or device should be dry all the time. While cleaning, do not use chemical or hot water.

COMPLICATION AND PREVENTIVE MEASURES

Drugs delivered as aerosols have been found to be extremely safe except certain complication which may require attention. For example, high doses of β-agonists may lead to arrhythmias; inhaled steroid may have local complications (oral or esophageal candidiasis, dysphonia and cough) and systemic complications (glaucoma, cataract, loss of bone density, fracture, hypothalamic-pituitary-adrenal axis suppression). Local complications can be avoided by rinse after inhalation, reduction in frequency of inhaled corticosteroids and use of spacer device. Cross-infection with use of nebulizers in hospitalized patients are also known to occur.

REFERENCES

1. Rubin BK. Air and soul: the science and application of aerosol therapy. Respir Care. 2010;55(7):911-21.
2. Global strategy for diagnosis, management and prevention of COPD. Global Initiative for Chronic Obstructive Lung Disease. Web site. http:/www.goldcopd.org. Updated 2013.
3. Global strategy for asthma management and prevention. Global Initiative for asthma web site. http://www.ginaasthma.org. Updated 2012.
4. Dolovich MB, Ahrens RC, Hess DR, Anderson P, Dhand R, Rau JL, et al. Device selection and outcomes of aerosol therapy: Evidence-based guidelines: American college of Chest Physicians/American College of Asthma, Allergy and Immunology. Chest. 2005; 127(1):335-71.
5. Khilnani GC, Banga A. Aerosol therapy. Indian J Chest Dis Allied Sci. 2008;50:209-19.
6. Sims MW. Aerosol therapy for obstructive lung diseases: device selection and practice management issues. Chest. 2011;140(3):781-8.
7. Dhand R. Basic techniques for aerosol delivery during mechanical ventilation. Respir Care. 2004;49(6):611-22.
8. Dhand R, Guntur VP. How best to deliver aerosol medications to mechanically ventilated patients. Clin Chest Med. 2008;29(2):277-96.
9. Ehrmann S, Roche-Campo F, Sferrazza Papa GF, Isabey D, Brochard L, Apiou-Sbirlea G, et al. Aerosol therapy during mechanical ventilation: an international survey. Intensive Care Med. 2013;39(6):1048-56.
10. Bishop MJ, Larson RP, Buschman DL. Metered dose inhaler aerosol characteristics are affected by endotracheal tube actuator/adapter used. Anesthesiology. 1990;73(6):1263-5.
11. Rau JL, Dunlevy CL, Hill RL. A comparison of inline MDI actuators for delivery of a beta agonist and a corticosteroid with a mechanically ventilated lung model. Respir Care. 1998;43:705-12.
12. Ari A, Areabi H, Fink JB. Evaluation of aerosol generator devices at 3 locations in humidified and non-humidified circuits during adult mechanical ventilation. Respir Care. 2010;55(7):837-44.

16
Prone Positioning

Puneet Khanna, Girija Prasad Rath

INTRODUCTION

Prone ventilation may be defined as the application of mechanical ventilation with the patient lying in prone position. It is effective in improving oxygenation by promoting alveolar recruitment, and has been used in patients ventilated mechanically for severe hypoxic respiratory failure. It also reduces ventilation-induced lung injury by homogeneous distribution of stress and strain in the lungs. The effect of prone positioning may be variable; some patients may not have any effect while the others might present with long-lasting effects persisting well after reverting to supine position.

INDICATION

- Severe acute respiratory distress syndrome (ARDS) with refractory and life-threatening hypoxemia
- Patients with wounds in posterior of body, burns and skin flaps.

CONTRAINDICATION

Absolute

- Increased intracranial pressure (ICP)
- Increased intra-abdominal pressure
- Chest and abdominal wounds
- Cervical spine fracture or instability
- Intestinal ischemia
- Peritoneal dialysis.

Relative

- Extreme obesity
- Hemodynamic instability
- Known case of difficult airway
- *Others:* Untrained staff, breast implants, penile prosthesis.

APPLIED ANATOMY AND PATHOPHYSIOLOGY

The improved oxygenation accompanying prone positioning appears primarily related to regional differences in functional residual capacity (FRC) in the face of a relatively unchanged distribution of dorsal-ventral perfusion.[1] The largest proportion of pulmonary blood flow is directed to the dorsal regions of lungs during both supine and prone positions. The possible reason is dependency of regional lung perfusion primarily on gravity leading to improved perfusion in the nonconsolidated lung with proning. However, this explanation has not been substantiated by research.[2] Whatever may be the patient position, perfusion to dorsal lung region predominates. With gravity accounting for less than half of the perfusion, heterogeneity seen in either position. The changes in regional pleural pressure are also of importance. The gradient of pleural pressure from negative ventrally to positive dorsally during the supine position is not completely reversed with placed prone. Hence, the distribution of positive pressure ventilation is not homogeneous in prone position. Thus, the recruitment of dorsal lung seems to be the predominant mechanism of improved oxygenation.

The dorsal lung recruitment with more homogeneous distribution of ventilation and perfusion seems to be one of the possible causes of increased oxygenation in the prone position. With patient in prone position, the densities in dorsal part of the lung decrease causing more homogeneous distribution of alveolar inflation and ventilation, whilst perfusion probably remains greatest in the dorsal regions. The ventilation/perfusion (V/Q) ratio, thus, improves with subsequent increase in oxygenation. The improvement in oxygenation possibly results from a redistribution of blood flow from poorly ventilated areas of the lung to the regions with better V/Q ratios. This process probably results from the alveolar recruitment in previously atelectatic, but well-perfused alveoli, hence, improving V/Q ratio.[3-7]

Physiological Effects of Prone Position

Prone position results in optimization of V/Q match (increased blood flow to the dependent lung) with an increase in FRC and less atelectasis. It facilitates drainage of secretion and less deformation of lung which helps in increased ventilation. Abdominal distension is reduced in prone position which causes increase in FRC. The heart sits against sternum (rather than left lung) and thus, the lung is less compressed. The transpleural pressure gradient between dependent and non-dependent lung is decreased during the prone position. The plateau pressure is more uniformly distributed in prone position which results in a uniform alveolar ventilation. The recruitment maneuvers are also more effective in prone position.

Baby Lung in ARDS

The "baby lung" concept is originated as an offspring of computed tomographic (CT) examinations. In most patients with acute lung injury (ALI) or ARDS, the normally aerated tissue acquires the lung-dimension of a 5–6 years old child with an approximately 300–500 mg of aerated tissue. The respiratory compliance is linearly related to the "baby lung" dimension suggesting that the ARDS lung is not stiff but small, with a near normal elasticity. Initially, it was thought that the "baby lung" is a distinct anatomical structure, in the nondependent region of lung.[8] However, the density redistribution in prone position showed that it is a functional concept and not anatomical, as believed.

CLINICAL ASPECT AND TECHNIQUE

Piehl and Brown (1976) first described improved oxygenation in patients with acute hypoxemic respiratory failure who were mechanically ventilated in prone position.[9] This was further confirmed in different studies which showed an improved overall oxygenation in majority of patients when such positioning was utilized.[10]

Gas Exchange and Mortality

Gattinoni et al. compared conventional treatment (in supine position) in patients with ALI or ARDS with a predefined strategy of placing the patients prone.[11] A significant improvement of pulmonary function in the form of improvement in $PaO_2 : FiO_2$ (partial pressure of oxygen: fraction of inspired oxygen) ratio was observed during the first 4 days in patients ventilated in prone position. The prevalence of ARDS and the number of days of ALI was reduced; the incidence of pneumonia was also reduced. These findings concerned the secondary end points. No differences was evident between the two groups with regard to various parameters of gas exchange even after 10 days. The lack of an associated reduction of ventilation time and mortality may be reflected by the small sample size in this study, and it is possible that with a larger sample size a significant reductions might be observed. Nevertheless, few recent studies on prone positioning claimed to reduce the mortality with ARDS by more than half.

Prone positioning in severe ARDS (PROSEVA) examined the role of prone positioning in patients with early, severe ARDS. 466 patients (mean $PaO_2: FiO_2$ 100 mm Hg) were randomized to undergo ventilation in supine or prone position.[12] Most of the patients (60%) had ARDS owing to pneumonia, and received vasopressors (73–83%), neuromuscular blockers (82–91%) and glucocorticoids (40–45%). Prone position significantly reduced 28-day mortality as compared to the patients in supine position (16% vs 32.8%, p <0.001). Prone position also reduced the incidence of 90-day mortality (23.6% vs 41%, p <0.001). This positioning can be done without purchasing a new bed or special equipment, and still can achieve reduced mortality by more than 50%, which is unheard in the ARDS literature. The results seem to be too good to be true, but it is difficult to ignore.

Reduction of Pneumonia

Immobility is an important risk factor for the development of atelectasis and nosocomial infections in critically ill patients. A reduction in the prevalence of nosocomial pneumonia has been observed in patients ventilated prone. It may be attributed to the enhanced mobilization of secretions with altered position of the patient and maintenance of airway patency. Guerin et al. observed the incidence of ventilator-associated pneumonia (VAP) to be significantly lower in patients treated with prone position.[9] However, other studies on intermittent prone positioning have not reported a reduced incidence of pneumonia. Several studies on continuous postural oscillation observed a decreased prevalence of pneumonia but comparable incidence mortality. These data suggest that although pneumonia and impaired gas exchange add to morbidity, they may not be the primary cause of mortality.

Kinetic therapy is defined as the use of a bed that turns slow but continuously more than 40° along its longitudinal axis. Its use significantly improves the $PaO_2 : FiO_2$ ratio in mechanically ventilated patients with ALI or ARDS. Nevertheless, none of the study, till date, demonstrated survival advantage with its use in patients with ALI or ARDS.[13,14]

Prone positioning has not been found to be advantageous over continuous lateral rotational therapy (roto-rest) in patients with ARDS.[15] Continuous rotation in the prone position, in multiple trauma patients, has been demonstrated to improve oxygenation and $PaO_2 : FiO_2$ ratio, and to reduce FiO_2 as compared to supine position. This study demonstrated a significant reduction in overall mortality with kinetic therapy in prone position.[14] Additionally, the duration of ventilatory support and length of hospital stay was decreased in patients who were nursed prone. The use of a prone oscillating bed was advantageous in trauma and surgical patients with ALI or ARDS and was superior to kinetic therapy in supine position.

Neurotrauma

Neurointensivists are usually hesitant to use prone position due to the risk of increased ICP during the procedure.[16] Supine position with 30° head-up tilt has been recommended to reduce ICP. In patients with severe respiratory insufficiency and hypoxemia, the scenario may be different. Theoretically, an improved gas exchange and arterial oxygenation result in reduction of ICP, owing to the beneficial effect of improved oxygen transport to the damaged brain. A study was undertaken to explore whether the advantages of the prone position outweigh the risk of intracranial hypertension in patients with reduced intracranial compliance.[17] An improvement of oxygenation, increase in ICP and mean arterial pressure (MAP) was observed during treatment of patients in prone position. As MAP increased to a greater extent than ICP, cerebral perfusion pressure (CPP) was observed to be improved. However, the patients with high ICP were not included in the study.

Methods

- *Manual:* Performed manually
- *Automated beds:* Rotoprone™ therapy system bed.

Timing of Proning

Early application of prone position in mechanically ventilated patients with severe ARDS has been found to be beneficial in reducing mortality.[12]

Duration of Proning

A 6 hours protocol is usually followed unless otherwise specified. After 6 hours, the patient is turned supine with lateral rotation. The patient should remain supine until the gain of improved arterial oxygen saturation (SaO_2), venous oxygen saturation (SvO_2) and arterial blood gases (ABGs) declines, but no longer than 6 hours. However, the PROSEVA trial suggests that the sessions of prone position should be at least 16 hours/day.[12]

Evidence suggests that doing prone ventilation for more than 12 hours results in a progressive improvement in gas exchange. The duration of prone ventilation used in most of the studies were based on scheduled patient care or the practicality of research implementation rather than a defined treatment rationale. McAuley et al. evaluated the effects of prone ventilation on respiratory parameters and extravascular lung water.[18] There was progressive improvement in gas exchange from 1–18 hours without an apparent plateau. In this study, all patients responded to ventilation in the prone position. Three patients initially found as nonresponders at 1 hour were later becomes as responders at the end of 12 hours.

Response to Proning

The primary goal of positioning a patient prone is to improve gas exchange by making ventilation more uniform and improving ventilation in previously dependent lung areas. Patients with 30% or more increase in oxygenation after prone position with a low end-expiratory lung volume (EELV) as compared to supine position are considered as responders.[19] Responder may also be defined as patients with a $PaO_2 : FiO_2$ ratio greater than 20 mm Hg or a decrease in partial pressure of carbon dioxide ($PaCO_2$) less than 2 mm Hg after 15 hours of prone position.[20]

Indications of a positive response to prone position broadly include:
- An increase in saturation of arterial oxygenation (SpO_2)
- Return of mixed SvO_2 to baseline within 5 minutes of the turn, and eventual increase in SvO_2
- Heart rate and blood pressure return to baseline
- Respiratory rate less than 30/minutes or return to baseline
- *Arterial blood gas:* Increase in PaO_2 and SaO_2 within minutes of the position change; no change in $PaCO_2$.

PREPARATION

- Standard institutional protocol for prone-positioning patients should be developed
- The procedure is to be explained to the patient and relatives
- Ensure the endotracheal tube (ETT) and tracheostomy tube are securely fastened
- Ensure patient's eyes are well lubricated and eyelids are held closed with adequate eyepads
- Attend to mouth care
- Dress the anterior wounds prior to turning, if any
- Ensure all lines and chest drains are slack enough to allow for the 180° turn

- Remove electrocardiograph (ECG) leads
- Anticipate problems with the airway, vascular access and other invasive devices
- Ensure adequate number of personnel during the turning process
- Reassess need of adequate sedation with or without paralyzing agents.

PROCEDURE

- Five persons are needed for turning the patient; one person, most experienced, should hold the head and airway. Two persons should be positioned on each side of the bed.
- Move intercostal drainage (ICD) tubes, bags, intravenous lines and catheters to the opposite side of the bed.
- Proning is done in three steps: (1) Place the arm that will go under the body during the turning process close to the body when the patient in supine position (Fig. 1A). The two staff members, who will be pulling the patient towards them, horizontally, to one side of the bed (Fig. 1B), place their hands in the same position as doing a log roll. (2) Then the patient is rotated laterally in side-lying position (Fig. 1C). The person holding the head gives the go ahead to turn the patient 90°. The other two staff members on the opposite side of the bed are responsible for ensuring safety of lines, tubes and legs during the turn. (3) The two persons who were previously guarding lines and tubes then position their arms under the patient ensuring that the patients arm closest to the bed is grasped. The other two staff members will assist in the lowering of the patient once the final positioning is done (Fig. 1D). A pillow is placed under the patients shoulders to give a small elevation to the upper part of body. Once again on the head holder/pillow command the patient is positioned prone.
- Once the patient is positioned prone, a pillow is placed over the patients face to protect the eyes and airways. The face may be turned to one side (Fig. 1D).
- The arms are positioned appropriately to allow for maintenance of normal anatomical alignment. A swimming position is recommended with changing of head and arm position every 2 hours. Abdomen should hang between two pillows/supports.
- Electrocardiograph monitoring then to be reconnected, posteriorly.
- Repositioning the patient is carried out in the similar manner as the above with a particular attention to all the points highlighted.

POST-PROCEDURAL CARE

- After the turn, all tubes and lines should be rechecked and secured; the ventilator parameters are reassessed as the changed compliance may lead to pressure changes in the airway.
- Pulmonary secretions may increase and require frequent suctioning.
- The whole bed should be tilted 15–30° to reduce conjunctival edema as the duration varies in different protocols (e.g. 6–16 hours a day for up to 10 days).
- Finally, the neck and extremities, particularly external fixators used for fracture stabilization, should be placed in appropriate physiologic positions to avoid compression neuropathy.

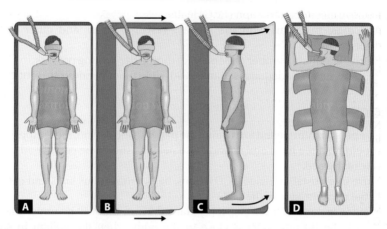

Figs 1A to D Various steps of proning. (A) Supine patient; (B) Patient shifted horizontally to the side of the bed; (C) Side-lying position; (D) Complete prone position

COMPLICATION/PROBLEM

Despite the encouraging results, the prone ventilation has not been widely accepted for the management of ARDS. It could possibly due to the complexity involved with this maneuver with potential life-threatening complications. However, reports to date suggest that it is a safe procedure in critically ill patients, though the details are lacking.[21]

- Critically ill patients with ARDS may frequently require insertion of multiple chest tubes, arterial and venous access catheters, and ETT or tracheostomy tubes. Obstruction or dislodgement of ETT, chest tube and abdominal drains may occur during this positioning.
- There is difficulty in carrying out cardiopulmonary resuscitation (CPR) in view of cardiac arrest.
- Development of peripheral nerve injuries or skin necrosis and damage to the eyes. An increased number of pressure sores, swelling and edema.
- Decreased enteral nutrition.
- Increased intrabdominal and ICPs.
- Difficulty in monitoring (e.g. placement of ECG leads).
- Labor intensive, difficult to perform various procedures and for reintubation, if required.
- Delays referral to other potentially lifesaving measures such as extracorporeal membrane oxygenation (ECMO).

REFERENCES

1. Glenny RW, Lamm WJ, Albert RK, Robertson HT. Gravity is a minor determinant of pulmonary blood flow distribution. J Appl Physiol (1985). 1991;71:620-9.
2. Glenny RW. Blood flow distribution in the lung. Chest. 1998;114(Suppl 1):8S-16S.
3. Douglas WW, Rehder K, Beynen FM, Sessler AD, Marsh HM. Improved oxygenation in patients with acute respiratory failure: the prone position. Am Rev Respir Dis. 1977; 115(4):559-66.

4. Pelosi P, Tubiolo D, Mascheroni D, Vicardi P, Crotti S, Valenza F, et al. Effects of the prone position on respiratory mechanics and gas exchange during acute lung injury. Am J Respir Crit Care Med. 1998;157(2):387-93.

5. Albert RK, Leasa D, Sanderson M, Robertson HT, Hlastala MP. The prone position improves arterial oxygenation and reduces shunt in oleic-acid-induced acute lung injury. Am Rev Respir Dis. 1987;135(3):628-33.

6. Pelosi P, Brazzi L, Gattinoni L. Prone position in acute respiratory distress syndrome. Eur Respir J. 2002;20(4):1017-28.

7. Nyrén S, Mure M, Jacobsson H, Larsson SA, Lindahl SG. Pulmonary perfusion is more uniform in the prone than in the supine position: scintigraphy in healthy humans. J Appl Physiol. 1999;86(4):1135-41.

8. Gattinoni L, Pesenti A. The concept of "baby lung". Intensive Care Med. 2005;31(6): 776-84.

9. Piehl MA, Brown RS. Use of extreme position changes in acute respiratory failure. Crit Care Med. 1976;4(1):13-4.

10. Guerin C. Ventilation in the prone position in patients with acute lung injury/acute respiratory distress syndrome. Curr Opin Crit Care. 2006;12(1):50-4.

11. Gattinoni L, Tognoni G, Pesenti A, Taccone P, Mascheroni D, Labarta V, et al. Effect of prone positioning on the survival of patients with acute respiratory failure. N Engl J Med. 2001;345(8):568-73.

12. Guérin C, Reignier J, Richard JC, Beuret P, Gacouin A, Boulain T, et al. Prone Positioning in Severe Acute Respiratory Distress Syndrome (PROSEVA). New Engl J Med. 2013;368(23):2159-68.

13. Stiletto R, Gotzen L, Goubeaud S. Kinetic therapy for therapy and prevention of post-traumatic lung failure. Results of a prospective study of 111 polytrauma patients. Unfallchirurg. 2000;103(12):1057-64.

14. Nelson LD, Choi SC. Kinetic therapy in critically ill trauma patients. Clin Intensive Care. 1992;3(6):248-52.

15. Staudinger T, Kofler J, Mullner M, Locker GJ, Laczika K, Knapp S, et al. Comparison of prone positioning and continuous rotation of patients with adult respiratory distress syndrome: results of a pilot study. Crit Care Med. 2001;29(1):51-6.

16. Mpe MJ, Mathekga K, Mzileni MO. The outcome of neuro-trauma: A 1-year retrospective study in an intensive care unit. Critical Care. 2001;5:P245-S116.

17. Sud S, Friedrich Jo, Taccone P, Polli F, Adhikari NK, Latini R, et al. Prone ventilation reduces mortality in patients with acute respiratory failure and severe hypoxemia: systematic review and meta-analysis. Intensive Care Med. 2010;36(4):585-99.

18. McAuley DF, Giles S, Fichter H, Perkins GD, Gao F. What is the optimal duration of ventilation in the prone position in acute lung injury and acute respiratory distress syndrome? Intensive Care Med. 2002;28(4):414-8.

19. Reutershan J, Schimitt A, Dietz K, Unertl K, Fretschner R. Alveolar recruitment during prone position: time matters. Clin Sci (London). 2006;110(6):655-63.

20. Charron C, Repesse S, Bouferrache K, Bodson L, Castro S, Page B, et al. $PaCO_2$ and alveolar dead space are more relevant than PaO_2/FiO_2 ratio in monitoring the respiratory response to prone position in ARDS patients: a physiological study. Crit Care. 2011;15(4):R175.

21. Taccone P, Pesenti A, Latini R, Polli F, Vagginelli F, Mietto C, et al. Prone positioning in patients with moderate and severe acute respiratory distress syndrome: a randomized controlled trial. JAMA. 2009;302:1977-84.

17

Manual Chest Physiotherapy in Ventilated Patients

Rajendra Kumar

INTRODUCTION

Chest physiotherapy (CPT) plays an important role in the treatment of mechanically ventilated patients. It requires thorough assessment of each patient. Commonly used CPT techniques in the intensive care by physiotherapist comprise of percussion, vibration, shaking, directed cough, postural drainage, suctioning, coughing and various breathing exercises. Appropriate CPT techniques one/two or with a combination to the patient depending on affected lobes/segments, nature of secretions, etc. CPT techniques facilitating the mobilization of secretions from the airways, which have impairment in mucociliary clearance or an ineffective cough mechanism. Routine CPT should avoid in intensive care unit (ICU), it should base on thorough assessment of the patient. The goals of CPT are to reduce airway obstruction, improve mucociliary clearance and ventilation, and optimize gas exchange. The airways of mechanically ventilated patients should be kept clear to ensure optimal ventilation of all areas of the lung.

INDICATION

- Retained secretions/mucus plugs in the airways which may interface with the exchange of oxygen [decrease in partial pressure of oxygen (PaO_2) or saturation of arterial oxygenation (SpO_2)].
- *Atelectasis:* The condition is caused by the collapse of an alveolar segment, often by retained secretions.
- Abnormal chest radiographs suggesting collapse of lung segment, mucus plugging or infiltrates.
- *Respiratory muscle weakness:* Because of this patients are unable to maintain adequate control of respiratory secretions and often have a weak and ineffective cough.

CONTRAINDICATION

Respiratory Conditions

- Frank hemoptysis
- Severe bronchospasm
- Undrained pneumothorax (tension pneumothorax)
- Severe hypoxemia
- Pulmonary edema.

Cardiac Conditions

- Cardiac arrhythmias
- Severe hypertension
- Hypotension
- Acute myocardial infarction.

Other Conditions

- Confirm or suspected elevated intracranial pressure (ICP), especially for postural drainage.
- *Vomiting and/or aspiration:* The head-down position or specific postural drainage positions are contraindicated in patients clearly at risk of aspiration.

APPLIED ANATOMY

Thorax

The bony thorax covers and protects the principal organs of respiration. The posterior surface is formed by the 12 thoracic vertebrae and the posterior part of the 12 ribs. The anterior surface is formed by the sternum and the costal cartilage. The lateral surfaces are formed by the ribs.

Sternum

The sternum or breastbone is divided into three parts: (1) Body, (2) Manubrium, and (3) Xiphoid process.

Ribs

Ribs are the bony thoracic cage is formed by 12 ribs located on either side of the sternum. The first 7 ribs connect posteriorly with the vertebral column and anteriorly through costal cartilages with the sternum. These are known as the true ribs. The remaining 5 ribs are known as the false ribs. The first three have their cartilage attached to the cartilage of the rib above. The last two are free or floating ribs. The ribs increase in length from the first to the seventh rib, and then decrease to the 12th rib. They also increase in obliquity until the 9th rib and then decrease in obliquity to the 12th rib. The ribs are separated from each other by the intercostal spaces that contain the intercostal muscles.

Muscles of Respiration

Inspiration is an active movement involving the contraction of the diaphragm and intercostals. In the disease, the role of the accessory muscles of inspiration may have an important role even at rest. The accessory muscles include the sternocleidomastoid (SCM), scalene, serratus anterior, pectoralis major and minor, trapezius and erector spinae. The degree to which these accessory muscles are used by the patient is dependent on the severity of cardiopulmonary disease.

Diaphragm

The diaphragm is the principal muscle of respiration. During quite breathing, the diaphragm contributes approximately two-thirds of the tidal volume in the sitting or standing positions, and approximately three-fourths of the tidal volume in the supine position. It is also estimated that two-thirds of the vital capacity in all position is contributed by the diaphragm. The position of the diaphragm and its range of movement vary with power, the degree of distention of the stomach, size of the intestine, size of the liver and obesity. The average movement of the diaphragm in quite respiration is 12.5 mm on the right and 12 mm on the left. This can increase to a maximum of 30 mm on the right and 28 mm on the left during increased ventilation. The posture of individual determines the position of the diaphragm. In the supine position, the resting level of the diaphragm rises. The greatest respiratory excursions during normal breathing occur in this position. In a sitting or upright position, the dome of the diaphragm is pulled down by the abdominal organs, allowing a larger lung volume.

Intercostals

There are 11 external intercostals muscles on each side of the sternum and these are help in inspiration. There are also 11 internal intercostals per side. These are considered primary expiratory in function.

Sternocleidomastoid

The sternocleidomastoids (SCMs) are strong neck muscles arising from two heads, one from manubrium and the other from the medial part of the clavicle. When the head is fixed, they assist in elevating the sternum increasing the anteroposterior (AP) diameter of the thorax. The SCMs are the most important accessory muscles of inspiration. Their contractions can be observed in all patients during forced inspiration and in all patients who are dyspneic.

Scalenes

The anterior, medial and posterior scalenes are three separate muscles that are considered a functional unit. When their superior attachment is fixed, the scalene act as an accessory respiratory muscles and elevates the first two ribs during inspiration.

Serratus Anterior

It is innervated by the long thoracic nerve (cervical nerves C5, C6 and C7). Normally, they assist in forward pushing of the arm (in boxing or punching). When the scapulae are fixed, they act as accessory respiratory muscles and elevate the ribs to which they are attached.

Pectoralis Major

It is a large muscle arising from the clavicle, the sternum and the cartilages of all the true ribs. In forced inspiration when the arms are fixed, it draws the ribs forward the arms, thereby increasing thoracic diameter.

Pectoralis Minor

During deep inspiration, they contract to elevate the ribs to which they are attached.

Trapezius

This large muscle is innervated by the external or spinal part of the accessory nerve and cervical nerves C3 and C4. Its ability to stabilize the scapulae makes it an important accessory muscle in respiration. This stabilization enables the serratus anterior and pectoralis minor to elevate the ribs.

Erector Spinae

In deep inspiration, these muscles extend the vertebral column, allowing further elevation.

Expiration

Expiration is a passive process, occurring when the intercostals and diaphragm relax. Their relaxation allows the ribs to drop to their preinspiratory position and the diaphragm to rise. These activities compress the lungs, raising intrathoracic pressure above atmospheric pressure and, thereby contributing to airflow out of the lungs. The most important muscles of expiration are the abdominal muscles. The external, internal oblique and transverses abdominis muscles compress the abdomen. The rectus abdominis muscles draw the anterior ribs to the symphysis pubis and compress the abdomen during expiration. Expiratory muscles are active at high rates of ventilation when movement of air out of the lungs is impeded, such as in respiratory failure.

TECHNIQUE

Percussion and vibration CPT techniques are commonly used for the patient with impaired coughing ability and on mechanical ventilation. Percussion and vibration are used to increase mucociliary clearance and mobilize the secretions from peripheral airways to central airways. These techniques are more effective when therapist using postural drainage position for specific lobes/segments to drain the secretions from central and peripheral airways; however, patient with mechanical ventilation postural drainage postures are compromised. To increase effectiveness of CPT, therapist applied percussion and vibration directly over bare skin, hence therapist can observe skin redness, position of chest tube or any other drains, electrocardiogram (ECG) electrodes and insertion site of central lines. Frequency and force of percussion and vibration are depending on the patient's body position and gender (male/female or child). Percussion can be done by one/two handed depending on the therapist experience and patient pain tolerance.

Percussion

Percussion can be used during inspiratory and expiratory phase of respiration. Position of the hand should be cupped and all fingers are adducted with flexion-extension at the wrist joint. The maximum frequency and force of chest percussion are not known. However, the rate of manual chest percussion is between 100 and 480 times/minute, and 58-65 N force on chest wall reported. Therapist should applied equal force on chest wall from each hand; and percussion over breast tissues should be avoided because of patient's discomfort and pain. The mechanism of chest percussion is the transmission of a wave of energy through the chest wall into the lung. The resulting motion loosens secretions from the bronchial wall and moves them proximally where ciliary motion and cough (or suction) can remove them.

Vibration

Vibration is a forceful and intermittent chest wall compression performed primarily during expiration. Vibration is the placement of both hands (placement of dominant hand first) along the ribs in the direction of expiration and vibrate chest wall in the expiratory phase of respiration. The frequency of manual chest vibration is between 12 and 50 Hz. Vibration is performed by co-contracting all the muscles of upper extremities to cause a vibration while applying pressure to the chest wall with the hands. In mechanically ventilated patient, the vibration techniques timed with ventilator-controlled expiration. Mechanical devices used to perform vibration differ from the manual method in that the mechanical device is continuously applied during both inspiration and expiration. Vibration technique used in both conditions whether patient is on mechanical ventilator or on spontaneous breathing. Vibration is not recommended to patients with rib's fractures these may cause perforation of pleura and cause pneumothorax, intrapleural bleeding or extrapleural hematoma.

Shaking

Shaking is the vigorous maneuver in which compressing the chest wall intermittently with high frequency during whole of expiratory phase of respiration. In shaking, mechanical energy transmitted through the chest wall to loosen secretions. Shaking is a bouncing maneuver against the thoracic wall in a rhythmic fashion throughout expiration. It is proposed to mobilizing the secretions from the small peripheral airways to larger central airways. Factors, such as pain and tolerance of the patient should be taken into account and the technique moderated accordingly.

Directed Cough

Directed cough is the technique to mobilize bronchial secretions from peripheral airways to central airways. Directed cough is used when a patient's coughing power is not effective and he is not able to bring the secretions out. Directed cough is maneuver that is taught, supervised and monitored. Directed cough is used in both patients who are mechanically ventilated or spontaneously breathing patients. For this method, first take deep inspiration, and then closure of glottis followed by increasing intrathoracic pressure by contracting the expiratory muscles against a closed glottis, which results in opening of glottis and forceful expulsion of gas with secretions.

Manual Hyperinflation

The technique of manual hyperinflation is used in patients with an artificial airway, who are mechanically ventilated or who have a tracheostomy or endotracheal tube (ETT). The method of airway clearance promotes mobilization of secretions and reinflates collapsed areas of lung. Three caregivers are necessary to provide this treatment. It may be necessary to premedicate the patient with a sedative or analgesic so that airway clearance may be better tolerated. The caregivers providing the treatment should be positioned on opposite sides of the bed to allow greater freedom of movement and improved observations of the patient's response to treatment. If secretions are tenacious or thick normal saline (1–3 mL) may be used before hyperinflation to assist in removal of thick secretions.

Postural Drainage

Postural drainage is accomplished by positioning the patient, hence the position of the lung segment to be drained permit gravity to have its greatest effect. Modified positions are used when a precaution or relative contraindication to the ideal position exists. For example, of an increase in ICP is a concern, the head of the bed should remain flat instead of being tipped into Trendelenburg (head-down) position. Different types of positions are used to drain the retained secretions from a specific lobe/segment. The supine lying with head-up or head-down position and side-lying positions are frequently using in ICU. In ICU, therapist mostly concentrated on bilateral lower lobes of the lung because of patient lie most of the time in head-up position. Patient should turn laterally on each side as frequently as 2 hourly to improve oxygenation and mobilization of secretions. Side-lying and prone-lying positions are more effective than supine and sitting position for better oxygenation of patient. Patient may have decrease oxygenation during treatment because of secretions mobilization to central airways and once secretions have been removed patient's oxygenation and tidal volume improved. Monitoring of vital signs tidal volume, heart rate (HR), respiratory rate (RR), blood pressure (BP) and oxygen saturation throughout the treatment is necessary to ensure safe and effective postural drainage. Collapse of lung lobe or segment may improve fast when patient positioned with affected lung uppermost. Increase oxygenation and adjustment ventilator settings, if required, before to start therapy. Once the patient respond favorably then continued the treatment further.

Suctioning

Suctioning is performed routinely in intubated patients to aid in secretion removal and cough stimulation. The frequency of suctioning is determined by the quantity of secretions. Suctioning is the standard part of CPT. Tracheal suctioning requires the insertion of a catheter into the upper airway, where it is passed down the trachea to the level of the carina. The carina is richly innervated by the vagus nerve. When the tip of the suction, catheter comes in contact with the carina, it can provoke a strong parasympathetic response, which in turn can trigger a sudden decrease in the heart rate and produce cardiac arrhythmias. Therapist should monitor their patients carefully for the appearance of such events and provide supplemental oxygen during the procedure.

Deep suctioning is sometimes required in mechanically ventilated patients, in which the catheter is inserted until an obstruction is felt (usually the carina or wall of the right main stem bronchus), then slightly withdrawn, suction is continuously applied while the catheter is withdrawn from the airway.

One of the complications of the tracheal suctioning is tracheal-laryngeal ciliary dysfunction due to irritation of the airway mucosa. The greatest mucosal damage has been noted with vacuum pressures above 120 mm Hg, although pressures as high as 170 mm Hg are used. Therapist should use the lowest pressure as possible for removal of secretions that is effective. Inline tracheal suction catheter was initially thought to be more beneficial than using a port adopter with a standard catheter to maintain positive end-expiratory pressure (PEEP) during the suctioning procedure. Currently, there is no evidence to support a reduction in ventilator-associated pneumonias decrease in hospital stay or a decrease in mortality with the inline devices.

The inline devices have been shown to have more colonization of the respiratory tract and should be changed every 24–48 hours to minimize pulmonary infection. The physical therapist may observe instilling saline in the tracheal tube to "loosen" secretions. However, saline does not reach the peripheral airways or change the rheological properties of the mucus.

Saline instillation may also cause nosocomial infection, and the fluid instilled is not all retrieved. No studies found that instillation of saline is beneficial, current recommendations are that instillation of normal saline should not be performed as a routine step with endotracheal or tracheal suctioning. Instead, use airway humidification and patient's adequate hydration. Before suctioning through an artificial airway, therapist should increase oxygenation to minimize complications of suctioning.

Suctioning should not be performed routinely, but only when clinical indications for suctioning exist (rhonchi, increased airway pressure, decreased lung volumes, increased work of breathing, visible secretions) with close monitoring of changes in vitals.

PREPARATION

Equipment-related Preparation

- A bed capable of Trendelenberg and reverse Trendelenberg positions
- Pillows for patient position and patient comfort
- Oxygen source, flowmeter and Bain's circuit
- Ventilator settings adjustment
- Suction chamber for sputum disposal
- Functional suction equipment including an appropriate size of catheter
- Cardiopulmonary monitor for SpO_2, ECG, BP, etc.
- Stethoscope to auscultate the area affected
- Emergency airway equipment including manual resuscitator bag
- Nebulization can help to brings out the thick and tenacious secretions from the peripheral airways to central airways.

Patient-related Preparation

- Explain the procedure to the patient
- Patient's gown or light towel to cover percussed area whenever required, otherwise keep the area bare
- Prior to CPT start, be sure that the patient is not experiencing nausea and has not just given feed
- Tube feeding should be discontinued a minimum of 15–30 minutes prior to start a CPT session
- Assess the patient's chest radiographs for pulmonary findings and assess the indications for bronchial hygiene therapy (suctioning) and CPT
- Determine which region (most affected region of lungs) of the lungs requires attention
- Consciousness level of the patient and ability to cooperate the procedure
- Pain management, i.e. is it adequate?
- The level of sedation, use for paralyzing agent, e.g. is adverse reactions to suction due to inadequate sedation?
- Check baseline vitals, arterial blood gas (ABG), SpO_2 and tidal volume.

Others

- Universal precautions by physiotherapists are required
- Clean the hands and wear hand glove to protect from cross contamination.

PROCEDURE

Percussion

- Percussion is performed with the patient positioned with affected lobe or segment in postural drainage position thought to be more effective than any other position.
- Position of the therapist hand should be cupped and all fingers should be adducted with rhythmical flexion-extension at wrist joint during inspiration and expiratory phases of respiration (Fig. 1).

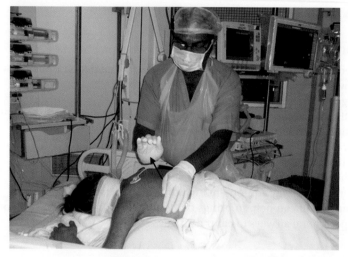

Fig. 1 *Percussion technique:* Cupped hand and rhythmic flexion-extension at wrist joint
Note: Patient is being ventilated in prone position

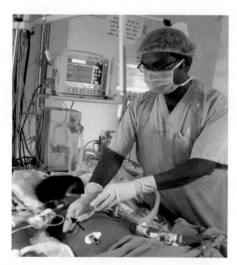

Fig. 2 *Percussion technique for child:* "Tenting" overlapping the second finger over the first and third

- Therapist cupped hand create an air pocket that traps air between hand and chest wall, and energy wave sent to bronchi to loosen the secretions.
- Therapist used one hand or two hands depending on area and available space on chest wall; in female patient, its more appropriate to use one hand to avoid discomfort.
- Vigorous and rapid chest percussion may avoid because it leads to bronchospasm, skin redness and petechiae and patient's discomfort.
- Percussion technique for neonates and infants is called "tenting". This consists of overlapping the second finger over the first and third (Fig. 2).

Vibration

- Vibration is the placement of both hands along the ribs in the direction of expiratory movement of the chest (Fig. 3).
- It may be initiated just before the expiratory phase and extended to the beginning of inspiratory phase.
- This technique can be used during mechanically ventilated patients in phase of expiration and should be performed over the involved area of the lung.

Shaking

- Patient must be in the appropriate postural drainage position then, place hands over the lobe of the lung to be treated.
- At the peak of inspiration, the physiotherapist should vigorously shake the chest using body weight and continue to shake throughout the expiratory phase.
- The hands follow the movement of the chest as the air exhaled.
- Technique must be timed with ventilator-controlled exhalation.
- If the patient has a rapid respiratory rate, it may be important to apply shaking only during every other exhalation.

Directed Cough

- Position the patient according to the affected lung lobe or segment.
- The expiratory phase is reinforced in this maneuver.
- The depth of the expiration is increased by brief firm pressure from the physio-therapist hand compressing the sides of the thorax (thoracic squeeze) just at the end of inspiration and throughout the expiratory phase (Figs 4A and B).

Manual Hyperinflation

- One caregiver (doctor) squeezes the ventilation bag slowly to inflate the lung. To enhance the clearance of airway secretions, manual hyperinflation was supposed to include the application of a larger than normal volume at a slow inspiratory

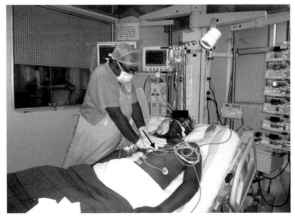

Fig. 3 *Vibration:* Using both hands keep dominant hand first then other, create force through upper extremities

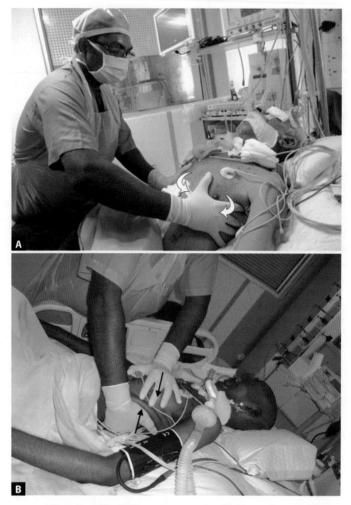

Figs 4A and B (A) Thoracic squeezing; (B) Directed cough

flow (achieved by a slow compression of the ventilator bag), an inspiratory pause (to allow complete distribution of the inflated air among all the ventilated parts of the lung), release of bag should be rapid, resulting in high expiratory flow rate.

- A second caregiver (physiotherapist) provides directed cough with shaking or vibration and percussion to assist with the mobilization of secretions. The compression phase should begin just before the inflation pressure has been released and continue until the end of the expiratory phase.
- After about six cycles of inspiration/expiration, the patient's airway is suctioned by third caregiver (nurse/physiotherapist) using sterile technique. The length of treatment is individualized and depends on the amount of secretions present in the airways and the areas of the lungs affected.
- Manual hyperinflation may be performed with intubated infants or children using an appropriately size of ventilation bag (Fig. 5). Care must be taken to apply slow inflation, so as to avoid a high peak inspiratory pressure, which carries the risk of barotraumas.

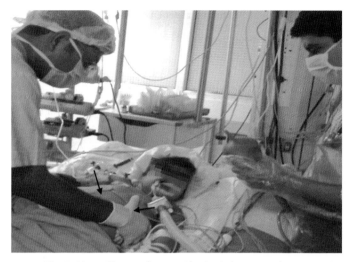

Fig. 5 Manual hyperinflation with physiotherapy technique

Postural Drainage

- Therapist positioned the patient's body in such a position in which permit gravity to facilitate drainage of mucus from the lung periphery to the segmental bronchus and upper airway. After determining the lobe of the lung to be treated, position the patient in appropriate position using Trendelenberg bed, pillows or bed rolls as needed to support the patient comfortably in the position indicated (Fig. 6).

Suctioning

- Check the amount of negative pressure produced by the suction apparatus and, if necessary adjusts to 100–160 mm Hg
- Note ventilator settings [increase fraction of inspired oxygen (FiO_2) if baseline SpO_2 <92–95%]
- Select an appropriate size of catheter of less than half the diameter of the ETT/TT (tracheal tube)
- Use only suction catheter that have multiple tip holes
- Attach the catheter to the suction source
- Expose the vent end of the catheter and connect it to the suction tubing; any part of the catheter that may contact the patient's trachea must be kept sterile
- Slide the catheter out of its packaging, taking care not to cause contamination
- Disconnect the patient from the ventilator
- Gently insert the catheter into the ETT/TT. No suction pressure (negative pressure) is applied during insertion of the catheter (Fig. 7)
- If resistance to the catheter is present, pull the catheter slightly approximately 1–2 cm back and apply suction pressure (negative pressure) by placing thumb over the vent (Fig. 8)
- Turn the catheter slowly while withdrawing it, so that the side holes of the catheter are exposed to a greater surface area
- Reconnect the patient to the ventilator.

Postural drainage postures

Both upper lobes (Apical segments)

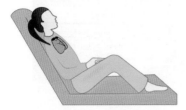

Left upper lobe (Anterior segment)

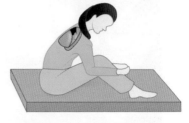

Right upper lobe (Anterior segment)

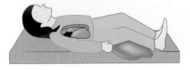

Left upper lobe (Posterior segment)

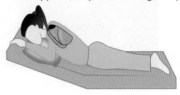

Right upper lobe (Posterior segment)

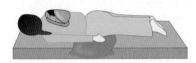

Left upper lobe (Lingula)

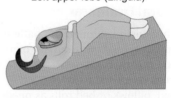

Right middle lobe

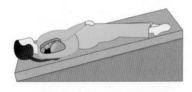

Both lower lobes (Anterior segments)

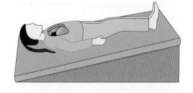

Both lower lobes (Posterior segments)

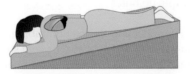

Left lower lobe (Lateral segment)

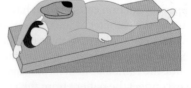

Right lower lobe (Lateral segment)

Both lower lobes (Superior
segments–Apical)

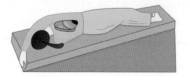

Fig. 6 Different postural drainage postures for different lobes and segments

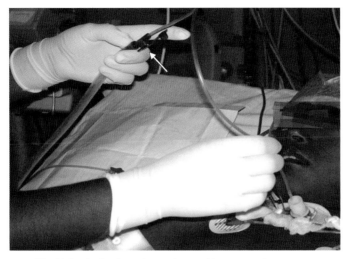

Fig. 7 *Suctioning:* Inserting catheter without negative pressure

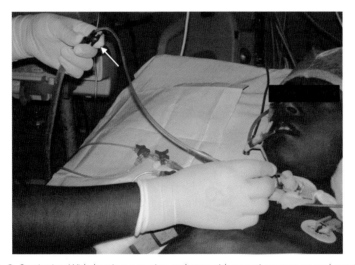

Fig. 8 *Suctioning:* Withdrawing a suction catheter with negative pressure and rotation

POST-PROCEDURE CARE

Respiratory Monitoring

- *Vitals:* Oxygen saturation by pulse oximeter, respiratory rate and pattern.
- *Examination:* Breathe sound, discomfort and dyspnea.
- *Airway secretion:* Cough and sputum production including color, quantity, consistency and odor.
- Blood gases.
- Ventilator parameter.

Hemodynamic Monitoring

- Blood pressure and heart rate
- Heart and rhythm.

Others

- *Patient related:* Skin color, mental status and patient's reaction to the therapy including subjective responses to pain.
- *Equipment related:* Disinfect all nondisposable equipment used and store appropriately.

COMPLICATION/PROBLEM

Respiratory

- Hypoxemia can be caused by the interruption of ventilation, reflex broncho-spasm and of the oxygen supply. Pre- and postoxygenation can minimize this effect.
- Atelectasis (collapse of the parts of lungs due to the removal of air during suctioning procedure).
- Mucosal trauma with increase secretions—mucosal trauma is reduced by using an atraumatic soft catheter, good suctioning technique and the correct suction pressure.
- Bronchospasm or bronchoconstriction.
- Cough paroxysms.
- Spontaneous pneumothorax, pneumomediastinum and subcutaneous emphysema.

Cardiac

- Cardiac dysrhythmia's direct tracheal stimulation causing a vasovagal reflex can cause dysrhythmias. Pre- and postoxygenation can minimize this effect.
- Hypertension or hypotension.
- Cardiac arrest.

Sepsis

- Nosocomial pulmonary tract infection
- Sepsis (airway infection).

Others

- Raised ICP-CPT has been proven to increase ICP dramatically, therefore suction and CPT should be used when indicated
- Gastroesophageal reflex
- Chest pain
- Ribs or costochondral junction fracture
- Central line displacement.

SUGGESTED READING

1. Adams A, Ball V, Brett G, Eddleston J, Russel G, Russel L. The intensive care unit. In: Smith M, Ball V (Eds). Cash's Textbook of Cardiovascular/Respiratory Physiotherapy, 1st edition. London, UK: Mosby. 2005.

2. Anderson JM, Innocenti DM. Techniques used in chest physiotherapy. In: Downie PA (Ed). Cash's Textbook of Chest, Heart and Vascular Disorders for Physiotherapists, 4th edition. UK. New Delhi: Jaypee Brothers Medical Publishers (P) Ltd. 1993.

3. Imle PC, Klemic N. Methods of airway clearance: coughing and suctioning. In: Mackenzie CF, Cristina P, Ciesla N (Eds). Chest Physiotherapy in the Intensive Care Unit, 2nd edition. USA: Williams and Wilkins. 1989.

4. Mejia-Downs A, Bishop KL. Physical therapy associated with airway clearance dysfunction. DeTurk WE, Cahalin LP (Eds). Cardiovascular and Pulmonary Physical Therapy an Evidence Based Approach, 2nd edition. USA: McGraw Hill. 2011.

5. Tecklin JS. The patient with airway clearance dysfunction. In: Irwin A, Tecklin JS (Eds). Cardiopulmonary Physical Therapy: A Guide to Practice, 4th edition. Missouri, USA: Mosby. 2004.

6. Woodard FH, Jones M. Intensive care for the critically ill adult. In: Pryor JA, Prasad SA (Eds). Physiotherapy for Respiratory and Cardiac Problems, 3rd edition. London, UK; Churchill Livingstone. 2002.

Vascular and Cardiac Procedures

18
Venous Cannulation: Peripheral

Nikhil Kothari, Arun Sharma

INTRODUCTION

Most of the patients we come across in hospital would have a little plastic tube called intravenous (IV) cannula lodged in a vein, and these little plastic devices have quietly revolutionized the entire medical practice. Intravenous cannula placed inside a vein allows us for administration of fluids (crystalloids and colloids), blood, blood products, medications, parenteral nutrition and chemotherapy.[1] It can also be used for sampling of blood, at the time of insertion. Veins are network of channels through which blood flows in our body, it has three-layered wall consisting of muscle fibers surrounded by a layer of connective tissue. Veins have valves, which ensure unidirectional flow of blood and prevent pooling of blood in the dependent portions of body; they can also obstruct passage of IV cannula into a vein. In general, smaller gauge of IV cannula should be preferred in order to avoid damaging the vessel wall and to ensure adequate blood flow around the IV cannula, thereby reducing the risk of thrombophlebitis. In an emergency situation when large volumes of fluid is to be infused over a short period of time, even the larger gauge IV cannula can be used.

INDICATION

- Intravenous drug delivery and chemotherapy.
- Intravenous fluid administration.
- Blood and blood components transfusion.
- Limited intravenous nutritional support.
- Administration of radiological contrast for computed tomography and magnetic resonance imaging.

CONTRAINDICATION

- Local site infection or cellulitis.
- Local site burn.
- Pre-existing vascular or lymphatic compromise.
- Presence of arteriovenous (A-V) fistulas, injured extremities or thrombosis.

APPLIED ANATOMY

The venous system consists of superficial and deep veins. The superficial or cutaneous veins are used for venipuncture. The pressure within veins is low and therefore a pulse will not be palpated in a vein, but sometimes the pulsations are visible in a thin patient with superficial veins. Knowledge of vein wall anatomy and physiology is necessary in understanding the potential complications of IV therapy. The vein wall consists of three layers: the outermost tunica adventitia, middle one tunica media and the innermost, tunica intima (Fig. 1).[2] Tunica adventitia (outer layer) consists of areolar connective tissue, which supports the vessel. It is thicker in arteries than in veins because of the greater blood pressure exerted on arteries. Tunica media (middle layer) consists of muscle and elastic tissue. This layer is thick and comprises the bulk of the vein. This layer is stronger in arteries than veins, to prevent collapse of the artery. Stimulation or irritation of the tissue may produce spasms in the vein or artery, which impedes blood flow and causes pain. The application of heat promotes vasodilation and reduces pain. If vasospasm occurs, apply heat above the IV site to help reduce spasm. Tunica intima (inner layer) is a smooth, elastic, endothelial lining which also forms the valves in veins (arteries have no valves). Valves may interfere with the withdrawal of blood, as they close the lumen of the vein when suction is applied. Slight readjustment of the IV needle will solve the problem. Complications including phlebitis or thrombus may arise from damage to this layer. Injury to this lining can result from tearing of the lining from a traumatic insertion or excessive motion of the IV catheter or caused by administering irritating medication and solutions. Bacterial contamination of IV site can also cause damage of tunica intima.[3]

Common sites for IV cannulation are dorsal veins over hand, median vein of forearm, medial cubital vein, cephalic and basilic vein (Fig. 2). Besides these veins, lower limb venous plexus like dorsal venous arch, lesser saphenous or great saphenous vein can also be used for placing an IV cannula (Fig. 3), other rare sites which could be used during emergency are femoral vein and external jugular vein. While using external jugular vein during hypovolemic shock, patient must be kept in Trendelenburg position for few minutes, head turned to opposite side after which slight pressure must be applied on the vein distal to puncture site as it may help in filling of the vein and makes the vein more prominent. The lower limb veins carry high risk of thrombophlebitis and thromboembolism, so routine cannulation of these veins should be avoided.[4]

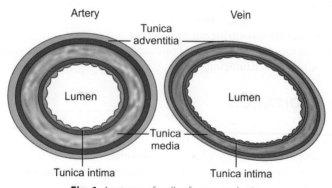

Fig. 1 Anatomy of walls of artery and vein

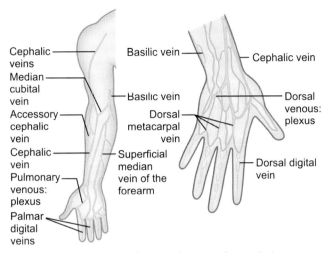

Cephalic veins
Median cubital vein
Accessory cephalic vein
Cephalic vein
Pulmonary venous: plexus
Palmar digital veins

Basilic vein
Basilic vein
Dorsal metacarpal vein
Superficial median vein of the forearm

Cephalic vein
Dorsal venous: plexus
Dorsal digital vein

Fig. 2 Anatomy of venous drainage of upper limb

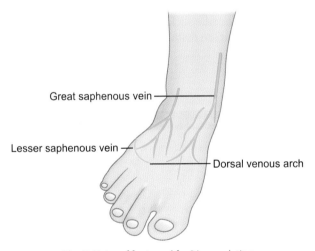

Great saphenous vein

Lesser saphenous vein

Dorsal venous arch

Fig. 3 Veins of foot used for IV cannulation

In neonates, vascular access can be obtained via the umbilical vein. In infants, scalp veins are often amenable complaisant to cannulation, and central catheters can also be inserted by this route. Intraosseous infusion can be used for fluid administration in case of emergency although care must be taken with needle placement in order to avoid injury to epiphyseal growth plates (see chapter on intraosseous cannulation).

TECHNIQUE AND EQUIPMENT

Intravenous therapy has evolved from the earliest attempts to transfuse blood and the first historic documentation of attempted IV therapy was in 1492, by a doctor caring for Pope Innocent VIII in Rome.[5] Later after one and half century, Christopher Wren (1632-1723) created the first working IV infusion device, using a quill and a pig's bladder.[6] The initial quills could not be easily fixed into blood vessels and were neither firm nor durable; silver which was more malleable and firm, gradually replaced quills, so that pipes of varying caliber could be designed. Problems associated with early IV drug delivery included migration of the silver needle and breakage. In order to prevent these devastating complications, it was important to invent a more reliable indwelling catheter. The mid-twentieth century was the golden era for the development of disposable medical devices. It began in 1950 with a landmark discovery by Dr David Massa, an anesthesiology resident at Mayo clinic. Dr Massa began by shortening a 16-gauge needle and inserting another steel needle as an inner stylet.[7] Over the top of the needle was fitted a plastic catheter which was attached to a metal hub. This resulted in an over-the-needle plastic tube configuration from which the present day cannula developed.

Present day IV canulae are available from sizes 14 gauge to 26 gauge with universal color coding for easy recognition of IV cannula (Table 1). Commonly used adult size is 20 gauge (Fig. 4). In cases of rapid fluid transfusion, even large gauge 18 (green) or 16 (gray) can be used in adult patient. Cannula size 22 (blue) is preferred in pediatric age group and size 24 (yellow) in infants and neonates.[8] The stylet of the cannula must be withdrawn carefully and disposed in needle cutter in order to prevent needle stick injury. Nowadays, protective cannulas are available with a plastic guard on distal end of needle stylet to prevent needle stick injury (Fig. 5).

Table 1 Universal color coding for IV cannula

Color	Gauge	External diameter (mm)	Length (mm)	Flow rate (mL/min)
Orange	14	2.0	45	300
Gray	16	1.6	45	150
Green	18	1.2	45	80
Pink	20	1.0	33	55
Blue	22	0.8	25	25
Yellow	24	0.7	19	15
Violet	26	0.6	19	14

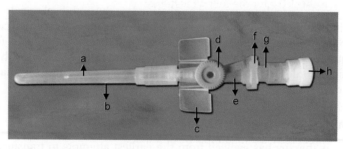

Fig. 4 Parts of modern day IV cannulae. (a) Catheter over needle; (b) protective covering; (c) catheter wings; (d) injection port; (e) luer connector; (f) needle grip; (g) flash chamber; (h) luer lock plug

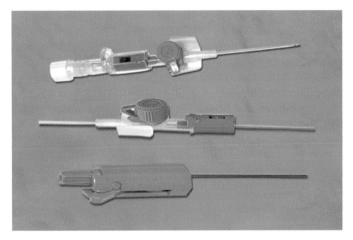

Fig. 5 Images of safety cannula to prevent needle stick injury

Source: With permission from Vygon (UK)

PREPARATION

While inserting IV cannula, proper aseptic precautions using non-touch technique must be practiced.

A surgical hand scrub is usually not required and a standard hand wash technique is adequate for this procedure; followed by decontamination with liquid soap after insertion of IV cannula.[9]

- Sterile gloves must be worn at the time of peripheral IV cannula insertion for infection control and to protect the practitioner.
- The site chosen should be preferably on nondominant hand and away from joint areas.
- Skin preparation at the site of insertion must be done using 2% chlorhexidine gluconate in 70% isopropyl alcohol, which is then allowed to dry completely for 30 seconds.[10]
- For patients sensitive to chlorhexidine gluconate an alternative agent like povidone iodine can be used
- Do not repalpate the peripheral IV cannula insertion site after applying disinfectant.
- Prepare a check list for the following items:
  Sterile gauze swabs, chlorhexidine gluconate 2% in 70% isopropyl alcohol, sterile gloves, sterile drape, sterile semipermeable transparent dressing, clean tourniquet, 10 mL syringe, 10 mL 0.9% sodium chloride for IV cannula flushing, topical local anesthetic if required (EMLA cream).

PROCEDURE

- Explain the procedure to the patient. The patient's verbal or implied consent for placement of IV cannula must be obtained.
- Ask the patient to hold the extremity firm until the completion of the cannulation.

- The patient should be in a reclining position or lying comfortably on bed to prevent any syncope.
- Immobilize the extremity, with the help of assistant, particularly for pediatric or uncooperative patients.
- After proper disinfection of tourniquet, it should be applied 3 to 5 cm above the IV cannula insertion site.
- Keep the extremity in full extension to make the vein prominent, and place the selected cannulation site in a dependent position to engorge the vein (Fig. 6A).
- Local anesthesia is not routinely administered for intravenous cannulation, its use should be considered in special situations. Topical anesthetics (EMLA cream, eutectic mixture of 2.5% lignocaine and 2.5% prilocaine) are often used for IV cannulation in children, to reduce anxiety and pain.[11] It is applied as a thick layer of cream at the site of cannulation and then covered with an occlusive dressing. It must remain on the skin for 60 minutes prior to the procedure to achieve maximum tissue penetration.
- Open the cannula carefully and ensure that the stylet within the cannula is positioned with the bevel uppermost.
- Hold the cannula inline with the vein at a 10–30° angle to the skin and carefully insert the cannula through the skin (Fig. 6B).
- As the cannula pierces the skin, a pop is felt and as it pierces the vein, second pop is felt and blood will be seen in the flashback chamber.
- Lower the cannula slightly to ensure it enters the lumen of the vein and does not puncture the posterior wall of the vessel, and advance the cannula for few millimeters into the vein (Fig. 6C).
- Then withdraw the stylet slightly and slowly advance the cannula sheath into the vein. The stylet must not be reinserted as this can damage the cannula, resulting in catheter embolus.
- While advancing the cannula into the vein, ensure that the vein remains anchored throughout the procedure, secure the wings of cannula and take care of accidental dislodgement of IV cannula (Fig. 6D), release the tourniquet (Figs 6D to F).
- Flush the cannula with 0.9% normal saline to check the patency and to ensure easy administration without pain, resistance or localized swelling.
- Secure the cannula with sterile, semipermeable, transparent dressing.
- The cannula is routinely replaced after 72 hours, or even earlier if clinically indicated.[12]
- Dispose of the stylet in the sharps' container at the bedside.

Difficult vascular-access algorithm: Deep brachial veins are paired veins present on either side of brachial artery, which can be easily accessed 1 to 2 cm above the antecubital crease.[13] Because these veins are neither palpable nor externally visible, they are often patent and untouched by untrained staff. The medial branch of deep brachial vein is preferred as the lateral branch lies directly posterior to the biceps tendon and is difficult to access.

POST-PROCEDURE CARE

- Hands must be decontaminated using 2% chlorhexidine solution, immediately before and after each episode of contact with IV cannula site.
- Documented review of cannula site for signs of infection daily.

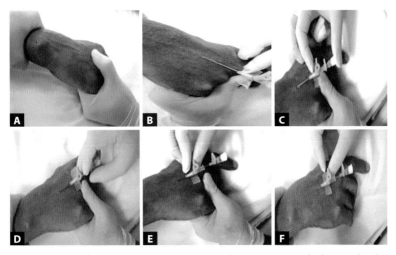

Figs 6A to F Steps for IV cannulation. (A) Proximal pressure is applied to make the vein prominent; (B) While inserting, the cannula is kept at 10–30° angle to the skin and bevel of the stylet should be kept facing up; (C) Cannula is lowered down to touch skin while sliding it into the vein and stylet removed as blood is seen in flash chamber; (D to F) While gradually withdrawing the stylet, the cannula is gently pushed forward in the vein

- A sterile, semipermeable, transparent dressing is used allowing observation of insertion site, if dressing is wet or soiled, it should be changed.[14]
- 2% chlorhexidine gluconate in 70% isopropyl alcohol is used to decontaminate port and surrounding area, and allowed to dry prior to the administering fluid or injections via the cannulae.
- Patency is maintained by heparin flush (10–100 units/mL).
- Drip sets used in line with local single use item policy or for intermittent administration must be replaced after 72 hours.
- Drip sets used for administration of blood, blood products, lipids and parenteral nutrition must be replaced immediately.
- Cannula can be replaced at 72 hours or before, if high-risk of infection is present or clinically indicated.
- Where venous access is limited, the cannula can remain in situ for longer duration, if there are no signs of infection and risk assessment undertaken.
- Document in notes, details of date and time of insertion and removal of cannula.

COMPLICATION/PROBLEM

- *Immediate complication*:
  - Extravasation of IV fluid occurs when the tip becomes dislodged from the vessel lumen, it appears as bleb at the cannula site, the patient complains of intense pain and the line is difficult to flush.[15]
  - *Arterial placement:* Peripheral catheters may accidentally be inserted into arteries instead of veins. Most common site is the antecubital fossa, with the catheter entering the brachial artery instead of the median cubital vein. In this situation the catheter should be removed, pressure should be placed over the site for 5–10 minutes.[16]

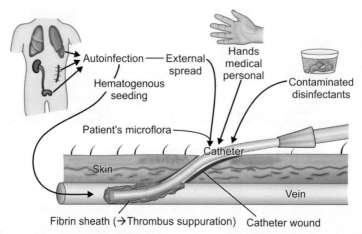

Fig. 7 Intravenous cannula as a source for blood stream infections

- *Late complication:*
  - Intravenous catheters can lead to local infection as well as bacteremia, arising from skin commensals (Fig. 7).
  - Peripheral venous thrombophlebitis, an extremely common complication, results from local damage to tunica intima followed by inflammation and thrombus formation. Thrombophlebitis causes pain, erythema, swelling and a palpable cord-like structure along the course of the vein.[17,18]
  - In neonates, use of umbilical vein for IV cannulation may be associated with portal vein thrombosis.
- *Rare:* Catheter embolism is a rare complication of IV cannula; occurs when the tip of IV cannula is sheared off. Once the needle is withdrawn from the catheter and then reinserted, sharp edge of stylet needle damages outer catheter, which may result in catheter embolization. Therefore, once the needle is removed it should never be reinserted.[19,20]

REFERENCES

1. Ortega R, Sekhar P, Song M, Hansen CJ, Peterson L. Videos in clinical medicine. Peripheral intravenous cannulation. N Engl J Med. 2008;359:e26.
2. Forauer AR, Theoharis C. Histologic changes in the human vein wall adjacent to indwelling central venous catheters. J Vasc Interv Radiol. 2003;14:1163-8.
3. Xiang DZ, Verbeken EK, Van Lommel AT, Stas M, De Wever I. Sleeve-related thrombosis: a new form of catheter-related thrombosis. Thromb Res. 2001;104:7-14.
4. Sansivero GE. Venous anatomy and physiology: considerations for vascular access device placement and function. J Intraven Nurs. 1998;21(5):S107-14.
5. Rivera AM, Strauss KW, van Zundert A, Mortier E. The history of peripheral intravenous catheters: how little plastic tubes revolutionized medicine. Acta Anaesthesiol Belg. 2005;56:271-82.
6. Deepak KK. Evolution of Medical application of syringe. Indian J Physiol Pharmacol. 2006;50(3):199-204.
7. Massa DJ, Lundy JS, Faulconer A, Ridley RW. A plastic needle. Proc Staff Meet Mayo Clin. 1950;25:413-5.
8. Tordoff SG, Sweeney BP. Intravenous cannulae colour coding A perennial source of confusion. Anaesthesia. 1990;45(5):399-400.

9. Zoutman DE, Ford BD, Bryce E, Gourdeau M, Hebert G, Henderson E, et al. The state of infection surveillance and control in Canadian acute care hospitals. Am J Infect Control. 2003;31(5):266-72.

10. Eiselt D. Presurgical skin preparation with a novel 2% chlorhexidine gluconate cloth reduces rates of surgical site infection in orthopaedic surgical patients. Orthop Nurs. 2009;28(3):141-5.

11. Romsing J, Henneberg SW, Larsen SW, Kjeldsen C. Tetracaine gel vs EMLA cream for percutaneous anaesthesia in children. Br J Anaesth. 1999;82(4):637-8.

12. Rickard CM, Webster J, Wallis MC, Marsh N, McGrail MR, French V, et al. Routine versus clinically indicated replacement of peripheral intravenous catheters: a randomised controlled equivalence trial. Lancet. 2012;380(9847):1066-74.

13. Wang R, Snoey E, Frazee B. Ultrasound-guided deep brachial and basilic vein cannulation in the emergency department. Cal J Emerg Med. 2005;2:38-40.

14. Morris W, Tay MH. Strategies for preventing peripheral intravenous cannula infection. Br J Nurs. 2008;17(19):S14-21.

15. Boyd S, Aggarwal I, Davey P, Logan M, Nathwani D. Peripheral intravenous catheters: the road to quality improvement and safer patient care. J Hosp Infect. 2011;77:37-41.

16. Tiru B, Bloomstone JA, McGee WT. Radial artery cannulation: A review article. J Anesthe Clinic Res. 2012;3(5):doi:10.4172/2155-6148.1000209209.

17. Crnich CJ, Maki DG. The promise of novel technology for the prevention of intravascular device-related bloodstream infection. Pathogenesis and short-term devices. Clin Infect Dis. 2002;34(9):1232-42.

18. Safdar N, Fine JP, Maki DG. Meta-analysis: methods for diagnosing intravascular device-related bloodstream infection. Ann Intern Med. 2005;142(6):451-66.

19. Bloom AI, Woolf YG, Cuenca A. Accidental embolization of an intravenous cannula in the upper limb: retrieval following computed tomography localization. Eur J Emerg Med. 1996;3(2):106-7.

20. Chopra V, Anand S, Hickner A, Buist M, Rogers AM, Flanders SA, et al. Risk of venous thromboembolism associated with peripherally inserted central catheters: a systematic review and meta-analysis. Lancet. 2013;389(9889):311-25.

19

Venous Cannulation: Central Venous Catheter

Afzal Azim, Abhishek Kumar

INTRODUCTION

Central line placement is a common procedure used for venous access and various other indications in intensive care unit. Its advantages over peripheral venous access include decreased phlebitis, availability of multiple ports for administration of drugs, nutrition, fluids and central venous pressure (CVP) monitoring. The technique needs expertise and training for proper placement, reduction in complications and safe medical practice.[1] The training for central line placements can be on-live demonstration on patients which is now being replaced by simulator-based training at various centers. Ultrasound-guided placement of central venous catheters (CVCs) placement should also be practiced to increase success rate and decrease complications.[2]

INDICATION

- Hemodynamic monitoring (CVP)
- Poor peripheral venous access
- Insertion of pulmonary artery catheter
- Infusion of vasoactive substances, chemotherapy or hyperalimentation
- Rapid resuscitation with fluids, blood and blood products
- Temporary dialysis access
- Transvenous pacing
- Aspiration of air embolism
- Plasmapheresis.

CONTRAINDICATION

Absolute

- Infection at site of insertion
- Anatomic variation or obstruction
- Superior vena cava (SVC) syndrome.

Relative

- Presence of coagulopathy
- Presence of pacing wires or any other indwelling catheters at insertion site
- Patient with right ventricular assist device.

APPLIED ANATOMY

The most common sites for central venous cannulation include internal jugular vein (IJV), subclavian vein (SCV) and femoral vein (FV). Other veins like external jugular vein (EJV), brachial vein and axillary vein may also be chosen in some select patient populations. Site selection is usually based on indication, operators experience, comfort of operator and presence of coagulopathy.

Internal Jugular Vein

- Location of vein is in between two heads of sternocleidomastoid muscle (SCM)
- Internal jugular vein lies just lateral to the carotid artery
- Right IJV has a straight course to right atrium
- The lower pleural dome on right side makes right internal jugular less vulnerable to trauma (pneumothorax), as compared to left IJV
- Right IJV cannulation avoids injury to thoracic duct.

Subclavian Vein

- It is located below the clavicle and passes over the first rib and apical pleura, parallel to the subclavian artery.

Femoral Vein

- Located in femoral triangle just medial to femoral artery
- Higher incidences of infection are reported as compared to SCV or IJV catheterization.[3]

TECHNIQUE AND EQUIPMENT

Early attempts to central venous access occurred in the early 1900s. Reports first described catheters using the cubital veins and FV. In 1956, Forssmann and others were awarded the Nobel Prize for their work in venous access techniques. Aubaniac was the first to describe his 10-year experience with the use of subclavian catheters for the rapid resuscitation with fluids in military casualties in 1952.[4]

Choice for insertion site and approaches:

Internal Jugular Vein

Advantage

- Bleeding can be recognized
- Malpositions are rare
- Less risk of pneumothorax
- High success rate.

Disadvantage

- Carotid artery puncture
- Not suitable for patients with tracheostomies
- Not preferred for patients with elevated intracranial pressure
- Uncomfortable for patients
- Difficult access during emergencies when airway control is also required.

Technique

Three techniques are commonly followed for IJV cannulation. *These include:*
1. Anterior approach
2. Central approach
3. Posterior approach

Anterior approach: The needle is inserted along the medial edge of the SCM just lateral to the carotid artery. The needle is directed towards clavicular head of SCM at an angle of 45° (Fig. 1).

Central approach: Also known as low or apex approach. The needle is inserted caudal to the junction of sternal and clavicular heads of SCM at an angle of 30° to the skin with the direction toward clavicular head of SCM or ipsilateral nipple.

Posterior approach: The needle is inserted at the posterior lateral margin of SCM muscle about 5 cm cephalad from the sternoclavicular joint near the margin of EJV and posterior margin of SCM. The direction of needle should be toward suprasternal notch or contralateral nipple (Fig. 2).

Subclavian Vein

Advantage

- Comfortable for patient
- Easier to maintain
- Less chances of infections

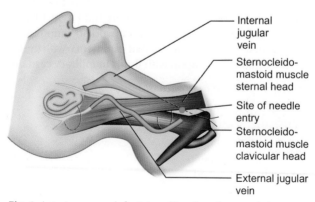

Fig. 1 Anterior approach for internal jugular vein cannulation

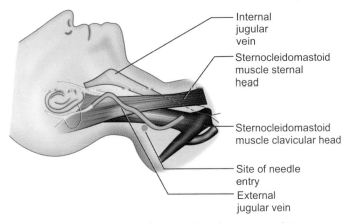

Internal
jugular
vein

Sternocleidomastoid
muscle sternal
head

Sternocleidomastoid
muscle clavicular head

Site of needle
entry

External
jugular vein

Fig. 2 Posterior approach for internal jugular vein cannulation

- Useful in patients with short neck and morbid obesity
- Unlikely to collapse in circulatory shock because of its fibrous attachment to clavicle hence it becomes the vein of choice in these clinical situations.

Disadvantage

- High chances of pneumothorax
- Difficult to compress inadvertent subclavian artery puncture
- Not a good choice in coagulopathic patients.

Technique

Subclavian vein is cannulated by two common approaches:
1. Supraclavicular approach
2. Infraclavicular approach

Supraclavicular approach: Insert the Pilot needle at 45°, bisecting the approximately 90° angle formed by the superior aspect of the clavicle and the lateral border of the SCM. The needle should be introduced parallel to the chest wall.

Infraclavicular approach
- Turn patients head away from the side which is to be cannulated and position his arms at the side
- Locate the midpoint of the clavicle and insert the pilot needle 1 cm lateral and inferior to the clavicle.
- Using an angle of 10–15° beneath the clavicle, aim medially in the direction of the suprasternal notch, and "walk" the needle below the clavicle.
- Once the clavicle is passed, further advancement should be almost parallel to the skin for approximately another 2–3 cm until you aspirate free-flowing venous blood.

Femoral Vein

Advantage

- Easy access
- Does not interfere with cardiopulmonary resuscitation (CPR)
- Does not interfere with airway access.

Disadvantage

- Infections
- Deep vein thrombosis
- Retroperitoneal bleed
- Difficult in ambulatory patients
- Delayed delivery of drugs during CPR.

Technique

The FV is cannulated 1–1.5 cm medial to the femoral arterial pulsations and 2–3 cm inferior to the inguinal ligament. If femoral arterial pulsations are feeble or weak then the FV is cannulated as follows: Divide the space between the anterior superior iliac spine and the pubic tubercle into three segments. The femoral artery lies where the medial segment meets the other two segments and the FV lies 1–1.5 cm medial to this point. The needle is inserted 2–3 cm below the inguinal ligament directed cephalic at 45–60° angle.

Less Preferred Sites for Central Venous Cannulation

External Jugular Vein

- Location variable in neck and left side is easier to access for right-handed person
- Usually difficult in hypotensive patient due to poor filling
- Difficult to pass guidewire to the SCV due to the presence of valve.

Axillary Vein

- Can be localized with arm in extended position
- Lies in axillary fossa just medial to axillary artery
- Localization is better with the use of ultrasound-guide
- There is limited data on infection rate associated with its cannulation.

Central Venous Catheter

Material and Properties

Central venous catheters are polyurethane (commonly used for catheter body) catheters with characteristics like:
- Tensile strength, which allows for thinner-wall construction and smaller external diameter

- High degree of biocompatibility, kink and thrombus resistance
- Ability to soften within the body.

Types of Catheter

- *Based on lumen of catheter:* Single or multiple lumen catheter
- *Drugs coated catheter:* Catheter coatings may include the bonding of the catheter surface with antimicrobial and/or antiseptic agents to decrease catheter-related infection and thrombotic complications. Heparin-bonding process is one example. Other agents reported in the literature include antibiotics such as minocycline, rifampin, antiseptic agents like chlorhexidine and silver sulfadiazine.
- *Choice of catheters:* It is based on the clinical assessment and needs of the patient. Usually depends on the basis of lumens, length, approach and the specialized coated catheters.
- *Flow rate of catheter:* It is important to remember that the flow in central lines is determined by the diameter of the catheter and the length of the line (Poiseuille's law). Thus a 16 gauge peripheral intravenous (IV) will have far greater flow rates (up to 220 mL/min) than a double or triple lumen CVC.

Length of Catheter to be Inserted

Incorrect positioning of catheter can manifest with serious complications. Ideally the correct position of the tip of CVC should be in the SVC above the level of pericardial reflection along the long-axis of SCV. Site chosen for insertion, patient's height and body habitus should decide the catheter length insertion. Length of insertion based on above factors may not be practical and hence catheter length insertion calculated for different sites may be used. McGee et al. suggested that an insertion depth of 16 cm is safe for IJV and SCV route[5] while Russel et al. suggested a length of 13 cm for the CVCs to be appropriate.[6] It has also been recommended that when using central approach for cannulating the right-sided IJV the catheters can be fixed at a length of 12–13 cm in males and 11–12 cm in females. Catheters can be fixed at a length of 13–14 cm in males and 12–13 cm in females in the left IJV for correct positioning of the tip of catheter.[7] Chest X-ray (CXR) is the gold standard to confirm the correct position of CVC (Fig. 3). Ideally the tip of the catheter should lie at the level of carina in CXR.

Ultrasound-guided Central Venous Cannulation

Bedside ultrasound not only displays us an image of patient's vascular anatomy, but also gives us real-time visualization of the needle as it enters the vein. *Advantages are:*[6,8]

- Real-time visualization and guidance for venous cannulation
- Success of cannulation with minimal attempts
- Decreased procedure-related complications.

It is important to understand the sonographic difference between veins and arteries. Veins appear as thin walled, nonpulsatile, and easily compressible structure (Fig. 4). This principle applies to both the central and peripheral veins. Also, it is essential to keep in mind that superficial vessels stand alone while

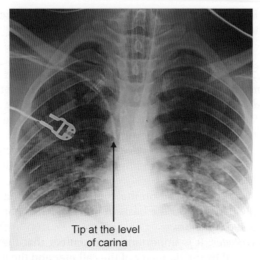

Fig. 3 Properly positioned central venous line

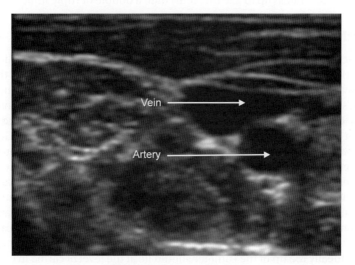

Fig. 4 Ultrasonography view

deeper vessels are paired (vein and arteries together). It is always safe to spend adequate time in vein scanning prior to needle puncture. The depth, direction and patency of the vein should be examined using ultrasound prior to needle insertion.

The choice of central vein for ultrasound-guided procedure is usually the IJV or SCV. The FV should only be considered if the above veins are not accessible. Since the SCV runs for a significant distance under the clavicle its ultrasound visualization is difficult due to high acoustic impedance from the clavicle. Only in a lateral or supraclavicular approach good imaging of SCV can be obtained. Hence it is a difficult choice for ultrasound-guided cannulation. On the contrary, the IJV does not have any bony interference, making it an ideal vessel to cannulate.

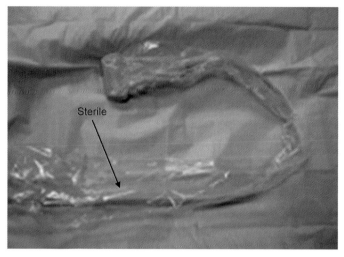

Fig. 5 Transducer

Probe selection: Transducer frequency ranging from 7.5 MHz to 10 MHz, and flat surface (linear array) is recommended for ultrasound-guided vascular access. Care must be taken to cover the probe with a sterile sheath prior to starting the procedure (Fig. 5).

PREPARATION

- Obtain consent from patient or next of kin when possible except in emergent conditions, explaining the risks and benefits of the procedure.
- Institute monitoring to the patient [pulse oximeter, blood pressure cuff, electrocardiogram (ECG)], if not previously attached.
- Review investigations like platelet count, international normalized ratio (INR) and activated partial thromboplastin time (aPTT). Coagulopathy may decide the site of cannulation or need for transfusion of blood products during or after cannulation and also the choice of ultrasound-guided cannulation.
- Obtain peripheral IV access whenever possible before attempting central venous cannulation.
- Give oxygen therapy, if procedural sedation is required for a conscious patient.
- Optimize patient position according to site and comfort of operator.
- Perform full asepsis for the procedure.
- *Equipment required:* Central venous catheter insertion tray, sterile gloves, antiseptic solution with skin swab, sterile drapes, sterile towels, sterile gown, sterile saline flush, (approximately 30–50 mL), lidocaine 1% (obtain additional vial of lidocaine 1%, if needed), gauze pieces, dressing and scalpel blade no. 11.

PROCEDURE

- *Site selection:* The procedure begins with identification of optimal site, identifying relevant landmarks and patient positioning for site access and operator comfort.

- *Maximal sterile barrier precautions (Figs 6 to 8):* Maximum sterile barrier constitutes use of a surgical cap, surgical mask, sterile gown and gloves, protective eye shield, and a large sterile drape that covers the patient's entire body from head to toe. This technique has shown significant reduction in the incidence of catheter-related bloodstream infections (CRBSI). Any deviation from these standard precautions, except in emergent life-threatening situation, should result in an immediate cessation of cannulation until the deviation is corrected.
- *Site preparation:* Chlorhexidine gluconate sterile preparation should be used for at least 30 seconds (e.g. if internal jugular cannulation is planned then prepare from external auditory meatus to clavicle and to the trachea). For children less than 2 months old, povidone iodine may be used.

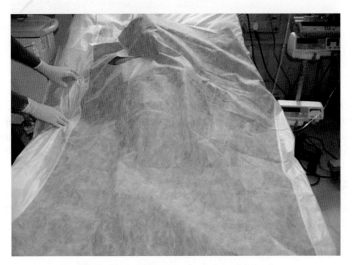

Fig. 6 Maximal barrier precautions (patient)

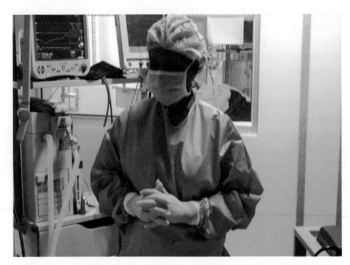

Fig. 7 Maximal barrier precautions (doctor)

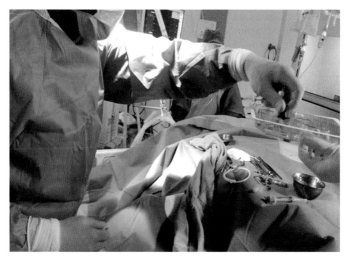

Fig. 8 Procedure assistant is essential to maintain sterility at all times

- Allow chlorhexidine site to dry (2 min).
- Prepare your procedure kit with the help of a nurse assistant who should be wearing a sterile gown, sterile gloves, cap and mask. It is important to keep in mind that the central venous line set should be opened only after site preparation and when you are ready to introduce the pilot needle to decrease the exposure time of central venous line to atmosphere.
- Position the patient according to the site of cannulation and comfort of operator. Trendelenburg position for IJV cannulation (15–30°) increases the venous return, increases intrathoracic pressure and decreases the chances of air embolization. The American Society of Anesthesiologists (ASA) task force (2012) recommends that when clinically appropriate use Trendelenburg position for IJV cannulation. Wedge support for SCV is not recommended and even turning of head for subclavian can decrease the diameter of SCV and pose difficulty in cannulation.
- Seldinger technique for cannulation, which is the guidewire dilatation technique has made the procedure safe and easy and should be always practiced.
- Give adequate local anesthesia (1%)
- The pilot puncture should be performed using an 18–20 gauge needle and syringe
- Free blood should be aspirated into the syringe
- Confirm that puncture is not arterial
  - If any doubt for arterial puncture then connect the high pressure tubing to the needle and look for the blood flow. Blood should not flow higher than the centimeter of CVP expected.
  - In certain conditions like tricuspid regurgitation, atrial fibrillation, even with venous cannulation the blood may appear to be pulsatile.
- If doubts still persist than blood gas analysis can also be done.
- After confirmation for vein with pilot puncture, puncture with CVP needle, and confirm free flow.

- The direction of bevel of the needle should be outward during IJV site and caudal during SCV cannulation.
- Direction of "J" tip of guidewire during insertion in IJV and SCV should always be caudally directed.
- Pass the guidewire through the needle keeping an eye on ECG for any arrhythmias.
- If the patient develops arrhythmia immediately withdraw the wire.
- *There are a couple of important safety points regarding guidewire insertion, enumerated below:*
    - The guidewire should not offer any resistance during its movement
    - Never force a wire
    - If you require force, the wire is in the wrong spot and can result in laceration of the vessel.
    - If you cannot advance the guidewire recheck your introducer needle and syringe aspirate for free flow of blood.
- If all of this fails, remove your needle, apply pressure to the site and consider placing your central line elsewhere or take an expert's help.
- Remove the pilot needle and leave the guidewire *in situ*
- Using a scalpel, make a stab incision at the junction of the wire with the skin.
- Now with the help of dilator provided in the kit widen the tract over the guidewire. Be cautious not to dilate the vessel.
- Remove the dilator and leave the guidewire in place
- Railroad the CVC over the wire
- Remove the wire and after confirming free flow of blood from each port clamp the ports.
- Suture the catheter to the skin
- Avoid antibiotic ointment for skin dressing.

Ultrasound-guided Internal Jugular Vein Cannulation

- Preparation for the procedure in terms of equipment, sterility and assistance is similar to the nonultrasound-guided cannulation.
- The patient's head can be placed in slightly rotated position or in a neutral head position (benefit of a neutral head position is that the IJV acquires a more lateral position to the carotid artery. It would rotate anterior and can even override the artery with head movement to the opposite side especially if too much rotation is done).
- Keeping the two vessels in a parallel alignment can minimize the risk of arterial puncture. This is especially important in patients with low venous filling pressures and vein collapse.
- Ultrasound should also be used to locate the SCM while choosing the puncture site.
- Needle insertion through the muscle should be avoided to prevent muscle hematoma.
- The indicator on the transducer should be oriented in the same direction as the indicator on the screen and located in the upper left hand side of the display. It is used as a reference point when directing the needle toward the vein.

- The transducer is placed in transverse orientation over the triangle formed by the two heads of the SCM.
- Gradually slide the probe distally, until you find, two dark and oval or round appearing vessels. Use the transducer to compress the vein to confirm it.
- Position the vein in the center of image on the screen and place the needle in the midline of the transducer (Fig. 9). Estimate or measure the depth of the IJV from the skin surface. You can use the same distance when determining how far from the transducer the needle should enter the skin when the angle of insertion is close to 45°. In this scenario it is also important to remember that the length of the needle should be at least 1.4 times as long as the measured depth of the vein. Align the needle with the longitudinal axis of the vein while advancing it.
- Advance the needle under direct vision (dynamic technique). The needle tip on the screen appears as a hyperechoic structure that casts a narrow shadow called "ring-down" artifact. Following cannulation of the vein standard Seldinger technique should be used to place the catheter during which ultrasound is usually not needed.
- The technique for central venous access of the FV is similar to the above described IJV approach.
- Preparation for the ultrasound-guided procedure in terms of equipment, sterility and assistance is similar to the nonultrasound-guided cannulation.

Key Points during Ultrasound-guided Procedure

- If we miss to identify the needle in the tissue then look at "ring-down" effect.
- Always look for the compressibility of vessel. Doppler flow can be used, if doubt still exists.
- If you angle the transducer toward the entry site of the needle on the skin you can visualize the needle earlier.
- Do not advance the needle if the needle tip is not visualized.

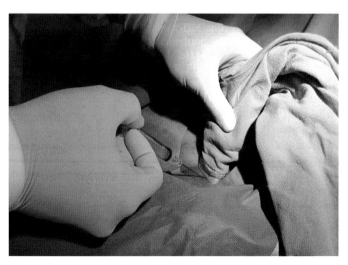

Fig. 9 Needle in the midline of transducer

- Supine and Trendelenburg is the most preferred position.
- Excessive head rotation should always be avoided.
- Carotid artery and IJV should be in the same window during cannulation. Use caution if using a long-axis approach for central venous cannulation due to the inability to maintain visualization of the carotid artery at all times.

POST-PROCEDURE CARE

- Enough evidence does not exist to evaluate whether catheter fixation with sutures, staples or tape is better. It should be determined by local or institutional policies. Suture the central line through the holes on the flanges and also take suture around the body of the catheter so that it should not slip out.
- Transparent or gauze dressing may be used for site dressing depending upon the patient's profile and unit policy. However, transparent dressings are to be preferred unless contraindicated.
- According to Centers for Disease Control and Prevention (CDC) guidelines 2011 transparent dressings can be changed every 7 days and gauze dressing can be changed every 2 days depending on clinical presentation of the patient.
- Asepsis should be maintained during handling of the hubs. For all stat medications, hub should be cleaned with alcohol swabs.
- Always order CXR to confirm tip of catheter and detection of complications.
- If position of catheter needs to be readjusted, then use full sterile technique as described for insertion of new central line.
- If IV therapy is urgent and catheterization was uncomplicated, catheter can be used prior to CXR confirmation.
- Documentation and notes of cannulation should be put in the patients file for medico-legal purposes and record.
- Examine the catheter insertion site daily for redness, induration and inflammation.
- Review the catheter daily for its need and remove if not necessary.

COMPLICATION/PROBLEM

Vascular

- Air embolus
- Artery puncture
- Pericardial tamponade
- Local hematoma
- Catheter embolus
- Infective
    - Local cellulitis
    - Bloodstream infection.

Pulmonary

- Pneumothorax
- Hemothorax

- Chylothorax
- Hemomediatinum
- Neck hematoma with tracheal obstruction.

Miscellaneous

- Arrythmias
- Catheter malpositioning
- Catheter knotting
- Nerve injuries.

Catheter-related Bloodstream Infection

Catheter-related bloodstream infection is a clinical definition for diagnosing and treating patients which requires laboratory confirmation to identify the catheter as the source of the bloodstream infection. *According to CDC guidelines (2011) diagnosing CRBSI requires fulfillment of one of the following criteria:*

- A positive semi quantitative [> 15 colony-forming units (CFU) or catheter segment] or quantitative (> 10^3 CFU or catheter segment) cultures whereby the same organism (species and antibiogram) is isolated from the catheter segment and peripheral blood.
- Differential period of CVC culture versus peripheral blood culture positivity of more than 2 hours.

An estimate has been made and shown in various studies that in United States approximately \$25,000–\$56,000 increase in excess healthcare cost or infection episode.[9-14] The reduction in central line related infections can be easily made by prevention techniques emphasized by CDC guidelines. Training and education of healthcare providers, who place and care catheters and utilization of maximum sterile precautions are some practices which reduce the burden of CRBSI. Use of checklist which includes central line bundle and nurse empowerment has shown to reduce incidence of CRBSI.

Central-line bundle: It includes the following elements:

- Adherence to hand hygiene
- Practice of maximal barrier precautions during central-line insertion
- Use of chlorhexidine (2%) for skin antisepsis
- Optimal-site selection depending upon patient profile for catheter insertion
- Daily review of central line with prompt removal of unnecessary lines.

REFERENCES

1. Centers for Disease Control and Prevention. National Nosocomial Infections Surveillance (NNIS) System report, data summary from October 1986-April 1998, issued June 1998. Am J Infect Control. 1998;26:522-33.
2. Hind D, Calvert N, McWilliams R, et al. Ultrasonic locating devices for central venous cannulation: meta-analysis. BMJ. 2003;327:361.
3. Burke JP. Infection control - a problem for patient safety. N Engl J Med. 2003;348:651-6.
4. Aubaniac R. Subclavian intravenous injection; advantages and technic. Presse Med. 1952;60(68):1456.
5. McGee WT, Moriarty KP. Accurate placement of central venous catheters using a 16-cm Catheter. J Intensive Care Med. 1996;11:19-22.

6. Russell WC, Parker JL. Thirteen centimetre central venous catheters, lucky for all? Anesthesia. 2003;58:388.

7. Kujur RS, Rao MS, Mrinal M. How correct is the correct length for central venous catheter insertion. Indian J Crit Care Med. 2009;13(3):159-62.

8. Slama M, Novara A, Safavian A, Ossart M, Safar M, Fagon JY. Improvement of internal jugular vein cannulation using an ultrasound-guided technique. Intensive Care Med. 1997;23:916-9.

9. Teichgräber UK, Benter T, Gebel M, Manns MP. A sonographically guided technique for central venous access. AJR. 1997;169:731-3.

10. Denys BG, Uretsky BF, Reddy PS. Ultrasound-assisted cannulation of the internal jugular vein. A prospective comparison to the external landmark-guided technique. Circulation. 1993;87:1557-62.

11. Orsi GB, Di Stefano L, Noah N. Hospital-acquired, laboratory confirmed bloodstream infection: increased hospital stay and direct costs. Infect Control Hosp Epidemiol. 2002;23:190-7.

12. Blot SI, Depuydt P, Annemans L, Benoit D, Hoste E, De Waele JJ, et al. Clinical and economic outcomes in critically ill patients with nosocomial catheter-related bloodstream infections. Clin Infect Dis. 2005;41:1591-8.

13. Mermel LA. Prevention of intravascular catheter-related infections. Ann Intern Med. 2000;132:391-402.

14. Burke JP. Infection control - a problem for patient safety. N Engl J Med. 2003;348:651-6.

20

Venous Cannulation: Peripherally Inserted Central Catheter

Vandana Agarwal, Atul P Kulkarni

INTRODUCTION

Peripherally inserted central catheters (PICC) provide reliable long-term central venous access with lower potential for complications. They are convenient for patients who require long-term venous access as it avoids repeated punctures and possible thrombophlebitis due to infusion of irritant medications. However, it also predisposes patients to increased risk of bloodstream infection, if not handled appropriately.

INDICATION

- Infusion of chemotherapeutic agents for treatment of malignancy, it can be used for up to a year, if properly maintained, as it prevents thrombophlebitis in peripheral veins
- For parenteral nutrition in patients who have high-output intestinal fistula
- In critically ill low birthweight or preterm babies to reduce the number of needle punctures to skin as every puncture increases the risk of infection.

CONTRAINDICATION

- Lack of peripheral venous access at possible insertion sites
- Venous thrombosis of upper extremity
- End-stage renal disease or patients with impending need of dialysis as upper extremity veins should be preserved for fistula formation.

APPLIED ANATOMY

Venous drainage of upper extremity, as commonly present, are depicted in Figure 1.

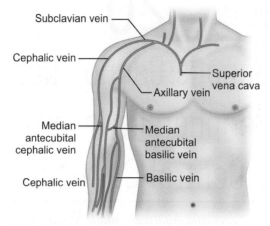

Fig. 1 Diagrammatic representation of upper extremity veins

TECHNIQUE AND EQUIPMENT

Prior to catheter insertion, one should take into consideration the type of intravascular device required. Catheter selection is based on the indication for insertion, type of catheter, site of insertion, number of luminal ports required, insertion site and patient factors.

There are two techniques that can be used:

1. *Peel-away cannula technique:* Venous access is established at the antecubital fossa like a peripheral venous cannula by inserting the cannula and stylet. The stylet is then removed and the catheter inserted through the cannula. Finally, the cannula is pulled back and peeled away from the catheter. This technique has a higher incidence of thrombophlebitis than the modified Seldinger technique.

2. *Modified Seldinger technique:* Vein is accessed by a needle or a cannula and a guidewire is threaded either through the needle or the cannula. The cannula or the needle is subsequently removed with the guidewire in place. A nick is made at the site of skin puncture and an introducer sheath with the dilator is advanced over the guidewire, thereafter the guidewire and dilator assembly is withdrawn. Central venous catheter is subsequently inserted through the introducer sheath, which is later pulled back and peeled off.

In patients with difficult venous access or patients with morbid obesity or history of previous difficult insertions ultrasound can be used to improve the success of cannulation. Ultrasound also facilitates access to larger veins higher in the upper arm. Upper arm insertions is associated with reduced rate of thrombophlebitis and thrombosis than antecubital fossa insertions. However, one has to be trained in using the ultrasound before attempting this procedure and maximum barrier precautions should be used for ultrasound machine and probe as well.

Selection of catheter: There are two types of catheter material: Polyurethane and silicone, available in various sizes, with single or multiple lumens (Fig. 2). Polyurethane catheter is a tougher material. This allows larger internal diameter

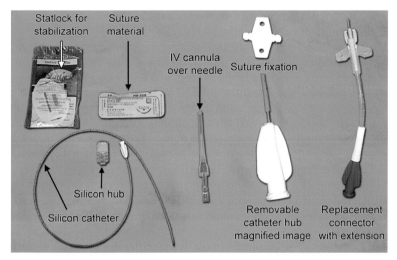

Fig. 2 Peripherally inserted central catheters set with single lumen catheter (60 cm, 4F) with radiopaque tip, silicon hub, IV introducer cannula over the needle (14 gauge), statlock for stabilization as shown in Figure 3, suture material, suture fixation device, removable hub (magnified image), if extension is required for fixation of replacement connector with extension available as single or double lumen

Abbreviation: IV, intravenous.

and thus higher flow rates as the walls are thinner compared to their silicon counterparts. However, because of the thin wall, they have the potential for breakage and rupture. Inherently polyurethane catheters are more thrombogenic. To minimize the risk of thrombophlebitis smallest gauge of catheter must be used. Catheter sizes vary depending on the brand chosen and provide a wide range from 3.5 Fr to 9.5 Fr, length varying from 35–68 cm available as single or multilumen.

PREPARATION

Certain pre-requisites are essential prior to insertion. It is very important to pay attention to asepsis as any compromises can lead to increased risk of catheter-related bloodstream infection and possible consequences.

- Peripherally inserted central catheters line should be inserted in a dedicated procedure room, a designated clean area with sterile conditions and facilities for portable radiograph or fluoroscopy, i.e. not in outpatient department (OPD) or in any corridor. Usually, this procedure is not recommended in intensive care unit (ICU) patient; conventional central lines are preferable in ICU, however, if someone is admitted in the ICU with PICC line in situ, it can be used till multilumen-catherter inserted.
- To minimize the risk of infection or other complications, PICC lines should be inserted preferably by competent staff or trainee staff under supervision by competent staff.
- Informed consent should be taken by the clinician with details of procedure, indication explained to the patient, parent or guardian.
- To improve adherence of the dressing, if catheter insertion site is hairy, then it should be clipped and not shaved prior to application of antiseptic.

- Peripherally inserted central catheters lines should be inserted preferably in the nondominant hand for ease of self-care
- *Skin preparation:* Insertion site should be prepared using a solution containing 2% chlorhexidine gluconate in more than or equal to 70% ethyl or isopropyl alcohol. Patients who are allergic to chlorhexidine, 10% povidone iodine can be used, however, the solution should be allowed to dry and not wiped away with a gauze. The antiseptic solution should be applied vigorously to a wide area of skin approximately 30 cm in diameter. Antiseptic solution should be applied with a fresh swab in a circular motion beginning in the center of the proposed site of insertion and moving outward, for at least 30 seconds. This step should be repeated three times or more, if the insertion site is dirty.
- Before placing a PICC line, operator or anyone assisting the procedure should scrub hands and forearms with antiseptic solution for at least 3 minutes and dry with a sterile towel. They should aseptically put on sterile gown and sterile gloves.
- Maximum barrier precaution should be used by the operator or any one assisting the procedure. This should include sterile gown, gloves, full body drape, cap and mask.

PROCEDURE

- *Catheter site selection:* Basilic and the cephalic veins in the antecubital fossa are the most common sites for insertion of PICC lines. Basilic vein has a nontortuous course and the largest diameter of veins in upper extremity. Cephalic vein on the contrary, is much smaller in diameter and terminates at an angle of 90º in the terminal axillary vein, this can sometimes cause difficulty in advancing the catheter.
- In infants or very small babies, catheter may be inserted through the saphenous vein with termination of the catheter tip above the level of diaphragm in inferior vena cava.
- For insertion in upper extremity, most appropriate catheter location is when tip of the catheter is close to the junction of superior vena cava and the right atrium. Position of line can be confirmed fluoroscopically in real time which obviates the need for post-procedure X-ray. If fluoroscopy is not available then post-procedure modified, chest X-ray should be taken to confirm location of the catheter. If X-ray is taken then the catheter should be visualized along its entire length in the arm across the axillary and subclavian veins and into the superior vena cava.
- After insertion using one of the two methods described above the catheter should be secured in place either by sutures (Fig. 3) or sutureless fixation (Fig. 4). The only advantage of sutureless fixation device is its quick but with added cost.
- The catheter-insertion site should be dressed with sterile, transparent, semi-permeable, self-adhesive, polyurethane dressing to allow visualization of the insertion site. In exceptional circumstances, if there is persistent ooze from puncture site after catheter insertion, a gauze dressing may be used, but it should be replaced by a transparent dressing at the earliest.
- It is not recommended to use prophylactic antibiotics or antifungal drugs (oral, parental or topical) or antibiotic lock to prevent catheter colonization or bloodstream infection at the time of catheter insertion or during use.

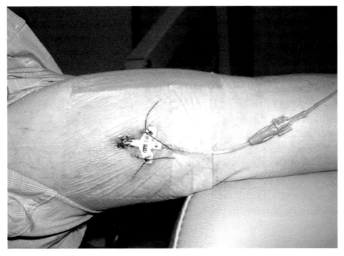

Fig. 3 Sutured fixation

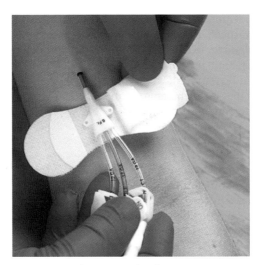

Fig. 4 Sutureless fixation

POST-PROCEDURE CARE

- *Documentation:* Accurate documentation is essential to track outbreaks of infection also for audit. This should include type of catheter used, brand, gauge of the catheter, length of catheter inserted, site of insertion, skin (preparation solution used, name of the operator, date and time of insertion). Similarly, if the catheter is removed date and time of removal and any site observations are made during follow-up.
- It is essential to educate patients or parent/guardian regarding self-care of PICC line in between treatment regimens. They should be explained theoretical and practical aspects of training with step-by-step instructions

in text and images. This should include hand hygiene, change of dressings, flushing techniques, frequency of flush needed and manipulation of catheter. They should be instructed to report any discomfort or changes in their catheter site at the earliest.

- It is not recommended to immerse or submerge catheter dressing in water.
- Strict hand hygiene precautions should be followed by healthcare workers before and after handling of catheters or dressing or palpation of insertion sites with an antiseptic-containing soap solution or use an alcohol-based antiseptic solution.
- Catheter insertion site should be monitored for pain, tenderness, redness, swelling, exudate, fever and for signs of sepsis during dressing changes or anytime the catheter is accessed.
- These catheters should be flushed periodically to maintain patency and also following injection to prevent mixing of incompatible medications. 70% alcohol swabs should be used prior to handling of ports. These catheters should be flushed with normal saline with 10 mL or larger syringes (to prevent catheter rupture because of excessive pressure generated with smaller syringes) in a pulsatile (push-pause or start-stop-start) manner.
- Catheter dressing should be changed every 7 days or as per manufacturer's guidance and definitely when it is visibly soiled or peeled off because of perspiration irrespective of the duration in place.
- Aspiration of blood for tests or blood cultures is not recommended as this can block the catheter and lead to catheter colonization.
- Catheter should be removed, when no longer needed. During removal, one must ascertain that the catheter is completely removed and no breakage has occurred and document it.

COMPLICATION/PROBLEM

- *Thrombus formation:* It can occur, if the PICC line is large for the vessel, or if the vascular endothelium is damaged, e.g. if the patient uses crutches or if the patient has a hypercoagulable. Prevention can be done by choosing an appropriate size and site of the catheter, and if the patient has a hypercoagulable state, then low dose warfarin may be required. If the thrombus formation occurs, patient may get swelling near and distal to the point of occlusion, peripheral collateral venous distention, periorbital edema or tearing of the eye on the affected side, or discomfort of the shoulder or jaw on the affected side.
- *Nonthrombotic occlusion:* It can occur, if a fibrin deposit occurs at the tip. This can lead to persistent withdrawal occlusion. Short infusion of alteplase over 2–4 hours can rescue this complication. Also, medications infused can get crystallized, if flushing is not done appropriately before and after infusion.
- *Bloodstream infection:* It is essential to maintain hand hygiene during and after insertion and everytime the catheter is accessed to prevent the risk of this complication.
- *Phlebitis:* Mechanical phlebitis is cause usually at catheter insertion in small veins in the antecubital fossa. It occurs due to mechanical irritation vascular endothelium due to movement of the catheter when bending and

straightening the arm. Sometimes fibrin sheath can form on the external surface of the catheter, resulting in infusate leak between the fibrin sheath and catheter. Leakage of infusate usually occurs at the point where the sheath ends causing chemical irritation of the vascular endothelium and thus causing chemical phlebitis.

- *Catheter malposition:* It can occur at the time of insertion or later on due to catheter migration. If the catheter is placed proximal in the superior vena cava, there is increased risk of thrombus formation. If it is too far in the right atrium, then it can cause arrhythmias. So it is prudent to confirm the integrity and position of the catheter prior to infusion. Also appropriate securing either with sutures or sutureless fixation device will prevent this complication.

- *Catheter damage:* It can get damaged due to improper flushing technique. If syringes smaller than 10 mL are used, greater pressure is generated than can be withstood by the catheter material and so the catheter can get damaged and may require replacement.

SUGGESTED READING

1. Guideline for Peripherally Inserted Central Venous Catheters (PICC) Centre for Healthcare Related Infection Surveillance and Prevention & Tuberculosis Control Version 2. [online] Available from *www.health.qld.gov.au/qhpolicy/docs/gdl/qh-gdl-321-6-1.pdf* [Accessed March 2013].
2. LA Bowe-Geddes, HA Nichols An Overview of Peripherally Inserted Central Catheters. Topics in Advanced Practice Nursing eJournal. [online] *www.medscape.com/view article/508939_5.*

21

Tunneling of
Central Venous Catheter

Dharmendra Bhadauria, Vivek Ruhela

INTRODUCTION

Mostly tunneled venous catheters are inserted for either hemodialysis in anticipation of need of long-term vascular access or chemotherapy. They are also used for the repeated administration of drugs, parenteral fluids and blood products and also for repeated blood sampling.[1] The patients who require central venous catheters (CVCs) tend to be prone to complications like infection due to the nature of their illness being a large percentage in settings such as intensive care units, undergoing cancer therapy and are therefore immunosupressed, or undergoing long-term treatment such as hemodialysis.[2] With use of tunneled catheters, the rates of infection, malfunction and thrombosis have significantly decreased in comparison to temporary catheters. Whenever patients required access for more than 1 month, tunneled catheter should be preferred.[3] Now, acceptability even for shorter duration has increased for these catheters. Catheters capable of rapid flow rates are preferred.

INDICATION

- As hemodialysis access when no other options exist
- When an arterio-venous fistula or graft is maturing
- When a continuous ambulatory peritoneal dialysis catheter is planned or during break-in period
- When a live donor transplant is scheduled and expected in few weeks
- In children weighing less than 20 kg or where the child's developmental level precludes safe cannulation of arteriovenous (AV) fistula
- When repeated and long-term administration of drugs such as chemotherapy, fluids and blood products is required.

CONTRAINDICATION

Absolute

- Bacteremia or sepsis
- Infection at the insertion site
- Disseminated intravascular coagulopathy

Relative

- Severe thrombocytopenia and coagulopathy
- Inexperience, unsupervised operator
- Local infection
- Distorted local anatomy
- Previous radiation therapy
- Suspected proximal vascular injury.

APPLIED ANATOMY

A specific knowledge of anatomy in addition to a working knowledge is required for safe and successful procedure. Anatomical misunderstanding may result in failure to insert the catheter or some complications such as a prolonged procedure, increased morbidity and mortality.

Venous anatomy: Walls of vein are relatively thin and fragile in comparison to arterial walls, rendering them at risk from iatrogenic injury. Structurally, there are three layers in venous wall: an inner endothelial layer (tunica intima), a middle muscular layer (tunica media) and an outer connective tissue layer (tunica adventitia). This connective tissue makes the venous system to be distensible and compliant, but is also the reason for their fragility comparing to arteries. These layers in venous wall are longitudinally organized; it means that injury in the wall of a vein has a tendency to extend along the long axis, leading to larger defects with the increased risk for serious bleeding.

Access site: The indication and type of catheter being inserted is needed to decide for site of access. However, usually first site of choice is the right internal jugular vein. Other veins in the neck may be chosen, if this vein is occluded or cannot be used for some other reason. Right internal jugular vein is preferred one for the access, followed by left internal jugular vein, right femoral vein and left femoral vein. Central venous catheterization should be avoided in subclavian veins due to development of early stenosis.

Anatomical Pitfalls

- *Internal jugular vein (IJV):* The IJV is most frequently used for CVC.[4] It lies in a straight line connecting the mastoid process and the medial end of the clavicle and is more distensible than the subclavian vein (SCV).[5] The diameter of the internal jugular vessel is greatest below the cricoid cartilage, reaching 2.0–2.5 cm.[6] A head-down tilt of 15° (Trendelenburg's position) causes the vein prominently distended. Excessive palpation of the neck and extensive rotation of the head causes difficulty in cannulation of the vein, therefore it is recommended that once you have located the artery stop further palpation because extensive palpation of the carotid artery may distort the anatomy.[6] Usually, the IJV is more collapsible compared to the SCV[7] and this may complicate catheterization because the advancing needle may press the anterior wall of the vein against the posterior wall. This may result in passing the needle through both walls without locating the lumen. If no blood is found after advancing the needle at a depth of 2.0–2.5 cm, the needle should be withdrawn and therefore re-establishing a lumen by drawing the anterior wall from the posterior wall. Right IJV is usually the preferred one because of its straight course, facilitating successful and correct placement of the catheter.[4] An anatomical study conducted by Botha et al.[8] showed that the IJV lies directly posterior to the apex of the triangle in 78.79% of the cases on the left and 97.14% of the cases on the right. Apex is formed when the sternal and clavicular heads of sternocleidomastoid meet which is also known as Sedilott's triangle (Fig. 1A).

- *Common carotid artery:* The common carotid artery usually medial to the IJV.[9] IJV is anterolateral in relation to the common carotid artery in approximately 92% cases. While in 2% of cases, IJV can lie anteromedially to the common carotid artery (Figs 1A and B).

TECHNIQUE AND EQUIPMENT

Type of catheter: 'One size does not fit all' also hold true for tunneled catheters. Patients on dialysis or plasmapheresis need catheters of relatively large lumen to allow high flow rates, whereas a patient on chemotherapy requires smaller luminal diameters for infusion.

Length of catheter: A thumb rule for right internal jugular hemodialysis catheter to determine length of catheter is 19 cm, if patient's height is less than 5.5 feet and 23 cm for height of more than 5.5 feet. These values are 23 cm and 29 cm, if you are planning for left internal jugular catheterization.

PREPARATION

- Informed consent is to be taken in all procedures.
- Coagulogram (PT and aPTT) and hematological parameters to be obtained and corrected, if deranged. Correction of underlying coagulopathies minimizes the risk of this problem. We use to administer prophylactic preprocedural antibiotics (1 g cefazolin) prior to tunnel catheter insertion unless the patient

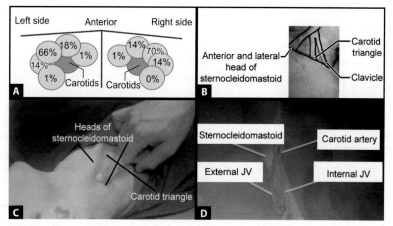

Figs 1A to D (A) Possible anatomy of IJV in relation to carotid artery at carotid triangle; (B to D) Relevant anatomy for venipuncture

is already on antibiotics for another reason. Sterility is to be maintained for tunneled catheter insertion and all personnel must follow standard surgical scrub protocol.

PROCEDURE

Venous Puncture

- It is very important to use maximum barrier protection for the placement of chronic dialysis catheters preferably in an operating room.
- The selected access site should be cleansed with a surgical scrub (chlorhexidine solution) and draped appropriately. The area to be scrub should extend from below the nipple line to the level of the ear and the line of the mandible (Fig. 2A).
- Patient is asked to turn his or her head away from the side of puncture. The puncture of the jugular veins should be guided by ultrasound as it may avoid most complications related to puncture site. Vein is larger and easily compressible than arteries on ultrasound (Fig. 2E). Local anesthesia should be obtained by subcutaneous lidocaine infiltration.
- Ideally, one should use a micropuncture set (21 gauge needle, 0.018 inch guidewire, coaxial 3 and 5 Fr dilators) for all venous access but as it increases the cost further, so we use the set, which is provided with the catheter kit by manufacturer. We used to attach the puncture needle to a 10 cc syringe. The ideal site of puncture is the carotid triangle (Figs 1B to D and 2A), the internal jugular vein between the medial and lateral heads of the sternocleidomastoid muscle 1 cm above the clavicle (Fig. 2A). Apical puncture site in triangle may lead to the catheter to kinking. Transverse orientation of probe is better than horizontal and the center of the probe is positioned above the target vein. The needle is then placed on the skin at the center of the probe and advanced on the same angle as the ultrasound probe toward the vein. Negative pressure in syringe should be taken as it pierces the skin. This will avoid through-and-through puncture. As we pass the needle into vein, the vein will tent (Fig. 2E). After venopuncture, there will be gush of dark red blood. The guidewire is then advanced into the vein (Fig. 2B).

Creation of Tunnel

- Expected course of the tunnel should be at least 8–10 cm and to be is infiltrated by subcutaneous lidocaine. A gentle curve of tunnel is preferable to avoid the risk of kinking and for better catheter flow rates. Catheter exit site should be at least 3–4 cm below and lateral to clavicle or can be measured by using the measuring wire. The incision should be at a right angle to the course that the catheter will take. A 11 size blade is then used to create a 5 mm incision on the chest wall at the desired exit site on the chest, only going through the skin and avoiding the muscle, as this will avoid more bleeding (Figs 2C and D).
- A trocar or tunneler included in the catheter kit is used to create a tunnel from exit site to the puncture site in the neck (Fig. 2F). It is important to enlarge the puncture site slightly to 5–10 mm using a scalpel to facilitate the entry of trocar to pass out of the skin adjacent to the venopuncture (Fig. 2D).

- The catheter is then attached to the trocar and pulled through the tunnel. It is best to pull the cuff of the catheter 5 cm into the tunnel (Fig. 2G).
- How the tunnel is approached from exit to venopuncture site is important to avoiding kinking. The chances of kinking are less, if the tunnel approached venopuncture site from above and laterally, then approached in a straight direct line. This depends upon how it is tunneled. The tunneling method which we follow is as:
  - After bending the trocar into a curved or 'L' shape (Fig. 2F), advance it with circular motion into a superior direction lying flat on the patient's chest wall. This maneuver leads to entry of trocar to the venopuncture site, from a lateral and slightly superior direction.
  - Raise the tip of trocar after reaching the venopuncture site to facilitate its exit from the incision.

Placement of Catheter

- Right or left side precut catheter are different in length. It is important to acquaint yourself with the nomenclature of the particular catheter used. The tip of distal end of guidewire should be in the inferior vena cava to decrease the risk of great vessel laceration, especially when you are dealing with left-sided catheter insertion.
- Predilation of catheter track with a smaller caliber dilator will facilitate the exchanged over the rigid wire for the peel-away sheath (Figs 2H and I). The sheath should be advanced with a slight twist at the skin with firm constant forward pressure into the vein.
- After removing the guidewire and dilator, catheter is pushed into sheath and vein as far as possible (Fig. 2J).
- The sheath is then slowly peeled apart by 'pull and apart method', while the catheter is held in position by pressure of thumb (Figs 2K and L). If there is no valve like flap in sheath, it can be occluded by pinching and still leaving enough room to allow for the tip of the catheter to be inserted up past its side holes. It will prevent bleeding or aspiration of air.
- The catheter needs to be retracted slightly to clear any kinks after full insertion.
- Then obtain a final fluoroscopic image to look for kink at curve of catheter and its position into heart (Fig. 2M). The tip should be at junction of superior vena cava and atrium or within the right atrium (preferable).
- The catheter is then sutured to the skin and the venopuncture site in the neck is closed. The ports of the catheter are flushed with saline. Both ports are aspirated with a 10 cc syringe to ensure good blood flow and then to be filled with prescribed amount of heparin on the ports.

COMPLICATION/PROBLEM

The following anatomically relevant complications can occur: Venous air embolism, cardiac tamponade, dysrhythmias, pneumothorax, thrombosis, catheter-related infection and catheter embolization.

- *Arterial puncture:* Because of its close anatomical relationship to the IJV, common carotid artery is the usual victim. The direct result of puncturing an artery is the formation of a hematoma,[10] which if large may result in the possible compression of the surrounding structures.

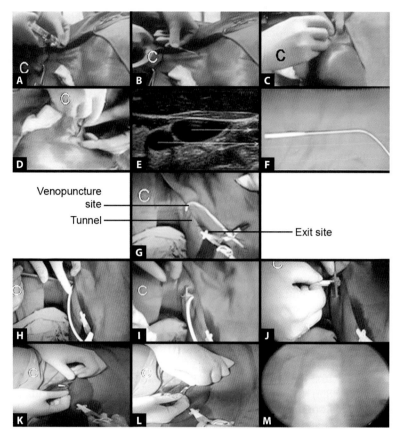

Figs 2A to M (A) Venopuncture at carotid triangle (blind method); (B) Insertion of guidewire; (C) Incision at exit site before start tunneling; (D) Widening of venopuncture site to facilitate tunneling; (E) Doppler appearance of artery and vein; (F) Curved tunneling device; (G) Catheter after tunneling and inserted guidewire; (H) Insertion of pull apart sheath on guidewire in vein; (I) Fully inserted pull apart sheath; (J) Insertion of catheter into sheath; (K and L) Pull and apart of sheath after catheter insertion; (M) Final position of catheter in right atrium on fluoroscopy

Note: C-cephalic end of patient.

- *Arterial pseudoaneurysms* have also been reported.[11] Pulmonary artery puncture[12] and puncturing of the ascending aorta,[13] within the pericardial reflection may cause a fatal hemopericardium.
- *Failure to locate the IJV:* The common cause in failure to locate the IJV is when there is common carotid arterial puncture leading to venous compression from hematoma formation.[5] Another possibility is due to the collapsible nature of the vein, the anterior wall of the vein may also be pushed against the posterior wall by the needle. The needle may therefore puncture both walls without reaching the lumen leading to failure to locate. Venous pseudoaneurysm with multiple attempts at puncturing the IJV has also been reported.[10]
- *Hemothorax:* Hemothorax is an uncommon complication in IJV cannulation.
- *Brachial plexus injury:* Brachial plexus injury is also less common complication in IJV cannulation but is more commonly associated with the cannulation of

the subclavian vein. Subclavian artery puncture is also associated with brachial plexus injury. When posterior access route is opted for IJV cannulation and the needle is aiming at the suprasternal notch, the upper trunk of the plexus may be injured. Especially when the needle is slightly posterior while entering the posterior triangle.[14] Therefore, if you have opted the posterior route then chances of injury to the upper trunk of the brachial plexus are there.

- *Phrenic nerve injury:* Phrenic nerve injury can occur in two ways, compression due to the formation of a hematoma[15] and direct injury because IJV and the phrenic nerve are closely related behind sternocleidomastoid. Direct injury to phrenic nerve may be irreversible.[16]
- *Horner's syndrome:* Horner's syndrome occurs due to lesions of the sympathetic chain.[17] Neurological injuries including damage to phrenic nerve, the sympathetic chain on the left, IX, X, XI and XII cranial nerves, and the anterior branches of the II, III and IV cervical nerves have been reported with IJV catheterization.[18]
- *Hoarseness:* Injury of the recurrent laryngeal branch posterior to the IJV during IJV puncture may result in this complication.[19]
- *Chylothorax:* Rare complication occurs due to injury to the thoracic duct, when placing a central venous catheter into the IJV on the left side.[20]
- *Accidental mediastinal entry:* Left IJV cannulation may lead to accidental mediastinal entry.[21,22] It indicates that one should be more cautious during left IJV catheterization.

Malpositioning of catheter tip: Following are the locations where malpositioning commonly occurs: IJV (43.4%), contralateral brachiocephalic vein (11.2%) and right atrium (9.8%).[23] Malpositioning may cause unusual chest pain syndromes.[24] Overall malpositioning appears to be more common via the left side, due to longer and oblique course of left brachiocephalic vein.

Prevention of complications: Following basic factors should be observed to keep the complications at the minimum:[25]
- The indications for CVC should be carefully considered.
- Thorough knowledge of the clinical anatomy of the SCV and IJV as well as their neighboring structures is required.
- Follow the technique meticulously.
- Most complications are found in the hands of inexperienced operators, means that there is no substitute for experience.
- Awareness of the complications, their frequency, and reason for occurrence is very important.
- The reason for the complications can in almost every instance be explained by the regional anatomy.
- Complications are more common in left side rather than right side cannulation.

REFERENCES

1. Bishop L, Dougherty L, Bodenham A, Mansi J, Crowe P, Kibbler C, et al. Guidelines on the insertion and management of central venous access devices in adults. Int J Lab Hematol. 2007;29(4):261-78.
2. Morales M, Mendez-Alvarez S, Martin-Lopez JV, Marrero C, Freytes CO. Biofilm: the microbial "bunker" for intravascular catheter-related infection. Support Care Cancer. 2004;12(10):701-7.

3. Schwab SJ, Buller GL, McCann RL, Bollinger RR, Stickel DL. Prospective evaluation of a dacron-cuffed hemodialysis catheter for prolonged use. Am J Kidney Dis. 1988;11: 166-9.
4. Mathers LH Jr, Smith DW, Frankel L. Anatomic considerations in placement of central venous catheters. Clin Anat. 1992;5:89-106.
5. Armstrong PJ, Sutherland R, Scott DH. The effect of position and different manoeuvres on internal jugular vein diameter size. Acta Anaesthesiol Scand. 1994;38:229-31.
6. Bazaral M, Harlan S. Ultrasonographic anatomy of the internal jugular vein relevant to percutaneous cannulation. Crit Care Med. 1981;9:307-10.
7. American Association of Clinical Anatomists, Educational Affairs Committee. The clinical anatomy of several invasive procedures. Clin Anat. 1999;12:43-54.
8. Botha R, van Schoor AN, Boon JM, Becker JH, Meiring JH. Anatomical considerations of the anterior approach for central venous catheter placement. Clin Anat. 2006;19: 101-5.
9. Edwards N, Morgan GA. How to insert a central venous catheter? Br J Hosp Med. 1989;42:312-5.
10. Chudhari LS, Karmarkar US, Dixit RT, Sonia K. Comparison of two different approaches for internal jugular vein cannulation in surgical patients. J Postgrad Med. 1998;44:57-62.
11. Luckraz H. Venous pseudo-aneurysm as a late complication of short-term central venous catheterisation. Cardiovasc Ultrasound. 2003;1:6.
12. Rosen M, Latto P. Handbook of Percutaneous Central Venous Catheterization, 2nd edn. London: WB Saunders Company. 1992.
13. Childs D, Wilkes RG. Puncture of the ascending aorta: a complication of subclavian venous cannulation. Anaesthesia. 1986;41:331-2.
14. Paschall RM, Mandel S. Brachial plexus injury from percutaneous cannulation of the internal jugular vein. Ann Emerg Med. 1983;12:58-60.
15. Depierraz B, Essinger A, Morin D, Goy JJ, Buchser E. Isolated phrenic nerve injury after apparently atraumatic puncture of the internal jugular vein. Intensive Care Med. 1989;15:132-4.
16. Armengaud MH, Trevoux-Paul J, Boucherie JC, Cousin MT. Diaphragmatic paralysis after puncture of the internal jugular vein. Ann Fr Anesth Reanim. 1991;10:77-80.
17. Milam MG, Sahn SA. Horner's syndrome secondary to hydromediastinum: a complication of extravascular migration of a central venous catheter. Chest. 1988;94:1093-4.
18. Briscoe CE, Bushman JA, McDonald WI. Extensive neurological damage after cannulation of internal jugular vein. Br Med J. 1974;1:314.
19. Moosman DA. The anatomy of infraclavicular subclavian vein catheterization and its complications. Surg Gynecol Obstet. 1973;136:71-4.
20. Kwon SS, Falk A, Mitty HA. Thoracic duct injury associated with left internal jugular vein catheterization: anatomic considerations. J Vasc Interv Radiol. 2002;13:337-9.
21. Tong MK, Siu YP, Ng YY, Kwan TH, Au TC. Misplacement of a right internal jugular vein haemodialysis catheter into the mediastinum. Hong Kong Med J. 2004;10:135-8.
22. Godwin JD, Chen JT. Thoracic venous anatomy. Am J Roentgenol. 1986;147:674-84.
23. Lum PS, Soski M. Management of malpositioned central venous catheters. J Intraven Nurs. 1989;12:356-65.
24. Webb JG, Simmonds SD, Chan-Yan C. Central venous catheter malposition presenting as chest pain. Chest. 1986;89:309-12.
25. Hegarty MM. The hazards of subclavian vein catheterization. Practical considerations and an unusual case report. S Afr Med J. 1977;52:240-3.

22

Intraosseous Cannulation

Nishant Verma, Rakesh Lodha

INTRODUCTION

Securing vascular access in critically sick patients can be challenging. Intraosseous (IO) access provides a rapid and safe means for delivery of medications, fluids and blood products during resuscitation. In addition, blood samples for laboratory analysis can be obtained from IO access. IO cannulation requires less skill and practice as compared to peripheral IV access, central lines or umbilical lines. Moreover, IO cannulation is rapid, safe, noncollapsible and associated with fewer complications as compared to central venous catheter placement.[1]

INDICATION

Initiation of IO access is indicated in acutely ill or injured infants and children who require an urgent vascular access but a peripheral or central venous access is not possible or feasible in a timely manner. Such scenarios include:
- Peripheral vascular collapse due to shock
- Small veins because of patient size
- Lack of expertise for obtaining a central venous catheter (CVC)
- Excessive time required to arrange for a CVC

    The use of IO access in adults is less popular than in children. It was thought that the less vascular yellow marrow of adults (red bone marrow is replaced by the yellow marrow at 5–6 years of age) would prevent drug absorption.[2] However, studies have demonstrated that although less vascular, yellow marrow still facilitates absorption. Therefore, this access can be safely and successfully used in older children and adults. Another limiting factor for IO use in adults was the inability to penetrate the dense bone cortex by the needle. This limitation has now been overcome with the availability of powered devices (e.g. EZ-IO device, Vidacare).

CONTRAINDICATION

As IO cannulation is primarily indicated in life-threatening emergencies, only few contraindications exist, which include:
- Fractured bone or previously penetrated bone: the administered drug will exit through the fracture/puncture site.
- Obvious overlying infection or osteomyelitis involving the cannulation site
- Patients with osteogenesis imperfecta.

APPLIED ANATOMY

An IO cannula provides access to the medullary cavity of the bone. The medullary cavity of long bones is composed of a network of venous sinusoids. These sinusoids drain into a central venous canal, which then empty via the emissary veins into the venous circulation (Fig. 1). The major vessels into which the emissary veins drain depend upon the insertion site. The following list provides the site and draining vessels for the most commonly used sites:

- Proximal tibia—Popliteal vein
- Femur—Branches of femoral vein
- Distal tibia (medial malleolus)—Great saphenous vein
- Proximal humerus—Axillary vein
- Manubrium (upper sternum)—Internal mammary and azygos veins.

TECHNIQUE AND EQUIPMENT

The concept of using the marrow cavity of a bone for administration of medications dates back to the 1920s, when liver extracts were transfused to adults suffering from pernicious anemia via their sternum. The IO access gained popularity in pediatric patients in 1940s, and it was used for infusion of medications, blood products and other fluids during situations of difficult venous access. The site of insertion in the pediatric population transitioned from sternum to the tibia because of risks involved in a sternal puncture.[3] The importance of prompt vascular access in critical care and resuscitation settings were recognized in the 1980s, which led to increased focus on IO access in various critical scenarios. Numerous studies till date have demonstrated that success rates for IO cannulation are much higher than for any other vascular access and the time required to obtain an IO access (only 1–5 minutes) is also lesser than that required for any other access.[4,5]

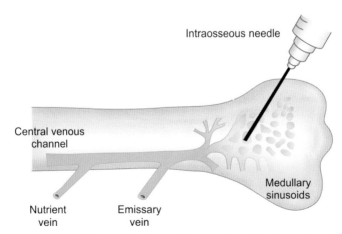

Fig. 1 Intraosseous needle located in the medullary cavity of the bone. Blood drains from sinusoids located in the medullary cavity to the central venous canal, and then into major vessels via emissary veins

Equipment

A variety of needles can be used for IO cannulation including butterfly needles, spinal needles, standard metal IV needles, bone marrow aspiration needles and the commercially available IO needles. However, needles with stylet should be preferred because stylet prevents occlusion of the needle lumen by bony spicules during IO insertion. Commercially available, single use needles should ideally be used for IO cannulation. Two types of IO cannulae are available commercially, the manual IO devices and the powered devices.

Manual IO devices: These devices require the operator to exert manual pressure to penetrate the bone and enter the marrow cavity. IO devices are comprised of a hollow metallic needle and a stylet to prevent obstruction or bending of the needle during insertion. The commonly used manual IO device is the disposable Jamshidi bone marrow aspiration needle (Fig. 2). Other frequently used manual devices are the Cook disposable IO needle (Fig. 3) and Jamshidi disposable IO needle (Fig. 4). The Cook needle has a circular handle, which facilitates holding and placement of this needle. It is available in two sizes 16G and 18G.

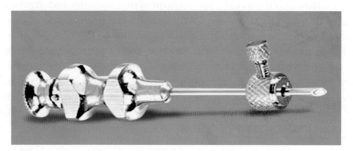

Fig. 2 Jamshidi disposable bone marrow aspiration needle

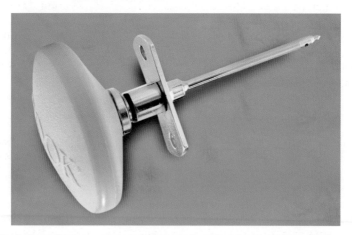

Fig. 3 Cook disposable intraosseous infusion needle with stylet. The circular needle provides a better grip and the stylet prevents obstruction by bony spicules

Source: Permission for use granted by Cook Medical Incorporated, Bloomington, Indiana

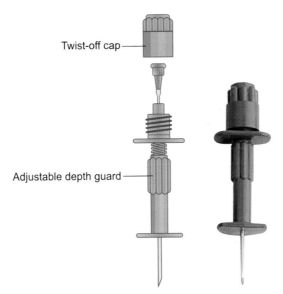

Twist-off cap

Adjustable depth guard

Fig. 4 Jamshidi disposable intraosseous infusion needle. Twist-off cap holds stylet securely in place and the adjustable depth guard controls the depth of entry into the bone

Powered devices: Apart from a metallic needle and stylet, the powered devices have a battery-operated driver and hence they do not require manual pressure for insertion. This is particularly important in adults, who have a thick bony cortex. The most commonly used powered device is the EZ-IO (Vidacare, San Antonio, Texas) which has a reusable lithium battery-powered driver (Fig. 5A). The driver works as a drill that rotates the needle into the IO space at a preset depth. The lumen of the needle is 15G and it comes in 3 lengths (15 mm for children weighing 3–39 kg, 25 mm for patients weighing < 40 kg and 45 mm length for the proximal humerus insertion site in patients weighing > 40 kg and patients with significant tissue or edema overlying the bone) (Fig. 5B). Other powered devices available for IO cannulation include (Figs 5C and D) the Bone Injection Gun (BIG, WaisMed, Kansas City, MO) and the FAST1 (First Access for Shock and Trauma, Pyng Medical, Vancouver, BC, Canada).

PREPARATION

- In most instances, IO cannulation occurs as part of care for a life-threatening emergency. Thus, informed consent is typically implied, however, whenever possible, the family members must be explained regarding the need for IO cannulation, the procedure, potential complications and duration of the procedure.
- No laboratory investigations are required prior to inserting the IO needle.
- Awake patients should receive local anesthesia prior to IO cannulation attempts. Apart from the local anesthetic, no other sedation or analgesia is administered.

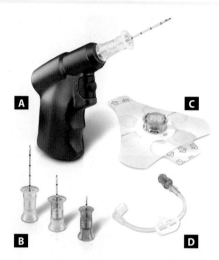

Figs 5A to D EZ-IO system (Vidacare). The lithium battery-powered, intraosseous driver (A); which when combined with an EZ-IO sterile needle set provides fast, safe and controllable intraosseous access. The EZ-IO needles (B); Come in three sizes: 15 mm needle set (pink hub), 25 mm needle set (blue hub), 45 mm needle set (yellow hub). Stabilizer dressing for fixing the needle (C), and IV extension tuning (D)

Source: Vidacare Corporation.

- As most of the patients undergoing IO cannulation are critically sick, the importance of monitoring vital parameters during this procedure cannot be overemphasized. Continuous pulse oximetry and electrocardiographic (ECG) monitoring (if available) should be done.
- The following equipment should be assembled prior to the procedure: povidone-iodine solution and alcohol-based skin preparation solution, surgical mask and apron for the clinician performing the procedure, sterile gloves, 5 mL and 10 mL syringes, syringe with saline flush, sterile 3-way tap with extension tubing, IO needle and/or device, 1% lidocaine for skin infiltration, specimen bottles (as required).

PROCEDURE

Site selection: In patients undergoing IO cannulation for life-threatening illnesses (like cardiac arrest), proximal tibia is the preferred site irrespective of the age of the patient.[6] Alternative sites vary based upon the age and skeletal maturity of the patient. The primary anatomic locations for IO cannulation are as follows:

- *Proximal tibia:* The proximal end of tibia has a flat wide surface and is covered by only a thin layer of subcutaneous tissue, thus allowing easy identification of landmarks. Moreover, this site is distant from the airway and chest, and hence will not interfere with any ongoing cardiopulmonary resuscitation (CPR). In children, the insertion site is approximately 2 cm below and 1 cm medial to the tibial tuberosity (Fig. 6). In skeletally mature adolescents and adults, the recommended site is 2 cm medial and 1 cm above the tibial tuberosity (Fig. 7).

Though, the proximal tibial insertion site can be used in children as well as adults, but in patients more than 6 years age a powered device is required to penetrate the thick bony cortex. If such a device is not available, then the clinician should attempt manual placement at an alternative site like the distal tibia.

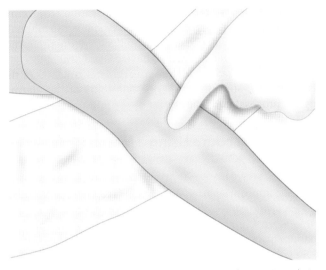

Fig. 6 Proximal tibial IO insertion site in children. It is located approximately 2 cm below and 1 cm medial to the tibial tuberosity

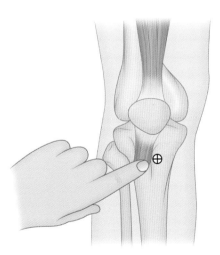

Fig. 7 Proximal tibial IO insertion site in older children and adults. It is located approximately 2 cm medial and 1 cm above the tibial tuberosity

- *Distal femur:* The distal femoral site is located approximately 2 to 3 cm above the superior border of the patella in the midline with the leg in extension (Fig. 8). The distal femur has much denser covering layers of fat, muscle and soft tissue, which make bony penetration difficult. So, this site is reserved for manual placement in infants and young children in whom the proximal tibial site is contraindicated or already punctured.
- *Distal tibia:* Either of the malleoli may be used for IO cannulation (medial malleoli preferred over lateral). The site of penetration is 1–2 cm superior to the malleoli in midline (Fig. 9). This site is available for manual or device-assisted IO placement in all age groups. Malleoli are the preferred site for IO cannulation in adults when a powered device is not available.
- *Other less commonly used sites:* Humerus (greater tubercle of the proximal humerus) (Fig. 10), sternum (superior one-third of the sternum), radius (radial styloid process) and iliac crest.

Performing the Procedure Using a Manual Device

Steps

1. Identify the age appropriate site of insertion (see site selection above).
   a. *Infants and children less than 6 years:* Proximal tibia.
   b. *Children more than 6 years and adults:* Distal tibia.
2. Put the patient in a safe position, which provides ready access to the insertion site without compromising the patient's condition.
3. Don an apron, a surgical mask and latex-free sterile gloves
4. Clean the selected insertion site area with the alcohol-based solution followed by povidone-iodine and allow it to dry.

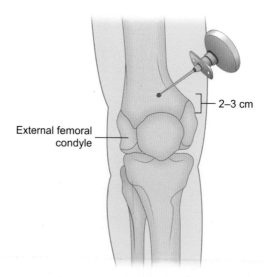

Fig. 8 Distal femoral IO insertion site. It is located approximately 2–3 cm above the superior border of the patella in the midline with the leg in extension

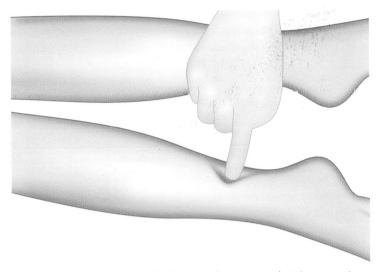

Fig. 9 Distal tibial IO insertion site. It is located approximately 1–2 cm superior to the malleoli in midline

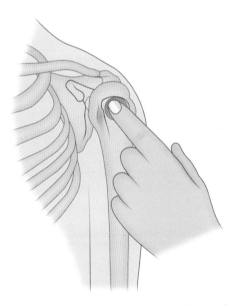

Fig. 10 Humeral IO insertion site. It is located at the greater tubercle of the proximal humerus

5. If the patient is conscious, use 1% lidocaine to infiltrate the skin, subcutaneous tissue and periosteum.
6. For the proximal tibial insertion site place the leg with knee extended in neutral position and then slightly externally rotate at the hip to expose the flat part of the tibial surface. Support the limb by placing a towel behind it during the insertion procedure (Fig. 11).

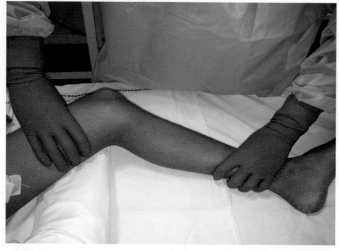

Fig. 11 Position of the patient for obtaining IO access at the proximal tibial site. Partially, flex the limb at knee joint and support it by placing a towel underneath it, then slightly externally rotate the limb at the hip joint

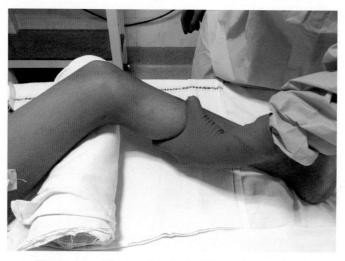

Fig. 12 Immobilization of the limb with non-dominant hand

Note: No portion of the stabilizing hand lies behind the insertion site

7. Check the device to ensure that the needle and the stylet are properly aligned and the stylet protrudes slightly beyond the end of the outer needle ready for insertion.

8. Immobilize the selected limb with the nondominant hand. Be cautious that no portion of the stabilizing hand should rest behind the insertion site (in order to avoid accidental injury to the practioner, if the IO needle passes through-and-through the bone) (Fig. 12).

9. Hold the needle in the dominant hand and position it at an angle of 90° to the skin at the marked site of insertion. In skeletally immature children, the needle is directed at a slight angle (10–15°) from vertical (caudad for the proximal tibia, cephalad for the distal tibia or femur) in order to avoid injury to the growth plate (Fig. 13).

10. Using a screwing action, apply pressure to the needle hub and gradually penetrate the skin, subcutaneous tissue and the periosteum. Avoid rocking the needle side-to-side, which may bend it or enlarge the access hole and lead to extravasation of fluid. Continue inserting the needle until a loss of resistance is felt, which indicates passage of needle through the cortex and into the marrow cavity.

11. Once the needle enters the marrow cavity, it will remain stable in an upright unsupported fashion. Now, remove the stylet, attach a 5 mL syringe and attempt aspiration. If blood/bone marrow is aspirated, then it indicates correct placement of the needle.

12. If no marrow is obtained on attempted aspiration, but the practitioner's clinical judgment is that the needle is correctly placed (loss of resistance was felt and the needle is standing in a stable unsupported position), then he/she should proceed to the next step and try flushing the needle.

13. Once proper placement is confirmed, a sterile 3-way tap is attached and the needle is flushed with 5–10 mL normal saline while observing for any extravasation (Some resistance to flushing is expected because, unlike a vein, the bone marrow cavity is not distensible).

14. Secure the needle with tape and a dressing that does not obscure the needle placement site so that infiltration can be rapidly detected.

15. Administer appropriate medications/fluids as prescribed.

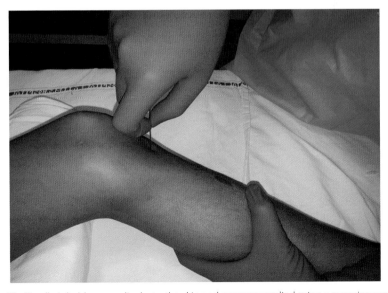

Fig. 13 Needle is held perpendicular to the skin and pressure applied using a screwing motion

Performing the Procedure Using a Powered Device Like EZ-IO

Steps

1–8 steps are same as in *Procedure using a Manual Device.*

9. Choose appropriate sized needle (mentioned in equipment section) and attach it to the drill.

10. Hold the drill with the attached needle at an angle of 90° to the skin. Apply pressure (without drilling) so that the needle penetrates the skin and reaches the bone (Fig. 14).

11. Now drill through the bone till there is a loss of resistance indicating penetration of the bony cortex.

12. Once the needle enters the marrow cavity, remove the drill and unscrew the stylet. Attach a 5 mL syringe and attempt to aspirate marrow.

Continue from stage 13 above.

POST-PROCEDURE CARE

The insertion site and the relevant limb should be observed frequently (at least hourly) for any signs of extravasation, leakage or development of compartment syndrome. If any of these complications are suspected, infusion or injection should be discontinued and removal of IO needle considered.

- *Duration of use:* IO cannulation provides rapid temporary vascular access. The optimal duration for which an IO access can be retained is a subject of controversy. However, it is advisable that the IO needle be replaced with a venous line as soon as possible and prolonged use beyond 24 hours should be avoided.

- *Removal of the IO needle*
  - Stop all the infusions through the IO needle and remove any device or dressing used to secure the needle to the skin.

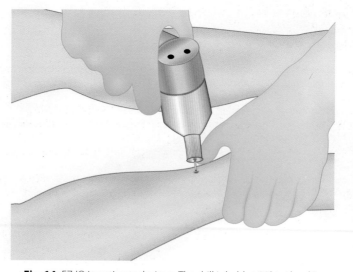

Fig. 14 EZ-IO insertion technique. The drill is held at 90° to the skin

 – Using gentle rotatory movements withdraw the needle smoothly.
 – Once the needle is removed, cover the insertion site with a sterile gauze pad and apply direct pressure.
 – After applying local pressure for several minutes, remove the gauze pad and cover the insertion site with a sterile dry dressing.

COMPLICATION/PROBLEM

- *Infection:* Osteomyelitis is a rare complication occurring in about 0.6% cases.[7] Most reported infections occur when the needle is left in situ for more than 24 hours.
- *Extravasation and compartment syndrome:* Through-and-through penetration of both anterior and posterior cortices caused by excess force after the needle has penetrated the cortex or rocking the needle side-to-side during insertion thus enlarging the access hole, in both these scenarios use of the needle will lead to fluid extravasation. Another cause of extravasation is incomplete placement of the needle or partial dislodgement of the needle. Extravasation, if unnoticed, may lead to a compartment syndrome.
  - *Prevention:* Care during insertion and avoiding excessive pressure and rocking movements during the insertion process. Proper fixation to avoid accidental dislodgement.
  - *Early recognition:* Careful evaluation of the access site and the limb after the saline flush and frequent reevaluations later during the use of the IO access.
  - *Management:* Immediate removal of the IO needle and careful observation of the limb.
- Use of excessive force or an inappropriately large needle or use of IO needle in an osteoporotic patient may rarely lead to fractures.
- There is a theoretical risk of injury to the growth plate during IO needle insertion in young children, if the needle is not appropriately directed.
- Other rare complications include skin necrosis, fat embolism, injury to mediastinal structures (in case of sternal needles).

REFERENCES

1. Voigt J, Waltzman M, Lottenberg L. Intraosseous vascular access for in-hospital emergency use: a systematic clinical review of the literature and analysis. Pediatr Emerg Care. 2012;28:185-99.
2. Fiser DH. Intraosseous Infusion. New Engl J Med. 1990;322(22):1579-81.
3. Tobias JD, Ross AK. Intraosseous infusions: a review for the anesthesiologist with a focus on pediatric use. Anesth Analg. 2010;110:391-401.
4. Fuchs S, LaCovey D, Paris P. A prehospital model of intraosseous infusion. Ann Emerg Med. 1991;20:371-4.
5. Banerjee S, Singhi SC, Singh S, Singh M. The intraosseous route is a suitable alternative to intravenous route for fluid resuscitation in severely dehydrated children. Indian Pediatr. 1994;31:1511-20.
6. Reades R, Studnek JR, Vandeventer S, Garrett J. Intraosseous versus intravenous vascular access during out-of-hospital cardiac arrest: a randomized controlled trial. Ann Emerg Med. 2011;58:509-16.
7. Rosetti VA, Thompson BM, Miller J, Mateer JR, Aprahamian C. Intraosseous infusion: an alternative route of pediatric intravascular access. Ann Emerg Med. 1985;14:885-8.

23
Umbilical Vascular Catheterization

Kirti M Naranje, Banani Poddar

INTRODUCTION

In neonates, especially in preterm babies, peripheral veins are commonly friable and finding an intravenous access is often difficult. Conventionally, placing a central line in a neonate is both exigent and difficult. Umbilical vascular catheterization provides potential surrogate site for vascular access in babies in first 14 days of life. The procedure of umbilical vascular catheterization is an imperative skill in the management of critically ill newborns. Both umbilical arterial catheter (UAC) and umbilical venous catheter (UVC) provide dependable and quick access to the vascular system of sick neonates.

INDICATION[1]

Umbilical Vein Catheterization

- Exchange transfusion
- Administration of fluids and parenteral nutrition especially hypertonic fluids
- Central venous pressure monitoring
- Administration of inotropes and other medications
- Delivery of blood and blood products
- Emergency vascular access during resuscitation
- Difficult to obtain peripheral access, babies less than 800 g
- Frequent blood sampling.

Umbilical Arterial Catheterization

- Exchange transfusion
- Frequent arterial blood gas sampling
- Continuous intra-arterial blood pressure monitoring
- Administration of fluid bolus and drugs (UVC preferred)
- Moderate-to-severe respiratory failure with more than 40% oxygen requirement.

CONTRAINDICATION

Contraindications are almost similar for both umbilical venous and arterial catheterizations.

Absolute

- Abdominal wall defects, e.g. omphalocele, gastroschisis, umbilical fistula
- Necrotizing enterocolitis (NEC), omphalitis, peritonitis
- Gastrointestinal surgery above the level of umbilicus.

Relative

- Vascular compromise in the lower limbs or gluteal region
- Hemorrhagic and thrombotic tendency
- Intestinal hypoperfusion
- Local infections.

APPLIED ANATOMY

During fetal development, umbilical arteries and vein form the major blood vessels that are responsible for circulation of blood from placenta to the fetus and vice versa. There are two umbilical arteries which wind around single umbilical vein and enter the abdomen at umbilicus. The umbilical vein is 2–3 cm in length and about 4–5 mm in diameter. It carries oxygenated blood from placenta to fetus. The umbilical arteries are smaller in size and carry deoxygenated blood from fetus to placenta. The umbilical vein travels alongside the falciform ligament upwards and reaches the base of liver. Here, it turns right and joins the left branch of portal vein after giving off several intrahepatic branches. The vein then connects with inferior vena cava (IVC) by means of ductus venosus which arises from the point where the umbilical and portal veins are united. The IVC then empties into right atrium. The umbilical arteries run caudally to enter internal iliac arteries prior to joining the aorta. Figure 1 illustrates the course of umbilical vessels.

The patency of the umbilical vein is maintained for approximately 7 days after birth. Umbilical arterial closure occurs before umbilical vein. They begin to constrict soon after birth and practically close within a few minutes of life. Nonetheless, they can be dilated and cannulated in the first few days of life. Consequently, the umbilical arteries transform into medial umbilical ligaments and the vein into the ligamentum teres hepatis.

TECHNIQUE AND EQUIPMENT

Umbilical vessels are embedded in Wharton's jelly (a gelatinous material present in the cord) and cannulation should be preferably attempted within first 3–4 days of life when umbilical stump is attached.

Umbilical Catheters (Fig. 2)

The size and material of catheter to be used should be determined. The size of catheter depends upon the birth weight of the baby (Table 1). For arterial catheterization, only single lumen catheters are used. Multilumen (double or

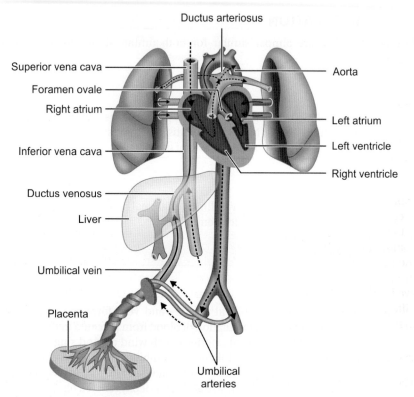

Fig. 1 Applied anatomy of umbilical vessels
Source: The Pediatric Anesthesia Handbook, 2nd edn.
Bell C, Kain ZN, Hughes C. Reprinted with permission. Copyright Elsevier

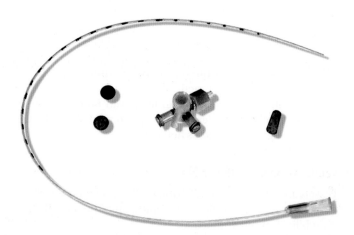

Fig. 2 A single lumen, 6 Fr umbilical catheter with tri-way connector
Courtesy: Vygon India Pvt Ltd

Table 1 Umbilical catheter size based on birth weight

Birth weight	UVC size
< 1500 g	3.5 Fr
1500–3500 g	5 Fr
> 3500 g	8 Fr
UAC size	
< 1200 g	3.5 Fr
≥ 1200 g	5 Fr

triple lumen) catheters are used exclusively for umbilical venous catheterization in critically ill neonates who require multiple simultaneous infusions. Multilumen catheters have the disadvantage of increasing the number of sites for possible contamination; hence the number of lumens should be restricted.[2] Except for the purpose of exchange transfusion, the catheters should not have side holes in order to lower the risk of thrombosis.[3] Most umbilical catheters currently available in market are made up of polyvinyl chloride (PVC). No clinically relevant differences were observed with heparin-bonded polyurethane over PVC catheters in reducing frequency of ischemia, NEC, aortic thrombosis or mortality.[4]

Depth of Insertion

There are various methods to determine the depth of insertion for umbilical catheter placement. These are mainly based on shoulder-umbilicus distance and baby's birth weight.[5,6]

Depth of Insertion for UVC

- *Based on shoulder-umbilicus distance:* The length in centimeters between infant's umbilicus and shoulder (from above the lateral end of clavicle) is measured and this length is applied to the graph shown in Figure 3 to obtain UVC insertion distance. Radiologically, the tip of the catheter should be located between 9th thoracic vertebrae and 10th thoracic vertebrae.
- *Based on birth weight:*
  $$\text{Depth for UVC insertion (cm)} = \frac{\text{Birth weight (kg)} \times 3 + 9}{2} + 1$$

Depth of Insertion for UAC

The tip of umbilical artery catheter can be high lying (when the tip of catheter is above the level of diaphragm) or low lying (when the tip of catheter is below the level of diaphragm). A high lying UAC is preferred over a low positioned UAC because of lower chances of ischemic and thrombotic events and longer duration of catheter use. Further, the incidence of intraventricular hemorrhage and NEC has not been found to be increased with a high positioned UAC.[7]

- *Based on shoulder-umbilicus distance:* The length in centimeters between infant's umbilicus and shoulder (from above the lateral end of clavicle) is measured and this length is applied to the graph shown in Figure 4 to obtain UAC insertion distance. A high lying UAC is located on a radiograph between

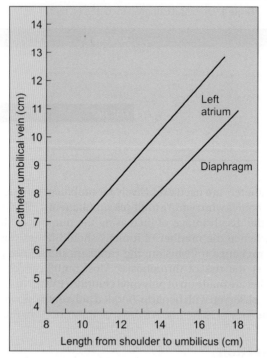

Fig. 3 Depth of insertion for umbilical venous catheterization. The tip of catheter should be located between the diaphragm and left atrium

Source: Adapted from Dunn PM. Localization of the umbilical catheter by postmortem measurement. Arch Dis Child. 1966;41(215):69-75. Reproduced with permission from BMJ Publishing Group

6th thoracic vertebrae and 9th thoracic vertebrae (in descending thoracic aorta above the origin of mesenteric and renal arteries), while a low positioned catheter is situated between 3rd lumbar vertebrae and 4th lumbar vertebrae.

- *Based on birth weight*
  High lying UAC:
  Depth of insertion (cm) = Birth weight (kg) × 3 + 9 + Length of umbilical stump
  Low lying UAC:
  $$\text{Depth of insertion (cm)} = \frac{\text{Birth weight (kg)} \times 3 + 9 + \text{Length of umbilical stump}}{2}$$

PREPARATION

- The parents should be explained about the procedure and written informed consent should be taken.
- Since the umbilical cord has no pain sensation, no specific sedation or analgesia is needed. Oral sucrose is an accepted option available to reduce pain during procedure. Lower limbs may be swaddled to soothe the baby. One should avoid skin while clamping or suturing.
- Continuous monitoring of the baby's cardiorespiratory status should be done throughout the procedure. The electrodes should be placed away from the abdomen.

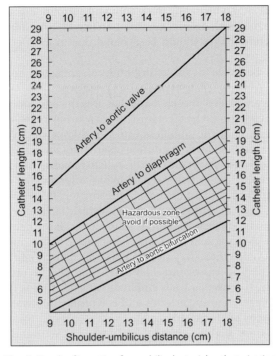

Fig. 4 Depth of insertion for umbilical arterial catheterization

Source: Adapted from Dunn PM. Localization of the umbilical catheter by postmortem measurements.
Arch Dis Child. 1966;41:69. Reproduced with permission from BMJ Publishing Group

- *Following equipment are required for the procedure:* Appropriate size umbilical catheter, curved iris forceps, straight artery forceps, surgical blade size 11, silk suture with needle size 3-0, needle holder, adhesive tapes, 2 cc and 5 cc syringes, three-way stopcock, sterile water, normal saline, sterile drape, sterile gauze pieces, heparin (10 units/mL), disinfectant of choice [chlorhexidine 0.1% solution (in babies < 1 kg); chlorhexidine 0.5% in alcohol 70% (in babies > 1 kg); povidone iodine], mask, gown and gloves.

PROCEDURE

- Baby's identity is confirmed before the start of procedure.
- Baby is kept in supine position and the arms and legs are restrained with the help of soft cotton ties or cloth. Care should be taken to avoid straining the baby's limbs.
- Absence of bruising of lower extremities and/or feet and toes should be ensured prior to placement of catheter.
- Insertion can be made easy by keeping saline soaked gauze on the umbilical stump for 30–60 minutes before the procedure. This is particularly useful when catheterization is tried after 24 hours of life.
- Strict aseptic technique must be adopted. Good hand hygiene along with maximum sterile barrier precautions must be employed.

- The umbilical stump including the clamp and surrounding skin of abdomen should be cleaned with disinfectant solution (e.g. chlorhexidine or povidone-iodine). Tincture iodine should be avoided due to its effects on neonate's thyroid gland.
- Care should be taken to avoid dribbling of antiseptic solution over the surrounding skin, especially in premature newborn.
- Sterile towels are placed in such a way that only the area around the stump is exposed and care should be taken to avoid obscuring infant's face.
- A tie is secured around the umbilicus with a loose knot which can be tightened, if there is unwarranted bleeding during insertion of the catheter.
- The cord is held tightly with the help of straight forceps just below the existing cord clamp. Using an 11 size surgical blade, it is then cut underneath the point of clasp with straight forceps, approximately 0.5–1 cm from the skin. This exposes a clean and smooth surface which facilitates visualization of umbilical vessels. Further, the cord is stabilized with the help of forceps. The lumen of the catheter is flushed with heparinized saline and air bubbles, if any, are removed. A three-way stopcock is applied to the end and locked.
- The three umbilical vessels are identified (Fig. 5). The arteries are small, round with thick, muscular walls and frequently protruding from the surface. The vein is bigger than the arteries and is typically thin-walled and often, a blood clot is seen on its cut surface.

Further steps are slightly different for umbilical vein and arterial catheterization.

Umbilical Vein Catheterization (Figs 6A to D)

- The opening of umbilical vein is dilated using iris forceps and blood clot, if any, is removed.
- The length of catheter to be inserted is predetermined and noted (Fig. 3). Using straight forceps catheter is grabbed 0.5–1 cm away from the tip and

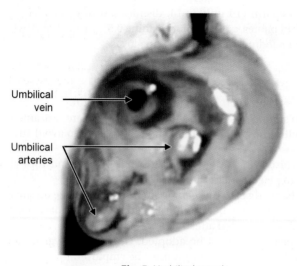

Umbilical vein

Umbilical arteries

Fig. 5 Umbilical vessels

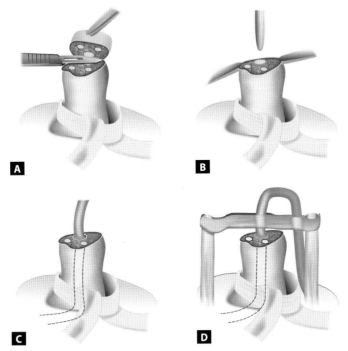

Figs 6A to D Schematic diagram showing umbilical vein catheterization
Courtesy: Dr Vibhor Borkar

introduced into the opening of vein. Further, the forceps is moved back to the catheter in the increments of 1–1.5 cm and the catheter is advanced into the vein in a cephalic direction.

- When the catheter is inserted up to approximately 4 cm, its intraluminal position is verified by drawing blood with syringe. The catheter is further advanced to the predetermined length. Once in position, patency is confirmed by good blood flow and absence of resistance to flushing with saline.
- For emergency resuscitative purpose, the catheter is advanced only 3–5 cm (in term infant), until there is good blood return.
- Care should be taken to avoid repeated probing and excessive pressure to prevent creation of false passage and damage to the vessel. If there is resistance, then catheter may be pulled back slightly and advanced by rotating clockwise.

Umbilical Arterial Catheterization

- The length of catheter to be inserted is predetermined depending upon high and low position (Fig. 4).
- The tip of toothless iris forceps is closed and inserted about 0.5 cm into one of the arteries in order to dilate its opening.
- The catheter is grasped with iris forceps and introduced into opening of the artery and advanced into the vessel using firm steady motion. It may be facilitated by applying mild gentle upward traction to the cord towards infant's head.

- As with UVC, once the catheter is inserted about 4–5 cm, its intraluminal position is checked by withdrawing the blood. The catheter is further advanced until desired length.
- Once in position, its patency is verified by good blood return, pulsatile blood flow and lack of resistance to flushing.
- Heparin may be added in low doses (0.5–1.0 U/mL) to the fluid infused through UAC. A solution of 0.45% NaCl with 0.5–1 IU heparin/mL is frequently used at the rate of 1 mL/hour for this purpose.

Securing the Umbilical Catheters

- Both the umbilical vein and artery catheters are secured separately with the help of silk sutures.
- The catheter is secured with the help of purse-string sutures going through Wharton's jelly and keeping away from skin. Both ends of suture are wrapped in opposite direction around the vessel and tied.
- Using tape, the catheter is secured using sleek "goalposts" method (Fig. 6D).[8]
- Finally, the correct position of the umbilical catheter is confirmed by radiographic examination prior to infusing fluids. A radiograph is not obligatory when catheterization is done in emergency situations for resuscitation of newborn.

POST-PROCEDURE CARE

- The baby`s vitals are noted post-procedure and hemodynamic stability is ensured. The baby is nursed in supine or lateral position.
- Care should be taken to avoid traction to the catheter at any time. Umbilical stump should not be covered.
- The umbilical tie is removed.
- Ongoing observation is required daily to note any signs of complications.
- Once the catheter is no longer required or when there is evidence of complications, it should be removed at the earliest. Optimal duration of umbilical venous catheter is up to 14 days while for arterial catheter it is 5–7 days.

COMPLICATION/PROBLEM

Umbilical vessel catheterization is an invasive procedure and a variety of complications are associated with it. The procedure of catheter insertion, catheter location, number of manipulations, catheter care, catheter size and type and the duration of catheter remaining in situ are some of the important factors affecting the occurrence of complications.[2]

With Both Umbilical Venous and Arterial Catheterization[9]

- Accidental line dislodgement
- Vessel perforation
- Air embolism
- Hemorrhage
- Catheter-related bloodstream infections
- Thrombosis and subsequent embolism.

Specific Complications Associated with Umbilical Venous Catheterization

- Hepatic necrosis related to infusions of hypertonic fluids to liver due to wrongly positioned line
- Perforation of peritoneum and colon
- Necrotizing enterocolitis
- Digital ischemia
- Portal vein thrombosis and portal hypertension
- Cardiac complications include arrhythmias, endocarditis and pericardial effusion and tamponade, if the catheter tip is wrongly placed high in right atrium.

Specific Complications Associated with Umbilical Arterial Catheterization

- Visceral infarction due to thrombosis of major branches of aorta
- Necrotizing enterocolitis
- Hypertension
- Intestinal perforation
- Vasospasm and lower limb ischemia
- Hypoglycemia or hyperglycemia
- Renal insufficiency
- *Less common complications:*[6] Intraventricular hemorrhage due to retrograde blood flow, sciatic nerve injury, paraplegia, transaction of omphalocele, Wharton's jelly embolus and injury to bladder.

REFERENCES

1. The College of Respiratory Therapists of Ontario [Online]. Ontario: Clinical best practice guidelines; Central Access: Umbilical Artery and Vein Cannulation; October 2008. Available from *www.crto.on.ca/pdf/PPG/Umbilical_CBPG.pdf* (Accessed 4th October 2013).
2. Nash P. Umbilical catheters, placement, and complication management. J Infus Nurs. 2006;29(6):346-52.
3. Barrington KJ. Umbilical artery catheters in the newborn: effects of catheter design (end vs side hole). Cochrane Database Syst Rev. 2002;(2):CD000508.
4. Barrington KJ. Umbilical artery catheters in the newborn: effects of catheter materials. Cochrane Database Syst Rev. 2000;(2):CD000949.
5. Dunn PM. Localization of the umbilical catheter by post-mortem measurement. Arch Dis Child. 1966;41(215):69-75.
6. Anderson J, Leonard D, Braner DA, Lai S, Tegtmeyer K, et al. Videos in clinical medicine. Umbilical vascular catheterization. N Engl J Med. 2008;359(15):e18.
7. Barrington KJ. Umbilical artery catheters in the newborn: effects of position of the catheter tip. Cochrane Database Syst Rev. 2002;(2):CD000505.
8. Umbilical Venous Catheterisation of the Newborn. The Royal Children's Hospital, Melbourne. [Online] Available from HYPERLINK *"http://www.rch.org.au/ uploadedFiles/Main/Content/neonatal_rch/clinical_practice_guidelines/UVC% 252525252520Newborn(2).pdf"* and *http://www.rch.org.au/uploadedFiles/Main/ Content/neonatal_rch/clinical_practice_guidelines/UVC%20Newborn(2).pdf* (Accessed 8th October 2013).
9. Roberts and Hedges. Clinical Procedures in Emergency Medicine. 4th edition. Saunders, An. Imprint of Elsevier. 2004.

24

Arterial Blood Sampling and Cannulation

Afzal Azim, Saurabh Saigal

INTRODUCTION

Invasive arterial line cannulation is most commonly inserted for beat to beat blood pressure (BP) measurement. It is a procedure performed frequently in critical care units and in patients undergoing surgery under anesthesia. Insertion of arterial line needs practice and experience. The radial artery is the most common site of arterial line insertion. This artery is preferred because of its superficial location, easily accessibility which makes it compressible for hemostasis. The brachial, ulnar, dorsalis pedis, axillary, posterior tibial and femoral arteries are other options.

INDICATION[1,2]

For Arterial Blood Gas Sampling

- Management of patients with severe acid/base disturbances
- Patients with respiratory distress
- In primary evaluation of any critically ill patient.

For Arterial Cannulation

- Continuous, beat-to-beat arterial BP measurement for hemodynamically unstable patients requiring vasoactive drugs
- Any patient who may require frequent (more than 4) blood gases in a day
- Measurement of cardiac output and functional hemodynamic parameters which are derived from the arterial waveform like pulse pressure variation (PPV), systolic pressure variation (SPV) or pulse contour analysis and stroke volume variation (SVV)
- Hypertensive emergencies (when patient on intravenous vasodilators)
- Situations associated with fallacies of pulse oximetry monitoring
- Difficult conditions for noninvasive BP monitoring (morbidly obese patient cuff too small for that limb; burned extremities)
- Patients on mechanical ventilation (may be relative indication)
- Transportation of sick patients (may be relative indication).

CONTRAINDICATION[1,2]

- Infection over the insertion site
- Severe peripheral vascular disease in the selected artery
- Severe coagulopathy
- Thromboangiitis obliterans
- Patients with history of Raynaud's phenomenon.

APPLIED ANATOMY

Before the insertion of a radial arterial line modified Allen's test is recommended. The test is used to determine collateral circulation of hand between the radial and ulnar arteries. The poor collateral perfusion is said to be present in 12% population.[1] If perfusion to ulnar artery is poor and a cannula occludes the radial artery, blood flow to the hand may be reduced. The test is performed by asking the patient to clench his hand. The ulnar and radial arteries are together occluded with digital pressure. The hand is subsequently unclenched and pressure over the ulnar artery is released. If there is adequate collateral circulation, the palm should flush in less than 6 seconds.[1,3] In practice the usefulness of this test is questionable in patients with altered sensorium and patients on sedation and paralysis. The Doppler ultrasound can be used for evaluation of collateral hand perfusion to stratify risk of potential ischemic injury from arterial cannulation.

TECHNIQUE AND EQUIPMENT

The first arterial blood vessel cannulation was performed by Stephen Hales in 1714. The first description of arterial cannulation was given in 1856 when femoral artery was cannulated for recording BP. Peterson et al. in 1949 first described the continuous recording of arterial blood pressure (BP) by plastic catheters for perioperative patients. In 1953, Sven Seldinger described the catheter-over-wire technique which is now widely practiced.[4]

Techniques of Radial Arterial Line Insertion

The most common arterial site cannulated for invasive BP monitoring is radial artery. In severe shock/hypotensive state, requiring high dose vasopressors, femoral artery could be considered for cannulation. The comparison between various sites can be seen in Table 1. There are three common insertion techniques.

Direct Cannulation

The wrist extension brings the artery closer to the surface, the wrist in this position is stabilized either with tape or with the aid of an assistant which makes the insertion easier. The radial artery is palpated. The cannula is inserted aiming to hit the middle of the artery at an angle of approximately 30–45° to the skin. When there is free flow of arterial blood back into the hub of the cannula, the cannula sheath is advanced over the needle into the artery.

Table 1 Comparison of sites for arterial cannulation

	Radial	Brachial	Femoral	Axillary	Dorsalis pedis artery
Ease	Relatively easy but difficult in hypotensive and vasoconstricted patients	Relatively easy in hypotensive patient	Easy cannulation even in hypotensive patient	Easy cannulation in hypotensive patients but may be technically difficult	Relatively easy
Neural injuries	Carpal tunnel syndrome	Damage to median nerve	Common femoral nerve injury	Brachial plexus injury	Deep peroneal nerve injury
Thrombus formation	High risk because of small lumen	High risk	Less risk	Less risk	High risk
Accuracy	Less accurate	Less accurate	More reliable	Most reliable due to proximity to aortic arch	Less accurate

Transfixation

After obtaining a blood flashback, cannula is further advanced through the posterior wall of the artery. The needle is removed and the cannula is slowly withdrawn while looking for free flow. Once free flow is achieved, the cannula is advanced proximally along the artery. The "transfixion technique" of deliberately advancing the needle/cannula through both sides of the artery and then withdrawing it again until blood flows up the cannula runs the risk of causing a false aneurysm or a hematoma around the artery and is usually not recommended.

Guidewire (Seldinger) Technique

In patients especially with atheromatous disease, a guidewire may be used. As advancement of cannula sheath over the needle proves difficult in such patients. The guidewire is inserted through the cannula sheath after removal of the cannula needle (or through needles which are provided in some arterial cannulation sets). The guidewire should freely advance along the artery. The cannula sheath is advanced along the artery, and the guidewire is then removed.

Interpretation of Arterial Pressure Waveform

Once inserted into the artery, a continuous arterial waveform trace is displayed at all times. This finally confirms that the invasive arterial BP monitoring is set up correctly (see details in chapter *Transducer and Pressure Monitoring*). *A typical waveform (Fig. 1) is described as follows:*

- *Peak systolic pressure:* Opening of the aortic valve leads to ejection of the blood from left ventricle into aorta which leads to a sharp uprising in the tracing which is referred as peak systolic pressure. Any changes noted in the stroke volume are reflected in the peak systolic pressure.

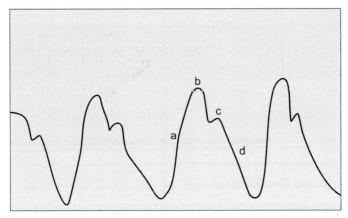

Fig. 1 Arterial waveform (a: Systolic upstroke; b: Peak systolic pressure;
c: Dicrotic notch; d: Diastolic run off)

- *Dicrotic notch:* As the pressure falls in the left ventricle, the aortic valve closes and the aorta subsequently relaxes. The closure and relaxation of the aorta is seen on the arterial tracing as dicrotic notch. This marks the end of systole and the onset of diastole.
- *Diastolic pressure:* The diastolic pressure represents the amount of vasoconstriction in arterial system. Any changes in vascular compliance are reflected in the diastolic pressure. During diastole, blood moves in the arterial system and onward into the smaller arteriole branches. There must be adequate time for this to occur, if the heart rate is faster and the diastolic time is shortened, there is less time for movement of blood into the smaller arteriolar branches.
- *Pulse pressure:* The difference between the systolic and diastolic pressure is called the pulse pressure.

  Apart from BP measurement, the shape of the waveform gives further useful information.
- *Myocardial contractility:* Myocardial contractility is indicated by the rate of change of pressure by unit time (dP/dt), i.e. the slope of the arterial upstroke.[1]
- *Hypovolemia:* This is characterized by a narrow arterial waveform and low dicrotic notch. If the patient is ventilated the peak pulse pressure wave varies with intermittent positive-pressure ventilation (IPPV) breaths (also called an *arterial swing*).[1]

Peripheral and Central Arterial Waveforms

Waveforms from a peripheral artery (the radial artery) are different from an aortic trace. A peripheral arterial trace has a higher peak systolic pressure, wider pulse pressure and prominent dicrotic notch. The systolic BP in the dorsalis pedis artery is higher than in the radial artery, which is higher than in the aorta. The primary reason is that peripheral arteries being smaller and less compliant are thereby less distensible than central arteries.[1]

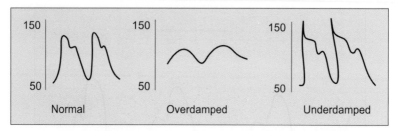

Fig. 2 Different types of arterial waveform

Damping and Resonance

The damping and resonance distorts the arterial waveform and leads to inaccurate recording of systolic and diastolic pressures. The mean arterial pressure (MAP) is constant and is not affected by the same. (See details in chapter on *Transducer and Pressure Monitoring* in this book).

- *Damping:* The restriction in the transmission of the arterial pulse pressure to the diaphragm of the transducer leads to damping. The waveform is smoothened without any sharp changes being displayed (Fig. 2). This type of trace underestimates the systolic BP but overestimates diastolic BP. Causes of damping are: air bubble, catheter kinks, overly compliant and distensible tubing, clots, injection ports, low flush bag pressure or no fluid in the flush bag, improper scaling.
- *Resonance:* The oscillating system which comprises of transducer, diaphragm and saline column in the arterial measurement system oscillates at maximum amplitude to an alternating external driving force (such as the arterial pressure). This trace over estimates systolic BP, and under estimate diastolic BP (Fig. 2). The causes of resonance includes: overly stiff noncompliant tubing, long tubing, increased vascular resistance, reverberations in tubing causing harmonics that distort the trace (i.e. high systolic and low diastolic).

Arterial Cannulae

Arterial cannulae are made of Teflon to minimize the risk of thrombosis. These are short and with narrow lumen to minimize the effect on blood flow distally. 20 G (pink) cannula is used in adult patients, a 22 G (blue) for children, and a 24 G (yellow) for neonates and small babies. The cannula is connected to an arterial pressure transducer kit (see details in chapter on *Transducer and Pressure Monitoring* in this book).

PREPARATION

- *Asepsis:* The Center for Disease Control and Prevention (CDC) and the Healthcare Infection Control Practices Advisory Committee (HICPAC) updated guidelines for the prevention of intravascular catheter-related bloodstream infections published in 2011. Use of a cap, mask, sterile gloves, and fenestrated drape is recommended.
- For femoral arterial cannulation full patient drapes should be used and the operator should wear full sterile gown similar to central venous cannulation.

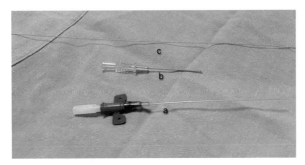

Fig. 3 Parts of arterial cannula: (a) Catheter; (b) Needle; (c) Guidewire

- *Equipment needed for arterial blood sampling:* Blood gas syringe, 5 mL syringe, needle size 23 G; liquid heparin flush: 0.05 mL of 1,000 IU/mL concentration of heparin for per mL of blood drawn (e.g. 0.1 mL of 1,000 IU/mL of heparin for 2 mL of blood sample).
- *Equipment for arterial cannulation:* Arterial cannulae (Fig. 3), arterial pressure transducing kit.
- *Other equipment:* Local anesthetic (1% lidocaine), suture material for femoral line (2-0 silk), scissors, chlorhexidine for site preparation, drapes to keep the site sterile, tapes for positioning of hand, towel or arm board for dorsiflexion of hand.

PROCEDURE

Arterial Blood Sampling

Sampling by an Arterial Puncture
- Explain procedure to patient
- *Site selection and position (radial/brachial/femoral):* Radial artery over the wrist is usually preferred site, due to ease of puncture due to underlying bone structures. Prefer nondominant hand for radial artery punctures. Modified Allen's test may be done to ensure patency of the ulnar circulation, before radial artery is punctured
- Part preparation with 2% chlorhexidine with 70% alcohol
- The hand is positioned in 30–60 degrees of dorsiflexion with the aid of a roll gauze and arm-band, avoiding hyperabduction of thumb
- Palpate the vessel
- Around 0.5 mL of lidocaine is infiltrated on both sides of artery through a 25 G or smaller needle. Aspirate prior to injection just to make sure that you have not entered the vessel
- *Puncture technique:* Hold the heparinized syringe-needle assembly (Fig. 4)
- Slowly insert the needle and after skin puncture. Once the artery is hit, the blood is seen in needle hub and then gently apply a slight negative pressure and the syringe fills in quickly
- Another technique to insert needle all the way till it hits the bone, and then to slowly retract it till syringe starts filling

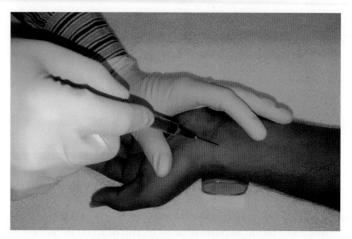

Fig. 4 Technique of arterial puncture

- *Is the sample obtained arterial:* Flashing pulsation when blood enters hub of the needle, syringe autofilling without withdrawal effort. Under normal conditions arterial blood is bright red in color, but color may be altered when oxygenation is poor
- *Sample handling:* After sampling, needle is quickly retracted, and sealed to prevent contact with air. Also, remove air/air bubble, if any from the syringe
- *Post-sampling compression:* Immediately after needle is withdrawn digital pressure is applied for 3–5 minutes.

Sampling by Existing Arterial Line

Prior to taking blood sample from the arterial line, ensure patency of arterial line, i.e. the pressure in pressure bag is raised up to 300 mm Hg, the tubing from the arterial cannula site to the three-way tap is clear and the arterial line flushes easily.

- *Universal precautions:* Sterile gloves has to be worn
- Insert a 5 mL syringe into the three-way tap, subsequently turn the tap OFF to the flush solution and slowly withdraw 5 mL of blood. Susequently discard both syringe and blood
- Next step turn the three-way tap OFF half way between transducer line and syringe (after doing this, the tap will be susequently closed to all directions)
- Insert a new empty syringe into three-way tap. Turn the tap OFF to flush solution, gently apply a negative pressure and blood will slowly fill into the syringe. At the same time observe for any perfusion changes in limb distal to cannula site
- Turn three-way tap OFF to patient and remove the syringe. Thereafter flush the line, using flushing device, with ensuring that the arterial line and three-way stopcock are clear of blood

- Replace the needle or stopper on the blood gas syringe
- Remove air/air bubble, if any from the syringe
- The sample has to be analyzed in arterial blood gas (ABG) machine.

Arterial Cannulation

- Always ensure that transducer along with pressure tubing is connected to the bedside monitor
- *Position of hand:* The wrist is extended and radial artery is palpated, over the distal radius where it is most superficial. For this position the arm is restrained in palm up position, with an arm-board to hold the wrist dorsiflexed (Fig. 5)
- It is prudent to place an absorbent pad underneath the arm, particularly if the Seldinger approach is going to be employed
- *Aseptic precautions:* Wash hands and wear sterile gown and gloves. Cleanse area selected for arterial line placement (0.5% chlorhexidine with alcohol or 2% chlorhexidine) (Fig. 6). Cover the area with sterile fenestrated sheet
- Apply anesthetic agent (local lignocaine 1–2%) (Fig. 7)
- Locate pulsating artery via palpation
- The artery is stabilized by pulling the skin taut
- The skin is punctured at 30–45 degrees for radial artery; 90 degrees for femoral artery (Fig. 8)
- As the flash of blood is observed in the catheter, gently insert the guidewire through the catheter (Fig. 9)
- Gently advance the catheter over the guidewire
- Once the catheter is advanced, gradually withdraw the guidewire
- Connect the catheter to high pressure tubing and thereafter check for arterial waveform on the bedside monitor
- Clean the concerned area of any blood and allow it to dry
- Secure the arterial cannula with suture (Fig. 10)
- All the intravenous sharps and other used materials are to be disposed off.

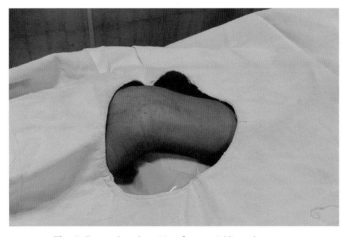

Fig. 5 Proper hand position for arterial line placement

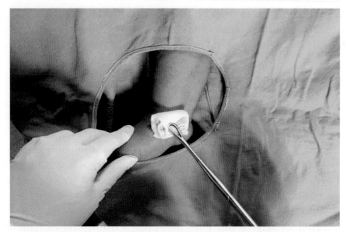

Fig. 6 Painting and draping at the site of radial arterial line insertion

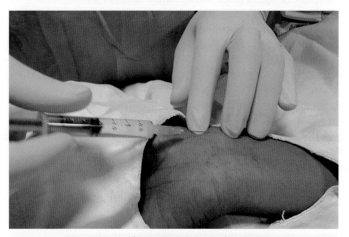

Fig. 7 Local infiltration at the site of cannulation

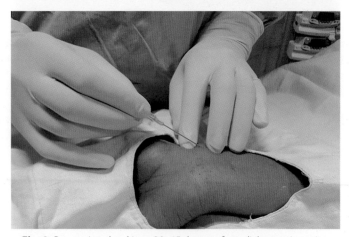

Fig. 8 Puncturing the skin at 30–45 degrees for radial artery insertion

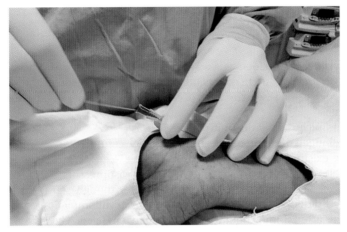

Fig. 9 Guidewire inserted through the arterial cannula

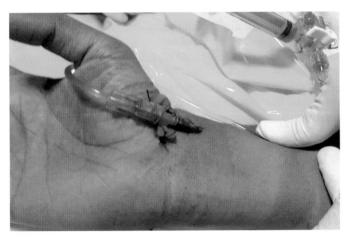

Fig. 10 Securing an arterial catheter

POST-PROCEDURE CARE

- Transparent dressing to be applied; dressing to be kept for 5–7 days but if any oozing, bleeding from site and if the dressing is soiled then it has to be removed
- Arterial lines are normally flushed with normal saline and in special circumstances heparin with concentration 2 U/mL which runs at 1–3 mL/hr. There is a three way-cock which regulates the flow from this pressurized bag to the arterial line, and has a sampling port through with sample is withdrawn
- Avoid contamination of the infusion system
- If catheter gets blocked due to clot it should not be flushed
- Daily inspection of site. If any indications, of compromised tissue perfusion in form of digital ischemia then it has to be removed
- Routine replacement of arterial catheters should be avoided
- Daily review must be there whether this patient needs an arterial line or not.

COMPLICATION/PROBLEM[1,2,5]

- *Inaccuracy:* Most common complication is inaccuracy as a result of damping effects
- *Hemorrhage:* Its incidence is 0.5%; this may occur if leaks in the system are there. To prevent this all connections must be tightly secured
- Partial occlusion is seen in (20%) of cases. The risk factors for partial occlusion include:
    - Multiple pricks at the time of insertion
    - Prolonged duration of use and large gauge cannula
    - Pre-existing vascular disease
    - Prolonged hypotension along with use of vasopressors.
- *Infection:* Local infection is common (0.7%), though sepsis secondary to infected radial arterial line is rare. Any sign of inflammation at the arterial site, the arterial line should be immediately changed. The risk of infection and permanent arterial occlusion becomes greater after an artery has been cannulated for more than 72 hours. The site chosen for arterial line placement does not seem to influence the rate of infection
- *Embolism:* Thrombo or air-emboli may occur. Extreme care should be taken to aspirate air bubbles and blood clots
- Accidental drug injection may cause severe, irreversible damage to the hand. *To prevent this:*
    - None of the drugs should be injected via arterial line
    - The arterial line should be labeled in red to reduce the likelihood of this occurring.
- Pseudoaneurysms are rarely reported (<0.1%). An important risk factor for these complications is the duration of use.

REFERENCES

1. Hignett R, Stephens R. Radial arterial lines: a practical procedure. Br J Hosp Med. 2006;67(5):M86-8.
2. Respiratory Therapy Services St. Joseph's Health Care London. (2000). Arterial Line Insertion Self Learning Package. [online] Available from http://rtboardreview.com/public/web_links/legacy/Artline_(St._Josephs_Health_Care_London).pdf. [Accessed March, 2015].
3. Wilkins RG. Radial artery cannulation and ischemic damage: a critical review. Anaesthesia. 1985;40(9):896-9.
4. RWD Nickalls. (2009). Supporting technologies—arterial line. [online] Available from http://www.nickalls.org/dick/papers/thoracic/hand-artline.pdf. [Accessed March, 2015].
5. Sheer BV, Parel A, Pfeiffer UJ. Clinical review: complications and risk factors of peripheral arterial catheters used for haemodynamic monitoring in anaesthesia and intensive care medicine. Crit Care. 2002;6:199-204.

25

Pulmonary Artery Catheterization

Puneet Goyal

INTRODUCTION

Pulmonary artery catheterization (PAC) is an easy and rapid technique for bedside hemodynamic monitoring in critically ill patients. Adequate training and expertise is required for this procedure to avoid associated complications and also for correct interpretation and analysis of hemodynamic data obtained with its use. Numerous randomized trials have shown that routine use of these catheters is not indicated and their use has been declining further with the availability and increasing use of noninvasive imaging modalities like transthoracic echocardiography, which can help in determining the cardiac preload and contractility and guide you in decision making for fluid therapy. However, clinical conditions and circumstances exist, which necessitate the use of pulmonary artery (PA) catheter, but only by physicians experienced in its use. Many clinicians are proficient in floating PA catheter; beginners should first observe PAC several times and then float first few catheters under supervision of a skilled and experienced clinician.

INDICATION

Cardiac Conditions

- Cardiogenic shock requiring inotropic or other supportive therapy
- Discordant left or right heart failure
- Severe chronic heart failure requiring inotropic, vasopressor or vasodilator therapy
- Potentially reversible heart failure like peripartum cardiomyopathy or myocarditis
- Evaluation and drug titration of severe pulmonary arterial hypertension
- Workup for heart transplantation

Non-cardiac Conditions

- Refractory acute respiratory distress syndrome or pulmonary edema, especially in presence of renal failure

- Refractory hypoxemia requiring high levels of positive end-expiratory pressure (PEEP)
- Refractory sepsis with hemodynamic instability
- Hemodynamically unstable patient unresponsive to conventional medical therapy.

CONTRAINDICATION

Absolute

- Tricuspid or pulmonic valvular stenosis
- Right atrial (RA) or right ventricular (RV) mass (e.g. tumor or thrombus)
- Tetralogy of Fallot (PA catheter in RV outflow tract can stimulate and produce infundibular spasm and, thereby hypercyanotic spell)

Relative

- High-grade arrhythmias, especially left bundle branch block, as PA catheter tip can cause transient right bundle branch block, thereby precipitating complete heart block
- Coagulopathy not only increases the risk of bleeding during central venous access but also increases the risk of endobronchial hemorrhage with catheter in PA
- Newly inserted pacemaker wires. Pacemaker wires get firmly embedded in endocardium/myocardium in 4–6 weeks after their insertion. Before this time, there is risk of dislodgement during PA catheter insertion or withdrawal.

APPLIED ANATOMY

Percutaneous central venous cannulation is a mandatory requirement before one can float PA catheter. An introducer sheath needs to be inserted into one of the major veins. Factors considered for preference of sites are as follows:

- *Right internal jugular vein (IJV):* It is the most preferred site for floating PA catheter for following reasons:
  - It has the shortest and the most straight path to enter into the right heart
  - Fairly constant relationship of anatomic structures, so high success rate
  - Right cupula of the lung is lower than left, so less chances of pneumothorax than on left IJV or subclavian vein.
- *Left subclavian vein:* Pulmonary artery catheter does not pass at an acute angle to enter inside superior vena cava (SVC), whereas if one chooses to use right subclavian or left IJV, the anatomy requires the catheter to bend at acute angle before entering SVC. This makes the left subclavian vein, the site of second choice for PA catheter insertion (remember cardiologists choosing this site for insertion of pacemaker wires).
- *Femoral veins:* These sites are distant from heart and passing a catheter into right heart may be quite difficult. They may be preferred, if the risk of bleeding is too high as vessels can be easily compressed at these sites.

TECHNIQUE AND EQUIPMENT

Werner Frossman, first demonstrated that right heart catheterization is possible in humans in 1929, by introducing a catheter into his own heart, although this was introduced only into right atrium. Andre Cournand and Dickinson Richards made catheter that was advanced into PA. Balloon tipped flow directed PA catheters were developed by HJC Swan and Dr William Ganz in 1970. These catheters could be floated into pulmonary arteries at bedside without the need of fluoroscopy. On their name, these balloon floatation PA catheters are popularly known as Swan-Ganz catheter.

Out of three described approaches to right IJV cannulation (middle, anterior or high and posterior) middle approach is preferred in most of the cases.

One has to locate the apex of the triangle formed by the lateral border of the sternal head of sternocleidomastoid (SCM) and medial border of clavicular head of SCM, also the medial one-third of clavicle forming the base of triangle. IJV is anterolateral to carotid artery at this point (Figs 1 and 2).

Equipment

Pulmonary artery catheter is a multi lumen catheter and is typically 110 cm long, with markings at every 10 cm interval (Fig. 3). The outer diameter of PA catheter can be 7.0, 7.5 or 8.0 Fr, depending upon the type of catheter and manufacturer (Fig. 4A). Distal most lumen is PA lumen which opens at tip of catheter. There is a balloon, situated just proximal to the tip, which has capacity of 1.5 mL. A thermistor is situated few centimeters proximal to the tip, which measures change in temperature to measure cardiac output. There are two additional lumens, opening at approximately 20 cm and 30 cm from tip, which open in right ventricle, right atrium or SVC, depending upon the size of right heart.

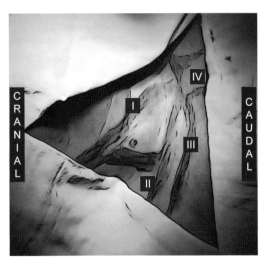

Fig. 1 Anatomic landmarks for right internal jugular vein cannulation, showing the triangle formed by sternal head of sternocleidomastoid (I), clavicular head of sternocleidomastoid (II), and medial one-third of clavicle (III). Also note the sternal notch (IV), and puncture site, marked by a dot at the apex of the triangle

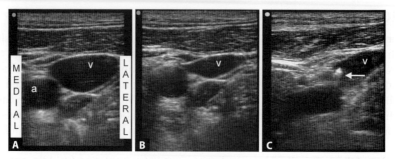

Figs 2A to C (A) Ultrasound image of right carotid artery "a" and right internal jugular vein "v", note anterolateral position of right internal jugular vein in relation to right carotid artery; (B) Internal jugular vein gets compressed with gentle pressure application by ultrasound transducer; (C) Guidewire (a bright white spot, shown as arrow) is seen inside right internal jugular vein

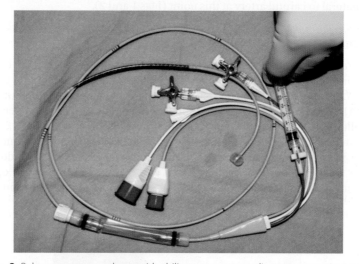

Fig. 3 Pulmonary artery catheter with ability to measure cardiac output continuously
Note that balloon is being checked by inflating with 1.5 mL safety syringe

These lumens can be used to measure central venous pressure (CVP) and RA pressures and to infuse vasoactive drugs and medications. Two additional ports have sensors attached to their proximal ends, which are connected to respective cables to calculate temperature change and cardiac output. Many PA catheters are especially equipped for monitoring cardiac output or mixed venous oxygen saturation continuously. Pacing PA catheter has a port or built in electrode for RV pacing (so far, not available in India) and other specialized catheters can provide data about RV function as well.

PREPARATION

- Written informed consent from patient or family members, if possible should be taken. Many a times, it is performed as an emergency procedure, in that scenario try to explain the risks and benefit of it to the family members. If consent is implied, it needs to be documented. An alternate venous access should be available before the procedure.

- *Monitoring and patient care during procedure:* Electrocardiogram (ECG), oxygen saturation (SpO_2) and blood pressure (BP) monitoring is mandatory during procedure. Oxygen supplementation should be provided to the patient, if on spontaneous breathing.
- *Arrangement of adjunct equipment:* Pressure transducer, connected to monitor with transducer lead at one end and to pressure monitoring line at other end. De-aired with heparinized saline, mounted in a stand at the level of heart and then zeroed.
- Wear cap, mask and eyeshield, scrub and, wear sterile gown and gloves. Maintain sterile technique throughout the procedure. Entire neck, clavicular area and shoulder are painted with povidone-iodine solution and left to dry for at least 3 minutes. Drape the area with adequate sized sterile sheet so as to cover the patient, bed and have optimum space to manipulate guidewire and PA catheter.
- Check the size of PA catheter and introducer sheath. Size of PA catheter is usually 7.5 Fr and that of introducer sheath is 8.5 Fr and they usually come together but in separate packages (Figs 4A and B). It is a good practice to check the sizes before opening the sterile packing.
- *Preparation of introducer and PA catheter:* Arrange introducer sheath with the dilator inside and a three ways attached to side port of sheath (Figs 5A and B). PA catheter, taken out of packing with its curvature undisturbed. Three ways attached to CVP and RA ports and flushed with heparinized saline. Pressure transducer attached to PA port (most distal) and flushed with heparinized saline to bring all the air bubbles out. Check balloon by inflating with 1.5 mL air with the help of safety syringe provided with pack (Fig. 3), and then allow it to deflate on its own, avoid pulling syringe plunger to deflate balloon. Locking mechanism is provided at the proximal end of balloon port to keep balloon inflated during catheter insertion. (*Note:* very important to inflate the balloon with the prescribed amount of air and only with the help of safety syringe provided for this purpose). Thread the protective sleeve over the distal end of catheter with paying attention that docking mechanism is facing in right direction so that it fits with the proximal end of sheath, as shown in Figure 3.

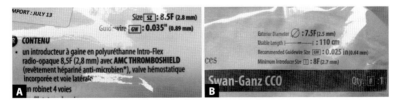

Figs 4A and B Snapshots from packages of introducer sheath and pulmonary artery catheter. (A) Size of introducer sheath (8.5 Fr); (B) Size of pulmonary artery catheter (7.5 Fr)

Note that minimum, 8 Fr sized introducer sheath is needed to float PA catheter of 7.5 Fr size

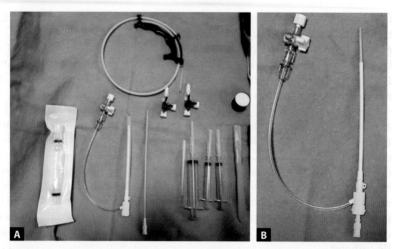

Figs 5A and B (A) Introducer kit with puncture needle, guidewire, introducer sheath and dilator and protective sleeve; (B) Position of dilator inside the sheath and three ways attached to side port

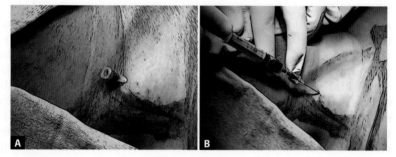

Figs 6A and B (A) Position of pilot needle at apex of triangle, note that venous blood is not oozing out of hub of needle; (B) Direction of puncture needle, pointing toward ipsilateral nipple (not shown in figure)

PROCEDURE

- *Position of the patient:* Supine or 15–20° Trendelenburg's position, with head turned to left side. Small pillow or a folded sheet underneath the shoulders is helpful in case of short neck individuals.
- Feel the carotid pulse at the apex of triangle (described above), in between two heads of SCM, try to retract the carotid artery little medially using fingers of left hand and make a pilot puncture just lateral to carotid using 22 G needle. Needle should be making an angle of 45° with the skin and directed toward ipsilateral nipple. If the dark venous blood is aspirated in the syringe, disconnect the syringe from the needle and look for the type of flow coming out of needle. (*Practical tip:* If RA pressure is not elevated, the venous blood usually does not come out of the hub of needle, as shown in Figure 6A)
- After locating the IJV with pilot needle, puncture is made with 18 G needle supplied with the kit (Fig. 6B) and guidewire is threaded through this needle

into right IJV. Length of the guidewire inside the vein should be such that the double mark on wire is just outside the puncture point on skin. Person performing the procedure should have his/her ears tuned to beeps of heart beat at monitor to diagnose any arrhythmias due to guidewire entering inside RA, in that case it needs to be withdrawn. Make a bold niche in skin and subcutaneous tissue with the blade. (*Practical tip:* Blade should be kept flat over the guidewire at entry point in skin and slide over the guidewire for about 1 cm deep from entry point).

- Introduce the sheath with dilator over the guidewire and advance it till dilator enters inside the vein for about 2–3 cm with tip of sheath also inside the vein (Fig. 7A). Keep the dilator fixed at this point and advance only the sheath over the dilator and guidewire. (*Practical tip:* Avoid inserting the dilator with sheath, inside vein as it can injure the vessel wall). Take the dilator and guidewire out. Always keep holding the proximal end of guidewire during entire procedure till you take it out completely, so as to prevent its loss inside the patient. Confirm the placement of sheath inside vein by aspirating venous blood from side port and then flush it with heparinized saline (Fig. 7B). Suture this sheath with the skin using 3–0 mersilk.
- Once the introducer sheath is in place, change the gloves and drape the head end of patient with fresh sterile sheet (usually supplied with introducer sheath package). Take the curled PA catheter in your hand without disturbing its preformed curvature as it helps in floating it into PA, as shown in Figure 8. Introduce the tip of catheter inside the sheath at 10–11 O'clock position with the concavity of catheter curl facing upward (Inset of Fig. 8).
- Advance the catheter to around 15–20 cm and then inflate balloon. (*Precautions:* Always inflate the balloon in slow and controlled manner. Always inflate balloon before advancing the catheter and deflate it before withdrawal). Keep monitoring pressure waveform from distal lumen (PA port) throughout the procedure. Be vigilant to make out changes in pressure waveform as you will identify entry of catheter in RV, PA and wedge position by changes in pressure waveform only (Figs 9 to 11). From right IJV approach RA is reached at around 20–25 cm. RV is reached at around 30–35 cm and catheter enters PA at 40–45 cm in case of normal sized cardiac chambers. If

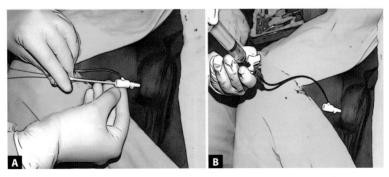

Figs 7A and B (A) Position of dilator while introducing sheath, dilator enters for 2–3 cm inside vein after piercing it and then sheath is advanced over it; (B) Blood is being aspirated from side port

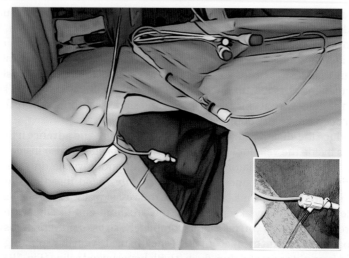

Fig. 8 Position of pulmonary artery catheter (at the time of floating) without changing its preformed curvature

Note the tip entering at 10–11 O'clock position of sheath with curl facing upward (inset)

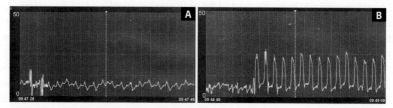

Figs 9A and B (A) Note the characteristic wave form of central venous pressure with three positive waves a, c and v; (B) Right ventricular waveform looks like square root sign

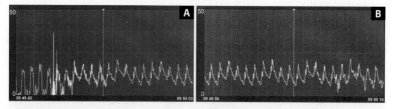

Figs 10A and B As the catheter tip enters main pulmonary artery, diastolic pressure becomes higher with systolic pressure remaining almost same as that of right ventricular. A dicrotic notch also appears in the pulmonary artery waveform

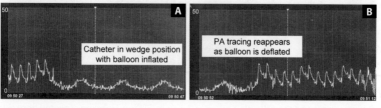

Figs 11A and B Tracing after catheter is wedged, loses systolic peak and is similar to right ventricular tracing in appearance, it reflects the back pressure from left atrium through capillaries

patient has cardiomegaly or any chamber enlargement then RV and PA may be reached at higher length. At any point of time if your catheter is inside RA or RV more than your anticipated length of catheter, it suggests that catheter is coiling inside that chamber without being advanced toward PA. In that case, deflate balloon, withdraw catheter and start afresh.

- Once pulmonary capillary wedge pressure (PCWP) waveform or pulmonary artery occlusion pressure (PAOP) is obtained, deflate the balloon and secure the protective sleeve over the catheter by docking its distal end into the proximal end of sheath. If you require less than 0.75 mL of air for balloon inflation to achieve PAOP waveform, it indicated that your catheter is too much inside the PA, consider withdrawing for few centimeters.

- *Practical tips:* If significant tricuspid regurgitation hinders floating PA catheter from RA into RV, try floating after head-up position. In case of difficulty in entering PA from RV, make head up and left side up and then float the catheter, as it may align origin of main PA with path of floating PA catheter.

- Confused between PAOP and RA/CVP tracing?
  - If catheter is in PA, PA tracing disappears after balloon is inflated and PAOP wave form appears. PAOP waveform changes to typical PA waveform with systolic and diastolic pressure once balloon is deflated.
  - Pulmonary artery occlusion pressure is lower or equal to PA diastolic pressure.

- In case of difficulty in floating PA catheter to its destination and if the patient is being monitored by transesophageal echocardiography (TEE) [in the settings of cardiac intensive care unit (ICU) or cardiac surgical operating rooms], one can be guided by the following views on TEE (Figs 12 to 16).

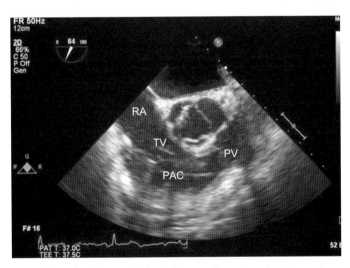

Fig. 12 Mid-esophageal right ventricular inflow outflow view showing pulmonary artery catheter inside right ventricle after crossing tricuspid valve and reaching up to pulmonic valve

Abbreviations: RA, right atrium; TV, tricuspid valve; PV, pulmonic valve; PAC, pulmonary artery catheter.

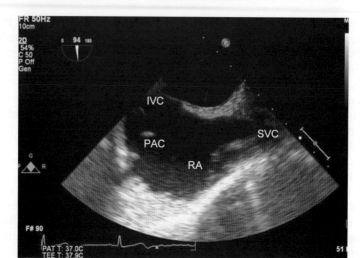

Fig. 13 Mid-esophageal bicaval view showing presence of pulmonary artery catheter inside right atrium

Abbreviations: RA, right atrium; SVC, superior vena cava; IVC, inferior vena cava; PAC, pulmonary artery catheter.

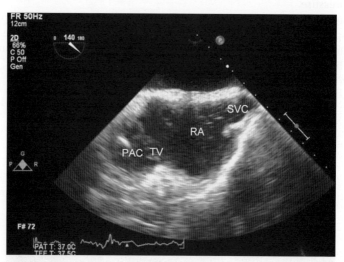

Fig. 14 Modified bicaval view, depicting entry of pulmonary artery catheter inside right ventricular after crossing tricuspid valve

Abbreviations: RA, right atrium; SVC, superior vena cava; TV, tricuspid valve; PAC, pulmonary artery catheter.

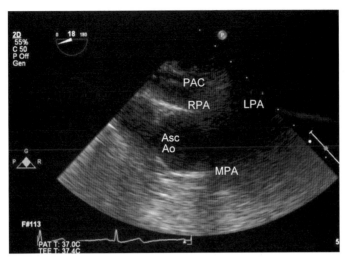

Fig. 15 Mid-esophageal ascending aortic short-axis view showing PA catheter in right PA (in majority of the instances catheter enters RPA because RPA is more in alignment with MPA)

Abbreviations: MPA, main pulmonary artery; RPA, right pulmonary artery; LPA, left pulmonary artery; Asc Ao, ascending aorta; PAC, pulmonary artery catheter.

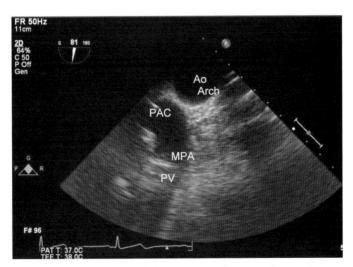

Fig. 16 Upper esophageal aortic arch short-axis view showing pulmonary artery catheter entering main pulmonary artery after crossing pulmonic valve

Abbreviations: PV, pulmonic valve; MPA, main pulmonary artery; Ao Arch, aortic arch; PAC, pulmonary artery catheter.

POST-PROCEDURE CARE

- After PA catheter has been floated to its place, note the amount of length inside. Attach the protective sleeve cover to the sheath with the docking mechanism (Figs 17A and B).
- It is important to maintain the catheter in its proper place and it can be secured with adhesive to the forehead of patient. In this way its length can be taken care of (Fig. 17C).
- Keep the balloon deflated and leave the catheter after withdrawing 1–2 cm from wedged position.

COMPLICATION/PROBLEM

All the complications related to central venous cannulation can happen during PA sheath insertion and are described in chapter on central venous cannulation. Complications pertaining to PA catheter can occur during its placement or because of its long-term presence in pulmonary artery and central circulation.

Complications During Its Placement

- *Conduction abnormalities:* Transient premature atrial or ventricular ectopies are common during its placement. If arrhythmias persist, medical or electrical therapy can be given, but is rarely required. Complete heart block develops in patients with pre-existing left bundle branch block.
- *Valvular damage:* Catheter withdrawal with inflated balloon may cause injury to tricuspid or pulmonic valve.
- *Catheter knotting or entrapment:* Catheter knotting can occur in right ventricle, if too much length of it is inserted without heading toward PA.
- *Malposition:* If patient has any atrial or ventricular septal defect, catheter may pass into left side of heart and then into aorta.
- *Cardiac perforation and tamponade:* Extremely rare
- *Endobronchial hemorrhage:* Balloon inflation in distal PA can cause this catastrophic complication.

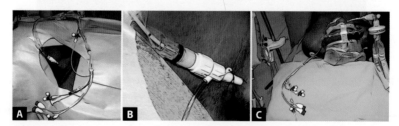

Figs 17A to C (A) Pulmonary artery catheter after floating to its destination and with protective sheath on it; (B) Attachment of docking mechanism on protective sleeve with its counterpart on introducer sheath. Also shown in the figure is 50 cm mark on pulmonary artery catheter just outside the sheath; (C) One suggested way to secure pulmonary artery catheter in place, post-procedure

Complications Because of Its Long Term Presence

- *Pulmonary infarction:* Keeping the balloon inflated for long in the wedge position, can block an artery and produce infarction
- *Thrombus formation:* Thrombus can be formed on PA catheter if left in situ for long. Risk is more, if patient is receiving antifibrinolytic therapy
- Endocarditis
- Infection and sepsis
- Balloon rupture or catheter fracture.

SUGGESTED READING

1. Schroeder RA, Barbeito A, Bar-Yosef S, Mark JB. Cardiovascular monitoring. In: Miler RD, Eriksson LI, Fleisher LA, Wiener-Kronish JP, Young WL (Eds). Miller's Anesthesia. 7th edition. 2009. Churchill-Livingston.
2. American Society of Anesthesiologists Task Force on Pulmonary Artery Catheterization. Practice guidelines for pulmonary artery catheterization: an updated report by the American Society of Anesthesiologists Task Force on Pulmonary Artery Catheterization. Anesthesiology. 2003;99(4):988-1014.
3. Chatterjee K. The Swan-Ganz catheters: past, present, and future. A Viewpoint. Circulation. 2009;119(1):147-52.
4. Binanay C, Califf RM, Hasselblad V, O'Connor CM, Shah MR, Sopko G, et al. Evaluation study of congestive heart failure and pulmonary artery catheterization effectiveness: The ESCAPE Trial. JAMA. 2005;294(13):1625-33.
5. Harvey S, Harrison DA, Singer M, Ashcroft J, Jones CM, Elbourne D, et al. Assessment of the clinical effectiveness of pulmonary artery catheters in management of patients in intensive care (PAC-Man): a randomised controlled trial. Lancet. 2005;366:472-7.
6. Connors AF, Speroff T, Dawson NV, Thomas C, Harrell FE, Wagner D, et al. The effectiveness of right heart catheterization in the initial care of critically ill patients. SUPPORT Investigators. JAMA. 1996;276(11):889-97.

26

Transducer and Pressure Monitoring

Jyoti Narayan Sahoo

INTRODUCTION

The purpose of pressure monitoring is to obtain information that will indicate whether the conditions that are required to maintain tissue perfusion are being maintained. Pressure monitoring is a basic tool in the armament of the clinician monitoring the critically ill patient. In patients with unstable cardio-circulatory status, physiological pressure measurements like blood, central venous, pulmonary artery, intracranial and intra-abdominal pressure are often the basis for therapeutic decisions. Targeting optimal perfusion pressure head and ensuring adequate nutrient to the tissues forms the basic part of management in the critically ill patient. Pressure transducers (PTs) is a device which convert mechanical physiologic signal [i.e. arterial, central venous, pulmonary artery and intracranial pressure (ICP)] to an electrical signal which is amplified, filtered and displayed on a bedside physiologic monitor in both a waveform and numeric value in mm Hg.

INDICATION

Monitoring of an organ system pressure head or a compartment pressure is indicated when there is decrease perfusion to the organ either due to decrease pressure head or increase surrounding compartmental pressure compromise the perfusion. Monitoring such pressures can help the clinician to optimize perfusion to the organ and to implement measure to decrease compartmental pressure.

Intravascular Pressure Monitoring

- For assessment of intravascular fluid status [central venous pressure (CVP), pulmonary capillary wedge pressure (PCWP)]
- Hemodynamic unstable (shock, hypertensive emergency) or anticipation of hemodynamic unstable patients (cardiovascular surgery, during anesthesia of high-risk surgical procedure)
- Patients on vasopressor or vasoactive medication
- Patients with end-organ damage such as CNS (intracranial hypertension) or intra-abdominal hypertension.

Intra-abdominal Pressure Monitoring

- Postoperative abdominal surgical patients
- Patients with blunt abdominal trauma
- Patients with an abdominal distension and signs and symptoms consistent with abdominal compartment syndrome (ACS) (e.g. oliguria, unexplained acidosis, mesenteric ischemia).
- Postoperative patients with close abdomen or abdominal pack after temporary abdominal closure for multiple trauma or liver transplantation.
- Patients with an underlying capillary leak syndrome (pancreatitis, septic shock, trauma, etc.), who have received large volumes of fluid resuscitation.

Intracranial Pressure Monitoring

- Severe traumatic brain injury [Glasgow Coma Scale (GCS) ≤ 8]
- Intracranial hemorrhage
- Cerebral edema
- Postcraniotomy (decompressive craniotomy)
- Space-occupying lesions (epidural and subdural hematomas, tumors and abscesses)
- Meningitis or encephalitis resulting in malabsorption of CSF.

TECHNIQUE AND BASIC PRINCIPLES OF PRESSURE TRANSDUCER

Pressure transducer was discovered by Rudolph H Sumpter in 1967 by using a diaphragm as strain-sensitive devices for measuring blood pressure (BP) and in 1973, an electric PT was introduced by Roger C Crites, but the major break came with the introduction disposal PT by Wallace et al. in 1986.

Pressure transducer equipment consists of:

- PT with or without flush device
- Noncompliant pressure tubing
- Fluid administration set
- Transducer housing
- Cable connection
- Pressure monitor

Pressure Transducer (Fig. 1)

The transducer is a device that converts the pressure waves generated by blood or fluid flow into an analog electrical signal that can be displayed on electronic monitoring equipment.

Mechanics of transducer: Transduction is the process wherein one form of energy is converted to another. The mechanical force (pressure) of the pulsed waveform (blood or body fluid) is converted to an electrical (voltage) signal. The conversion of pressure signal into an electrical signal is achieved by the physical deformation of strain gages which are bounded into the diaphragm of the PT. An input current is continuously passed from the bedside monitor to the transducer via a connecting cable. Within the transducer, a set of wires is wired in a Wheatstone bridge configuration, functioning as a resistor for current flow within

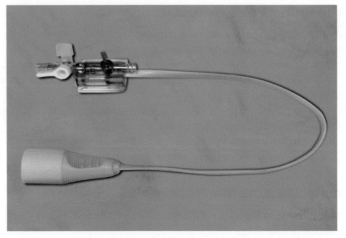

Fig. 1 Pressure transducer with flush device
(*Courtesy:* Edwards Life Sciences, India)

the transducer. As pressure (blood or fluid) is felt from the pulsed waveform against a sensing diaphragm, the electrical resistance inside the transducer changes proportional to the pressure received and flow of the input electrical current through the transducer is increased. The new output current from the transducer is returned, amplified, filtered and displayed in the bedside monitor. In this way, the biological signal of blood or body fluid pressure is converted to an electrical impulse. The resistance changes within the transducer replicate the physiological pulse amplitude variations throughout the input of the physiological waveform and its conduction through the tubing to the transducer. The returned electrical impulse, therefore varies as a reflection of the waveform changes during each cardiac cycle, and the configuration of the pressure waveform ideally is faithfully duplicated by the electrical signal.

Concepts of Natural Frequency and Damping of a Transducer System

Dynamic response of a system is characterized by its natural frequency and damping coefficient. A simple way of evaluating dynamic response can be done by performing a square wave test and by observing the resultant oscillations.

Frequencies: Natural frequency at which an object or system tends to vibrate with when hit or disturbed is called the natural frequency of the system or object. Most transducers have high frequencies of several hundred Hz (> 200 Hz). Natural frequency is important because the natural frequency of the commonly used measuring system (approximately 16–24 Hz) must exceed the natural frequency of the pressure measures (arterial pulse). If the monitoring system has a natural frequency that is too low and if the natural frequencies of the measurement system approach the frequency of the measuring system than the system will resonate, and pressure waveforms recorded on the monitor will be amplified (overshoot, ringing, or resonance). The pressure waveform that is displayed will not correlate with the original pressure.

Damping: Implies how an oscillations in a system decay after a disturbance. The damping ratio is a measure of describing how rapidly the oscillations decay from one disturbance to the next. The transducer monitoring system must have an appropriate damping coefficient. This is relevant because a system should be undamped (the system oscillate at its natural frequency) to give accurate reading. In an overdamped system, the system returns to equilibrium without oscillating giving a falsely narrowed pulse pressure, although mean arterial pressure (MAP) may remain reasonably accurate. In an underdamped system, the system oscillation amplitude gradually decreases in size until it come to stop. This underdamped system gives systolic pressure overshoot and contain additional artifacts produced by the measurement system that are not part of the original pressure wave. An optimal damping coefficient of a system is around 0.6–0.7 and can be determined by examining oscillatory wave after a high-pressure flush.

Pressure Tubing

It is a semi-rigid pressure tubing attaching the catheter to a transducer set-up (less than 3–4 feet). The pressure tubing is more rigid than standard IV tubing in order to prevent distortion of the pressure wave by the tubing.

The transducer cable attaches the transducer to the monitor, which displays a pressure waveform and numeric value.

The flush system consists of a pressurized bag of normal saline (with or without heparin). The pressure inside the flush system is maintained at 300 mm Hg to prevent back flow of blood from the arterial system into the pressure tubing. An intraflow valve is part of the transducer set-up (except for ICP transducer) and maintains a continuous flow of flush solution (approximately 3–5 mL/hour) into the monitoring system to prevent clotting at the catheter tip. A fast-flush device (except for ICP transducer) (Fig. 2) connected to the flush

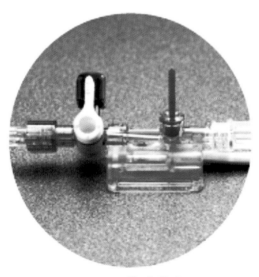

Snap-tab
flush device

Fig. 2 Flush system
(*Courtesy:* Edwards Life Sciences, India)

system allows for general flushing of the system and rapid flushing following withdrawal of blood from the system or when performing a square wave test.

Flush or Square Wave Test

The flush test is performed to test the accuracy of the system dynamics (natural frequency and dynamic coefficient). An invasive pressure monitoring system should accurately reflect patient's pressure, as it is used to titrate drugs therapy and any inaccuracies in measurement can lead to inappropriate treatment strategies and potential harm to the patient.

The flush test is assessed by observing the resultant oscillations when the flush device is activated rapidly for 1–2 seconds and released. Normally, the PT is kept patent by a pressurized solution (300 mm Hg) connecting with an integral flush device of the transducer with a flow rate to approximately 3 mL/hour. The flush device is activated by pulling the snap tab for 1–2 seconds (Fig. 3). The waveform sharply rise and square off at the top and when the snap tab is released the waveform return to baseline after few oscillation. The behavior of the waveform as it return to baseline reflects the dynamics of the system and indicates the accuracy with which it is reflecting the patient's pressures.

The ideal square-wave waveform: The system response to pressures, determine how fast the oscillations (the frequency) and how high (amplitude) the waves are. The amplitude ratio is calculated by measuring the size of the first and second oscillation. Ideally, the second oscillation should be about 1/3 the height of the first one (Fig. 4). This indicates that the system have an adequate damping coefficient when subjected to pressure. The first two oscillations are the primary focus. An optimally damped system (Fig. 5) will have 1.5–2 oscillations before returning to baseline tracing. Overdamping system (Figs 6A and B) will cause reduced waveform amplitude and loss of some waveform components.

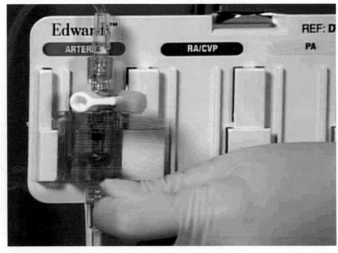

Fig. 3 Activation of fast-flush device by pulling the snap-tab
(*Courtesy:* Edwards Life Sciences, India)

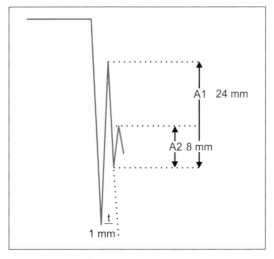

Fig. 4 The ideal square-wave waveform. Amplitude of the second oscillation should be about 1/3rd height of the first one

(*Courtesy:* Edwards Life Sciences, India)

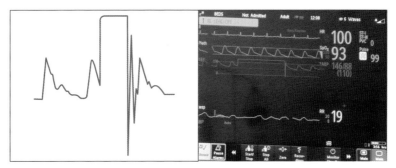

Fig. 5 Graphical representation of optimal damped system (Optimally damped system: 1.5–2 oscillations before returning to tracing)

(*Courtesy:* Edwards Life Sciences, India)

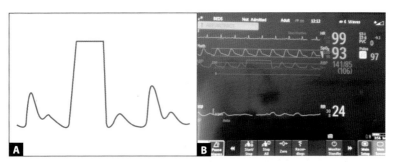

Figs 6A and B (A) Graphically representation of overdamped system; (B) Monitor display of overdamped arterial pressure monitoring system (Overdamped: less than 1.5 oscillations before returning to baseline tracing)

(*Courtesy:* Edwards Life Sciences, India)

Usually, have less than 1.5 oscillations before returning to tracing. These systems lead to a false low systolic pressure and a false high diastolic pressure reading. Potential sources of overdamping are distensible tubing, overly long extension tubing (>3–4 feet), air bubbles in the circuit and small diameter catheter. Clinically, such overdamping monitoring system can have disastrous consequences for patient on treatment for optimal BP control (hypertensive crisis or aortic aneurysm). In an underdamping system (Fig. 7), the square wave will be followed by multiple large oscillations. This pressure monitoring system will show false high systolic pressure reading and a false low diastolic pressure reading. Underdamping occurs when the natural frequency of the system is equal or less than the pressure waves which is transmitted. In this condition, the tubing vibrates along with pressure waveform, producing overshoots and undershoots waves or oscillation. Clinically, underdamping of monitoring system can delay identification of hypovolemia in critically ill patients by not identifying narrow pulse pressure which is the earliest indicator before hypotension develops.

TRANSDUCER PREPARATION AND PRESSURE MEASUREMENT

Pressure Transducer System Set-up (Figs 8A to C)

- The majority of pressures monitoring systems are set-up in a similar manner with few exceptions or modifications. Assemble all components of the system prior to set-up. The components include:
    - Preassembled disposable pressure tubing and disposable transducer with or without flush device.
    - Pressure cuff for IV bag (only for flush system transducer)
    - 500 mL bag of normal saline (only for flush system transducer)

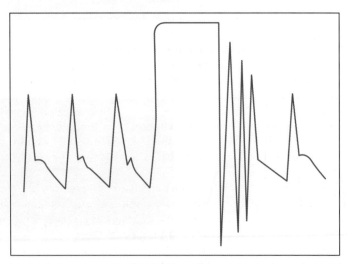

Fig. 7 Graphically representation of underdamped system (Underdamped: more than two oscillations before returning to baseline tracing)

(*Courtesy:* Edwards Life Sciences, India)

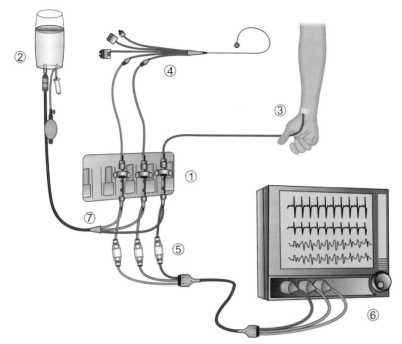

Fig. 8A Pressure transducer system set-up for intravascular pressure monitoring. (1) Transducers; (2) Normal saline flush bag in pressure bag; (3) Radial arterial line; (4) Swan-Ganz catheter PA and RA ports; (5) Pressure cable or trifurcated; (6) Bedside monitor; (7) Trifurcated fluid administration line

(*Courtesy:* Edwards Life Sciences, India)

- – IV stands with transducer mount (manifold)
- – Carpenter's level or laser leveling device
- – Pressure monitor, pressure module and monitor cable
- *Priming of the system*
  - – Perform hand hygiene and follow universal precautions.
  - – Obtain a 500 mL bag of saline (0.45 or 0.9); invert the bag and spike it with IV tubing, then turn it upright and fill the drip chamber, until it is completely full.
  - – *Priming the tubing:* Position all stopcocks so the flush solution will flow through the entire system. Ensure to flush all the stopcock ports.
  - – Activate the fast flush device and flush the saline through the entire set-up one more time (flush device is absent in ICP monitoring transducer device).
  - – Check to be sure that all air has been purged from the system. Examine the transducer and each stopcock for small bubbles cling to these components.
  - – Replace all vented port caps with closed (dead-end) caps, making sure to maintain the sterility of each cap's insertion end.
  - – Place the bag of saline into the pressure cuff, and built the pressure to at least 300 mm Hg. This pressure is required to maintain a continuous flow of 3–5 mL/minute through the intraflow valve, which prevent clotting of the catheter and backflow of blood into the tubing.

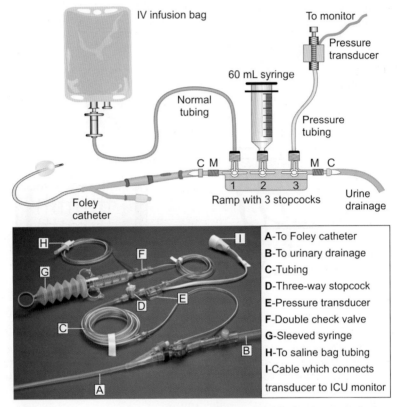

Fig. 8B Pressure transducer system set-up for intra-abdominal pressure monitoring
(*Courtesy:* Convatec India Private Limited)

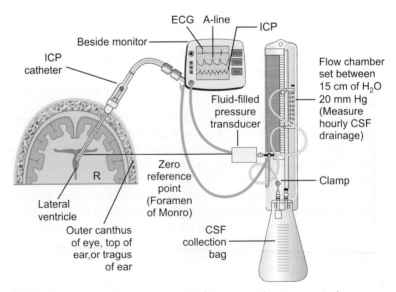

Fig. 8C Pressure transducer system set-up for intracranial or intraventricular pressure monitoring

- In ICP monitoring system, priming of the system (NO FLUSH) are performed as described previously in transducer set-up and the intraventricular transducer kit (with no flush device) is assemble as instructed per the package insert.
- *Zeroing the transducer to atmospheric pressure*
    - Zeroing the transducer helps to eliminate the effect of atmospheric pressure on the pressure readings. Zeroing make sure the monitor reads zero when there is no pressure is against the transducer (Fig. 9A).
    - To zero the transducer, open the stopcock between the transducer and air (Fig. 9B) and press the zero button on the monitor.
    - No particular point or patient position is required to perform this step and zeroing should be done, whenever the reading is in doubt or anytime the monitor has been disconnected from the transducer set-up.
- *Leveling*
    - The transducer is leveled to a particular position in the body where pressure is measured relative to atmosphere pressure. Correct leveling of transducer is essential to obtain accurate pressures reading and should be checked during routine monitoring and troubleshooting of the monitoring system.
    - All PT are leveled by a carpenter or laser leveler to the phlebostatic axis (Fig. 10A) except intracranial PT which is leveled to the outer canthus of the eye or the tragus of the ear corresponding to the foramen of Monro (Fig. 10B).
    - Phlebostatic axis is located at the fourth intercostal space, halfway between the anterior and posterior chest (mid-chest). The midaxillary line which is the midpoint is not accurate point in all patients especially in patients with barrel chests or severe chest deformities (Fig. 10C).
    - Mark the position of the phlebostatic axis on the patient chest and make sure the stopcock is precisely leveled with this landmark.
    - Relevel the transducer when the patient changes position, reading is in doubt or outside of prescribed parameters.
    - In correct leveling of transducer can give a wrong reading. A low or high position of the transducer relative to phlebostatic point gives a falsely high or low reading respectively (Figs 11A to C).

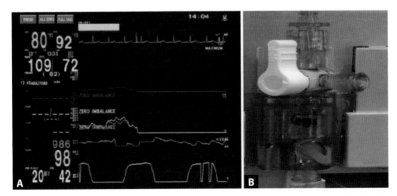

Figs 9A and B Zeroing the transducer to atmospheric pressure. (A) Monitor display of flat graph during zeroing; (B) Stopcock open between the transducer and air during zeroing

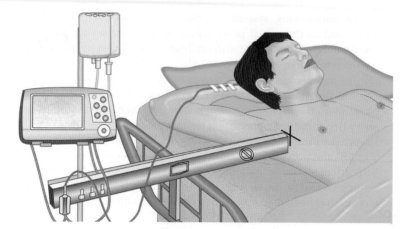

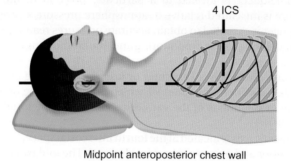

4 ICS

Midpoint anteroposterior chest wall

Fig. 10A Leveling to phlebostatic axis (Fourth intercostal space, midway between the anterior and posterior chest)

(*Courtesy:* Edwards Life Sciences, India)

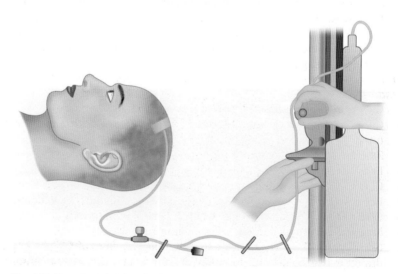

Fig. 10B Transducer level to the foramen of Monro (Eliminate the effects of gravity on intra-cranial pressure monitor)

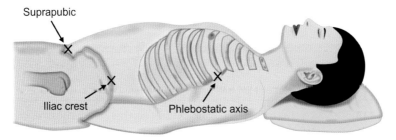

Fig. 10C Midpoint of iliac crest corresponds to phlebostatic axis in supine position
(*Courtesy:* Convatec India Private Limited)

Monitoring Pressure

- After the transducer kit set-up, zeroing and leveling, the transducer is connected to the intravascular catheter or intraventricular catheter or Foley's catheter.
- For intravascular pressure monitoring, the patient can be positioned in supine or semirecumbent position and pressure are measured directly at the phlebostatic point.
- In intracranial pressure measurement, the patient is usually in semirecumbent position with the transducer leveled at the outer canthus of the eye or tragus of the ear, and if the patient is in lateral position level the transducer to the midsagittal line (between the eyebrows).
- In IAP monitoring, patient should be placed in the supine position and there should not be any active abdominal muscle contraction. If this is not clinically feasible, ensure all subsequent reading is measured in the same position (head up position will have high IAP reading).
- At end of measurement return, all patients to head up position to reduce risk of ventilator-associated pneumonia (VAP).
- ICP monitoring and IAP monitoring (see details elsewhere in this book).

TROUBLESHOOTING

Troubleshooting of abnormal or dampened waveform and/or negative pressure reading:
- Check pressure monitoring system (set-up) for loose connection
- Check system for air bubbles, clots, and in ICP monitoring brain tissue in tubing
- Zero the transducer to atmospheric pressure
- Level the transducer to phlebostatic point.
- Check scale and labels in monitor for accuracy
- Perform flush test to determine the system dynamic (not in ICP monitoring)
- Check filter on drainage bag for wetness (in ICP monitoring)
- Maintain patient position as in previous measurements
- Check patency of the catheter by observing for flow of CSF by lower the drainage bag below the foramen of Monro or observe the response by compression to jugular vein. A transient rise in ICP will rule out occlusion of the catheter.

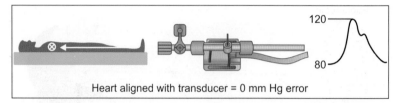

Fig. 11A Transducer level to the phlebostatic axis (accurate pressure measurement with no effect of hydrostatic pressure on transducer sensor)

(*Courtesy:* Edwards's Life Sciences, India)

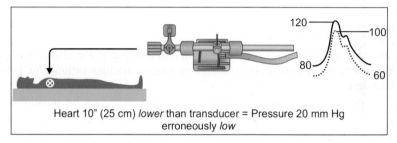

Fig. 11B Transducer position above the phlebostatic axis (for each inch the air fluid interfaces higher than the phlebostatic point, the pressure will be erroneously low by 2 mm Hg)

(*Courtesy:* Edward Life Sciences, India)

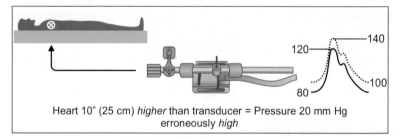

Fig. 11C Transducer position below the phlebostatic point (each inch the air fluid interfaces below than the phlebostatic point, the pressure will be erroneously high by 2 mm of Hg)

(*Courtesy:* Edwards Life Sciences, India)

- If there is greater variation in upper and lower peak of pressure due to respiratory variation, measure the pressure at end expiration or use mild sedation, and if possible neuromuscular blockade (NMB) in mechanical ventilated patients.
- In IAP monitoring fill, the bladder with no more than 25 mL of saline and allow 30–60 seconds for equilibrium and observe the pressure wave with respiratory variations and by gently applying oscillations to the abdomen before recording.

ACKNOWLEDGMENTS

- Edwards Life Sciences, India for allowing to reproduce Figures (1, 2, 3, 4, 5, 6, 7, 8A, 10A, 11A to C)
  Source: From McGee WT, Headley JM, Frazier JA. Quick guide to cardiopulmonary care, 2nd edition. Edwards Critical Care Education. 2008.
- ConvaTec India Private Limited for providing Figures 8B and 10C.

SUGGESTED READING

1. Bhatia A, Gupta AK. Neuromonitoring in the intensive care unit. I. Intracranial pressure and cerebral blood flow monitoring. Intensive Care Med. 2007;33(7):1263-71.
2. Fawcett J. Hemodynamic Monitoring Made Easy, 1st edition. Baillere Tindall. 2005.
3. Kirkpatrick AW, Roberts DJ, De Waele J, Jaeschke R, Malbrain ML, De Keulenaer B, et al. Intra-abdominal hypertension and the abdominal compartment syndrome: updated consensus definitions and clinical practice guidelines from the World Society of the Abdominal Compartment Syndrome. Intensive Care Med. 2013;39(7):1190-206.
4. Malbrain ML. Different techniques to measure intra-abdominal pressure (IAP): time for a critical re-appraisal. Intensive Care Med. 2004;30(3):357-71.
5. McGee WT, Headley JM, Frazier JA. Quick guide to cardiopulmonary care, 2nd edition. Edwards Critical Care Education. 2008.
6. Powner DJ, John AM. Technical aspects of intravascular pressure monitoring during donor care. Progr Transplant. 2010;20(1):22-6.

27
Pericardiocentesis

Jugal Sharma, Aditya Kapoor

INTRODUCTION

Pericardiocentesis is the name given to the procedure whereby pericardial fluid is drained either via needle aspiration or by creating a pericardial window and is an emergency lifesaving procedure for patients with pericardial tamponade. Echocardiographic guidance is important to enhance the safety and minimize potential complications. Availability of adequately trained personnel to perform pericardiocentesis is extremely important. *Whenever possible, it should be performed by a physician trained in invasive bedside techniques, an interventional cardiologist or a surgeon.*

INDICATION

- *Therapeutic*
  - *Emergency procedure:* Cardiac tamponade (most common indication)
  - *Elective procedure:* Large effusion not responding to medical treatment.
- *Diagnostic*
  - Clinical suspicion of infected or neoplastic pericardial pleural effusion.

CONTRAINDICATION

- *Absolute contraindication*
  - No absolute contraindications to pericardiocentesis except for the obvious one of absent effusion on echocardiography or other alternative imaging modalities
  - In absence of clinical evidence of tamponade, echocardiographic signs of right-sided cardiac chamber diastolic collapse do not warrant emergency pericardiocentesis.
- *Relative contraindication*
  - Aortic dissection
  - Bleeding diathesis
  - On anticoagulation therapy or following thrombolysis.

APPLIED ANATOMY AND PHYSIOLOGY

The pericardium is an avascular fibrous sac that surrounds the heart and extends cranially to cover the pulmonary trunk, superior vena cava and ascending aorta.

It comprises of an inner visceral and outer parietal layer and the space between these two layers constitutes the pericardial cavity. The pericardial space usually contains 15–50 mL of serous fluid, which serves as a lubricant between the two layers (visceral and parietal) of the pericardium and is primarily distributed over the atrial-ventricular and interventricular grooves. Apart from serving as a protective barrier, pericardium also modulates cardiac reflexes, coronary tone and facilitates mechanical coupling and interactions of cardiac chambers.

Pathophysiology of Pericardial Effusion

Accumulation of pericardial fluid leading to a pericardial effusion may be secondary either to increased production or reduction in drainage and may occur as an isolated problem or as a manifestation of underlying systemic disease. Accumulated material may include serous or infectious purulent material, fluid, blood, air or gas. Although any cause of acute pericarditis can potentially lead to development of a pericardial effusion, common causes include tuberculosis, bacterial or viral infections, malignancy, postradiation pericarditis, renal failure, collagen vascular diseases and hypothyroidism. Hemopericardium can occur secondary to coagulation abnormalities (either primary or in patients on anticoagulation therapy), postsurgical, myocardial rupture following acute myocardial infarction or penetrating chest trauma and in patients with dissecting aortic aneurysm. Chylopericardium (with accumulation of chyle) may be seen following pericarditis, postradiation, postsurgical, lymphatic obstruction, subclavian thrombosis and in patients with malignancy or tuberculosis. Pneumopericardium is a rare finding, and may occur following chest trauma, fistula formation, gas-forming infections or following medical interventions.

The extent of symptoms produced, more often depend on how rapidly the fluid accumulates within the pericardial sac. A gradual collection of fluid is usually well tolerated due to the accompanying pericardial stretch and distensibility, which accommodates the fluid and delays the onset of cardiac compression. This is especially common in patients with chronic kidney disease, malignancy and hypothyroidism, who may have fluid up to 1 liter without being overtly symptomatic. However, rapid accumulation of as much as 250 mL is sufficient to cause an increase in the pericardiac/cardiac silhouette and development of pericardial compression and tamponade. The normal intrapericardial pressure is subatmospheric (approximately 1–2 mm Hg) and cardiac compression occurs when the pressure rises and become positive. As long as the ventricular filling pressure exceeds the intrapericardial pressure, cardiac output is maintained since ventricular filling is not affected to a significant effect. However when the intrapericardial pressure becomes higher than the ventricular filling pressure, chamber filling is compromised, cardiac output falls and clinical features of tamponade appear. This generally happens when intrapericardial volume reaches a level high enough to cause the pericardium to reach the noncompliant portion of its pressure-volume curve, leading to tamponade. Due to increased intrapericardial pressure and resultant higher right ventricular filling, there is a reversal of the normal curvature of ventricular septum, leading to further compromise of left ventricular filling and volume. The consequent hemodynamic effect is the pulsus paradoxus, defined as decrease of systolic blood pressure more than or equal to 10 mm Hg with inspiration. However this sign may be difficult to ascertain in patients with severe hypotension and may even be absent in those with coexisting left ventricular dysfunction, atrial septal defect and aortic insufficiency.

Presence of hypotension, jugular venous distention due to increased venous pressure, and a quiet heart form part of the classical Beck's triad to describe the clinical picture of cardiac tamponade, most commonly produced by acute intrapericardial hemorrhage. Other clinical signs include tachycardia, tachypnea, dyspnea and Kussmaul's sign, in which there is increased jugular venous distention on inspiration. Presence of a pericardial friction rub usually indicates an inflammatory cause; its presence is not dependent on the size of the effusion and it may occasionally be absent in large effusions. The electrocardiography (ECG) may show low-voltage QRS complexes with electrical alternans (a beat to beat change in the QRS amplitude).

However, not all of these typical findings may be seen in patients with cardiac tamponade and therefore the decision to perform a pericardiocentesis often needs to be individualized on a case to case basis. Since cardiac tamponade can be fatal if not recognized and treated in a timely fashion, it needs to be considered in the differential diagnosis of all patients with shock especially if they have raised jugular venous pressure or pulseless electrical activity.

TECHNIQUE

Percutaneous pericardiocentesis was first described by Frank Schuh in 1840s, and was initially performed using a blind subxiphoid approach. Needle aspiration is now usually performed under echocardiographic, ultrasonographic, fluoroscopic or less commonly computerized tomographic visualization.

Different techniques for performing pericardiocentesis include:

- *Percutaneous needle aspiration:* Use of an aspiration needle which is inserted into the pericardial cavity to remove the fluid.
- *Open pericardiocentesis:* Wherein an incision is made in the subxiphoid area on the anterior chest and fluid is removed after dissection of tissues down into the pericardial sac. "Pericardial window" is the procedure during which a part of the pericardium and mediastinal pleura is resected via a right or left anterolateral thoracotomy creating a wide communication (window) between the pericardial and pleural cavity. The pericardial fluid gets evacuated into the pleural cavity from where it is slowly reabsorbed.
- *Thoracoscopic pericardial drainage* is a minimally invasive method of evacuating the pericardial fluid wherein a thoracoscope is introduced through thoracic incision and the pericardial space directly visualized. It is often possible to completely lyse adhesions with complete evacuation of clots and collection of biopsies.

Of all described techniques, at present, percutaneous needle pericardio-centesis under echocardiographic guidance has become the procedure of choice for the treatment of patients with large/compressive pericardial effusions or for diagnostic aspiration of pericardial fluid.

Although there is no significant difference in mortality between open surgical drainage and percutaneous pericardiocentesis for drainage of pericardial effusions, the choice of technique often depends on the underlying hemodynamic status of the patient and the size and type of effusion.

- In patients with symptomatic tamponade and severe hypotension, emergency needle aspiration is often life-saving and stabilizes the hemodynamics sufficiently to consider open drainage later, if required.
- Larger effusions are more effectively aspirated using needle pericardiocentesis while smaller, organized or loculated posterior effusions and post-traumatic cardiac tamponade may require open surgical drainage. Although needle pericardiocentesis may be used as a temporary measure to stabilize patients with traumatic cardiac tamponade, most of these patients will need emergent thoracotomy or creation of a pericardial window because rapid reaccumulation of blood can occur due to ongoing bleeding.

As a general rule, drainage of pericardial fluid with pericardiocentesis is associated with greater number of repeat procedures, while procedural complications may be higher following surgical drainage.

In hemodynamically stable patients where there is a high clinical suspicion of effuso-constrictive pericarditis, a right heart catheterization study should be performed prior to the pericardiocentesis. The right heart catheter should remain in-situ during the pericardial fluid aspiration and right heart and pericardial pressures should be recorded simultaneously throughout. After pericardiocentesis, the right atrial and pulmonary capillary wedge pressures should be normal in magnitude and waveform and higher than the recorded pericardial pressure. If these hemodynamic end points are not achieved, the patient warrants further evaluation for constrictive pericarditis.

Although usually performed under echocardiographic guidance, in the absence of on-site echocardiography, a wire with sterile alligator clips is attached to the spinal aspiration needle and connected to a precordial lead with continuous ECG monitoring. A blind approach may be attempted if neither echocardiography nor ECG monitoring is immediately available and the patient has severe hemodynamic compromise, but since this is often associated with a high complication rate, it should be avoided as far as possible.

PREPARATION

- It is mandatory to perform an echocardiogram in all cases, prior to the pericardiocentesis. This not only serves to diagnose the presence of pericardial fluid but also confirms that the effusion is at large enough to require aspiration (Figs 1A and B). Supporting echocardiographic signs of tamponade (including right atrial and right ventricular collapse) and presence/absence of loculations in the pericardial fluid need to be looked for carefully in all cases. An echocardiography machine should be available on site, since echocardiography guided pericardiocentesis has the advantage of permitting direct visualization of the aspiration needle as it enters the pericardial cavity.
- A clotting profile should be obtained in all cases prior to the procedure, except in patients with hemodynamic collapse where an immediate pericardiocentesis is warranted to be life-saving.
- Facility for continuous monitoring of blood pressure, ECG and oximetry should be available.
- Although bedside echocardiography guided pericardiocentesis is safe and effective, the procedure should be performed at a site which is equipped with good quality fluoroscopy, preferably in a cardiac catheterization laboratory where appropriate equipment is available for hemodynamic monitoring and any additional interventions.

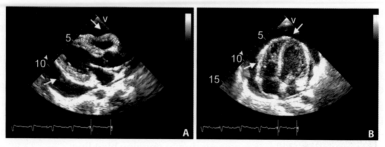

Figs 1A and B Echocardiography images showing large pericardial effusion: (A) Long-axis parasternal view; (B) Apical 4 chamber view

PROCEDURE

- The patient is best positioned in a semirecumbent position at a 30–45° angle so as to facilitate the heart to be closer to the anterior chest wall and allowing the fluid to gravitate inferiorly. The supine position is also an acceptable alternative.
- A standard pericardiocentesis kit should be available (this should contain aspiration needles, syringes and standard surgical drapes)
  - Needles, 18 G, 1.5 inch; 25 G, 5/8 inch or a spinal needle, 18 G, 7.5–12 cm. Needles used for pericardial aspiration should have a short bevel to reduce the risk of cardiac or coronary vessel injury. An 18 G, 10 cm needle is adequate for most patients. While a larger bore needle is preferable for purulent or organized pericardial effusions, for most such cases, an open drainage may be a better alternative.
  - Syringes: 10 mL, 20 mL, 50 mL
- A secure intravenous line should be ensured in all patients. On occasion, placement of a nasogastric tube may be required to decompress the stomach and decrease the risk of gastric perforation, especially in cases where the abdomen is distended or the patient is on positive pressure ventilation.
- Anatomic landmarks (xiphoid process, 5th and 6th ribs) are identified and the potential site for needle insertion is marked. The most frequently used sites are the left sternocostal margin or the subxiphoid approach.
- The site of needle entry is cleaned using antiseptic solution, surgical drapes applied and the area infiltrated with local anesthetic solution (lidocaine 1%) till the subcutaneous and deeper tissues (Figs 2A and B). In patients with severe hemodynamic compromise, a brisk cleaning of the local area followed by quick needle aspiration is recommended, rather than spend time in elaborate cleaning, draping and injecting the local anesthetic.
- A small skin puncture is performed using a No. 11 blade scalpel at the chosen site.
- A syringe filled with approximately 5 mL normal saline is connected to the aspiration needle and the needle is inserted through the skin incision, until the needle tip is posterior to the rib cage. (If a spinal needle is used, remember to insert it with the stylet in place to prevent dermal tissue from plugging the needle).
- The needle should be directed towards the left shoulder, while maintaining a 45° angle to the abdominal wall and 45° off the midline sagittal plane.

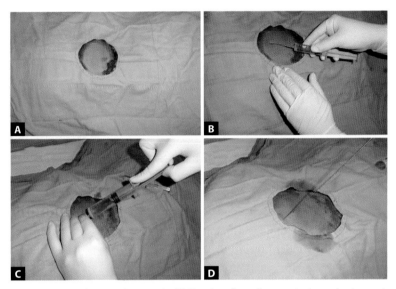

Figs 2A to D Steps of pericardiocentesis: (A) The site of needle entry is cleaned using antiseptic solution and surgical drapes applied; (B) The area is infiltrated with local anesthetic solution; (C) The needle is slowly advanced to a depth of 4–5 cm, with continuous negative pressure on the syringe until a return of fluid is visualized; (D) A soft floppy tip guidewire is advanced through the needle into the pericardial space

While advancing the needle, one may occasionally inject 1-2 mL of the prefilled normal saline to ensure that the needle lumen remains patent. If time and patient hemodynamics permit, needle insertion should be performed under direct echocardiographic guidance.

- The needle is slowly advanced to a depth of 4–5 cm, with continuous negative pressure on the syringe until a return of fluid is visualized (Fig. 2C), cardiac pulsations are felt, or a change in the ECG waveform is noted. Appearance of an injury pattern characterized by ST segment elevation on the ECG, suggests that the aspiration needle is in direct contact with the myocardium and needs to be withdrawn slightly until the ECG returns to normal.
- As the initial pericardial fluid is aspirated, the needle may move closer to the heart and an injury pattern may appear on the ECG waveform. The needle should be slowly withdrawn and repositioned if this happens. Hence it is important that once the operator is sure that the needle tip is intrapericardial, and some fluid has been removed (enough to stabilize the hemodynamic status), a soft floppy tip guidewire is advanced through the needle into the pericardial space (Fig. 2D) and an indwelling catheter inserted (described later).

Insertion of a Pericardial Drain or Indwelling Catheter

A single needle pericardiocentesis may not completely evacuate the effusion and in most cases active fluid accumulation may continue leading to recollection. Placing an indwelling pericardial catheter is therefore especially useful for patients with large or recurrent pericardial effusions, since this ensures continuous fluid aspiration as well as "buys time" if an immediate open drainage is logistically not feasible (Figs 3A to D).

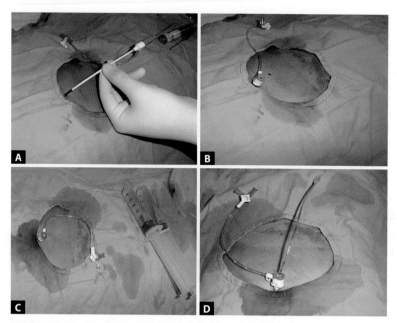

Figs 3A to D Steps of inserting an indwelling catheter: (A and B) Once the guidewire is inside the pericardial space, a sheath is inserted over the guidewire and placed inside the pericardial space; (C and D) Some fluid may also be aspirated via the sheath (C) followed by placement of an indwelling catheter (D)

- Once the needle tip is inside the pericardial space, a soft floppy-tip guidewire is passed through the needle. The guidewire is inserted till it wraps around the heart, and its tip comes to lie posteriorly at the level of the left atrial appendage. This confirms the wire to be intrapericardial. The needle is removed and a catheter with multiple side holes is passed over the wire followed by removal of the wire. Presence of side holes ensures adequate drainage and reduces the chances of catheter clogging.
- The catheter is flushed with 1–2 mL of fluid to prevent blockage and one should attempt to withdraw as much fluid as possible either by successively removing the filled syringe, and replacing it with another one or using a three-way stopcock and intravenous tubing connected to a collection bag.
- Although gravity assisted drainage may be useful, remember that negative suction should be avoided in an effort to increase the drainage.
- The catheter is secured with a dressing and a stay suture to prevent displacement.
- Indwelling catheters should not be left in-situ for longer than 24 hours as it may increase the possibility of infection. However, occasionally catheters may need to be kept in for longer periods especially in cases where pericardial fluid rapidly reaccumulates.

Other Approaches

- Although the subxiphoid approach is the most commonly used, alternative sites including an apical approach may be used, especially when performing the procedure under echocardiographic guidance. The needle is inserted

approximate 1 cm lateral to the apical impulse, gently advanced along the cardiac long axis and toward the aortic valve, aiming towards the right shoulder.
- Less commonly echocardiography guided parasternal approach may be used. The needle is inserted perpendicular to the chest wall in the fifth intercostal space, just lateral to the sternum and inserted into the largest portion of the effusion close to the body surface.
- In patients where routine approaches have failed and the echocardiographic window is poor (e.g. morbidly obese patients), CT guided approach may be used.

Precautions for Confirmation of Pericardial versus Intracardiac Needle Tip Placement

If hemorrhagic fluid is aspirated, and one is not sure whether the needle is intrapericardial or within a cardiac chamber, the following steps are useful:
- The position of the needle can be confirmed by injecting agitated saline through the needle and visualizing on echocardiography whether the agitated saline appears in the pericardial space or in one of the cardiac chambers.
- While maintaining the tip of the needle in-situ, inject a few milliliters of radiographic contrast medium through the needle under fluoroscopic guidance. If the needle tip is in the pericardial space, the contrast is seen around the cardiac silhouette and then gravitates to the dependent portion of the pericardial space. If the contrast immediately swirls and disappears, then the needle is in one of the cardiac chambers and needs to be repositioned. A guidewire may also be inserted via the needle and its course observed as outlined earlier: if it encircles the cardiac border the needle is likely to be intrapericardial.
- The hemorrhagic aspirate is transferred to a plain vial and observed for a few minutes. If it forms a clot, it is from one of the cardiac chambers, since a pericardial aspirate should not form a clot. This is because intrapericardial fibrinolytic activity prevents blood clotting especially in subacute and chronic pericardial effusions. However, in patients with acute hemorrhage into the pericardium, the pericardial fibrinolysis may be overwhelmed leading to blood clotting even in the aspirated pericardial fluid.
- Although hematocrit or hemoglobin measurement can also differentiate between the two (the pericardial aspirate should have a lower hemoglobin concentration than the patient's peripheral blood), this is obviously time consuming and impractical in an emergent situation.

POST-PROCEDURE CARE

- One should aim to remove the pericardial fluid till hemodynamics normalize and no further fluid can be aspirated.
- An echocardiogram should be repeated to confirm complete removal and/or reaccumulation.
- It is important to obtain a chest X-ray to rule out complications, e.g. pneumothorax, pneumopericardium, pleural effusion, etc.

- The patient should be continuously monitored in the ICU for new onset hemodynamic instability or other physical signs suggesting reaccumulation of the pericardial fluid (e.g. raised jugular venous pressure, tachycardia, muffled heart sounds and hypotension).

COMPLICATION/PROBLEM

Pericardiocentesis performed by experienced operators, especially under echocardiographic guidance has a low complication rate. Reported complications include the following:
- Dysrhythmias
- Cardiac perforation
- Coronary artery laceration
- Left internal mammary artery puncture
- Hemothorax, pneumothorax, pneumopericardium
- Hepatic laceration
- Bowel perforation.

Rarely, pericardiocentesis may be complicated by exacerbation of acute left ventricular failure and pulmonary edema, especially in patients with underlying left ventricular dysfunction. Hence the need for close peri- and postprocedure hemodynamic monitoring in all patients undergoing pericardiocentesis cannot be overemphasized.

SUGGESTED READING

1. Callahan, JA, Seward, JB, Tajik, AJ. Cardiac tamponade: pericardiocentesis directed by two-dimensional echocardiography. Mayo Clin Proc. 1985;60:344.
2. Harper RJ. Pericardiocentesis. In: Roberts JR, Hedges JR (Eds). Clinical procedures in emergency medicine, 5th edition. Philadelphia: Saunders Elsevier. 2010. pp. 287-307.
3. Salem K, Mulji A, Lonn E. Echocardiographically guided pericardiocentesis: the gold standard for the management of pericardial effusion and cardiac tamponade. Can J Cardiol. 1999;15(11):1251-5.
4. Saltzman AJ, Paz YE, Rene AG, Green P, Hassanin A, Argenziano MG, et al. Comparison of surgical pericardial drainage with percutaneous catheter drainage for pericardial effusion. J Invasive Cardiol. 2012;24(11):590-3.
5. Tsang TS, Freeman WK, Barnes ME, Reeder GS, Packer DL, Seward JB, et al. Rescue echocardiographically guided pericardiocentesis for cardiac perforation complicating catheter-based procedures. The Mayo Clinic experience. J Am Coll Cardiol. 1998;32(5): 1345-50.
6. Tsang TS, Freeman WK, Sinak LJ, Seward JB. Echocardiographically guided pericardiocentesis: evolution and state-of-the-art technique. Mayo Clin Proc. 1998;73:647.
7. Uemura S, Kagoshima T, Hashimoto T, Sakaguchi Y, Doi N, Nakajima T, et al. Acute left ventricular failure with pulmonary edema following pericardiocentesis for cardiac tamponade—a case report. Jpn Circ J. 1995;59:55.
8. Vandyke WH, Cure J, Chakko CS, Gheorghiade M. Pulmonary edema after pericardiocentesis for cardiac tamponade. N Engl J Med. 1983;309:595.
9. Vayre F, Lardoux H, Pezzano M, Bourdarias JP, Dubourg O. Subxiphoid pericardiocentesis guided by contrast two-dimensional echocardiography in cardiac tamponade: experience of 110 consecutive patients. Eur J Echocardiogr. 2000;1(1):66-71.
10. Wolfe MW, Edelman ER. Transient systolic dysfunction after relief of cardiac tamponade. Ann Intern Med. 1993;119:42.

28

Electrical Cardioversion

Saurabh Taneja, Sumit Ray

INTRODUCTION

Cardioversion is a technique, used to convert an abnormal tachycardia, i.e. heart rate more than 100/minutes to a normal sinus rhythm. Electrical cardioversion is usually used when patients suffering from tachyarrhythmia are clinically symptomatic or chemical cardioversion is ineffective. The direct current discharge is synchronized with the QRS complex (particularly the R wave), thereby minimizing the chances of triggering ventricular fibrillation. This therapy can be delivered by applying pads/paddles on the patient's bare chest and is usually effective immediately with minimal side effects.

INDICATION

Synchronized Cardioversion

- Hemodynamically unstable atrial fibrillation
- Hemodynamically unstable atrial flutter
- Hemodynamically unstable supraventricular tachycardia (SVT) arrhythmias
- Hemodynamically unstable ventricular tachycardia with a pulse
- Hemodynamically stable ventricular tachycardia unresponsive to pharmacologic therapy.

Unsynchronized Defibrillation

- Ventricular fibrillation
- Pulseless ventricular tachycardia.

CONTRAINDICATION

Absolute

- Patient in cardiac arrest due to asystole
- Severe electrolyte disturbances
- Digitalis toxicity
- Left atrial thrombus (for elective cardioversion).

Relative

- Large left atrial diameter (>4.5 cm) in patients with atrial fibrillation
- Sick sinus syndrome
- Ectopic or multifocal atrial tachycardia
- Junctional or sinus tachycardia
- Minimal hemodynamic or clinical improvement while in sinus rhythm
- Atrial fibrillation duration greater than 6 months
- Inadequate anticoagulation and more than 48 hours duration of atrial fibrillation [unless transesophageal echocardiography (TEE) negative for thrombus].

APPLIED PHYSIOLOGY AND ANATOMY

Each heart beat normally originates in the specialized "pacemaker" cells located in the right atrium. With each discharge (usually 1–2 times/second) in these cells, an organized electrical signal is sent through the heart that finally results in a coordinated rhythmic heart beat. Cardiac dysrhythmia or arrhythmia is a group of conditions in which the usually organized electrical activity of the heart becomes irregular, faster or slower than normal. Patients can have symptoms like rapid heart beat, shortness of breath or fatigue or may remain asymptomatic. The arrhythmias may cause hemodynamic instability. Delivering a synchronized cardioversion to restore the normal electrical activity of the heart may terminate such hemodynamically unstable arrhythmias.

In order to perform this technique of synchronized electrical cardioversion, two electrode pads or hand-held paddles are placed on the chest of the patient or one is placed on the chest and other on the back to encircle the heart. This ensures the delivery of maximal current to the myocardium. These pads/paddles are connected to a machine, which delivers a selected amount of energy at the optimal time in the cardiac cycle to revert the electrical rhythm to normal sinus rhythm.

The energy delivered is also influenced by the size of the chest wall and the electrode size. Thicker chest walls create more impedance and larger pad size decreases the impedance.

TECHNIQUE AND EQUIPMENT

The rapid expansion of commercially available electric power in the early 20th centuries led to an increase in the incidence of accidental electrocution and most deaths were caused due to ventricular fibrillation. The credit of introducing direct current shock for purpose of defibrillation should go to Gurvich and Yuniev of the Soviet Union, who, in 1939, proposed that ventricular fibrillation can be defibrillated using a single discharge from a capacitor. Defibrillation of the exposed human heart was first reported at Ohio in 1947 by a famous cardiothoracic surgeon, Claude Beck. Cardioversion of atrial fibrillation using a direct current shock was first reported in the Soviet Union in February 1959 by Vishnevskii and Tsukerman. Restoration of sinus rhythm in this patient having atrial fibrillation for 3 years was achieved during mitral valve surgery. They also reported the first successful transthoracic cardioversion using direct current cardioversion in 20 patients in 1960. Bernard Lown of Boston, USA, coined the term "cardioversion" for delivering a synchronized shock for an arrhythmia other than ventricular fibrillation. He also combined defibrillation and cardioversion with portability and safety. The Lown-Berkovits investigation group introduced the novel concept of synchronizing delivery of the shock with the QRS complex sensed from the electrocardiogram (ECG).

Types of Cardioversion

It is of two types:
1. Chemical cardioversion using drugs or medicines
2. Electrical cardioversion using direct electrical current across the patient's chest to terminate the tachyarrhythmia.

Electrical Cardioversion

- Synchronized cardioversion is state when the delivery of energy is synchronized with the large R wave or QRS complex so as not to shock during the vulnerable ventricular repolarization phase of the cardiac cycle.
- Unsynchronized cardioversion/defibrillation is a nonsynchronized delivery of energy during any phase of the cardiac cycle. In case of defibrillation, there is no concern about the timing of the charge as there is no coordinated intrinsic electric activity in the heart.

Application of shock during the relative refractory period (the T wave) can simulate the "R on T" phenomenon and induce ventricular fibrillation. Hence, it is essential to synchronize the delivery of electrical current to the myocardium with the peak of the QRS complex, the R wave. Cardioverters highlight or flag the QRS peak or R wave after one applies the pads/paddles and press the synchronization button. Synchronization reduces the energy requirements and complication rates of elective cardioversion. If the cardioverter-defibrillator is unable to identify the peak of QRS complex, it will not discharge the current as a safety feature, as happens in rapid ventricular rates.

Description of Equipment

The equipment consists of the manual external cardioverter-defibrillator with paddles or self-adherent electrode pads (size 8–12 cm diameter) and electrode gel to be applied to the paddles (Figs 1 and 2).

Paddle and Electrode Selection and Placement

Self-adherent pads 8–12 cm in diameter/paddles may be used for cardioversion. Pads/paddles can either be applied in their standard position, right upper parasternal and left fourth or fifth interspace midaxillary line (Fig. 3) or in the anteroposterior position (anterior over the sternum and posterior between the scapulae or both slightly to the patient's left, on the left side of the sternum and beneath the left scapula) to make the current travel through the heart.

Gel applied to the paddles minimizes electrical resistance (Fig. 2), but avoid excessive gel application to minimize smearing and hence, current travel along external chest wall.

Anteroposterior positioning may reduce energy requirements for cardioversion (through reduced electrical resistance) by up to 50% and may increase cardioversion success.

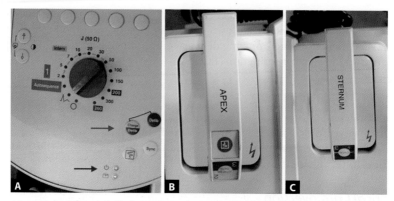

Figs 1A to C (A) Manual defibrillator-cardioverter; (B) The selections dial in the center with the energy levels to be selected in joules. Lower down, the indicator lights (green: machine is on; yellow: machine is charging) can be seen (blue arrow). In between, the knobs (color coded) for charging, defibrillation and synchronization can be seen (red arrow); (C) The two paddles, marked "apex" and "sternum" respectively to specify their respective positions on the chest while giving shock

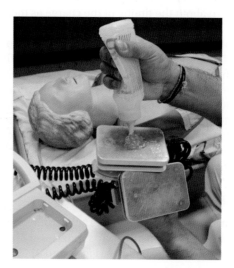

Fig. 2 Applying jelly before applying pads to the patient is essential

Selection of Energy Levels

The following are the energy levels for synchronized cardioversion and defibrillation as suggested by the American Heart Association (AHA).

- *Adult atrial fibrillation:* 120–200 J (biphasic); 200 J (monophasic); if unsuccessful, energy levels to be increased in a stepwise fashion.
- Other SVTs including adult atrial flutter generally require less energy. An initial shock with energy of 50–100 J is often enough. In case of failure of the shock, dose should be increased in a stepwise fashion.
- Unstable monomorphic (regular) ventricular tachycardia with pulse: treat with synchronized cardioversion (monophasic or biphasic), using initial

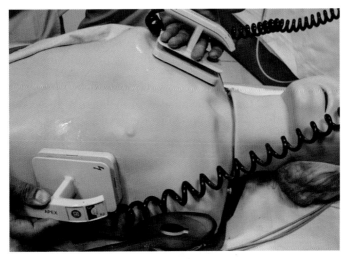

Fig. 3 Position of paddles while providing cardioversion. Paddle "apex" around 5 cm below the left axilla and paddle "sternum" to the right of the sternum below the right clavicle

energy of 100 J. Incase of no response to the initial shock, dose may be increased in a stepwise fashion.

- For unstable polymorphic ventricular tachycardia, i.e. irregular ventricular tachycardia, with or without pulse an unsynchronized high energy shock (monophasic 360 J, biphasic 200 J) should be given.
- In case of any doubts regarding monomorphic or polymorphic ventricular tachycardia in an unstable patient, shock delivery should not be delayed to perform a detailed rhythm analysis and high energy unsynchronized shock should be delivered.
- To cardiovert SVT in pediatric age group, an initial dose of 0.5–1 J/kg should be used. The dose may be increased up to 2 J/kg, if required. For monomorphic ventricular tachycardia with regular form and rate in pediatric age group, the initial energy dose is 0.5–1 J/kg which may be increased to 2 J/kg, if required.

PREPARATION

- *Fasting and consent (for elective cardioversion):* Solids and milk-containing drinks should not be consumed within 6 hours but the person may drink clear fluids up to 2 hours prior to the start of the procedure. Cardioversion can be elective (patient hemodynamically stable) or urgent (lifesaving).
- Resuscitation equipment should include an airway management kit, a supplementary oxygen source and suction equipment including suction tubing and catheter.
- A patent intravenous line should be there to administer sedative and resuscitative drugs, if required.
- *Drugs needed:* Emergency drugs and sedatives for elective cardioversion. Procedural sedation during elective cardioversion depends upon anticipated energy levels for cardioversion, patient factors (e.g. airway, obesity, hepatic

and renal disorders) and desired length of sedation. The more the energy levels used, more the depth of sedation required. Usual agents used are:
-   Short-acting benzodiazepines, such as midazolam or lorazepam
-   Opioids like fentanyl, a narcotic with less hemodynamic effects than morphine
-   Propofol with rapid onset and emergence but risk of hypotension.

• *Monitoring needed:* Monitor the following throughout the procedure—ECG, heart rate, blood pressure, saturation of arterial oxygenation (SpO$_2$) and neurologic checks.

• *Investigation needed (for elective cardioversion):* Chest X-ray, complete blood count, thyroid function tests, renal function and electrolytes, erythrocyte sedimentation rate, renal function and electrolytes, liver function tests and coagulation screen.

• *Anticoagulation in chronic atrial fibrillation:* Recent guidelines suggest that for patients with chronic atrial fibrillation (for >48 hours), adequate anticoagulation for 3 weeks should be done before elective cardioversion to minimize the risk of intra-arterial thrombi embolization on re-establishing the sinus rhythm. International normalized ratio (INR) should be maintained between 2 and 3 for at least 3 weeks before and 4 weeks after the cardioversion. TEE may be performed to detect small atrial thrombi, especially in the left auricular appendage, that are not visible with transthoracic echocardiography (TTE).

PROCEDURE

• Ensure the indication
• Obtain a resting 12-lead ECG and confirm the persistence of the rhythm disturbance
• Is the patient clinically symptomatic?
• Switch on the machine
• Placement of appropriate sized pads/paddles with gel applied at predefined sites with maximum skin/body contact of paddles (Figs 2 and 3)
• Recheck the rhythm and select the appropriate energy level (Fig. 4A)
• Synchronize with the patient's ECG and look for the flags on the R wave (Fig. 4B; yellow arrow)
• In case of unsynchronized defibrillation, the energy selected is usually the maximum level available and there is no need to synchronize the shock
• Charge the cardioverter and look for "energy available" signal (Fig. 4B; green arrow)
• Announce "all clear" and recheck visually confirming there is no physical contact with the patient or the bed
• Announce "delivering shock" and press the discharge buttons on both paddles simultaneously. There is often a brief delay. Keep buttons depressed until the shock is delivered).
• Recheck the rhythm on the monitor.

POST-PROCEDURE CARE

Continue monitoring the vitals (ECG and SpO$_2$ continuously, blood pressure at 15–30 minutes intervals) and the neurological status of the patient for at least 2-4 hours after the procedure (Figs 4C; Orange arrow).

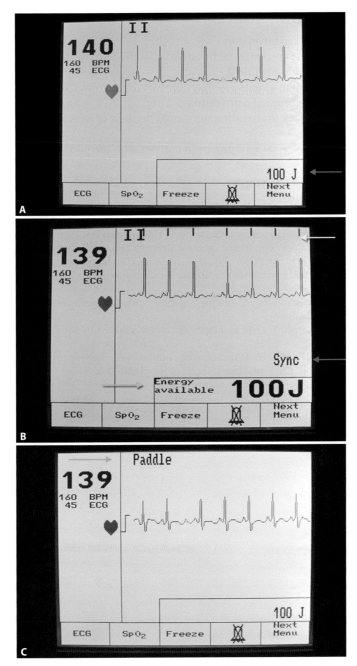

Figs 4A to C (A) Lead II of the ECG showing a heart rate of 140 beats/minute with 100 J of energy selected (seen in the lower right corner, red arrow); (B) The same screen with "synchronization" on, depicted by "Sync" written in the left lower corner of the screen and with 100 J energy available (blue arrow). The flags (depicted by yellow arrow) can be seen on top of each R wave. Also look for the energy available signal (green arrow); (C) The screen depicts the source of ECG recording is paddle as seen in the top right corner (orange arrow)

COMPLICATION/PROBLEM

- Unsuccessful cardioversion
- Conversion to ventricular tachycardia or ventricular fibrillation
- Localized cutaneous burns
- Thromboembolic events
- Recurrence of original arrhythmia
- Accidental shock to attending personnel because of contact with the patient or bed
- Damage to electrical equipment in contact with the patient or bed.

SUGGESTED READING

1. Cakulev I, Efimov IR, Waldo AL. Cardioversion: past, present, and future. Circulation. 2009;120(16):1623-32.
2. Link MS, Atkins DL, Passman RS, Halperin HR, Samson RA, White RD, et al. Part 6: electrical therapies: automated external defibrillators, defibrillation, cardioversion, and pacing: 2010 American Heart Association Guidelines for Cardiopulmonary Resuscitation and Emergency Cardiovascular Care. Circulation. 2010;122(18 Suppl 3): S706-19.
3. Shea JB, Maisel WH. Cardiology patient pages. Cardioversion. Circulation. 2002;106(22):e176-8.
4. Sucu M, Davutoglu V, Ozer O. Electrical cardioversion. Ann Saudi Med. 2009;29(3): 201-6.
5. Trohman RG, Parrillo JE. Direct current cardioversion: indications, techniques, and recent advances. Crit Care Med. 2000;28(10 Suppl):N170-3.

29

Temporary Cardiac Pacing

Saswata Bharati, Nirvik Pal, Devesh Dutta

INTRODUCTION

Cardiac pacing is a method where a small electrical current is delivered to the heart to initiate myocardial contractions artificially, when the intrinsic stimulation of myocardium is insufficient to maintain hemodynamic stability due to disturbances in the conduction system. A temporary pacemaker is used to treat a bradydysrhythmia or tachydysryhthmia when the condition is short lived or to bridge until a permanent pacemaker is placed. There are various methods of performing temporary cardiac pacing: transvenous pacing, transcutaneous pacing, transesophageal pacing, transthoracic pacing, pacing through pulmonary artery catheter and pacing by epicardial wires. The transvenous pacing is by far the most commonly performed technique for temporary cardiac pacing, particularly in the ICU set up. Transcutaneous pacing is another commonly performed temporary pacing method in the ICU set up particularly during emergency situation when little time is available (for example, during cardiopulmonary resuscitation).

INDICATION[1-3]

Temporary pacemakers are indicated as a bridging procedure in almost all the conditions where permanent pacemakers are indicated. There are certain other conditions where temporary pacemakers are used alone for brief period till the underlying risk subsides.

The various indications for temporary cardiac pacing are:

Therapeutic

- Treatment of different types of cardiac conduction abnormality following acute myocardial infarction
  - Asystole
  - Complete heart block (CHB)
  - Mobitz type II second degree atrioventricular block with anterior myocardial infarction
  - Bilateral bundle branch block (BBB) (alternating BBB or RBBB with alternating left anterior hemiblock/left posterior hemiblock) with or without first degree atrioventricular block
  - New BBB with transient CHB

- New bifascicular block
- Symptomatic alternating Wenckebach block
- Symptomatic bradycardia (sinus bradycardia or Mobitz type I second degree atrioventricular block with hypotension) not responsive to atropine
- Treatment of drug toxicity resulting in arrhythmias
- Second or third degree atrioventricular block causing hemodynamic instability or syncope at rest
- Asystole not related to acute myocardial infarction (AMI)
- Treatment of intraoperative bradycardia caused by β-blocker use in hemodynamically unstable patients
- Treatment of bradycardia dependent of ventricular tachycardia
- Termination of paroxysmal supraventricular tachycardia (PSVT) or type I atrial flutter by atrial overdrive pacing
- Treatment of atrioventricular junctional pacing following cardiopulmonary bypass by atrial or atrioventricular sequential overdrive pacing
- Long QT syndrome
- Torsade de pointes
- Augmentation of cardiac output postoperatively in low cardiac output condition following cardiac surgeries.

Prophylactic

- Pulmonary artery catheter placement and right ventricular endomyocardial biopsy in a patient with pre-existing left bundle branch block (LBBB). These procedures may produce short-lasting right bundle branch block (RBBB), which in these patients may lead to complete heart block
- Patients with bifascicular block with or without type II second-degree atrioventricular block or a history of unexplained syncope, undergoing general anesthesia
- Cardioversion in the setting of sick sinus syndrome
- During pharmacological treatment with drugs that worsen bradycardia
- New atrioventricular or bundle branch block with acute endocarditis
- Various cardiac surgeries, e.g. aortic surgery, tricuspid valve surgery, ventricular septal defect closure, ostium primum repair
- For neurosurgical procedures involving the brainstem and surgical resection of neck and carotid sinus tumors.

CONTRAINDICATION

There are no absolute contraindications to the use of temporary pacing as a means to control the heart rate. Few relative contraindications do exist for a particular type of temporary pacing, which however, can be overcome by using different method of temporary pacing.

- Patients with severe hypothermia
- Distortions of vascular anatomy or bleeding disorders are relative contraindications for transvenous pacing
- Cardiac glycoside toxicity, as well as other drug ingestions, can cause myocardial irritability, which increases the risk of ventricular fibrillation during the pacing lead insertion

- Presence of tricuspid valve prostheses is a relative contraindication for transvenous pacing
- Atrial pacing is contraindicated in the presence of atrial fibrillation and multifocal atrial tachycardia.

TECHNIQUE AND BASIC PRINCIPLES

In 1952, Paul Zoll first applied temporary pacemaker successfully in two patients with ventricular standstill using a pulsating current applied through two electrodes attached via hypodermic needles to the chest wall.[4] Since then, various types of pacemaker models came into use. Technological developments produced endocardial, epicardial and esophageal approaches to pace the heart in addition to the external pacing. All the approaches, however, use an external pulse generator along with electrode or electrodes, through which the electrical impulse is delivered to the myocardium either internally via endocardium or externally via epicardium.

Different Types

Transvenous pacing: Transvenous pacing involves intracardiac placement of the pacing wire through central venous access (Fig. 1). The preferred route for central venous access is the internal jugular vein followed by subclavian and femoral veins. However, other major veins (e.g. external jugular vein, brachial vein) can also be used. The leads are placed into endocardium of atrium and/or ventricle. The right atrial appendage and right ventricle apex provide the most stable positions for lead placement and, therefore, should be the target. The electrodes are placed under ultrasound or fluoroscopic guidance. For insertion of electrodes, flow-directed catheter can also be attempted using pressure or electrocardiography (ECG) guidance. Temporary transvenous pacing is dependable and well tolerated by patients. Both the atrium and ventricle can be paced in a synchronized way

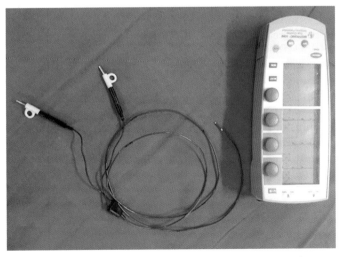

Fig. 1 Transvenous pacing leads with dual chamber pacemaker

leading to improve cardiac output. However, this procedure needs expertise as in inexperienced hands it could be a time consuming process and a higher incidence of complications is found.[5]

Transcutaneous pacing: This is by far the simplest and quickest technique where the heart is paced by the application of external pads over the chest wall. The large external pads are typically placed anteriorly (negative electrode or cathode) over the palpable cardiac apex and posteriorly (positive electrode or anode) at the inferior aspect of the scapula. The anode can also be placed at the anterior right chest below the clavicle. Sedation may be required as this procedure is often uncomfortable to the patients. This technique is commonly used in an emergent condition until temporary transvenous pacing can be instituted. Transcutaneous pacing facility is now available on most modern defibrillators. The Advanced Cardiac Life Support (ACLS) guidelines recommend transcutaneous external cardiac pacemakers for symptomatic bradycardia as a temporary measure and as a consideration for treatment of asystole. Use of transcutaneous external cardiac pacemaker may also be of benefit for overdrive pacing in treatment of certain tachycardias.

Pacing through pulmonary artery catheter:[6] Temporary pacing can be performed using pulmonary artery catheter (PAC) either with integrated atrial and ventricular electrodes or via Paceport through which pacing lead is inserted. In patients with aortic insufficiency or mitral regurgitation where slow heart rate can cause left ventricular dilatation, PAC with atrial and ventricular pacing capabilities can be useful.

- *Thermodilution pacing PAC:* This multifunctional PAC is integrated with atrial and ventricular electrodes, which produce atrial, ventricular and atrioventricular sequential pacing. The electrodes are attached to the outer surface of the catheter. These pacing PAC can perform all other functions that can be done using standard PAC such as measurement of right heart pressures, pulmonary arterial and pulmonary artery wedge pressures, blood sampling, solution infusion and cardiac output measurements by thermodilution technique. Using pacing PAC eliminates the need for separate insertion of temporary transvenous pacing electrodes. Varying success, relatively high cost as compared with standard PACs and chance of detachment of the electrodes are the disadvantages of these catheters. A *bipolar pacing catheter* (Fig. 2) is available for temporary right ventricular endocardial pacing when hemodynamic monitoring is not needed. It has two electrodes, one at the catheter tip and one 1 cm proximal, providing capabilities for bipolar pacing. An additional port is sometimes present to facilitate blood sampling or solution infusion. This probe can also be used for intra-atrial or ventricular ECG monitoring.

- *Paceport PAC:* This multifunctional five lumen PAC (Fig. 3) is provided with a Paceport (right ventricle port), through which a separate bipolar pacing lead can be inserted to produce stable ventricular pacing whenever necessary. This type of catheters is used when a condition for temporary cardiac Pacing cannot be diagnosed at the time of catheter selection and insertion. The Paceport PAC catheter provides for rapid ventricular pacing along with hemodynamic monitoring when the patients with LBBB develop complete heart block during its insertion. The pacing port can be used for pressure

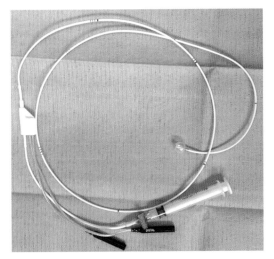

Fig. 2 Swan-Ganz bipolar pacing catheter

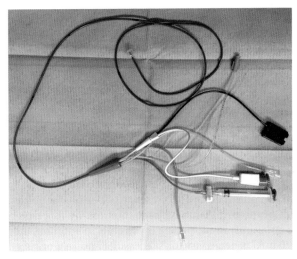

Fig. 3 Thermodilution Paceport PAC

measurement or fluid infusion when the pacing lead is not inserted. This type of catheters, however, lack the advantages associated with atrial pacing capability. The newer pulmonary artery A-V Paceport catheters possess a sixth lumen to accommodate an atrial pacing lead.

Pacing by epicardial wires: This is a commonly practiced technique for intraoperative and postoperative management of dysrhythmias associated with cardiac surgeries. The epicardial wires are placed during intraoperative period under direct vision (Fig. 4). This is a very reliable short-term technique where atrium and/or ventricle can be paced. Development of an inflammatory reaction around the wire and myocardium interface, and failure to sense and capture

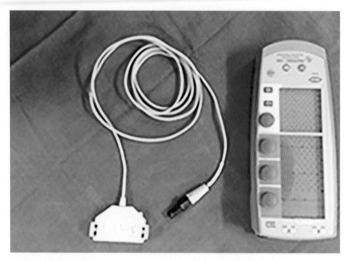

Fig. 4 Pacing cable for epicardial pacing wires with dual chamber pacemaker

after few days (typically after 5 days) are the major problems associated with this technique.[7]

Transthoracic pacing: In this method, a pacing wire or needle is directly introduced to the ventricular wall through the thorax by piercing the thoracic wall. Transcutaneous pacing has replaced this method. This is a useful technique during cardiac arrest, prophylaxis during catheter placement, and as a standby method in case of high risk of bradycardia.

Transesophageal pacing: This is the newest technique available. This relatively noninvasive and well-tolerated technique requires introduction of pacing lead through oropharynx to the esophagus where the electrodes are placed against left atrium. A modified esophageal stethoscope is used for this purpose. Pacing capture should be confirmed by the presence of peripheral pulse as detected by plethysmogram or invasive hemodynamic monitor. By this type of pacing only asynchronous atrial-only mode pacing is possible. In addition, the higher pacing threshold (8–20 mA) is necessary for successful capture. For successful capture, the pacing output should be set at 2–3 times the pacing threshold. A special generator, that must produce 20–30 mA of current output and a pulse width up to 10–20 milliseconds, is needed. This technique has been shown to be especially useful for diagnostic purposes in pediatric age group.

The transvenous temporary pacemaker is the most commonly done procedure for temporary pacemaking that needs technical skills involving few steps and an adequate set up. Steps for transcutaneous, transthoracic and transesophageal pacemaker insertion are very straightforward and simple to perform, although, the indications may vary for each of these methods. Choice of pacing technique is often influenced by the clinical setting, e.g. flow-guided balloon tipped catheter is less optimal in the setting of cardiac arrest due to no or minimal circulation is available, where transcutaneous pacemaker is indicated as it can be applied quickly and easily just by applying two external chest pads. After cardiac surgery, it is likely to have epicardial electrodes as they can be inserted directly under vision before the chest closure, eliminating the need for transvenous pacing subsequently. Pacing PAC (Swan-Ganz catheter), being less stable, is better avoided in conditions where temporary pacemaker has to be continued for some time and in pacemaker-dependent patients. Insertion of pacemaker leads using PAC catheter is similar to insertion of normal PAC catheter using Seldinger technique.

Pacemaker

- *Components of a temporary pacemaker unit:* Pulse generator, leads or wires and electrodes.
- *Types*
    - *Single chamber (Fig. 5):* This simple, easy to operate pacemaker is used when only one pacing electrode is available and can sense and stimulate only one chamber (atrium or ventricle) at a time. The pacing modes available with this model are synchronous (AAI, VVI) and asynchronous (AOO, VOO). Single chamber atrial-based pacing can be used in sick sinus syndrome with intact atrioventricular nodal function. There are three dials present for determining pacing rate, pacing threshold/output and sensitivity. In addition, there are buttons for 'rapid atrial pacing', which can be used to manage atrial flutter.
    - *Dual chamber (Fig. 6):* It can pace both right atrium and right ventricle using two separate pacing leads. The biggest advantage of this type of pacemaker is capability of atrioventricular sequential pacing which is more physiological and maintains better cardiac output. The different temporary pacing modes available are atrial (AOO, AAI), ventricular (VVI, VOO), or dual chamber (DDI, DDD, DOO, or DVI) and rapid atrial pacing (80–800 ppm). In comparison to single chamber pacemaker, dual chamber device is more complicated and needs more expertise in terms of optimizing the device to the patient, and requires more understanding of device timing cycles.
    - *Sensitivity:* Sensing is the ability of the pacemaker to detect natural (intrinsic) depolarization by measuring changes in electrical potential

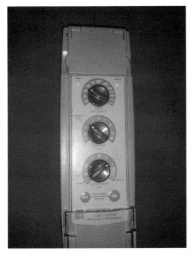

Fig. 5 Single chamber pacemaker

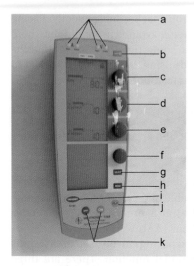

Fig. 6 Dual chamber pacemaker (a: Pace/Sense LEDs; b: Lock/Unlock key; c: Rate dial; d: Atrial output dial; e: Ventricular output dial; f: Menu parameter dial; g: Parameter selection key; h: Menu selection key; i: Emergency/Asynchronous pacing key; j: Pause key; k: Power On/Off key)

of myocardial cells. Sensitivity is the minimum current at which the pacemaker is able to sense intrinsic rhythms. It is represented numerically in millivolt (mV) on the pacing generator. The greater the number, the less sensitive is the device to intracardiac events. The sensitivity is adjusted to detect appropriate intrinsic electrical signal and at the same time filtering out the unwanted signals. A pacemaker is said to be 'oversensing' when it detects electrical signals other than the intended P or R wave, which may inappropriately inhibit pacing leading to underpacing. This happens when the sensitivity value of the pacemaker is kept low. A pacemaker will 'overpace', if the sensitivity value is set too high (making it less sensitive) leading to inability to recognize the intrinsic beat, and thus responding inappropriately. To determine the sensing threshold, the pacemaker rate is first set below (by 10 ppm) the endogenous rate if present, the pacing output is set to 0.1 milliampere (mA) and the mode is fixed to AAI, VVI or DDD. Then, the sensitivity number is increased (thereby, making the pacemaker less sensitive) until the sense indicator stops blinking. At this moment, the pacemaker starts pacing asynchronously. Once this is achieved, the sensitivity number is turned down until the sense indicator starts blinking with each intrinsic rhythm. The value at which this occurs is the threshold value. The sensitivity value is usually set at half the threshold value due to the possibility of peri-lead fibrosis over the course leading to reduction of the current transmitted to the pacemaker and also for small electrical signals.

- *Capture threshold and pacing output:* The capture threshold is the minimum pacing output at which an action potential is generated leading to myocardial contraction. To determine the capture threshold, the pacemaker rate is set above the endogenous rate. Following this, the pacing output is gradually decreased until a QRS complex is not preceded by a pacing spike seen in the ECG. The output at which this occurs is called the capture threshold. Typically, the pacing output is set at twice the capture threshold for safety margin. If the capture threshold is found to be more than 10 mA, then the safety margin is kept low as higher pacing output for long time may lead to myocardial fibrosis at the lead and myocardium interface.

– *Pacing rate:* The objective of setting a pacing rate is to get the maximum cardiac output. This, however, increases the myocardial oxygen consumption in an already compromised heart. A standard protocol is to set the heart rate around 80–90 per minute unless indicated otherwise.

– *Pacing mode:* Almost all type of pacing modes, which are present in permanent pacemaker, are also available in temporary pacemaker. The mode is commonly represented by three letters (e.g. VVI, DDD, etc.) according to the NBG codes. The first letter represents the chamber(s) paced. It can be A (Atrium) or V (Ventricle) or D (Dual; both atrium and ventricle). The second letter represents the chamber sensed. It can be A (Atrium) or V (Ventricle) or D (Dual; both atrium and ventricle) or O (None). The third letter represents response to sensing. It can be I (Inhibited; demand mode) or T (Triggered) or D (Dual; both triggered and inhibited) or O (None; asynchronous). For example, VVI pacing mode indicates ventricle is the chamber, which is both paced and sensed, and inhibition is the action when sensed an event. There are two more letters in the nomenclature, which are not frequently used. The fourth letter represents programmability and is either O (None) or R (Rate modulation). The fifth letter represents multisite pacing. This can be A (Atrium) or V (Ventricle) or D (Dual; both atrium and ventricle) or O (None).

- *Pacing leads and electrodes*
  - *Temporary transvenous pacing lead:* This smooth tipped, atraumatic, bipolar pacing leads are available in various sizes and lengths. The tip of the lead is either straight or curved at different angles. The atrial lead is J-shaped.
  - *Balloon-tipped:* This bipolar temporary pacing lead with balloon is suitable for both recording intracardiac signals and temporary pacing. The usual length of this lead is 105 or 110 cm. The balloon at its tip helps in accurate flow-directed placement. These are stiff with a performed atrial "J" wire with a balloon at the tip to help floating.
  - *Endocardial screw-in lead:* This bipolar lead is available in different lengths: 60, 90, 100, 140, 200 cm. This lead can also be used for intracardial ECG recording. The greatest advantage of this lead is full mobility of the patient without dislocation of the electrode due to firm anchoring of the electrode tip.
  - *Epicardial wire:* This is available in unipolar, bipolar or quadripolar configurations and is available in various lengths.
  - *Transthoracic patches:* These self-adhering, noninvasive stimulation leads are indicated for transcutaneous pacing, ECG monitoring and defibrillation and cardioversion. Modern transcutaneous external pacemakers use long electrical pulse duration (40 milliseconds) and large electrodes (80 cm^2). These features reduced the current required for capture as well as patient discomfort.
  - *Esophageal lead:* It is available in both pediatric as well as adult sizes. The number of electrodes at the tip could be 2, 4 or 8. The curved electrodes produce good tissue contact in esophagus. The transesophageal stimulation is pain free.

Temporary transvenous pacemaker insertion involves obtaining central venous access followed by intracardiac placement of the pacing wire. Here, the steps for insertion of transvenous pacemaker are described.

PREPARATION

Standard aseptic precautions are to be taken. Before initiating the procedure ensure defibrillator and resuscitation equipment are present along with monitor capable of monitoring vitals parameters such as ECG, pulse oximetry, invasive or noninvasive blood pressure.

PROCEDURE[8-12]

- Position of the patient: supine.
- The skin at the site of central venous access should be infiltrated with local anesthetic (lignocaine).
- Standard technique for central venous catheter placement should be followed. Seldinger's technique is used for vascular access. 6 or 7 Fr size sheath is inserted through femoral vein or internal jugular vein or subclavian vein.
- Ensure the electrode tip is J-shaped (for correct positioning in the heart). Balloon catheters usually have this curvature.
- The electrode is advanced under ultrasound or fluoroscopic guidance (Figs 7 and 8).
- The electrode should be advanced in such a way that the tip is directed toward the free wall of right atrium.
- Pass the wire with the help of rotation movement between thumb and index finger through the tricuspid valve to position it along the apex of the right ventricle.
- If difficulties are encountered during positioning of the electrode tip at right ventricle apex, then slide the wire into the right ventricle outflow tract and pull the wire backward to push it again toward the apex with the tip is at a downward angle.
- If unable to capture satisfactorily, then pull back the pacing catheter to right atrium and start over.
- Inconsistent ventricular capture needs fluoroscopy to reveal tip direction: correct it by directing the tip posteriorly or toward left shoulder. Lateral view is helpful along with AP view to see the proper position of lead tip.
- *Pacemaker setting:* Set the ventricular rate to 10/minute above patient's own ventricular rate or 70/minute. Start with pulse of 5 V and once the capture is established (spikes followed by QRS), gradually drop the voltage until capture is lost (usually at 0.7–1.0 V). Once the pacing threshold is determined, the pacemaker is set to deliver a pulse of at least twice the threshold. Normally, the sensitivity is set to 1–2 mV so that intrinsic ventricular depolarization can be sensed by lead and no current/spike will be generated from pulse generator. Output parameters of temporary pulse generator of some manufacturer are in ampere instead of voltage. So keep the output at 5 mA or 5 V even the threshold is 0.5 or 1 V. Because the temporary pacing lead is not fixed and position may get changed on movement of patient. So, this can provide extra safety and prevent noncapture. Unlike permanent pacing, we are not bothered about battery life (high output voltage = less battery life)

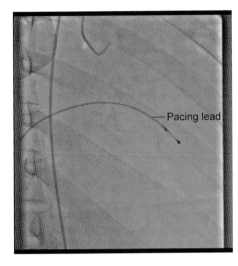

Fig. 7 Fluoroscopic right anterior oblique (RAO) view of temporary pacing lead

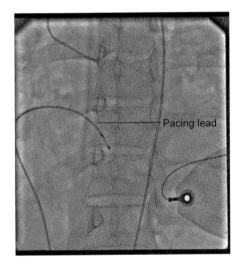

Fig. 8 Fluoroscopic left anterior oblique (LAO) view of temporary pacing lead

as it can be replaced as and when required. After the procedure and lead placement, ask the patient to take deep breath and cough to see any capture loss. Lastly, check for diaphragmatic pacing at 10 V output. In both the cases, minimal change of pacing lead tip is required to get consistent capture without diaphragmatic pacing.

- If neither spikes nor output is seen, then check the pacemaker connection along with the normal functionality of the pacing generator. If spikes are seen without any output, then check the position of the pacing wire and reposition it if necessary.
- Fix the wire to the skin by suturing close to the point of insertion once the position of electrode is confirmed with satisfactory capture and output. The area must be covered with antiseptic dressing.

Some important points to be remembered:
- Continuous ECG monitoring is recommended for endocardial lead placement
- Fluoroscopy is desirable but not necessary
- Site of pacing lead insertion: Preferred sites are right internal jugular vein or subclavian when it is done as a bedside procedure in ICU, and right femoral vein when it is done as a catheterization laboratory procedure under fluoroscopy.

POST-PROCEDURE CARE[4,8]

- Patient is advised to keep the lower limb immobilized and not to sit if temporary pacemaker lead insertion was done through groin (e.g. right leg for right groin access).
- At least one ECG after placement (Fig. 9) should be done. QRS complex should appear like LBBB morphology with leads placed at the apex of right ventricle.
- Immediate chest X-ray to ensure lead placement and to rule out pneumothorax.
- Daily threshold check to ensure proper capture and sensing.
- Separate IV access if drugs need to be administered in central line.
- Daily physical examination should be done to rule out pericardial rub (perforation), asymmetrical breath sounds (pneumothorax), hypotension, jugular venous distension (tamponade/pacing problem), fever (infection).
- Daily dressing change with antibiotic ointment.
- Battery status of the pulse generator is very important. Pacemaker-dependent patients who are not on cardiac monitor may die unattended if battery is exhausted and not replaced timely. Usually fully-dependent patient needs replacement of battery at around 48 hours. Some of the pulse generator shows light signal when battery is at low level and indicates replacement is urgent.

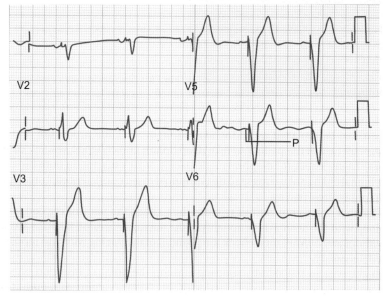

Fig. 9 ECG showing pacemaker spike (P) followed by successful ventricular depolarization as represented by QRS wave

- On fully dependent patient, the change of battery should be very quick or else, attach another pulse generator with full battery and start at a rate of 60 beat per minute at 5–7 mAmp or volt output with a sensitivity of 1.5 mV. The connector pins of the leads are to be immediately removed from old pulse generator and reattached to the new one. A transcutaneous pacing may be required if delay in change of battery is anticipated.
- If there is no contraindication, injection Heparin 5000 IU SC twice daily is given to prevent deep vein thrombosis (DVT) particularly when femoral venous route is chosen. If permanent pacing is required, discontinue heparin 12 hours prior to the procedure.

COMPLICATION/PROBLEM[5,8,13-15]

- *Failure to capture* is a common problem, which can be solved either by increasing the pacing output or by repositioning (if the pacing output requires more than 10 milliamps) the leads.
- *Failure to pace* happens when the pacemaker fails to deliver a stimulus which is manifested by absence of pacemaker spikes on the ECG. This can happen due to oversensing, pacing lead problems, battery or component failure and electromagnetic interference. Among these, oversensing is most frequently encountered. Oversensing occurs due to inappropriate sensing of electrical signals (may or may not be seen on the ECG), that inhibits the pacemaker from pacing.
- *Dislodgment* of pacing wires is another frequently encountered problem. Knotting of lead wire may also happen.
- *Ventricular arrhythmias* particularly after post-AMI temporary pacemaker insertion, which may occasionally require removal of the lead or repositioning. These arrhythmias, however, subside when manipulation of the lead has ceased.
- Development of *septicemia* (most frequently by *Staphylococcus epidermidis*) occurs when the pacing wire is left in situ for more than 48 hours, which may require treatment with antibiotics. Strict asepsis should be maintained when the leads are placed in situ. Signs of early infection require prompt intervention.
- *Thromboembolism* may occur in patients susceptible to deep venous thrombosis. Avoidance of femoral route along with DVT prophylaxis should be considered.
- *Pneumothorax* and/or *hemothorax* during vascular (subclavian) access for transvenous pacing.
- Transcutaneous pacing is painful, also the ventricular capture is often erratic in this method.
- *Cardiac perforation* (of right ventricular wall) can be produced by the pacing leads, which may rarely produce cardiac tamponade. Increase in pacing threshold and occasional pericarditis pain are the manifestations. Withdrawing the lead and repositioning it may solve the problem. Cardiac tamponade needs urgent appropriate management.
- Local trauma and hematoma formation.

REFERENCES

1. Gammage MD. Temporary cardiac pacing. Heart. 2000;83:715-20.
2. Antman EM, Anbe DT, Armstrong PW, American College of Cardiology, American Heart Association Task Force on Practice Guidelines, Canadian Cardiovascular Society, et al. ACC/AHA guidelines for the management of patients with ST-elevation myocardial infarction: a report of the American College of Cardiology/American Heart Association Task Force on Practice Guidelines (Committee to Revise the 1999 Guidelines for the Management of Patients with Acute Myocardial Infarction). Circulation. 2004;110:e82-292.
3. Fitzpatrick A, Sutton R. A guide to temporary pacing. BMJ. 1992;304:365-9.
4. Zoll PM. Resuscitation of the heart in ventricular standstill by external electric stimulation. N Engl J Med. 1952;247:768-71.
5. Rajappan K, Fox KF. Temporary cardiac pacing in district general hospitals—sustainable resource or training liability? QJM. 2003;96:783-5.
6. Risk SC, Brandon D, D'Ambra MN, Koski EG, Hoffman WJ, Philbin DM. Indications for the use of pacing pulmonary artery catheters in cardiac surgery. J Cardiothorac Vasc Anesth. 1992;6:275-9.
7. Reade MC. Temporary epicardial pacing after cardiac surgery: a practical review: part 1: general considerations in the management of epicardial pacing. Anaesthesia. 2007;62:264-71.
8. Jafri SM, Kruse JA. Temporary transvenous cardiac pacing. Crit Care Clin. 1992;8:713-25.
9. Austin JL, Preis LK, Crampton RS, Beller GA, Martin RP. Analysis of pacemaker malfunction and complications of temporary pacing in the coronary care unit. Am J Cardiol. 1982;49:301-6.
10. Overbay D, Criddle L. Mastering temporary invasive cardiac pacing. Crit Care Nurse. 2004;24:25-32.
11. Goldberger J, Kruse J, Ehlert FA, Kadish A. Temporary transvenous pacemaker placement: what criteria constitute an adequate pacing site? Am Heart J. 1993;126:488-93.
12. Ezeugwu CO, Oropello JM, Pasik AS, Benjamin E. Position of temporary transvenous pacemaker after insertion. J Cardiothorac Vasc Anesth. 1994;8:367-8.
13. Murphy JJ. Current practice and complications of temporary transvenous cardiac pacing. BMJ. 1996;312:1134.
14. Betts TR. Regional survey of temporary transvenous pacing procedures and complications. Postgrad Med J. 2003;79:463-5.
15. McLeod AA, Jokhi PP. Pacemaker induced ventricular fibrillation in coronary care units. BMJ. 2004;328:1249-50.

30

Intra-aortic Balloon Pump Counterpulsation

Virendra K Arya

INTRODUCTION

The intra-aortic balloon pump (IABP) is most commonly employed temporary circulatory-assist device to improve coronary and systemic perfusion. It is being widely used in hemodynamically unstable critically ill patients with coronary artery disease and heart failure since its introduction into clinical practice in the 1960s. It is important to understand the basic principles, physiological effects, appropriate set-up and potential problems of IABP use for better patient outcome and safe use of this device.

INDICATION

As per existing literature following are evidence-based indications for use of IABP therapy:

Indications with Proven Benefit[1-3]

- Cardiogenic shock secondary to acute myocardial infarction refractory to medical therapy
- Mechanical complications of acute myocardial infarction: acute mitral regurgitation and ventricular septal defect
- Refractory ventricular arrhythmias
- Refractory unstable angina
- Decompensated systolic heart failure (as a bridge to definitive treatment).

Indications with Probable Benefit[4]

- Perioperative support for high-risk coronary artery bypass surgery
- Perioperative support for high-risk cardiac patients undergoing noncardiac surgery
- Decompensated aortic stenosis

Indications with No Evidence to Suggest Benefit[5]

- Sepsis
- Routine use in high-risk patients undergoing percutaneous coronary intervention (PCI).

Perera et al. in 2010 published one large randomized controlled trial showing no significant benefit in reducing the incidence of major adverse cardiovascular and cerebral events at 4 weeks by elective IABP insertion before high-risk PCI. Hence, at present routine IABP therapy in high-risk patients undergoing PCI is not recommended and is only preserved to patients who are unstable or likely to become unstable during PCI.

CONTRAINDICATION

Absolute

- Significant aortic regurgitation and aortic dissection
- Aortic stent
- End-stage cardiac disease with no viable other treatment options
- Bilateral femoral-popliteal bypass grafts (femoral route only contraindicated).

Relative

- Uncontrolled sepsis
- Abdominal aortic aneurysm
- Severe bilateral peripheral vascular disease
- Uncontrolled bleeding disorder
- Prosthetic ileofemoral grafts/iliac artery stents
- Distal aortic arch and descending aorta having grade 4 to 5 atheroma on TEE examination.

TECHNIQUE: BASIC PRINCIPLES

It was shown historically that removing a certain amount of blood volume from the femoral artery during systole and replacing this volume rapidly during diastole could increase coronary perfusion, decrease cardiac workload and reduce myocardial oxygen consumption.[6] In 1953, Kantrowitz first proposed that by increasing aortic diastolic pressure one could improve coronary blood flow and benefit patients with ischemic heart disease;[7] however, this technique had limitations due to problems with access (need for arteriotomies of both femoral arteries), turbulence and development of massive hemolysis by the pumping apparatus. In the early 1960s, Moulopoulos, Topaz and Kolff developed an experimental prototype of the intra-aortic balloon whose inflation and deflation were timed to the cardiac cycle.[8] By 1968, Kantrowiz and colleagues first applied IABP in clinical setting.[9] In 1973, two different groups[10,11] reported the successful use of the IABP in patients who could not be weaned from cardiopulmonary bypass and a new era in the perioperative care of patients with ventricular dysfunction was started. Initially, an open surgical insertion and removal were required for an IABP catheter that was 15 Fr gauge in size; later on with 8 Fr gauge catheter made available commercially, percutaneous IABP insertion becomes possible with less complications.[12] The first prefolded IAB was developed in 1986.

Basic Principles of Counterpulsation

Counterpulsation describes of balloon inflation in diastole and deflation in early systole. Balloon inflation in diastole causes displacement of blood within the aorta, both proximally and distally leading to an increase in coronary blood flow and also potential improvements in systemic perfusion by augmentation of the intrinsic elastic recoil of the aortic root. Deflation of balloon during early systole creates extra space in aorta thus reducing afterload and improving ventricular ejection of failing heart against reduced afterload.

Equipment

The IABP console (Fig. 1) includes the following: (1) A helium gas cylinder—helium has advantage over other gases of being least viscous and inert gas so that the lag time in inflation and deflation of balloon is least; (2) a gas supply unit; (3) a monitoring system for recording the ECG and blood pressure; (4) a control unit that processes the ECG and generates a triggering signal. This regulates timing of inflation and deflation of the balloon via either opening a valve to supply gas or closing it to interrupt the gas flow. Description of the circuit between the patient and the IABP is shown in Figure 2 and description of the IABP catheter is shown in Figure 3.

Latest fiberoptic IABP catheter does not require re-zeroing or flush system. Electrical interference, patient movements or anything interfering with quality of pressure waveform signal does not affect it. Following the principle of counterpulsation, the IABP remains deflated during systole that coincides with the QRS-T interval (the R wave triggers deflation of the balloon). Subsequently, it is inflated during diastole, which corresponds to the T-P interval (Fig. 4).

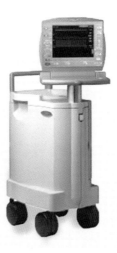

Fig. 1 Intra-aortic balloon pump console

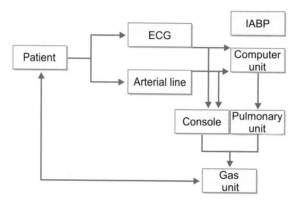

Fig. 2 Arrangement of circuit between patient and intra-aortic balloon pump (IABP)

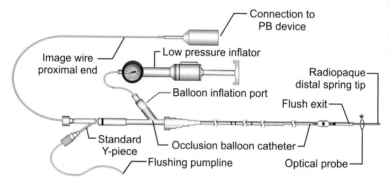

Fig. 3 Fiberoptic intra-aortic balloon pump catheter assembly and components

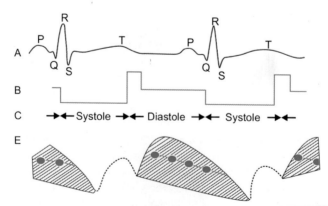

Fig. 4 Function of the intra-aortic balloon pump balloon. (A) ECG; (B and C) Balloon deflation—corresponding to systole, and inflation—corresponding to diastole; (E) Aortic pressure waveform during balloon function

Hemodynamic Changes during Intra-aortic Balloon Pump Therapy

Intra-aortic balloon pump primarily manipulates preload and afterload to produce its cardiovascular effects. Mechanical inflation of the balloon during diastole in aorta causes "volume displacement" that improves the coronary circulation, with a redistribution of blood flow and an alteration in oxygen consumption.[13] Deflation of the balloon takes place at the end of diastole, precisely at the start of isovolumic contraction. As a result, resistance to left ventricular output is reduced, thus reducing afterload.[14] In addition following hemodynamic effects of IABP therapy are observed:

- *Reduction in systolic pressure:* The systolic pressures of beats following IABP diastolic augmentation are about 10% less as compared to nonaugmented beats implying a reduction in afterload.[15]
- *Fall in presystolic (end-diastolic) aortic pressure:* During IABP therapy, the end-diastolic aortic pressure is reduced by up to 30%, implying systolic unloading.
- *Shortening of the isometric phase of left ventricular contraction:* Due to IABP deflation, the aortic valve opens prematurely, thus shortening the isovolumic phase of left ventricular contraction and thereby reducing myocardial oxygen consumption.[16]
- *Reduction of left ventricular wall tension and rate of increase in left ventricular pressure (dP/dT):* The rate of increase in left ventricular pressure is reduced by IABP therapy by up to 20% in comparison with control values.[17]
- *Effects on ejection fraction, cardiac output and the Frank-Starling law for the left ventricle:* Left ventricular ejection fraction is improved during IABP therapy. In addition, cardiac output is increased between 0.5 and 1.0 L/min, or up to 30%. The Frank-Starling curve is displaced toward the left, indicating an improvement in left ventricular function.[18]
- *Reduction in preload and afterload:* The left ventricular diastolic volume is reduced because of systolic unloading. In addition, the relation between the change in left ventricular diastolic pressure and the change in left ventricular diastolic volume shows a tendency toward lower values, which translates into an improvement in left ventricular compliance.[19]
- Increase in diastolic pressure time index (DPTI)/tension time index (TTI) ratio is seen.

Intra-aortic Balloon Pump and Myocardial Oxygen Supply and Demand

The analysis of arterial waveform for the DPTI and the TTI depicts effect of the IABP in improving myocardial oxygen supply via an improved DPTI/TTI ratio (Fig. 5). The DPTI reflects the diastolic and subendocardial blood flow and depends on the aortic diastolic pressure, the left ventricular end-diastolic pressure and the duration of diastole. IABP increases DPTI by raising the diastolic blood pressure and reducing the end-diastolic pressure. The TTI represents the area under the left ventricular systolic pressure curve that in turn reflects myocardial oxygen consumption. The TTI is reduced during balloon deflation because of the reduction in systolic blood pressure.

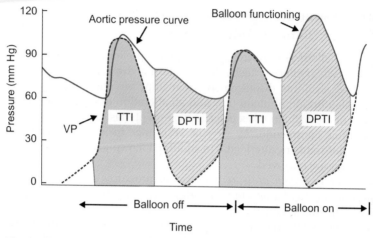

Fig. 5 Effect of the intra-aortic balloon pump on myocardial oxygen supply (DPTI) and demand (TTI)

The ratio DPTI/TTI is called the endocardial viability ratio (EVR) and it represents the relationship between myocardial oxygen supply and consumption. A normal balance between myocardial oxygen supply and demand is equivalent to the maximum EVR value of one. An EVR value of less than 0.7 indicates severe myocardial ischemia. IABP use has been shown to result in an increase in EVR.[20] The EVR index is a useful criterion for deciding on the prompt use of IABP in cases of intraoperative heart failure.

Intra-aortic Balloon Pump and Perfusion of the Coronary Circulation

IABP balloon inflation during diastole causes displacement of the surrounding blood and an increase in diastolic pressure. This increases coronary perfusion via an increase in the diastolic perfusion pressure gradient. In animal studies with normal systemic blood pressure, the IABP reduced myocardial oxygen consumption without causing a significant change in the overall coronary flow. In ischemic animal models with hypotension, the myocardial oxygen consumption depended on coronary flow. The IABP had a small effect on the perfusion of myocardial regions supplied by obstructed coronary vessels.[21] It has been seen that the blood flow peripheral to the stenosis remained unchanged during IABP therapy and it causes an increase in prestenotic as opposed to poststenotic flow.[22,23] However, relief of angina symptoms in patients with coronary artery disease and severe aortic disease have been observed with IABP use indicating that there must have been improvement in coronary flow.[24] It has been proposed that the balloon action to increase in diastolic pressure stimulates the collateral circulation in the region around the ischemic core of the myocardial lesion. Hence, IABP therapy is also described as "artificial myoconservation".[25,26] Kern et al. recorded the velocity time integral of diastolic flow to measure the intracoronary flow velocity during catheterization in 12 patients who were undergoing IABP treatment.[27] They observed greatest increase diastolic blood flow in patients with baseline systolic pressure less than 90 mm Hg and concluded that the IABP increased the proximal coronary flow velocity via a doubling of the velocity time integral of diastolic flow. During IABP therapy, the end-diastolic pressure is reduced and this according to Laplace's Law will reduce the wall stress caused before the opening of the aortic valve, thus reducing myocardial oxygen demand. In a study, done to determine the effects of IABP therapy on systolic unloading, independently of the increase in diastolic pressure; it was found that the systolic unloading was apparent under normotensive conditions, but not under hypotensive conditions (coronary perfusion pressure < 80 mm Hg).[28] Hypotension increases aortic compliance causing expansion of the aortic wall during balloon inflation, hence no displacement of blood volume. Furthermore, at the instant of balloon deflation, aortic pressure is not reduced, and consequently there is no reduction in either static work or myocardial oxygen consumption.

Intra-aortic Balloon Pump and the Peripheral Circulation

Pressure, resistance, and rheological properties of blood determine peripheral blood flow. Balloon inflation during diastole increases diastolic blood pressure, with a consequent increase in arteriovenous pressure gradient and an improvement in diastolic blood flow. In addition, this also causes activation of the aortic baroreceptors due to displacement of the stroke volume, and in turn blocks the medullary vasoconstrictive reflex. This reduces peripheral vascular resistance, thus improving blood flow. During prolonged hemorrhagic shock, the IABP appears to improve the vasokinetic control of splanchnic blood flow. It eliminates the phenomenon of hyperemic reperfusion and thus reduces reperfusion injury.[29] The effects of the IABP on postoperative renal function were shown to improve renal perfusion during counterpulsation;[30] however, a mean reduction of 66% in renal blood flow was found while the lower end of IABP balloon was placed opposite to the origin of renal arteries.[31] A reduction in urine output after insertion of IABP is highly suggestive of the possibility of juxtarenal balloon positioning.

Intra-aortic balloon pump causes hemolysis from mechanical damage to the red blood cells and the hemoglobin levels and the hematocrit often decrease up to 5%. Thrombocytopenia can also result from mechanical damage to the platelets, heparin administration, or both.[32]

The cerebral autoregulation is not adversely affected by the use of fully augmented IABP. However, cerebral autoregulation efficiency worsens with the potential risk of cerebral hypoperfusion when progressive reductions in inflation ratio are made during counterpulsation weaning. Patients with cardiogenic shock and inflation ratio reduction often show reduction in electroencephalogram (EEG) chaotic activity at end-diastole that may be indicating impairment of cerebral blood flow (CBF) dynamics. In a study that measured cerebral blood flow velocities using transcranial Doppler (TCD) at the middle cerebral artery showed that the end-diastolic velocities became negative. These were known as "reversal flow" and were considered to be the result of a steeling phenomenon from the deflation of the IABP in the aortic root.[33] However, clinically relevant effects of this phenomenon are still not clear.

The variables that influence the increase in diastolic pressure during balloon inflation are shown in Box 1. The aortic elasticity is an important factor and it

---

Box 1 Variables that affect the increase in diastolic pressure with intra-aortic balloon pump[34]

- *Balloon position:* Nearer to the aortic valve causes greater increase in diastolic pressure.
- *Volume:* When balloon volume equals the stroke volume, diastolic pressure augmentation becomes maximized.
- *Diameter and obstructive capability of the balloon:* The greatest possible increase is seen during complete aortic obstruction.
- *Heart rate:* LV and aortic diastolic filling times are inversely proportional to heart rate; shorter diastolic time produces lesser balloon augmentation per unit time.
- Optimal regulation of balloon gas flow and timing.
- *Stroke volume:* When stroke volume is < 25 mL, no significant diastolic increase occurs. In hypovolemia stroke volume reduces, hence IABP become ineffective.
- *Aortic compliance:* As aortic compliance increases (or SVR decreases), the magnitude of diastolic augmentation decreases.
- *Blood pressure:* It is indirectly related to the aortic elasticity. Aortic volume doubles when mean blood pressure increases from 30 mm Hg to a normal 90 mm Hg.

Abbreviations: LV, left ventricle; SVR, systemic vascular resistance.

has been shown that the balloon is restricted by the aortic blood volume shortly before inflation, and any further increase in the pump volume results only in swelling of the aorta and not in effective distribution of the blood.[34]

TECHNIQUE: INSERTION AND OPERATION

Preparation

Intra-aortic balloon pump insertion is most of times an emergency rescue procedure and only require echo to rule out cardiac contraindications and ultrasound vascular scan of the artery from where it is intended to be inserted, if moderate-to-severe aortic regurgitation or vascular occlusion of artery is suspected. The site is prepared by routine antiseptic solutions like betadine or chlorhexidine solutions as for any cut-down or central venous access procedure. Baseline blood work should be sent before or soon after insertion to rule out subsequent hemolytic and renal effects of IABP.

Device Insertion

It is important to always review the instruction booklet supplied with IABP catheter before use. The size of the IABP balloon is chosen based on the height of the patient. The usual range for an adult patient is between 25 cc (for patients under 5 feet tall) to 50 cc (for patients over 6 feet tall) but operator must follow individual manufacturer's guidance manual. The IABP is usually inserted percutaneously through femoral artery using the Seldinger technique under strict aseptic precautions in supine position. Alternative access sites include brachial and axillary artery percutaneous insertion techniques and open surgical aortic approach. A Seldinger technique is used after successful puncture of the chosen artery to insert a dilator and sheath combination on a J-shaped guidewire that is inserted to the level of the aortic arch through puncture cannula. Then dilator is removed and the sheath allows the balloon to be fed over the guidewire into the descending aorta, usually under fluoroscopic guidance. The tip of the IABP catheter should be 1–2 cm distal to the origin of the left subclavian artery. This corresponds to the level of the second rib (Fig. 6). In the case of blind placement, the take-off of the left subclavian artery can be identified using the second rib as a landmark. The caudal end of the balloon should be positioned above the origin of the renal arteries. In most patients, the right and left renal arteries arise between the first and second lumbar vertebral bodies.

Alternative methods used for guiding IABP catheter placement are trans-esophageal echocardiography or open sheath less insertion during cardiac surgery. Percutaneous sheath less insertion can be used in patients with peripheral vascular disease but this method is associated with an increase in minor bleeding and infection.

Initial Set-up (Triggering and Timing)

Following insertion, the balloon catheter is connected to the console and the system is purged with helium. The central lumen of the catheter is then connected to a pressure transducer. An aortic pressure waveform should be visible after this is done. Most important precaution is not to take blood samples from this line. Systemic anticoagulation (unfractionated heparin 2,500–5,000 IU 6–8 hourly) is usually now given, aiming for a target activated partial thromboplastin ratio of 2 or activated clotting time (ACT) between 250–300.

Precise timing of balloon inflation and deflation during the cardiac cycle is essential to ensure optimal effects of counterpulsation whilst minimizing possible

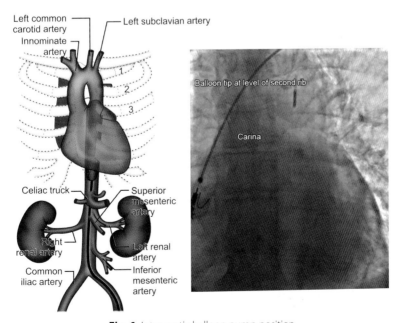

Fig. 6 Intra-aortic balloon pump position

harmful effects related to mistiming. Most commonly, the ECG waveform is used to trigger balloon inflation and deflation. In case of poor ECG trace or cardiac arrhythmias, the arterial pressure waveform is an alternative technique; however, damping of arterial pressure line could be a problem. Modern machines allow either method to be easily selected. The balloon starts to inflate at the onset of diastole, which corresponds to the middle of T-wave on the ECG waveform and the dicrotic notch of the arterial pressure trace. The balloon inflation causes a sharp upstroke on the arterial pressure waveform at the aortic valve closure followed by a tall peak that represents the assisted diastolic pressure. Deflation occurs at a point just before the upstroke of systole on the arterial pressure trace (immediately before opening of the aortic valve) corresponding with the peak of the R-wave on the ECG trace. As the balloon deflates, the assisted aortic end-diastolic pressure dips down to create the second deep wave, usually U-shaped on the arterial pressure waveform. IABP timing in relation to the cardiac cycle is monitored by display of arterial pressure waveform, the ECG trace and an intraballoon pressure trace as shown in Figures 7 and 8.

While IABP augmentation is optimal the diastolic augmented pressures goes higher than the systolic pressures, hence the radial artery invasive pressures will be showing diastolic augmented pressures as systolic pressures that may be higher than actual systolic pressures. Similarly, the postaugmented dip, which is deeper than actual diastolic pressures will be read as diastolic pressures. This means that both systolic and diastolic pressures displayed by radial artery pressure line are actually diastolic phase pressures with optimally functional IABP (Fig. 8). IABP monitor display console should be monitored for actual display of all pressures.

The number of augmented beats per cardiac cycle is referred to as augmentation frequency ratio. This is selected based on the hemodynamic status and the presence of myocardial ischemia. In practice, an augmentation ratio of 1:1 is initially used provided heart rate is less than or equal to 100. The volume of balloon inflation can be adjusted to adjust level of augmentation. Initially, full augmentation is applied. Inaccurate early timing of inflation leads to increased afterload for left ventricle and premature early deflation may lead to coronary artery steal thus worsen hemodynamic instability and further compromise coronary perfusion.

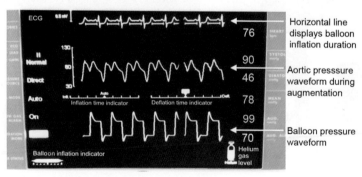

Fig. 7 Intra-aortic balloon pump display screen during ECG triggered 1 : 1 augmentation

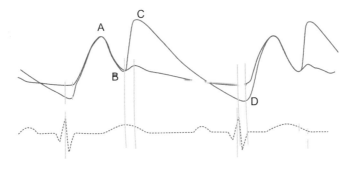

— Arterial pressure waveform during IABP therapy
— Arterial pressure waveform without IABP therapy
····· ECG waveform
A-Systolic pressure
B-Dicrotic notch (balloon inflation)
C-Augmented diastolic pressure
D-Reduced end diastolic pressure (balloon deflation)

Fig. 8 Intra-aortic balloon pump arterial waveform in relation to cardiac cycle (1:1 augmentation)

Selection of Timing Method on the Basis of the Goals of Counterpulsation

It is important to determine the goals of counterpulsation therapy before the timing method or settings are chosen since it has been found that maximizing inflation time and left ventricle unloading cannot be done simultaneously.[35] For example, in patients with acute ischemia, who have not undergone revascularization, IABP therapy may prove beneficial, if the goal is to improve perfusion to the heart. In this situation, conventional timing set to achieve the maximum inflated time, without compromising systole, may be appropriate. In revascularized patients, an IABP is primarily used with aim to assist in left ventricle recovery and healing. In such cases, timing should be more focused on deflation and real-time or R-wave deflation should be used to optimize unloading of the left ventricle and reduce cardiac work. Fully automatic IABP timing can be accurate, reducing timing errors and improving the ease of use of IABPs. However, the effect on clinical outcomes has not been examined, so the clinical benefit is unclear. Table 1 summarizes risks and benefits of various timing practices.

Intra-aortic Balloon Pump Arterial Waveform Analysis

Two waveforms need to be set for the IABP to "pump" effectively: (1) The ECG signal to "trigger" the balloon and, (2) The arterial pressure signal to "time" the counterpulsation. The arterial waveform is a less reliable trigger and uses the systolic upstroke. IABP arterial waveform analysis on the console monitor display can be used for the detection and correction balloon inflation and deflation timings errors. During normal augmentation, assisted systolic and diastolic pressures are always less than unassisted systolic and diastolic pressures and augmentation starts from dicrotic notch and ends just before next systole (Fig. 9).

Table 1 Benefits and risks of various timing practices for intra-aortic balloon pump

Timing method	Benefits	Risks
• Conventional inflation	Improved oxygen supply	None
• Conventional deflation	↓ afterload	↓ augmentation
• Real time deflation (R-wave deflation)	↑ stroke volume/cardiac output	↑ myocardial oxygen demand
		↑ left ventricular stroke work
Timing errors		
• Early inflation	None	↓ stroke volume
		↑ left ventricular stroke work
		↑ dyssynchrony
• Late inflation	None	↓ augmentation time
• Early deflation	None	↓ augmentation time
• Late deflation	None, extremely dangerous, left ventricle eject against afterload imposed by balloon	↓ stroke volume/cardiac output
		↑ myocardial oxygen demand
		↑ left ventricular stroke work

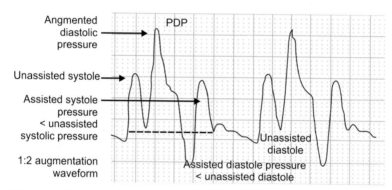

Fig. 9 Optimal inflation and deflation timings of intra-aortic balloon pump in 1 : 2 augmentations

If the IABP balloon is inflated early, the upstroke of peak diastolic pressure occurs early on the descending portion of unassisted systolic pressure waveform (Fig. 10A). In case of early deflation, the U-shape rather than V-shape of the arterial waveform is noted and a brief shelf before the next systole is formed (Fig. 10B). In case of late deflation, the balloon remains partly or completely inflated at the beginning of the next systole and the balloon-assisted aortic end-diastolic pressure becomes greater than the unassisted end-diastolic pressure (Fig. 10C). This situation is extremely dangerous and modern IABP consoles have inbuilt mechanism to prevent it. A significant portion of the dicrotic notch is visible in case of late balloon inflation (Fig. 10D).

IABP Balloon Pressure Waveform Analysis

IABP balloon pressure waveform analysis can be used to set the balloon inflation level as well as for diagnosis of balloon inflation-related problems. Figure 11 shows normal balloon pressure waveform.

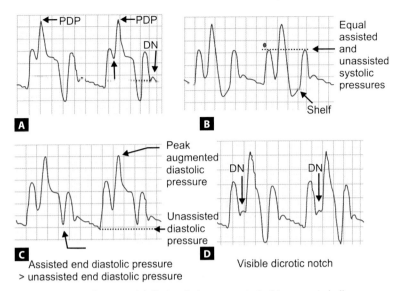

Figs 10A to D Inflation and deflation timings errors in 1 : 2 intra-aortic balloon pump augmentations

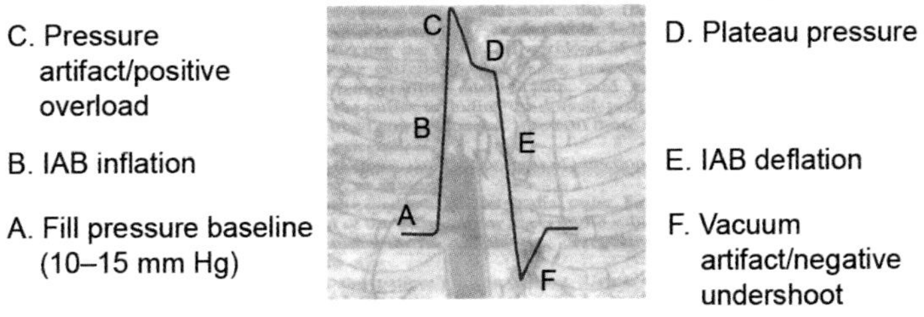

C. Pressure artifact/positive overload

B. IAB inflation

A. Fill pressure baseline (10–15 mm Hg)

D. Plateau pressure

E. IAB deflation

F. Vacuum artifact/negative undershoot

Fig. 11 Normal IABP balloon pressure waveform and its components

Low balloon pressure plateau could be seen in hypotension, hypovolemia, low systemic vascular resistance, low balloon inflation volume, a balloon sized too small for the patient or positioned too low in the aorta (Fig. 12A). High balloon pressure plateau may be caused by hypertension, a balloon too large for the aorta, or a restriction to gas flow within the system. The top of the plateau may be square or rounded (Fig. 12B). Balloon pressure baseline elevation may be caused by a restriction of gas flow or gas system over pressurization (Fig. 12C). A helium leak is usually indicated by balloon pressure baseline depression. Other possible causes not related to helium leak include inappropriate timing settings (early inflation or late deflation) that do not permit enough time for gas to return to the console or a mechanical defect that causes failure to autofill (Fig. 12D).

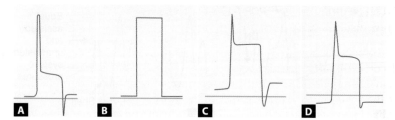

Figs 12A to D Various waveforms of intra-aortic balloon pump balloon: (A) Low balloon pressure plateau; (B) High balloon pressure plateau; (C) Balloon pressure baseline elevation; (D) Balloon pressure baseline depression

MAIN POINTS OF CARE

It is recommended that hospitals should have patient care protocols with an IABP in situ. These protocols should include the following:

- Patients should be managed in a suitable area by staff conversant with IABP management.
- Ensure reliable triggering and correct timing.
- Monitor vital signs and the need for augmentation regularly. Very high systolic pressures on radial arterial line indicate high augmentation and need to be adjusted. These high pressures should never be treated with vasodilators; in fact, vasodilators should not be used while patient is on IABP.
- Despite another arterial line is in situ, always record patient's blood pressure from IABP console.
- Patients should be anticoagulated as per unit protocol unless there is a contraindication.
- Do not take blood samples from the balloon arterial pressure line.
- It is important to perform hourly assessment for signs of peripheral hypoperfusion or limb ischemia in the limb distal to the IABP catheter insertion site. This should include assessment of color, capillary refill, sensation and presence of pulses by palpation or Doppler studies.
- It is not unusual for left upper limb circulation to become compromised in the event of proximal migration of the catheter obstructing left subclavian artery blood flow. Hence, hourly perfusion assessment of the left upper limb should be performed.
- Presence of limb ischemia should be a prompt consideration for removal of the IABP and sheath and urgent vascular surgical review.
- The end of the patient bed should not be elevated to more than 30 degree to minimize proximal catheter migration.
- Regularly assess insertion site for oozing, bleeding, swelling and signs of infection.
- Regularly check hemoglobin (risk of bleeding or hemolysis)
- Regularly check platelet count (risk of thrombocytopenia)
- Regularly check renal function (risk of acute kidney injury secondary to distal migration of IABP catheter)
- The balloon pump must not be left in standby by mode for any longer than necessary and never longer than 20 minutes in view of high-risk of device-related thrombus formation.

WEANING FROM INTRA-AORTIC BALLOON PUMP COUNTERPULSATION

Once the patient is not in cardiogenic shock and have an adequate blood pressure whilst on minimal or no inotropic support, weaning from IABP should be started. Reasonable target values to aim for prior to weaning are a mean arterial pressure more than or equal to 65 mm Hg, reasonably warm extremities and, if monitored, a cardiac index of more than or equal to 2 l/min/m², no lactic acidosis and mixed venous saturation more than or equal to 60%. IABP counterpulsation weaning is usually started by reducing the ratio of augmented to nonaugmented beats. This can be done by reducing the augmentation frequency every 1–6 hours, from the ratios of 1:1 to 1:2 to 1:3. If a ratio of 1:3 is tolerated for 6 hours by the patient, this is an indication for IABP to be put into the standby mode and remove. An alternative weaning method is to decrease the balloon filling volume (augmentation level) by 10 mL every 1–6 hours until a filling volume of 20 mL is reached. The balloon pump should not be left in situ once IABP is switched off as this is associated with a high chance of thrombus formation on the balloon and distal embolization. A ratio of 1:3 should also not be used for prolonged periods as this is also associated with a significant increase in thrombosis risk.

COMPLICATION/PROBLEM

Problems

Common problems, their causes and recommended action are described in Table 2.

Table 2 Troubleshooting while intra-aortic balloon pump counterpulsation

Problem	Cause	Action
ECG troubleshooting		
Interference in ECG	Faulty lead/electrodes	Check electrode contact/replace
Intermittent ECG	Faulty lead/electrodes/cable	Check electrode contact/replace
Weak ECG signal	Wrong electrode position/ poor quality electrodes	Try alternate lead configuration/ adjust gain setting
Trigger troubleshooting		
Does not trigger	ECG signal too small	↑ ECG gain
Triggers erratically	Large A-pacer tails/demand pacer in V/AV mode	Select A pacer trigger
		Select ECG or pressure trigger
Alternate in pressure mode	Pressure trigger needs resynchronization	Start resynchronization
Balloon troubleshooting		
Requires frequent preloading	Leak in safety disc or balloon/ loose attachment	Check and replace
Poor augmentation		Check and tighten/replace balloon
Cannot autofill	Clogged/faulty filter	Call service engineer
	No helium/fill malfunction	Replace helium/manual fill
Power troubleshooting		
No function in portable mode	Low battery charge	Charge/replace battery

Complication

The incidence of one or more major complications (defined as death, major limb ischemia, severe bleeding or balloon leak) was reported 2.8% by the Benchmark Counterpulsation Outcomes Registry. The incidence of minor complications was found in 4.2% of the patients. This registry published data on nearly 1,700 patients who underwent IABP therapy between 1996 and 2000.[3]

The most common complications of IABP therapy arise either from the intravascular presence of the device itself or the technique used for its insertion. Red blood cells and platelets are mechanically injured from rapid inflation and deflation of the balloon that commonly results in anemia and/or thrombocytopenia. IABP catheter-related thrombus formation and subsequent embolization are also significant risks involved. Consequently, patients with an IABP in situ are usually anticoagulated systemically, resulting in an increased risk of bleeding from the catheter insertion site.

The most common vascular complication is limb ischemia as many patients requiring IABP therapy will also have established peripheral arterial disease or multiple risk factors. All patients must therefore be monitored on an hourly basis for their peripheral pulses, capillary return and skin temperature till an IABP catheter is in situ. In case of unresolved persistent limb ischemia, IABP catheter may require removal and urgent vascular surgical review.

Balloon rupture is a rare complication that is usually indicated by a sudden loss of inflation pressure or the presence of blood in the balloon line. This is associated with a risk of intraballoon thrombus formation and intravascular helium embolization. The inbuilt safety mechanism in IABP device is that in case of balloon rupture the console will alarm and withdraw helium from the balloon before shutting down. In such situation, balloon should be removed to ensure complete removal of helium gas. The complications of IABP are listed in Table 3.

SPECIAL SITUATIONS

* *Cardiac arrest:* Pressure triggering should be selected with reduction in the pressure threshold on the IABP console. Internal mode should be used if there is no arterial pressure trace; however, this increases the chance of asynchronous counterpulsation.

Table 3 Complications of intra-aortic balloon pump[36]

Vascular	Balloon-related
• Limb ischemia	• Misplacement or migration of the balloon (may lead to occlusion of renal or subclavian arteries or perforation of the aortic arch)
• Vascular laceration and local vascular injury at time of insertion	
• Aortic dissection	• Balloon perforation or rupture leading to gas embolization
• Spinal cord and visceral ischemia	
• Peripheral thrombotic embolization	• Thrombocytopenia
• False aneurysm and AV fistula formation	• Anemia
Miscellaneous	
• Infection	
• Entrapment	

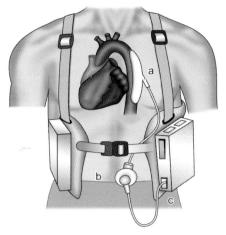

Fig. 13 Components of the Kantrowitz CardioVAD (KCV): (a) Blood pump,
(b) Percutaneous access device (PAD), (c) Mobile drive console
Source: Reproduced with permission from: Circulation 2002;106:i-183-8.

- *Defibrillation:* IABP counterpulsation does not need to be discontinued during defibrillation, but staff must remain clear of the IABP console and connections when a shock is delivered.

PERMANENT INTRA-AORTIC BALLOON PUMP

In 2002, Jeevanandam and colleagues implanted permanent IABP known as the Kantrowitz Cardio Ventricular-assist-device (KCV) in patients with end-stage cardiomyopathy refractory to medical treatment and who were not transplant candidates.[37] They reported hemodynamic and functional improvement in the status of these patients and the ability of the device to be used intermittently without anticoagulation.

The KCV drive consoles consist of the microprocessor that automatically analyzes electrical signals from the heart and actuates shuttling of compressed air to the device (Fig. 13). Patient can turn-off the KCV at will and also disconnect it allowing more patient comfort without increasing the risk for thromboembolism. This device has no valves or internal electronics and requires no anticoagulation.

The main drawback of KCV is that it provides only "partial" support and increases cardiac output by approximately 40% depending on the afterload condition of the patient. It depends on native heart activity to function and cannot be placed in patients with severe biventricular dysfunction, uncontrolled tachyarrhythmias, or with native valvular disease. Because of these shortcomings, this device is not popular at present as bridge to transplant in end-stage cardiac failure patients.

REFERENCES

1. Ryan TJ, Antman EM, Brooks NH, Califf RM, Hillis D, Hiratzka LF, et al. 1999 Update: ACC/AHA Guidelines for the Management of Patients With Acute Myocardial Infarction: Executive Summary and Recommendations A Report of the American College of Cardiology/American Heart Association Task Force on Practice Guidelines (Committee on Management of Acute Myocardial Infarction). Circulation. 1999;100: 1016-30.
2. Fotopoulos GD, Mason MJ, Walker S, Jepson NS, Patel DJ, Mitchell AG, et al. Stabilisation of medically refractory ventricular arrhythmia by intra-aortic balloon counterpulsation. Heart. 1999;82:96-100.
3. Ferguson JJ 3rd, Cohen M, Freedman RJ Jr, Stone GW, Miller MF, Joseph DL, et al. The current practice of intra-aortic balloon counterpulsation: results from the Benchmark Registry. J Am Coll Cardiol. 2001;38(5):1456-62.
4. Rubino AS, Onorati F, Santarpino G, Abdalla K, Caroleo S, Santangelo E, et al. Early IABP following perioperative myocardial injury improves hospital and mid-term prognosis. Interact Cardiovasc Thorac Surg. 2009;8:310-5.
5. Perera D, Stables R, Thomas M, Booth J, Pitt M, BCIS-1 Investigators, et al. Elective intra-aortic balloon counterpulsation during high-risk percutaneous coronary intervention: a randomized controlled trial. JAMA. 2010;304:867-74.
6. Moazami N, McCarthy PM. Temporary circulatory support. In: Cohn LH, Edmunds LH Jr (Eds). Cardiac Surgery in the Adult. New York: McGraw Hill. 2003. pp. 495-520.
7. Kantrowitz A. Origins of intraaortic balloon pumping. Ann Thorac Surg. 1990;50:672-4.
8. Moulopoulos SD, Topaz S, Kolff WJ. Diastolic balloon pumping (with carbon dioxide) in the aorta—a mechanical assistance to the failing circulation. Am Heart J. 1962;63: 669-75.
9. Kantrowitz A, Tjonneland S, Krakauer JS, Phillips SJ, Freed PS, Butner AN. Mechanical intraaortic cardiac assistance in cardiogenic shock. Hemodynamic effects. Arch Surg. 1968;97:1000-4.
10. Buckley MJ, Craver JM, Gold HK, Mundth ED, Daggett WM, Austen WG. Intra-aortic balloon pump assist for cardiogenic shock after cardiopulmonary bypass. Circulation. 1973;48:III90-4.
11. Housman LB, Bernstein EF, Braunwald NS, Dilley RB. Counterpulsation for intraoperative cardiogenic shock. Successful use of intra-aortic balloon. JAMA. 1973;224:1131-3.
12. Kuki S, Taniguchi K, Masai T, Yoshida K, Yamamoto K, Matsuda H. Usefulness of the low profile "True 8" intra-aortic balloon pumping catheter for preventing limb ischemia. ASAIO J. 2001;47:611-4.
13. Williams DO, Korr KS, Gewirtz H, Most AS. The effect of intraaortic balloon counterpulsation on regional myocardial blood flow and oxygen consumption in the presence of coronary artery stenosis in patients with unstable angina. Circulation. 1982;66:593-7.
14. Folland ED, Kemper AJ, Khuri SF, Josa M, Parisi AF. Intraaortic balloon counterpulsation as a temporary support measure in decompensated critical aortic stenosis, J Am Coll Cardiol. 1985;5:711-6.
15. Schottler M, Schaefer J, Schwarzkorpf HJ, Wysocki R. Experimentally induced changes of arterial mean and aortic opening pressure by controlled variation of diastolic augmentation. Basic Res Cardiol. 1974;69:59-67.
16. Mullins CB, Sugg WL, Kennelly BM, Jones DC, Mitchell JH. Effect of arterial counterpulsation on left ventricular volume and pressure. Am J Physiol. 1971;220:694-8.
17. Urschel CW, Eber L, Forrester J, Matloff J, Carpenter R, Sonnenblick E. Alteration of mechanical performance of the ventricle by intraaortic balloon counterpulsation. Am J Cardiol. 1970;25:546-51.

18. Nichols AB, Pohost GM, Gold HK, Leinbach RC, Beller GA, McKusick KA, et al. Left ventricular function during intraaortic balloon pumping assessed by multigated cardiac blood pool imaging. Circulation. 1978;58:I176-83.

19. Diamond G, Forrester JS. Effect of coronary artery disease and acute myocardial infarction on left ventricular compliance in man. Circulation. 1972;45:11-9.

20. Nanas JN, Nanas SN, Kontoyannis DA, Moussoutzani KS, Hatzigeorgiou JP, Heras PB, et al. Myocardial salvage by the use of reperfusion and intraaortic balloon pump: experimental study. Ann Thorac Surg. 1996;61:629-34.

21. Kern MJ, Aguirre FV, Caraccido EA, Bach RG, Donohue TJ, Lasorda D, et al. Hemodynamic effects of new intra-aortic balloon counterpulsation timing methods in patients: a multicenter evaluation. Am Heart J. 1999;137:1129-36.

22. Berne RM, Levy MN. Cardiovascular Physiology, 6th edition (chap. 8). St Louis: Mosby-Year Book. 1992. pp. 225.

23. MacDonald RG, Hill JA, Feldman RL. Failure of intra-aortic balloon counterpulsation to augment distal coronary perfusion pressure during percutaneous transluminal coronary angioplasty. Am J Cardiol. 1987;59:359-61.

24. Folland ED, Kemper AJ, Khuri SF, Josa M, Parisi AF. Intraaortic balloon counterpulsation as a temporary support measure in decompensated critical aortic stenosis. J Am Coll Cardiol. 1985;5:711-6.

25. Ohman EM, George BS, White CJ. Kern MJ, Gurbel PA, Freedman RJ, et al. Use of aortic counterpulsation to improve sustained coronary artery patency during acute myocadial infarction. Results of a randomized trial. The Randomized IABP Study Group. Circulation. 1994;90:792-9.

26. Fuchs RM, Brin KP, Brinker JA, Guzman PA, Heuser RR, Yin FC. Augmentation of regional coronary blood flow by intra-aortic balloon counterpulsation in patients with unstable angina. Circulation. 1983;68:117-23.

27. Kern MJ, Aguirre F, Penick D. Enhanced intracoronary flow velocity during intra-aortic balloon counterpulsation in patients with coronary artery disease. Circulation. 1991; 84(Suppl II):II-485.

28. Akyurekli Y, Taichman GC, Keon WJ. Effectiveness of intraaortic balloon counterpulsation and systolic unloading. Can J Surg. 1980;23:122-6.

29. Landreneau R, Horton J, Cochran R. Splanchnic blood flow response to intraaortic balloon pump assist of hemorrhagic shock. J Surg Res. 1991;51:281-7.

30. Hilberman M, Derby GC, Spencer RJ, Stinson EB. Effect of the intra-aortic balloon pump upon postoperative renal function in man. Crit Care Med. 1981;9:85-9.

31. Swartz MT, Sakamoto T, Arai H, Reedy JE, Salenas L, Yuda T, et al. Effects of intraaortic balloon position on renal artery blood flow. Ann Thorac Surg. 1992;53:604-10.

32. Walls JT, Boley TM, Curtis JJ, Silver D. Heparin induced thrombocytopenia in patients undergoing intra-aortic balloon pumping after open heart surgery. ASAIO J. 1992;38:M574-6.

33. Bellapart J, Geng S, Dunster K, Timms D, Barnett AG, Boots R, et al. Intraaortic balloon pump counterpulsation and cerebral autoregulation: an observational study. BMC Anesthesiol. 2010;10:3-13.

34. Weber KT, Janicki JS. Intra-aortic balloon counterpulsation. A review of physiology principles, clinical results and device safety. Ann Thorac Surg. 1974;17:602-36.

35. Zelano JA, Li JK, Welkowitz W. A closed-loop control scheme for intraaortic balloon pumping. IEEE Trans Biomed Eng. 1990;37:182-92.

36. Parissis H, Soo A, Al-Alao B. Intra-aortic balloon pump: literature review of risk factors related to complications of the intraaortic balloon pump. J Cardiothorac Surg. 2011;6:147-52.

37. Jeevanandam V, Jayakar D, Anderson AS, Martin S, Piccione W Jr, Heroux AL, et al. Circulatory assistance with a permanent implantable IABP: initial human experience. Circulation. 2002;106:I183-8.

31

Tourniquet for Vascular Injuries

Sushma Sagar, Kamal Kataria

INTRODUCTION

A tourniquet is a device, which occludes blood circulation of upper and lower limb for a desired period of time. It is not only responsible for temporary occlusion of the bleeding vessels in emergency setting but also provides a bloodless operative field by exerting sufficient pressure on arterial blood flow during elective surgeries. During emergency, use of a tourniquet cannot reverse shock but it may lessen the intensity of shock and can provide vital time to start effective resuscitation.

Currently, there are two types of tourniquets in use, i.e. non-inflatable (non-pneumatic) tourniquets and pneumatic tourniquet. Non-pneumatic tourniquets are usually made of rubber or cloth with very few indications like phlebotomy, intravenous infusion and prehospital care of injured extremity. A pneumatic tourniquet constricts blood flow by air-inflated cuff. The amount of cuff pressure is controlled by a regulating device on the tourniquet machine.

INDICATION

A tourniquet may be useful in following conditions:
- Traumatic or non-traumatic amputations
- Intravenous regional anesthesia (Bier's block)
- Isolated limb perfusion for malignancies
- Injuries that do not allow direct control of bleeding
- Failure to control bleeding by direct pressure bandaging
- Reduction of fractures in the extremity
- Minor surgical procedures over hand, wrist or elbow
- Joint replacement surgeries
- Fasciotomy.

CONTRAINDICATION

The tourniquet should be used carefully in following conditions:
- Bleeding lesions, which can be controlled by simpler, safer means like direct wound pressure, a pressure dressing, and limb elevation

- Skin grafts (to help distinguish all bleeding points)
- Open fractures of the leg
- Severe peripheral vascular disease
- Sickle cell disease
- Severe crush injury
- Diabetic neuropathy
- Patients with history of deep vein thrombosis and pulmonary embolism.

APPLIED PHYSIOLOGY

Tourniquets when used judiciously prove very useful, whereas, if used for a wrong indication, they may lead to complications. For example, ischemic reperfusion injury can occur following the use of tourniquet in a wrong way. Here tissue damage occurs when the blood supply is returned after a period of ischemia. During the ischemic period, there is lack of nutrients and oxygen derived from the blood. This leads to creation of an environment in which reperfusion causes oxidative damage and inflammation.

TECHNIQUE

Earliest use of tourniquet dates back to 199 BCE–500 CE by Romans for controlling the bleeding during amputations. They used narrow straps of bronze.[1] Initially, a simple garrote, tightened by twisting a rod was used as tourniquet. The "tourniquet" derives its name from "tourner" which literally means turn. Later a French surgeon Jean Louis Petit in 1718 made a screw device for occlusion of blood flow during surgical procedures.[2] Subsequently, in 1864, Joseph Lister used for the first time a tourniquet device to create bloodless surgical field. He advocated limb elevation for exsanguination prior to use of tourniquet.[3] Friedrich von Esmarch developed a rubber bandage for control of both bleeding and exsanguinate in 1873, which came to be known as Esmarch's bandage or Esmarch's tourniquet. This device was better than earlier devices made with cloth or screws.[4] However, Richard von Volkmann showed that use of Esmarch's tourniquet can result in limb paralysis.[5] In 1904, Harvey Cushing developed a pneumatic tourniquet, which used compressed gas source to inflate cylindrical bladder and compress the blood vessels. This overcame the limitations of Esmarch's tourniquet as it could be applied and removed very quickly. Moreover, the chances of nerve paralysis were minimal.[6] James McEwen, a biomedical engineer in Vancouver, Canada invented the modern microcomputer based tourniquet.[7] Most of the modern systems are automated and estimate limb occlusion pressure with individualized setting of safe tourniquet pressures.

Limb Occlusion Pressure

The minimum pressure required to stop the flow of arterial blood into the limb distal to cuff, at a specific time by a specific tourniquet cuff applied to a specific location on the limb of a specific patient. Risk of nerve-related injury can be minimized by setting of tourniquet pressure on the basis of limb occlusion pressure. The Association of perioperative Registered Nurses (AORN) recommended that in adults, the tourniquet pressure may be set at limb occlusion pressure measured by a validated method, plus a safety margin of 40 mm Hg for limb occlusion pressure less than 130 mm Hg, 60 mm Hg for those of 131–190 mm Hg and 80 mm Hg for those of more than 190 mm Hg.[8] For children, an addition of 50 mm Hg to measured limb occlusion pressure has been recommended by the 2009 AORN.

Duration

It is patient's age, physical health and integrity of blood supply to the limb that determines the safe inflation time for tourniquet. Safe inflation time for a healthy adult is 1.5–2 hours.[9] It is recommended that tourniquet should be deflated for 10–15 minutes, if inflation time is more than safe limit. This deflation will restore oxygenated blood supply to distal part of limb as well as will allow the metabolic waste products to be removed.

PREPARATION AND PROCEDURE

The tourniquets to be applied by trained and knowledgeable persons who know about the uses and potential complications of pneumatic tourniquets. Before applying a tourniquet, following points should be kept in mind:
- The whole system should be leak proof.
- The tourniquet cuff should be kept away from skin antiseptic solutions.
- Cuff width should be of appropriate size (Fig. 1).
- Length of cuff should be 7–15 cm longer than circumference of limb.
- Cuff should be tied at a point of maximum circumference of limb.
- There should be adequate padding under the tourniquet.
- The cuff should not be rotated into a new position once it is applied over limb.
- Esmarch bandage exsanguination technique may prove to be effective in decreasing blood flow to the extremities (Fig. 2).
- Pressure gauges should be continually monitored to detect pressure variations (Fig. 3).

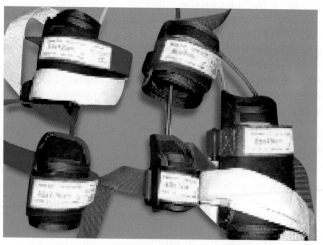

Fig. 1 Pneumatic tourniquets; correct cuff size depends on shape, length and width of the limb

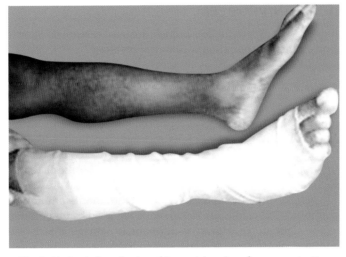

Fig. 2 Method of application of Esmarch bandage for exsanguination before application of tourniquet

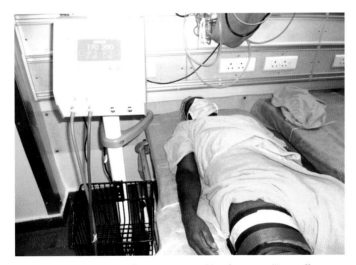

Fig. 3 Regulating device of tourniquet machine for controlling cuff pressure

- The cuff pressure and inflation time should be kept minimum after keeping in mind the age and comorbidities of patient.
- Surgeons should be kept informed of inflation times.

POST-PROCEDURE CARE

- Whenever possible disposable tourniquets should be encouraged otherwise reusable cuffs should be thoroughly cleaned.
- The affected limb should be thoroughly inspected for any complication.

COMPLICATION/PROBLEM

Complications are rare when the tourniquets are used carefully. Following are the complications, which are common with tourniquets use.

Local Complications

- *Muscle injury:* Very rarely, rhabdomyolysis has been reported due to tourniquet use. Sometimes, post-tourniquet syndrome can be seen which is characterized by subjective numbness of the limb without objective anesthesia. This is caused by ischemia, microvascular congestion and edema.
- *Nerve injury:* Neurological injuries ranging from paraesthesia to paralysis are common complications. These result due to mechanical pressure and faulty aneroid gauges. Large diameter nerve fibers are more commonly involved. Most commonly affected is the radial nerve followed by ulnar nerve, median nerve and sciatic nerve. However, permanent damage is rare and most of these injuries resolve spontaneously within 6 months.
- *Skin injury:* Chemical burns can result through use of cleaning solutions meant for skin preparation, which can percolate beneath the tourniquets thus causing chronic exposure. Pressure necrosis or friction burns can result in skin injury due to movement of badly applied tourniquets. However, this is an uncommon complication.
- *Vascular injury:* Tourniquet usage may exert mechanical pressure to the atheromatous plaques in the blood vessels thereby causing plaque rupture, a rare complication. This can even lead to requirement of amputation. Hence, precautions should be undertaken in patients with severe peripheral vascular disease.
- *Intraoperative bleeding:* Increased bleeding may result from poorly fitted cuff, incomplete exsanguination of the limb, incompletely inflated cuff, increased intravascular coagulation or fibrinolysis.

Systemic Complications

- *Cardiovascular:* Tourniquet usage may cause side effects in patients with cardiac insufficiency due to mobilization of blood volume and fluid shift by exsanguination of lower limbs. This increases the circulating blood volume and subsequent transient rise in central venous pressure and systolic blood pressure.
- *Temperature:* Tourniquet inflation raises the core body temperature and its release is associated with a drop in temperature. In children, the rise in temperature is higher, thus, precaution must be taken during surgery against their warming.
- *Ischemic reperfusion injury:* Reperfusion injury is the set of complications resulting from the restoration of blood flow after a period of ischemia. Due to ischemic damage, cells sustain sublethal damage. This is followed by reperfusion induced oxidative damage resulting in lethal injury. Basically, reperfusion exacerbates the local ischemic damage and may cause systemic organ failure. Increased microvascular permeability may result in acute respiratory distress syndrome (ARDS), renal and cardiac complications.

- *Pulmonary embolism (PE):* Pulmonary embolism is a very rare complication that may occur in patients with history of deep vein thrombosis. It may occur during both inflation and deflation.

REFERENCES

1. Thigh tourniquet, Roman, 199 BCE-500 CE. (online) Available from Web address *www.sciencemuseum.org.uk.* [Accessed July, 2009].
2. Gross SD. A Manual of Military Surgery, or Hints on the Emergencies of Field, Camp and Hospital Practice. Philadelphia: JB Lippincott. 1862.
3. Lister JB. Collected papers. Vol 1. Oxford: Clarendon Press. 1909. p 176.
4. Von Esmarch F. First aid to the injured: six ambulance lectures. HRH Princess Christian, translator, 6th edition. London: Smith, Elder and Co. 1898.
5. Klenerman L. The Tourniquet Manual. London: Springer. 2003.
6. Cushing H. Pneumatic tourniquets: with special reference to their use in craniotomies. Med News. 1904;84:557.
7. McEwen JA. Complications of and improvements in pneumatic tourniquets used in surgery. Med Instrum. 1981;15:253-7.
8. AORN, recommended practices for use of the pneumatic tourniquet. In: Perioperative Standards and Recommended Practices, 2009 edition. Denver, CO: AORN Inc. 2009. pp 373-85.
9. Horlocker TT, Hebl JR, Gali B, Jankowski CJ, Burkle CM, Berry DJ, et al. Anesthetic, patient and surgical risk factors for neurologic complications after prolonged total tourniquet time during total knee arthroplasty. Anesth Analg. 2006;102:950-5.

SECTION 3

Neurological Procedures

32

Jugular Venous Oximetry

Hemant Bhagat

INTRODUCTION

Jugular venous oximetry or jugular bulb oxygen saturation (SjO_2 or $SjVO_2$) is a tool which represents a balance between the supply [cerebral blood flow (CBF)] and the need [cerebral metabolic requirement of oxygen ($CMRO_2$)]. This is achieved by locating the tip of the catheter at the jugular venous bulb which measures the jugular venous oxygen saturation using the fiber-optic sensors or by intermittent sampling of the venous sample. The jugular venous bulb drains approximately two-thirds of the ipsilateral and one-third of the contralateral cranial compartment. Consequently, its measurement is representative of global CBF.

INDICATION

- Acute neurological deterioration (traumatic brain injury, subarachnoid hemorrhage, etc.)
- Initiation of hyperventilation for raised intracranial pressure
- Status epilepticus
- Neurological deterioration due to systemic illness
- Prognostication following cerebral injury
- Institution of barbiturate coma
- As a research tool for understanding the cerebral physiology.

CONTRAINDICATION

- Coagulopathy
- Thrombosis of jugular veins
- Cervical spine injury
- Presence of a tracheotomy.

APPLIED ANATOMY

The jugular venous bulb lies opposite to the anterior arch of first and second cervical vertebra as visualized on the radiograph. As per the surface anatomy, the mastoid process lies at the same level. The judgment for right location of catheter tip will be based on relying on these anatomic landmarks (Fig. 1). The tip of the catheter should usually be placed within the jugular bulb at the same side as that of the lesion in the brain. If there is a bilateral lesion of brain or no obvious

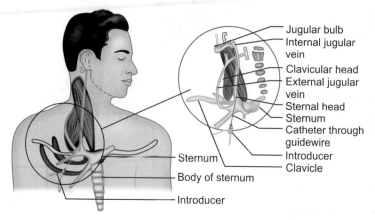

Fig. 1 Anatomical landmarks for retrograde cannulation of internal jugular vein

lesion of brain, then the dominant jugular vein should be cannulated which is commonly the right side.

TECHNIQUE AND BASIC PRINCIPLES

The technique for placement of jugular venous oximetry catheter consists of retrograde cannulation of the internal jugular vein (IJV) and locating the tip of catheter into the jugular bulb using the anatomic landmarks (Figs 2 and 3). The normal values of SjO_2 are 55–75%. This is derived from the following formula:

$$SjO_2 = \text{arterial oxygen saturation (SaO}_2; 97\%\text{–}100\%) -$$
$$\text{cerebral oxygen extraction (25\%–45\%)}$$

Decrease in SjO_2 values (less than 50%) indicates one of the following:
- Decreased supply (CBF)
    - Cerebral ischemia
    - Hyperventilation
- Increased demand [cerebral metabolic rate of oxygen ($CMRO_2$)]
    - Seizures
    - Fever

Increase in SjO_2 (more than 75%) indicates one of the following:
- Decreased demand ($CMRO_2$)
    - Cerebral infarction/brain death
    - Hypothermia
    - Use of sedatives
- Increased supply (CBF)
    - Cerebral hyperemia

Recording of Values

Continuous Monitoring

- *Real time:* The jugular venous oximetry catheter which uses three wavelength of light can calculate the hemoglobin value from the absorption system and allows real time continuous monitoring of SjO_2.

- *Non-real time:* The SjO_2 catheter which uses two wavelengths of light, the hemoglobin value has to be manually entered to calculate jugular venous oxygen solutions. Though it is continuous, the values are not estimated in real time.

Intermittent Monitoring

In the situation where central venous catheter is used intermittent venous sampling has to be done and venous oxygen saturations have to be measured by an arterial blood gas (ABG) analyzer.

PREPARATION

The basic equipment required for its placement are as follows:
- *Fiber-optic catheter for monitoring the SjO_2:* Several catheters have been used in IJV for jugular venous oximetry. The Oximetrix system uses a 4 Fr gauge Shaw Opticath which needs to be calibrated in vivo after placement. This should be recalibrated after every 12 hours of use. Another 4 Fr gauge catheter by Baxter healthcare has been used which requires recalibration only after 24–48 hours. These catheters are not freely available in India. We use single-lumen central venous catheter (5 Fr/5.5 Fr) for retrograde cannulation of IJV.
- Ultrasonography (USG) machine
- Fluoroscope
- Sterile drapes.

PROCEDURE

- *Positioning of patient:* Jugular bulb oxygen saturation monitoring is usually done in patients with deranged intracranial physiology or/and raised intracranial pressure (ICP). So it is advised not to advocate the head-down position which may risk the increase in ICP. In case of short neck it may be reasonable to use a sand bag in the interscapular region to allow extension and adequate exposure of neck. Avoid extreme neck rotation which may carry risk of obstruction to the contralateral cerebral venous outflow.
- *Preparation of skin:* Disinfect the skin over the IJV with antiseptic solutions as per the hospital policy.
- Sterile draping of the area of interest.
- Use aseptic precautions to identify the IJV using a USG machine or a finder needle.
- Puncture the IJV with a introducer needle in the retrograde direction (Fig. 2)
- Insert the J tipped guidewire through the introducer needle for few centimeters beyond the needle insertion site (Fig. 3).
- Place the catheter over the guidewire under fluoroscopic guidance so that the tip of catheter lies over the anterior arch of C_1-C_2 vertebra or the mastoid process.
- If fluoroscope is not available then place the catheter tips estimating a length approximately measuring the distance between the skin puncture site to the ipsilateral mastoid process or till a resistance is met. This can be confirmed later using the radiographs and readjusting the tip if necessary (Fig. 4).

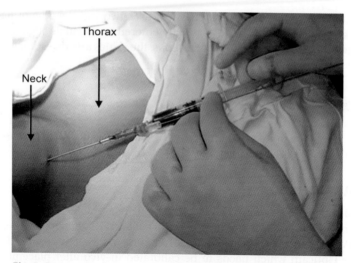

Fig. 2 Retrograde placement of guidewire through the introducer needle

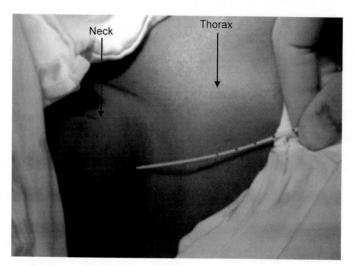

Fig. 3 Retrograde introduction of catheter in internal jugular vein

- *Secure the catheter:* The catheter should be firmly secured to the skin with the help of sutures.
- *Aseptic dressings:* The surrounding skin underlying the catheter entry point should be cleaned and covered with a sterile dressing (Fig. 5).

POST-PROCEDURE CARE

- Follow-up for the correct location of the tip of catheter
- Asepsis of the catheter and the underlying skin.

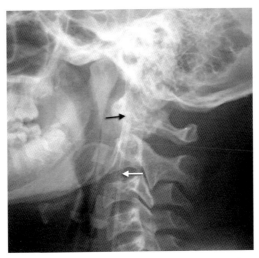

Fig. 4 Radiograph of placement of jugular bulb oxygen saturation catheter in internal jugular vein (white arrow) and catheter tip at the level of anterior arch of first cervical vertebra (black arrow)

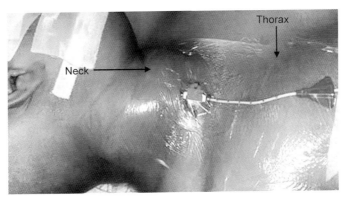

Fig. 5 Securing the skin entry point of catheter with sterile dressing

COMPLICATION/PROBLEM

- *Catheter misplacement:* This can occur in the form of placement of catheter tip either proximal to the jugular bulb. This can be prevented by using the fluoroscope during the catheter positioning (Fig. 6).
- Inadvertent puncture of carotid artery and arterial cannulation can occur. USG-guided catheter placement can avoid this complication.
- *Catheter migration:* Catheter migration can occur from its position area giving erroneous readings (Fig. 6). This can be prevented by properly securing the catheter at the skin entry point. Follow-up radiograph will help in early recognition and management of catheter migration.
- *Extracranial contamination of venous sample:* Extracranial contamination of venous sample can occur when the catheter tip is below the jugular bulb or when venous sampling is done very fast. This can be prevented by ensuring

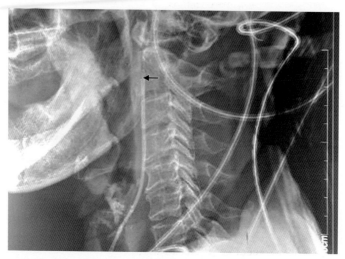

Fig. 6 Radiograph of catheter tip malposition below the jugular bulb (black arrow)

correct placement of catheter tip and sampling the venous blood a rate less than 2 mL/minute.

- Relatively insensitive to brainstem and cerebellar lesions as these areas contribute little to cerebral venous outflow.
- *Catheter blockage:* Whenever intermittent sampling is done via a venous catheter there is a possibility of its lumen being blocked. This can be prevented by continuous flushing of the catheter lumen with heparin added saline using keep the vein open (KVO) mode of the syringe infusion pumps.
- *Catheter-related sepsis:* Through data is scarce, there is a theoretical possibility of introducing bloodstream infection. Prevention should aim at placement of SjO_2 catheter under strict aseptic precautions and maintaining a sterile dressing and aseptic handling throughout the days of indwelling catheter.

ACKNOWLEDGMENT

I gratefully acknowledge the contribution of Dr S Saranya Vishnumathy for the sketch and thankful to the residents of neuroanesthesia for helping me in acquiring rest of the figures.

SUGGESTED READING

1. Andrews PJD. Jugular venous oximetry. Eur J Anaesthesiol. 1998;15:61-3.
2. Gopinath SP, Robertson CS, Constant CF, Hayes C, Feldman Z, Narayan RK, et al. Jugular venous desaturation and outcome after head injury. J Neurol Neurosurg Psychiatry. 1994;57:717-23.
3. Schell RM, Cole DJ. Cerebral monitoring: jugular venous oximetry. Anesth Analg. 2000;90:559-66.
4. Tisdall MM, Smith M. Multimodal monitoring in traumatic brain injury: current status and future directions. Br J Anaesth. 2007;99:61-7.

33

Lumbar Puncture

Bhaskar P Rao, Neha Singh

INTRODUCTION

Lumbar puncture in intensive care unit (ICU), otherwise known as spinal tap, involves insertion of a needle intrathecally, either to obtain cerebrospinal fluid (CSF) for diagnostic studies for varied life-threatening conditions or to instill some drug as a therapeutic measure. Being invasive in nature and that too in close proximity to spinal cord and numerous nerves, there is always a possibility to develop iatrogenic neurological complications leading to significant post-procedure morbidity. Thus, it is prudent to obtain the very knowledge of proper anatomy, indications, contraindications and management of procedure-related complications for all involved in patient care. Although, it is still considered a blind procedure, inclusion of ultrasound for the identification of the pertinent intervertebral space can definitely alter the safety issues associated with the technique, especially in patients with difficult landmarks.[1,2]

INDICATION

Lumbar puncture is essential in the diagnosis of varied infective and noninfective conditions in ICU patients. These conditions can be broadly classified into acute, non-acute and supportive situations. Similarly, it is often utilized or extremely useful as a therapeutic measure for various conditions enlisted below.

Diagnostic

Acute Conditions

- Suspected central nervous system (CNS) infections
- Clinical suspicion of subarachnoid hemorrhage not supported by computed tomography (CT) scan[3,4]
- To diagnose and differentiate bacterial and viral meningitis in symptomatic patients.

Non-acute Conditions

- Idiopathic intracranial hypertension (pseudotumor cerebri)
- Carcinomatous meningitis

- Tuberculous meningitis
- Normal pressure hydrocephalus
- Central nervous system syphilis
- Central nervous system vasculitis.

Supportive Conditions (Non-diagnostic but Still Useful)

- Multiple sclerosis
- Guillain-Barré syndrome
- Paraneoplastic syndromes.

Therapeutic

- Intrathecal administration of chemotherapy
- Intrathecal administration of antibiotics
- Injection of contrast media for myelography or for cisternography.

CONTRAINDICATION

There is no absolute contraindication to perform lumbar puncture except for patient refusal. But, there are many conditions where this procedure is relatively contraindicated where it can be weighed for the benefits against the risks. These are:

- Suspected raised intracranial pressure
- Coagulopathy/thrombocytopenia
- Epidural abscess
- Cardiovascular instability
- Respiratory instability
- Local infection
- Vertebral anomalies, etc.[5-9]

APPLIED ANATOMY

Procedure of lumbar puncture requires an intimate understanding of the functional anatomy of the spinal column, spinal cord and spinal nerves along with their surface markings. The vertebral column consists of 33 vertebrae: seven cervical, twelve thoracic, five lumbar, five sacral and four coccygeal segments (Fig. 1). The part of the body of concern during lumbar puncture is lumbar vertebrae, which along with other vertebrae forms a hollow ring-like structure to accommodate and provide a protective enclosure for the spinal cord. The ring is formed anteriorly by the vertebral body, laterally by the pedicles and transverse processes, and posteriorly by the lamina and spinous processes.

The spinal cord lies inside the spinal canal being covered by three layers or membranes, namely dura mater, arachnoid mater and pia mater. Dura mater is the outermost layer, followed by the arachnoid mater, and the pia mater. The space between pia mater and arachnoid membrane is known as subarachnoid space, containing CSF.

Besides these, as the needle passes into the subarachnoid space, the following ligaments come across: supraspinous ligament (connecting the tip of the spinous

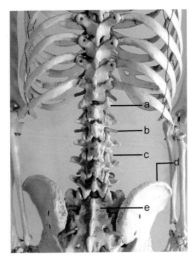

Fig. 1 Vertebral column showing vertebral body and spinous processes (a: Vertebral column, b: Spinal nerve emerging out of intervertebral foramina, c: Lumbar segment, d: Highest point of the iliac crest, e: Sacrum)

processes), interspinous ligament (connecting the body of the spinous processes together), and ligamentum flavum (holding the laminae together).

The main issue during lumbar puncture is needle insertion and possible spinal cord damage. Hence, the length of the spinal cord where it ends matters and varies as per the age. At birth, the spinal cord ends at approximately L_3 and in 60% adults, it ends at L_1.[10]

Surface Anatomy

Being a blind procedure, the importance of the surface landmarks on the patient cannot be ignored. The line joining the spinous processes of the vertebral column forms the midline and serves as the reference. The spinous processes of the lumbar spine are either horizontal or slightly slant in a caudal direction, which necessitates a mild cephalad angulation of insertion of the lumbar puncture needle. The line joining the highest points of both the iliac crests (Tuffier's line) passes through the interspace between fourth and fifth lumbar vertebrae. This forms a major anatomical landmark for lumbar puncture (Fig. 2). As the spinal cord ends at L_1 or L_2 level, it is prudent to avoid needle insertion at or above these interspaces, making L_3–L_4 and L_2–L_3 as the most preferred interspaces for needle insertion.

TECHNIQUE AND EQUIPMENT

Historically, in 1889, London physician Walter Essex Wynter was the first to enter into dural space, following a bit crude technique in order to reduce the raised intracranial pressure.[11]

But, the credit of first needle lumbar puncture goes to Quincke, a German physician, who first reported his findings in a conference and later a specific type of spinal needle has been named after.[12]

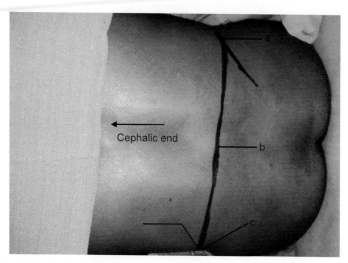

Cephalic end

Fig. 2 Anatomical landmark for lumbar puncture: Tuffier's line (a: Highest point of the right iliac crest, b: Tuffier's line, c: Highest point of the left iliac crest)

Different methods of lumbar puncture: Subarachnoid space can be entered either via the midline or through the paramedian approach.

1. *Midline approach:* This is the most commonly utilized approach in which the needle is introduced along the midline in the proposed interspinous space (space between the spinous process of the vertebra above and below), with a slight cephalad direction. Here, the needle pierces through the following layers: skin, subcutaneous tissue, supraspinous ligament, interspinous ligament, ligamentum flavum and dura mater, from superficial to deep inside (Fig. 3). When a bone is contacted quite superficially, in all likelihood, the needle is probably hitting the lower spinous process, whereas in depth, it would be hitting either the upper spinous process or lamina. In both the cases, the needle needs to be redirected to enter into the subarachnoid space.

2. *Paramedian approach:* In cases with difficult spine, or in patients where positioning is a bit restricted resulting in difficult or impossible midline approach, paramedian technique is the alternative choice. Here, the site of puncture is approximately 2 cm lateral to the inferior aspect of the superior spinous process of the proposed interspinous space with an angle of 10–25° toward the midline. Being paramedian in nature, both the ligaments encountered in midline approach are bypassed and the paraspinal muscles come onto the way, comparatively reducing the overall degree of resistance. When bone is encountered superficially, the needle has probably hit the medial part of the lower lamina and should be redirected upward and laterally. On the other hand, when bone is encountered deep inside, probably it is hitting the bony lamina and should be redirected only slightly upward and medially.

All these approaches are usually done either in sitting or in lateral decubitus position. Although, the preferred position varies from one operator to other and it is well known that anatomical midline is easier to appreciate in sitting than in the lateral decubitus position; sitting position is usually neither possible nor advisable in ICU patients.

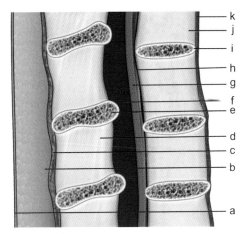

Fig. 3 Layers traversed (a–g) during spinal needle insertion (a: Skin, b: Subcutaneous tissue, c: Supraspinous ligament, d: Interspinous ligament, e: Spinous process, f: Ligamentum flavum, g: Spinal cord covered with meninges, h: Posterior longitudinal ligament, i: Intervertebral disc, j: Vertebral body, k: Anterior longitudinal ligament)

USG-guided Lumbar Puncture

Lumbar puncture is usually considered as a blind procedure until difficulty arises out of either obesity or difficult spine itself. Alternatives available in such a scenario are either fluoroscopy or ultrasonography-guided procedure. Although, fluoroscopy-assisted lumbar puncture is a proven method of help, it has got many disadvantages like limited availability, cumbersome transport of the patient out of the ICU along with inherent risk of radiation exposure.[13] In contrast, ultrasonography has been found to be a better alternative as it is devoid of all such hindrances[1] and known to reduce both attempts and rate of complications,[14] being particularly true in obese.[2] Required equipment are ultrasound machine, one high-frequency (5–10 MHz) probe and one low-frequency (2–4 MHz) probe for patients with elevated body mass index (BMI), transducing gel, sterile marker pen and equipment needed for the lumbar puncture itself. The ultrasound probe is placed horizontally over the midline on the back of the patient with the probe marker toward the operator's left at the level of the iliac crests (Fig. 4). This shows the spinous processes as characteristic crescent-shaped, hyperechoic structure with posterior acoustic shadowing (Fig. 5).

Although, these ultrasound images are obtained in the transverse plane, these markings are made and connected in the sagittal plane. All the spinous processes identified should be marked with a marker pen. Identifying the spinous processes above and below the space along the back defines the midline. Then, the transducer is moved into the longitudinal plane with the probe marker pointing toward the patient's head (Fig. 6). The probe is to be placed parallel to the direction of the spine between the spinous processes, and the gap seen between the hyperechoic convexities is the interspinous space. Once detected, the center of the interspinous space is to be marked with pen on both sides of the probe. As the ultrasound probe is removed, the transverse and the sagittal skin markings are extended until they intersect. The point where these lines intersect makes the point for the insertion of the lumbar puncture needle.

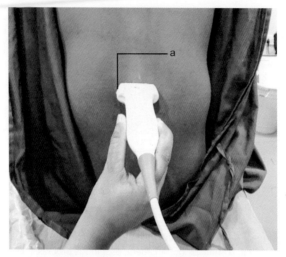

Fig. 4 Horizontal placement of the ultrasound probe (a: Probe marker)

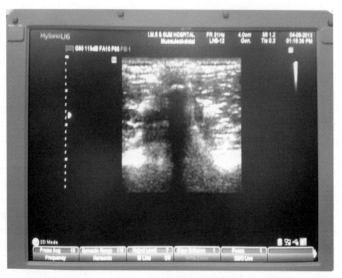

Fig. 5 Spinous process seen as characteristic crescent-shaped, hyperechoic structure with acoustic shadowing

The Needle

Although, lumbar puncture needles of different sizes, lengths, bevel and tip designs are available in the market, Quincke-Babcock needle (popularly known as Quincke's needle) is the one in common use (Figs 7 and 8). *Some important features of these needles are:*

- *Sterile hollow metallic needle with a transparent hub:* For better CSF visibility
- *Available sizes:* 16–30 gauge (higher the gauge, thinner the needle)
- *Length:* 3.5 inch

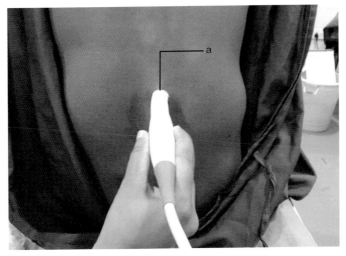

Fig. 6 Vertical placement of the ultrasound probe (a: Probe marker)

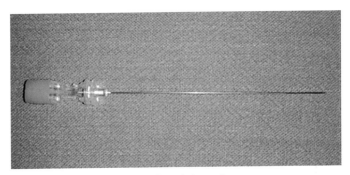

Fig. 7 Quincke's needle

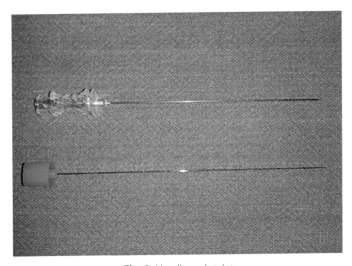

Fig. 8 Needle and stylet

Table 1 Depicting color coding of the different size of lumbar puncture needles

Size (in gauge)	Color
18	Pink
19	Beige
20	Yellow
21	Green
22	Black
25	Orange
26	Brown
27	Gray

- Stylet (prevents unintended tissue blocking into the lumen and occluding the path of CSF flow) with color-coded distal end according to the gauge/size of the needle (Table 1).
- Key/slot arrangement of stylet and the hollow needle hub for better handling and manipulation.

PREPARATION

- *Consent:* Obtaining an informed consent is a must for any patient-related ICU procedure, as for lumbar puncture, either from the patient or from the relatives or next of kin.
- *Monitoring:* Patient should be continuously monitored for the vital parameters as it may not be prudent to alter patient position much in a hemodynamically unstable patient.
- *Hand wash:* Washing hands with soap and water is an essential component of any ICU procedure just like for lumbar puncture along with wearing cap, mask and sterile gown.

PROCEDURE

- *Position:* Although, both sitting and lateral recumbent positions are described for the procedure, lateral decubitus (left or right) with neck and both knee fully flexed (fetal position) is the preferred one (Fig. 9). Sitting position is usually not a possible scenario in ICU patients and it is said to overestimate the CSF pressure.
- *Asepsis:* The overlying skin around the intended site of puncture is cleaned and disinfected utilizing an alcohol-based antiseptic, and a disinfectant such as povidone-iodine or alcohol-based chlorhexidine (Fig. 10). The antiseptic solution is usually applied in a centrifugal manner starting at the proposed injection site and proceeding outward in a gradually widening circle and should be allowed to dry before the procedure is begun. Although, there is a concern for arachnoiditis with chlorhexidine-containing solutions, evidence is very limited and additionally, literature speaks in favor of chlorhexidine for its faster onset, better efficacy and potency[15] over povidone-iodine. Once the

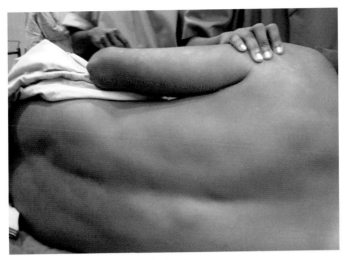

Fig. 9 Fetal position for lumbar puncture procedure

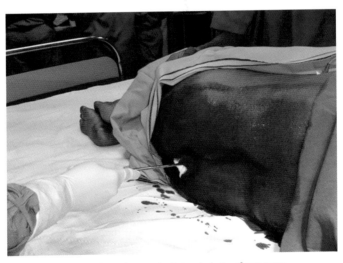

Fig. 10 Asepsis over the intended site of puncture

skin is prepared, a sterile drape sheet with a hole in the center is placed over the back of the patient.

- *Entry point:* The entry site of spinal needle is very crucial in determining the overall outcome and complication out of the procedure. After palpation of both the highest points of iliac crests, an imaginary line is drawn joining these points is a guide, usually to the body of fourth lumbar vertebra. The spinous processes of L_3, L_4, and L_5, and the interspaces in between can usually be directly identified by palpation (Fig. 11). The spinal needle can be safely inserted into the subarachnoid space at the $L_{3/4}$ or $L_{4/5}$ interspace, since this is well below the termination of the spinal cord.

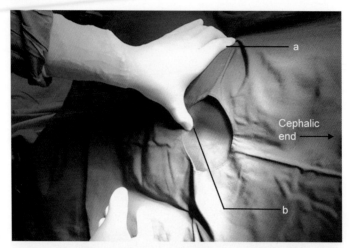

Fig. 11 Entry point selection with the help of anatomical landmarks (a: Fingers over the upper iliac crest palpating for the highest point, b: Thumb over the corresponding intervertebral space)

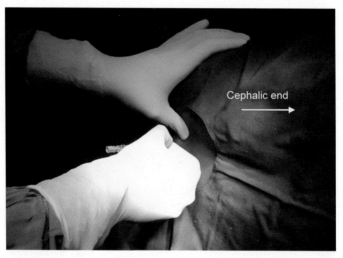

Fig. 12 Spinal needle insertion technique

- *Pre-procedure anesthesia (for conscious patient):* Once the position and entry point have been decided upon, local anesthetic (2–3 mL of 2% lignocaine with or without adrenalin) is infiltrated into the skin, subcutaneous tissue and along the expected entry path of the spinal needle. Sedoanalgesia can also be considered for some of the patients.
- *Needle insertion:* A spinal needle is inserted into the interspinous space between the lumbar vertebrae L_3/L_4, L_4/L_5, or L_5/S_1 interspace.[16] It is advanced slowly, directed upward toward the umbilicus with the bevel of the needle positioned toward flank so as to avoid cutting the fibers of the dura which run parallel to the spinal axis, thus may theoretically reduce the incidence of post-puncture headache (Fig. 12).

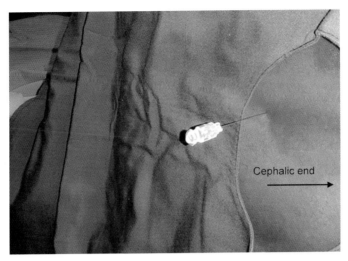

Fig. 13 Clear cerebrospinal fluid seen at the hub end

- The technique of needle advancement is either to move in the needle in a stepwise fashion with intermittent withdrawal of the stylet to check for CSF flow[17] or to feel for the two successive "give-way", one after ligamentum flavum and other after the puncture of dura and arachnoid membrane. On removing the stylet from the spinal needle, drops of CSF should be seen and collected in the specified vials (Fig. 13). The opening CSF pressure may be measured during this collection by using manometer.
- Usual volume of CSF collected for analysis is 8–15 mL except for situations where a higher volume is required, e.g. cytological or culture study.

POST-PROCEDURE CARE

- While collecting, one should avoid attempting negative pressure aspiration of CSF through syringe which may complicate into subdural hemorrhage or root herniation. After collection, the stylet has to be fully replaced into the needle again before final withdrawing, which has to be done in one single smooth motion to avoid any nerve retraction and injury. A gauze piece is placed at the insertion site as the needle is retracted out.
- When feasible, CSF should be sent for analysis within an hour of collection. Instead, it can be stored at 4–8°C for a short period and at –20°C for a relatively longer period. But, only the RNA and protein components are possible to be analyzed from a long-stored sample.
- Another recommendation is to divide 12 mL of CSF into three or four sterile containers before sedimentation. One of these should be stored at 4–8°C for general and microscopic investigation of bacteria and fungi, antibody testing, polymerase chain reaction (PCR) and antigen detection, etc. A larger volume of CSF is usually needed to identify pathogens like *Mycobacterium tuberculosis*, fungi and parasites. Those meant for culture should be sent to the laboratory as early as possible, preferably within an hour at room temperature and should never be refrigerated or exposed to extreme cold, heat or sunlight.[18]

COMPLICATION/PROBLEM

Although, lumbar puncture is often considered a small and safe procedure, many complications are possible ranging from mild transient neurological deterioration to even death. These are:

- *Post-dural-puncture headache:* Incidence of post-dural-puncture headache (PDPH) is about 10–40%. This headache occurs secondary to traction on the neural structures as CSF leaks through the dura after lumbar puncture. The usual presentation is headache in the frontal or occipital region starting after 24–48 hours of the procedure and typically, it gets aggravated in upright position and gets relieved in supine position. The symptoms commonly associated with headache are nausea, vomiting, dizziness, tinnitus and visual disturbances. This can last from a few hours to a week or more. Although, much practiced, none of the trials could prove bed rest to have any significant prophylactic benefit over early ambulation.[19] ICU patients on sedation or sedoanalgesia usually may not experience PDPH at all unless the patient is conscious.

- *Backache or discomfort:* Some patients experience low backache or discomfort following lumbar puncture which radiates down the legs.

- *Bleeding:* It can occur at the site of puncture or later into the epidural space. The CSF is normally acellular, and a red blood cells (RBCs) count of five is considered normal after lumbar puncture. Subarachnoid hemorrhage or other true intracranial bleed can be differentiated from a traumatic puncture on the grounds of an altered ratio of white blood cell (WBC) to RBC ratio and the presence or absence of xanthochromia.[20] Patients who have thrombocytopenia (e.g. platelet count <50,000/μL), or other coagulopathy [international normalized ratio (INR) >1.4], or those on anticoagulant medications have an increased risk of bleeding after lumbar puncture.[8] Situations where lumbar puncture is necessary but there is associated coagulopathy, the procedure may be undertaken under imaging guidance. Although rare, bleeding into the spinal canal can result in neural compromise requiring laminectomy for removal, and diagnosis is usually difficult which requires high index of suspicion.[5,21]

- *Brainstem herniation:* Tonsillar herniation or cerebellar herniation is the most dreaded complication arising out of lumbar puncture in a patient with elevated intracranial pressure, which can lead to immediate death or other neurological manifestations. Hence, a pre-procedure CT scan is advisable in patients with the following risk factors: altered sensorium, focal neurological signs, papilledema, history of recent seizure episode.

- *Infective complications:* Out of all varieties of infective complications possible, meningitis is one of the most dreaded one. The routes of entry of organisms causing meningitis are multimodal: skin flora, contaminated instruments, aerosolized oropharyngeal secretions of the operator or persons around, hematogenous spread in bacteremic patients.[22]

  Commonly isolated organisms in case of post-puncture meningitis are *Streptococcus salivarius*, *Streptococcus viridans*, alpha-hemolytic streptococci, *Staphylococcus aureus* and *Pseudomonas aeruginosa*.[6] The only way to prevent such infections is to follow utmost caution before, during and after procedure, and to observe hospital infection control protocol and surveillance. Although, literature and Centers for Disease Control and

Prevention (CDC) do not support routine use of gown, face mask, etc.; to be able to reduce the rate of infective complications in lumbar puncture patients, it is still prudent to follow such practices as until proven otherwise. Although there is a theoretical risk of inducing meningitis in a patient with bacteremia while doing lumbar puncture, the clinician should weigh the risk against its beneficial role in diagnosing or ruling out the disease.[23] Other types of infections arising possibly from direct inoculation into the vertebra are diskitis and vertebral osteomyelitis.[24]

- Local infections (spinal epidural or subdural empyema)
- Transient cranial nerve palsies
- Intraspinal epidermoid tumors of thecal sac.

REFERENCES

1. Dietrich AM, Coley BD. Bedside pediatric emergency evaluation through ultrasonography. Pediatr Radiol. 2008;38(Suppl 4):S679-84.
2. Nomura JT, Leech SJ, Shenbagamurthi S, Sierzenski PR, O'Connor RE, Bollinger M, et al. A randomized controlled trial of ultrasound-assisted lumbar puncture. J Ultrasound Med. 2007;26(10):1341-8.
3. Marton KI, Gean AD. The spinal tap: a new look at an old test. Ann Intern Med. 1986; 104(6):840-8.
4. Sternbach G. Lumbar puncture. J Emerg Med. 1985;2(3):199-203.
5. Ruff RL, Dougherty JH Jr. Complications of lumbar puncture followed by anticoagulation. Stroke. 1981;12(6):879-81.
6. Baer ET. Post-dural puncture bacterial meningitis. Anesthesiology. 2006;105(2):381-93.
7. Swartz MN, Dodge PR. Bacterial meningitis—a review of selected aspects. I. General clinical features, special problems and unusual meningeal reactions mimicking bacterial meningitis. N Engl J Med. 1965;272:898-902 contd.
8. Choi S, Brull R. Neuraxial techniques in obstetric and non-obstetric patients with common bleeding diatheses. Anesth Analg. 2009;109(2):648-60.
9. van Veen JJ, Nokes TJ, Makris M. The risk of spinal haematoma following neuraxial anaesthesia or lumbar puncture in thrombocytopenic individuals. Br J Haematol. 2010;148(1):15-25.
10. Fong B, VanBendegom JM, Reichman E, Simon RR. Emergency Medicine Procedures, 1st edition. McGraw-Hill Professional. 2003.
11. Wynter WE. Four cases of tubercular meningitis in which paracentesis of the theca vertebralis was performed for the relief of fluid pressure. Lancet. 1891;1(3531):981-2.
12. Quincke H. Verhandlungen des Congresses für Innere Medizin. Proceedings of the Zehnter Congress. Wiesbaden, Germany. 1891. pp. 321-31.
13. Stiffler KA, Jwayyed S, Wilber ST, Robinson A. The use of ultrasound to identify pertinent landmarks for lumbar puncture. Am J Emerg Med. 2007;25(3):331-4.
14. Peterson MA, Abele J. Bedside ultrasound for difficult lumbar puncture. J Emerg Med. 2005;28(2):197-200.
15. Arendt KW, Segal S. Present and emerging strategies for reducing anesthesia-related maternal morbidity and mortality. Curr Opin Anaesthesiol. 2009;22(3):330-5.
16. Greenberg BM, Williams MA. Infectious complications of temporary spinal catheter insertion for diagnosis of adult hydrocephalus and idiopathic intracranial hypertension. Neurosurgery. 2008;62(2):431-5; discussion 435-6.
17. Ellenby MS, Tegtmeyer K, Lai S, Braner DA. Videos in clinical medicine. Lumbar puncture. N Engl J Med. 2006;355(13):e12.
18. Ajello GW, Feeley JC, Hayes PS, Reingold AL, Bolan G, Broome CV, et al. Trans-isolate medium: a new medium for primary culturing and transport of *Neisseria meningitidis*, *Streptococcus pneumoniae*, and *Haemophilus influenzae*. J Clin Microbiol. 1984;20(1): 55-8.

19. Thoennissen J, Herkner H, Lang W, Domanovits H, Laggner AN, Müllner M. Does bed rest after cervical or lumbar puncture prevent headache? A systematic review and meta-analysis. CMAJ. 2001;165(10):1311-6.

20. Vermeulen M, van Gijn J. The diagnosis of subarachnoid haemorrhage. J Neurol Neurosurg Psychiatry. 1990;53(5):365-72.

21. Glotzbecker MP, Bono CM, Wood KB, Harris MB. Postoperative spinal epidural hematoma: a systematic review. Spine (Phila Pa 1976). 2010;35(10):E413-20.

22. Rubin L, Sprecher H, Kabaha A, Weber G, Teitler N, Rishpon S. Meningitis following spinal anesthesia: 6 cases in 5 years. Infect Control Hosp Epidemiol. 2007;28(10):1187-90.

23. Williams J, Lye DC, Umapathi T. Diagnostic lumbar puncture: minimizing complications. Intern Med J. 2008;38(7):587-91.

24. Wald ER. Risk factors for osteomyelitis. Am J Med. 1985;78(6B):206-12.

34

Epidural Analgesia

Sanjay Dhiraaj

INTRODUCTION

Critically ill patients in intensive care units (ICUs) suffer from numerous physiological and psychological stresses with pain being one of the most common and important contributor to either causing or increasing the quantum of this stress.

Pain at rest has been found to occur in more than 30% patients admitted to ICU with more than 50% having significant pain during routine care, such as endotracheal suctioning, positioning and wound care.[1]

With the advances in pain management intensivists have with them an armamentarium of approaches and techniques which can result in reduction of pain. This reduction may improve organ functioning and reduce morbidity. Regional analgesia is one of the methods to control pain in critically ill patients. It refers to techniques that use needles, catheters and infusion devices to deliver drugs in close proximity to peripheral nerves, plexuses, nerve roots, ganglia or directly into spinal fluid.[2] One of the most commonly used regional analgesic technique in the management of critically ill patients is epidural analgesia and used along with other pain alleviating drugs or techniques, as part of multimodal analgesia it can achieve better pain control with decreased side effects.[3]

INDICATION[4-6]

- Thoracic surgery
- Chest trauma and rib fractures
- Major upper and lower abdominal surgery. Vascular surgery of the lower extremities
- Major breast reconstructive surgery
- Orthopedic surgery, total knee replacement surgery
- Trauma of lower extremities, amputation of the lower limbs
- Pancreatitis
- Paralytic ileus
- Intractable angina
- Prevention or reduction in pain of a chronic pain syndrome, such as phantom limb pain. Complex regional pain syndromes
- Cancer pain.

CONTRAINDICATION[6,7]

Absolute

- Patient refusal
- Infection at the catheter site
- Allergy to local anesthetic or opioids
- Hypovolemia
- Severe aortic and mitral stenosis.

Relative

- Coagulopathy
- Increase in intracranial pressure
- Spine deformity
- Neurological disease
- Obstructive ileus.

APPLIED ANATOMY

Anatomy of the Epidural Space

Epidural space extends from the foramen magnum to the sacral hiatus and is bounded anteriorly by the posterior longitudinal ligament, intervertebral disks and bodies of vertebrae; laterally by the pedicles and intervertebral foramina and posteriorly by the ligamentum flavum and laminae of the vertebrae. Its contents include of nerve roots traversing it from foramina to peripheral locations, fat, areolar tissue, lymphatics and blood vessels (Fig. 1).[8]

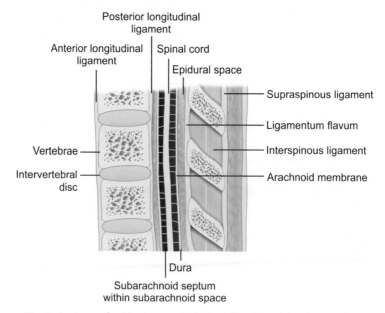

Fig. 1 Anatomy of epidural space. Sagittal section through lumbar vertebrae

Dermatomal Distribution of Sensory Analgesia

Dermatomal distribution of nerves is important for determining the level of analgesia that is required to achieve to provide adequate pain relief. Figure 2 shows the distribution of dermatomes.

TECHNIQUE AND BASIC PRINCIPLES OF EPIDURAL ANALGESIA

Selecting the Right Candidate

All patients undergoing epidural analgesia must be properly screened for the risk: benefit ratio and counseled with regards to side effects and complications of epidural analgesia. Epidural analgesia may be delivered by either a single injection, by continuous administration via an indwelling catheter or by patient-controlled epidural technique (PCEA).

In single injection technique epidural boluses are administered. Continuous epidural infusion provides steady state analgesia as it is administered through an indwelling catheter.

Patient-controlled epidural technique provides pain control in the hands of the patient as it allows the patient to himself administer additional doses of analgesics as an when he has pain.

Both continuous epidural technique and PCEA are used in management of critically ill patients and the choice of technique depends upon the status of the patient. A patient having pain but fully conscious and communicable would benefit

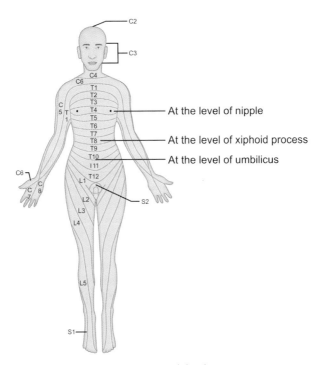

Fig. 2 Dermatomal distribution

from PCEA as opposed to a patient on ventilator with limited communicability for whom; continuous epidural technique would be a better option.

Drugs Administered for Epidural Analgesia

Drugs for epidural administration must always be tailored to individual patient's needs with respect to pain control, hemodynamic stability, and side effect profile of the drug.[6]

Most of the drugs are coadministered so as to achieve a rapid and prolonged analgesic effect, when compared with single-agent infusions as they work synergistically and have different sites of action which results in improved pulmonary function, decreased cardiovascular effects and decrease in incidence of paralytic ileus.[5,9-13]

Epidural analgesia is usually achieved through the administration of local anesthetics (lignocaine, bupivacaine and ropivacaine), opioids or a combination of both these agents.

Acting at the spinal root level, local anesthetics interfere with the voltage-gated sodium channels preventing the influx of sodium ions in the cell causing impediment or elimination of axonal impulse propagation. This in turn leads to inhibition of nerve impulse transmission.

They antagonize the release of prostaglandins resulting in inhibition of inflammatory response which help in the reduction of overall stress response activated in times of critical illness.[11,12]

Bupivacaine is most commonly used to provide analgesia in critically ill patients as it has a longer duration of action compared to lignocaine.[5,11]

Opioids produce analgesic effect by binding to the opioid receptors in the brain and the dorsal horn of the spinal cord. They modify the pain perception and reaction to the noxious stimuli.[4,11,12] They have no effect on sensory, motor or sympathetic nerve function. Morphine and fentanyl are the most frequently administered epidural opioids. Both of them are μ-receptor agonists.

Preservative free morphine is hydrophilic (water-soluble and lipid-insoluble) in character and so it permeates slowly through the dura to bind at the opioid receptor located in the dorsal horn of the spinal cord. As a result of this, it has a delayed onset of action (30–60 minutes) and a long duration of action (12–24 hours). As it remains in the cerebrospinal fluid (CSF) for a longer duration of time they tend to spread in the cephalad direction and so result in a wider segment of analgesia but may also result in late respiratory depression (8–24 hours after opioid administration) more so with bolus doses.[11,13,14] In contrast to this; fentanyl which is lipophilic in character has a rapid onset of action (5–15 minutes) but shorter duration of action (2–3 hours). Also it results in a narrower segment of analgesia as compared to morphine.

Adrenaline is often added to local anesthetic agents to reduce intravenous uptake and to prolong the effects of the block. The alpha 2 agonists like clonidine have antinociceptive properties and have been used as adjuncts to local anesthetic agents at various anatomic levels. Clonidine potentiates opioid analgesia when applied neuraxially.

Epidural Analgesia and Anticoagulation

The incidence of neurological dysfunction resulting from hemorrhagic complications associated with neuraxial block estimated to be, 1 in 150,000 epidurals and, 1 in 220,000 spinal anesthetics.[15,16]

Oral Anticoagulants

Anesthetic management of patients' anticoagulated perioperatively with warfarin depends on dosage and timing of initiation of therapy. The prothrombin time (PT) and international normalized ratio (INR) of patients on chronic oral anticoagulation require 3–5 days to normalize after discontinuation of the anticoagulant therapy.[17]

Regional Anesthetic Management of the Patient on Oral Anticoagulants[18]

- Before neuraxial block, discontinue oral anticoagulants and normalize PT
- Assess and monitor PT and INR daily
- Remove indwelling neuraxial catheters when the INR is 1.5
- If INR is greater than or equal to 3, withhold warfarin
- At present no definitive recommendation can be made regarding the management to facilitate removal of neuraxial catheters (e.g. discontinuation of warfarin therapy with spontaneous recovery of hemostasis or partial or complete reversal of anticoagulant effect). Individual factor may have to be taken in account.[19]

Regional Anesthetic Management of the Patient Receiving Unfractionated Heparin[18]

Regional anesthesia and intravenous (IV) heparinization for patients undergoing vascular surgery is acceptable with the following recommendations:
- Administer IV heparin 1 hour after needle/catheter placement
- If systematic anticoagulation therapy is already begun with an epidural catheter in place, then catheter should be removed after 2–4 hours of heparin discontinuation and after evaluation of coagulation status.
- Remove indwelling catheters 1 hour before a subsequent heparin administration.
- There is no contradiction to the use of neuraxial techniques during subcutaneous standard heparin at total doses less than or equal to 10,000 units daily.
- The risk of spinal hematoma with larger daily subcutaneous doses of heparin is unclear and so one needs to assess on an individual basis with more frequent neurological monitoring
- Serial platelet counts are indicated for patients receiving subcutaneous heparin for more than 5 days.[19]

Regional Anesthetic Management of the Patient Receiving Low Molecular Weight Heparin[18]

- Neuraxial techniques should be performed at least 10–12 hours after a thromboprophylaxis dose and 24 hours after a high therapeutic dose of low molecular weight heparin (LMWH)[18]
- With twice daily dosing, administration of the first dose of LMWH should be administered after 24 hours of operation regardless of anesthetic technique, and in the presence of adequate hemostasis
- Indwelling catheters should be removed before initiation of LMWH thrombo-prophylaxis
- The first dose of LMWH should be administered 2 hours after catheter removal or 24 hours after needle/catheter placement, whichever is later
- Patients who are on once daily dosing of LMWH require 6–8 hours between needle/catheter placement and the first dose of LMWH. Subsequent dosing should occur no sooner than 24 hours late.[19]

Epidural Needles[20]

The standard epidural needle is 17–18 G, 3 or 3.5 inches long, and has a blunt bevel with a gentle curve of 15–30° at the tip (Figs 3A to C). The Tuohy needle is most commonly used. The blunt, curved tip helps in pushing away the dura after passing through the ligamentum flavum instead of penetrating it.

Epidural Catheters[20]

Mostly 19- or 20-gauge catheter is introduced through a 17- or 18-gauge epidural needle for either patient-controlled or continuous analgesia. It is usually advanced 26 cm into the epidural space. Catheters have either a single port at the distal end or multiple side ports close to a closed tip (Figs 4A and B). In addition

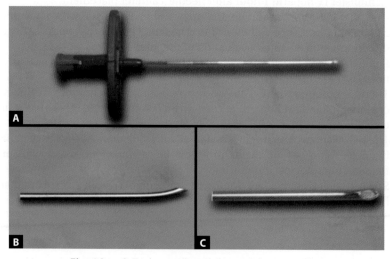

Figs 3A to C Tuohy needle with its curved tip magnified

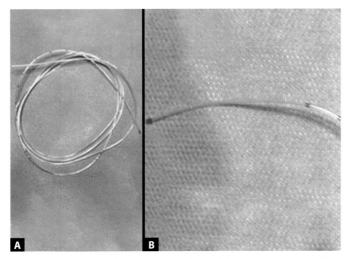

Figs 4A and B Epidural catheter with tip of the catheter magnified

to extending the duration of the block, it allows for lower total dose of anesthetic to be used.

PREPARATION[21]

- The first step is to communicate with the patient about the technique and taking an informed consent about the procedure
- Ensure adequate monitoring is in place [pulse, blood pressure, saturation of arterial oxygenation (SpO_2)]
- Ensure a wide bore cannula in place so that adequate fluid replacement may be possible, if required
- Ensure adequate resuscitation facilities in place
- *Disposable epidural tray/kit may containing the following[21] (Figs 5A and B):*
  - Appropriate prep solutions, swabs and sterile 4 × 4 gauze pads
  - Epidural catheter, threading assist guide, and syringe adapter attachment
  - Syringes
  - Luer-Lock procedural syringe (5 mL) filled with saline for loss-of-resistance technique
  - Tuohy epidural needle (18 gauge)
  - Filter (0.2 μm)
  - Lidocaine 1% (5 mL vial) for local infiltration
  - Test dose lidocaine 1.5% injectable, with epinephrine 1:200,000 (5 mL vial)
  - Epidural medications.

PROCEDURE

- Epidural catheter insertion may be undertaken in the sitting or lateral position with the back flexed. Usually an assistant helps the patient to remain in that position during the procedure.
- Under strict aseptic precautions appropriate skin preparation and draping is performed (Fig. 6).

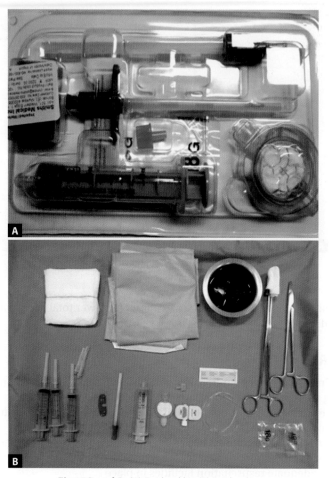

Figs 5A and B (A) Epidural kit; (B) Epidural tray

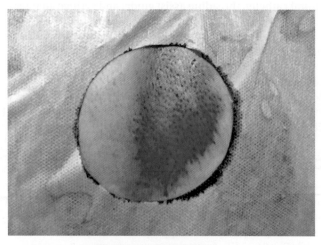

Fig. 6 Prepping and draping

- Locate the appropriate intervertebral space. This is done by using the knowledge of dermatomes as they relate to a level appropriate to the anatomical site of pain. Local anesthesia (lidocaine 1%) is then administered to the interspace area by first making a skin wheal, then injecting into the deeper tissues at the angle the epidural needle will follow (Fig. 7).
- The Tuohy epidural needle is then negotiated in such a way as to pass through the intervertebral space. As the Tuohy needle passes through the interspinous ligament is becomes firmly griped to it. Using the loss-of-resistance technique (with air or saline) or the hanging-drop method the needle is now advanced into the epidural space (Figs 8A and B).
- When the epidural placement of the needle is confirmed then the epidural catheter is placed in the epidural space by passing it through the epidural needle. The needle has to be rotated either cephalad or caudad before catheter placement so that the catheter passes either cephalad or caudal into the epidural space (Fig. 9).
- Advance the catheter about 3–5 cm into the epidural space. *Note:* Never attempt to withdraw the catheter while the needle is in place. The catheter may shear off, leaving the distal segment in the epidural space. Never readvance the needle after the catheter is in place, for the same reason.
- The needle is then slowly withdrawn over the catheter. The proximal end of the catheter is secured with an adapter filter (Fig. 10).
- Administer the test dose through the catheter. This is performed to detect either intravascular or subdural placement of the catheter. Aspirate to check for the presence of blood or CSF. After negative aspiration administer 3 mL of 1.5% lidocaine with 1:200,000 epinephrine. If the needle is intravascular, a noticeable increase in heart rate, blood pressure or both will usually be detected within 3 minutes after the injection. The patient may note tinnitus. Sensory and motor function of the lower extremities will be affected after 5 minutes if the catheter or needle is in the subdural space (Fig. 11).

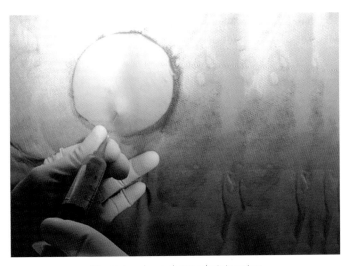

Fig. 7 Local anesthetic administration

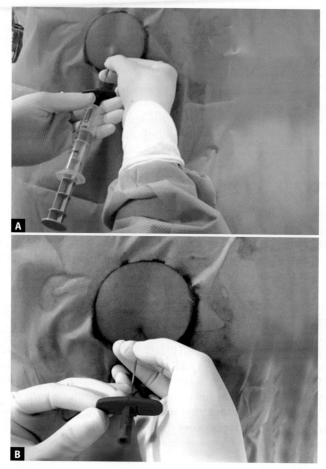

Figs 8A and B Advancement of needle with "loss of resistance" technique

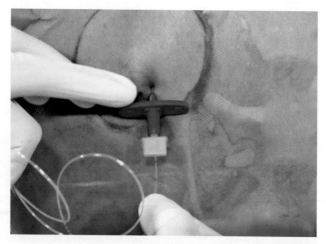

Fig. 9 Threading of catheter

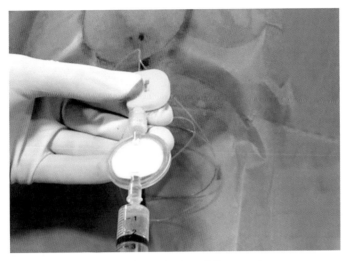

Fig. 10 Attaching adapter and filter to catheter

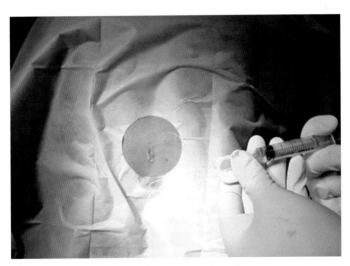

Fig. 11 Administration of test dose

- After a negative result the catheter is secured at the puncture site and along the back with tape.
- The patient is now ready for epidural analgesia. Aspirate to check for the presence of blood or CSF before each injection or before placing the patient on an infusion pump or PCEA pump. Continuous epidural infusion can usually provide analgesia for five to seven consecutive dermatome areas.
- Label the catheter "for epidural use only".
- *Fixing catheter:* Fixing of the epidural catheter is important in ICU patients as they need frequent change in positions. This may lead to inadvertent removal of the catheter. The method of fixing is illustrated in the Figures 12A to G.

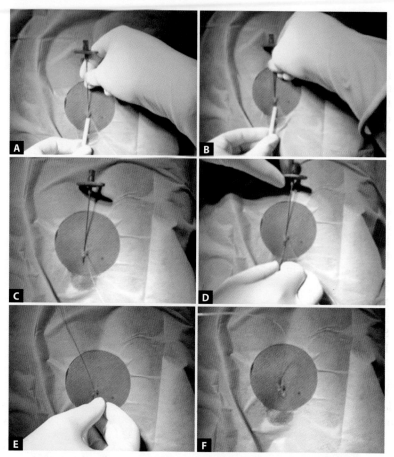

Figs 12A and F (A and B) Tunnelling the skin with Touhy needle; (C and D) Threading the catheter through needle; (E and F) Making a loop

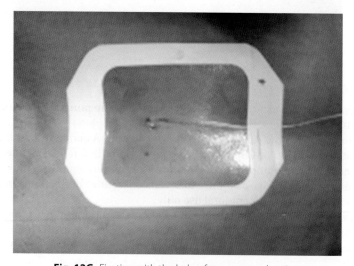

Fig. 12G Fixation with the help of transparent dressing

POST-PROCEDURE CARE

Patient Monitoring

All patients on epidural analgesia should be monitored every hour for 4 hours, then every 4 hours, if the patient is stable. *Monitoring should include:*
- *Cardiorespiratory monitoring:* Heart rate, blood pressure, respiratory rate, oxygen saturation and temperature
- Monitoring of drug distribution
  - Dermatomal level of sensory analgesia
  - Bromage scale for motor function
  - Level of sedation
  - Side effects and complications.

The acute pain service (APS) team should be notified, if:
- Inadequate analgesia
- Patient difficult to arouse
- Respiratory rate less than or equal to nine breaths/minute
- Persistent nausea and vomiting
- Systolic blood pressure above or equal to 90 mm Hg
- Motor assessment reveals an inability of the patient to bend their knees on motor evaluation
- Sensory level is above T4/T6 (unless thoracic epidural)
- Itching.

Drugs to be Ready

Naloxone and ephedrine are to be kept ready to manage oversedation and hypotension, if needed.

Catheter Care

The epidural catheter insertion site should be inspected every shift. If the dressing has drainage, it may indicate either CSF drainage or epidural solution drainage then the APS team should be informed to evaluate the integrity of the catheter.

COMPLICATION/PROBLEM[9]

Procedure Related

- *Subarachnoid injection:* Injection of large volumes of anesthetic solution into the subdural or subarachnoid space may result in a high or total spinal block, with respiratory arrest, severe hypotension and possibly cardiac arrest. These conditions must be recognized and treated immediately.
- *Postspinal headache:* Subdural puncture, always a risk when performing epidural anesthesia, carries a high risk for spinal headache, particularly in younger and pregnant patients. Give IV fluids, lying down position, CO_2 retention techniques. For severe or persistent headache, a blood patch may be necessary.
- *Migration of epidural catheter:* Epidural catheters may be inadvertently inserted into a blood vessel or into the subarachnoid space. The test dose is

used to avoid this possibility and to prevent placing a large dose of anesthetic into either the circulation or the subarachnoid space.

- *Catheter damage:* The distal portion of the catheter may break off in the epidural space. This may occur, if an attempt is made to withdraw the catheter through the epidural needle. It may also occur, if the needle is readvanced after the catheter is deployed. If the catheter will not advance through the needle, remove the needle and catheter together and repeat the procedure at another interspace.

Opioid Related

- *Respiratory depression:* Early phase depression is mostly seen due to opioid absorption through the epidural vessels (within 1 hour) and late phase depression seen mostly with hydrophilic drugs like morphine due to accumulation of drug in the CSF and its cephalad spread (mostly 8–24 hours). Regular monitoring and assessment for the first 24 hours is necessary.
- *Nausea and vomiting:* Occurs due to stimulation of chemoreceptor trigger zone (CTZ). Use antiemetics.
- *Constipation:* Due to decrease in intestinal motility, increased absorption of intestinal fluids. Stimulant laxatives could be used.
- *Pruritus:* Due to histamine release. Consider 5-HT3 antagonists.
- *Urinary retention:* May be because of inhibition of micturition reflex. Assess for bladder distension.

Local Anesthetic Related

- *Toxicity:* Intravascular absorption of local anesthetic due to inadvertent vascular injection resulting in circumoral numbness, muscular twitching, cardiac arrhythmias and seizures. Supportive measures with treatment of symptomatic arrhythmias. Treatment of seizures and provision of supplemental oxygen and consider for ventilatory support, if needed.
- *Hypotension:* Vasodilation occurs due to blockade of sympathetic nervous system. Monitoring of blood pressure and administration of fluids, vasoconstrictors as needed.

Needle/Catheter Related

- Trauma which may result in backache
- Neural injury to nerve or cord
- Bleeding
- *Epidural hematoma:* Bleeding in epidural space. Stop epidural infusion. Assess and monitor for any numbness or weakness of the limbs. If present, urgent decompression required
- *Epidural abscess:* Infection in epidural space. Inspect epidural site for evidence of infection. Antibiotic therapy as per institutional protocol

REFERENCES

1. Schulz-Stübner S, Boezaart A, Hata JS. Regional analgesia in the critically ill. Crit Care Med. 2005;33(6):1400-7.
2. Novak-Jankovic V. Regional anaesthesia in the ICU. Periodicum Biologorum. 2009; 3(2):285-8.
3. Mehta Y, Arora D, Vats M. Epidural analgesia in high risk cardiac surgical patients. HSR Proc in Intensive Care and Cardiovasc Anesth. 2012;4(1):11-4.
4. McCaffrey M, Pasero C. Pain Clinical Manual. 2nd edition. Philadelphia, PA: Mosby. 1999.
5. Cousins MJ, Bridenbaugh PO. Neural Blockade in Clinical Anesthesia and Management of Pain. 2nd edition. Philadelphia, Pa: Lippincott Williams & Wilkins. 1998. pp.129-75.
6. Schulz-Stubner S. The critically ill patient and regional anesthesia. Curr Opin Anaesthesiol. 2006;19:538-44.
7. Ryder E, Ballantyne J. Postoperative pain in adults. In: Ballantyne J (Ed). The Massachusetts General hospital handbook of pain management. 3rd edition. Philadelphia, Pa: Lippincott Williams & Wilkins. 2005. pp. 283-305.
8. David L. Brown. Spinal, Epidural and Caudal Anesthesia. In: Miller RD (ed). Miller's Anesthesia, 7th edition. Churchill Livingstone. 2009. pp. 2619-66.
9. Faut-Callahan M, Hand WR. Pain management. In: Nagelhout J, Zaglaniczny K (Eds). Nurse Anesthesia, 2nd edition. St. Louis, Mo: Elsevier Saunders. 2005. pp. 1157-74.
10. Clark F, Gilbert HC. Regional analgesia in the intensive care unit. In: Vender J, Szokol J, Murphy G (Eds). Critical Care Clinics. Philadelphia, Pa: WB Saunders Co. 2001. pp. 943-64.
11. De Benedittis G. Management of postoperative pain in neurosurgery. In: Burchiel KJ (Ed). Surgical Management of Pain. New York: Thieme Medical Publishers. 2002. pp. 257-64.
12. Casey Z, Wu CL. Epidural opioids for postoperative pain. In: Benzon H, Raja S, Molloy R (Eds). Essentials of pain medicine and regional anesthesia. Philadelphia, Pa: Elsevier. 2005. pp. 246-52.
13. Practice guidelines for acute pain management in the perioperative setting: an updated report by the American Society of Anesthesiologists Task Force on Acute Pain Management. Anesthesiology. 2004;100(6):1573-81.
14. Rothly BB, Therrien SR. Acute pain management. In: St. Marie B (Ed). Core curriculum for pain management nursing. Philadelphia, PA: WB Saunders Co. 2002. pp. 264-6.
15. Tryba M. Epidural regional anesthesia and low molecular heparin: Pro. Anasthesiol Intensivmed Notfallmed Schmerzther. 1993;28:179-81.
16. Stafford-Smith M. Impaired haemostasis and regional anaesthesia. Can J Anaesth. 1996; 43(5 Pt 2):R129-41.
17. Heit JA. Perioperative management of the chronically anticoagulated patient. J Thromb Thrombolysis. 2001;12(1):81-7.
18. Horlocker TT. Regional anaesthesia in the patient receiving antithrombotic and antiplatelet therapy. Br J Anaesth. 2011;107(Supp 1):i96-106.
19. Practice advisory for the prevention, diagnosis, and management of infectious complications associated with neuraxial techniques: a report by the American Society of Anesthesiologists Task Force on infectious complications associated with neuraxial techniques. Anesthesiology. 2010;112(3):530-45.
20. Morgan GE, Mikhail MS, Murray MJ. Morgan and Mikhail's Clinical Anesthesiology, 4th edition. McGraw-Hill. 2005. pp. 383-434.
21. Pfenninger JL, Grant C. Pfenninger and Fowler's procedures for primary care. 3rd edition. Elsevier. 2010. pp. 13-8.

35

Cranial Burr Hole

Rabi N Sahu, Kuntal Kanti Das, Arun K Srivastava

INTRODUCTION

Burr hole is a surgically created opening in the calvarial skull to gain access into the dura, underlying brain and the ventricular system for a given purpose. The practice of making holes into the skull to access various intracranial pathologies has a long history that dates back to prehistoric times. Evidence from the human remains from Neolithic times and various cave paintings of that era indicate that trephination, i.e. the process of making burr holes into the skull, was practiced for curing various ailments like epilepsy, mental symptoms and migraine. History also suggests that the bone that had burr holes would often be kept as a charm by prehistoric people to keep the evil forces away. Even in the modern era where more and more technological advances are being adapted into the field of neurosurgery, burr hole remains a basic and a very useful neurosurgical procedure having a diverse applications in different clinical settings.

INDICATION

Burr hole remains a widely used procedure in neurosurgery. *Some of its common applications are enumerated below:*
- As a preliminary step to perform craniotomy or craniectomy for accessing intracranial pathologies (meninges, brain parenchyma and ventricles)
- Access for intracranial pressure monitoring in intensive care setting
- To drain brain abscess, hematomas (extradural/subdural/intraparenchymal)
- For ventricular drainage to relieve hydrocephalus (either external drainage or various shunt procedures)
- To enable brain biopsy (either free hand or through frame-based/frame-less stereotaxy)
- For creating granulation tissue in extensive scalp loss due to trauma
- For elevating a surrounding depressed fracture segment
- To provide access to dural venous sinus for transvenous endovascular procedures like coil or glue embolization.

CONTRAINDICATION

- Presence of active infection at the intended site of burr hole
- Uncontrolled coagulopathy.

APPLIED ANATOMY

Structures that are traversed while creating the burr hole include scalp and bony calvarium. Scalp consists of five layers. These are (from outside inward) skin, subcutaneous tissue containing scalp vessels, galea aponeurotica, loose areolar tissue and pericranium that is tightly adherent to the underlying bone. Scalp bleeding is easily controlled by compressing the vessels in the connective tissue layer by Raney clips or by applying Dandy forceps/artery forceps on cut margin of the galea and everting it. Galeal layer provides strength to the scalp and prevents cerebrospinal fluid (CSF) leakage from the wound. Hence, the wound is closed in two layers.

Calvarial skull represents flat bone and is formed by membraneous ossification. It is composed of two tables with an intervening diploic space. Intradiploic space is composed of spongy bone while inner and outer tables are made of compact cancellous bone. In certain areas, the intradiploic space is aerated giving rise to the air sinuses. At suture lines, both tables meet and diploic space is usually absent. Diploic space contains venous channels, which sometimes communicate with extracalvarial vasculature (emissary veins). Because of different nature of the tables and the diploic space, surgeon gets a different feel during the creation of burr hole. Bleeding occurs from diploic veins during the process which may at times be a cause of air embolism unless these areas are properly sealed with bone wax.

PREPARATION

- Preparations for burr hole would depend on the indication for which it is being created. The foremost is an informed and written consent. It is important that the operating surgeon explains the need for the procedure and the possible complications. The consent should clearly state chances of intracranial hematoma, infection and meningitis in addition to risks particular to the procedure.
- Preoperative investigations like hemogram, blood chemistry, coagulation profile, chest X-ray and electrocardiogram (ECG) would be required just like any other surgery.
- When the procedure is being done under general anesthesia, the standard anesthetic monitoring is carried out like any other general anesthesia. End-tidal carbon dioxide monitoring is especially useful when burr hole is being created for transvenous interventional procedures, posterior fossa surgery or when burr holes are made around the venous sinuses as these cases may be complicated by air embolism. Even when the burr hole is being created under local anesthesia, basic monitoring like blood pressure, heart rate, pulse oximetry is desirable especially in elderly with cardiorespiratory comorbidities.
- Prophylactic antibiotic is usually administered before marking the incision. For supratentorial procedures, prophylactic antiepileptic and for lesions with cerebral edema, injectable steroid is administered before the procedure.
- Equipment required are basic and simple. We need scalpel to make incision, self-retaining retractor to keep skin margins away while exposing bone. For making the burr hole, we need a perforator and a burr mounted on the Hudson's brace or a drill, if available. Bone curette or scoop is used to remove thin shells of bone. Instruments used have been shown in Figure 1.

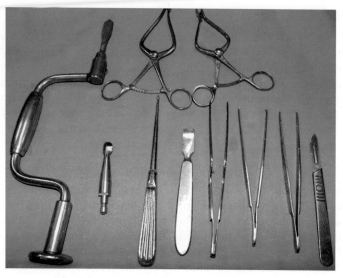

Fig. 1 Instruments required for making a burr hole

PROCEDURE

- The procedure is simple and can be performed either under local anesthesia or general anesthesia depending on the actual indication. It can be accomplished either with conventional Hudson's brace with perforator and burrs of various sizes or with an electrically/pneumatically operated drill/burr.
- *Position:* The patient is positioned in such a way that the site of interest is at the top of the surgical field. Head may be rested on a horseshoe frame and immobilized with an adhesive tape or it can be rigidly fixed with three or four point skull fixation device. The head is elevated at least 30 degrees above the level of the heart so as to promote venous drainage from cranial sinus toward the heart.
- *Site of burr hole:* It depends on the indication for the procedure. When it is being created to access ventricle for CSF drainage or external ventricular drainage, there are some points that are of interest to us. *Some of them are:*
  - *Kocher's point:* 2 cm lateral to midline and 1 cm anterior to coronal suture
  - *Keen point:* 3 cm above and behind top of pinna
  - *Dandy point:* 3 cm above inion and 2 cm lateral to midline
  - *Double Dandy point:* 6 cm above inion and 4 cm lateral to midline.
- Right side is favored for ventricle access as majority of individuals are left hemisphere dominant.
- *Surgical site preparation:* Surgical site is cleansed twice before making incision. After positioning of the head, skin is prepared with savlon-ether-spirit-betadine used sequentially then incision is marked and finally the preparation is repeated before placing drapes. Surgical drapes are placed all around the skin mark, so as not to expose any additional skin except the incision line. Finally, povidone-iodine impregnated adhesive sheet is applied across drapes and skin incision mark.
- *Making the burr hole:* Skin incision is made with no. 15 blade right up to the pericranium after local anesthetic mixed with adrenaline has been injected

into the planned skin incision site. Minor bleeding from the skin margin is controlled with bipolar cautery and self-retaining retractors are placed to expose the underlying bone. Pericranium is separated from the bone before making burr hole. If one is making the burr hole by conventional method then initially the skull is perforated with a perforator mounted on Hudson's brace. Once the inner table of the calvarium is breached by the perforator, surgeon stops immediately. There is a sense of give away at this time and inexperience at this juncture may lead one to inadvertently enter into the dura or brain parenchyma. Once both the tables are breached by the perforator, burr is mounted onto the Hudson's brace and the opening is widened. The burr is withdrawn when the inner table becomes so thin that underlying dura starts becoming visible. This portion of the bone can then be removed with a bone scoop. Figures 2 and 3 show creation of burr hole. When one is using a drill, the entire process can be accomplished with the same drill unlike the conventional technique of using perforator before the burr.

POST-PROCEDURE CARE

Post-operatively, antibiotics are continued for 1–2 days, analgesics with antacids are administered for pain relief and other medications, as per indication of surgery, are continued. Dressing is changed on post-operative days 1st, 3rd and 7th unless there is any discharge or CSF leak from the wound. Sutures are removed on 7th post-operative day.

Closure

Once the procedure, for which the burr hole was made, is over, these holes can be managed by different ways during closure. These include leaving the holes as such, packing the hole with the bone dust obtained during creation of the hole, using burr hole buttons or by placing bone substitutes like

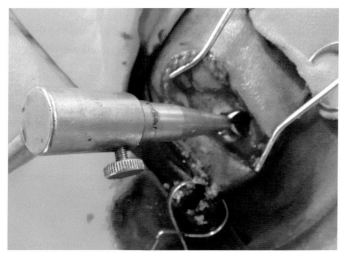

Fig. 2 Making a burr hole with Hudson brace burr

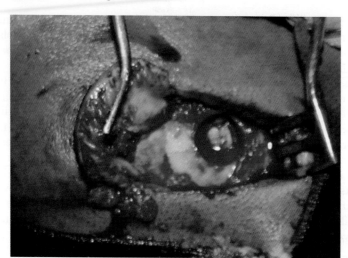

Fig. 3 Burr hole ready for procedure

polymethylmethacrylate (PMMA). Skin is closed in two layers, galea aponeurotica is closed with absorbable suture 2-0 and skin is closed with monofilament suture like nylon.

COMPLICATION/PROBLEM

Complications are inseparable part of any surgery and burr hole is no exception to it. However, most such complications are minor and with increasing experience of the operator, tend to reduce to negligible level. Some of the complications are enumerated below:
- Infection/osteomyelitis
- Accidental entry beyond inner table leading to dural tear/brain contusion and hematoma
- Injury to the underlying dural venous sinus
- Air embolism through the opened up intradiploic veins
- Extradural hematoma, if bone wax is not properly applied to the oozing bony walls of the hole
- Cosmetic deformity
- Trephination syndrome, a rare complication seen mainly after large craniectomies. It is characterized by progressive headache and neurological deficit from dynamic movement of the brain through the bony defect. Replacing the bone (cranioplasty) usually ameliorates such symptoms.

SUGGESTED READING

1. Donovan DJ, Moquin RR, Ecklund JM. Cranial burr holes and emergency craniotomy: review of indications and technique. Mil Med. 2006;171(1):12-9.
2. Furlanetti LL, de Oliveira RS, Santos MV, Farina JA, Machado HR. Multiple cranial burr holes as an alternative treatment for total scalp avulsion. Child's Nerv Syst. 2010; 26(6):745-9.
3. McLaughlin N, Martin NA. Effectiveness of burr holes for indirect revascularization in patients with moyamoya disease-A review of the literature. World Neurosurg. 2014; 81(1):91-8.

36
External Ventricular Drainage

Devesh K Singh, Arun K Srivastava, Kuntal Kanti Das, Rabi N Sahu

INTRODUCTION

External ventricular drainage is a temporary procedure, often done in emergent conditions, for letting out the ventricular cerebrospinal fluid (CSF) into a closed collection apparatus outside the body as a means of reducing the intracranial pressure. "EVD" is the popular acronym referring to this procedure, in which a small catheter is inserted through the skull through predefined bony landmarks into the dilated lateral ventricles of the brain. It is a life-saving procedure in dire situations with acceptable risks to the patient. Although a neurosurgical procedure, EVD can be done by general surgeons, emergency physicians or interventionists provided they have been properly trained.[1] Unlike CSF shunt procedures, it does not make the patient shunt dependent and also allows controlled and monitored CSF drainage.

INDICATION

- *Trauma*
  - Severe head injury (Glasgow coma scale, GCS ≤ 8) with raised ICP and ventriculomegaly. It not only acts therapeutically but also allows for simultaneous monitoring of the ICP.
- *Pure intraventricular hemorrhage/intracerebral hemorrhage with intraventricular extension*
  - EVD is usually placed into the lateral ventricle housing lesser amount of blood. It can be the only intervention done or it can follow endoscopic evacuation of the intraventricular hematoma. One may instill thrombolytics through the catheter in order to hasten the process of clot resolution.
- *Subarachnoid hemorrhage (SAH)*
  - Usually in poor grade SAH (Hunt and Hess grade IV and V). EVD allows some clinical improvement to occur after admission. Once they improve to better grades, surgical clipping or endovascular coiling of the aneurysm is done. In better grade patients, EVD may be placed intraoperatively after dural opening to make the brain lax. It will ensure easy dissection of the subarachnoid cisterns facilitating aneurysm clipping. At times, depending on the assessment at the time of dural closure, the surgeon decides to leave EVD in situ. Such EVDs are later on removed (discussed later). Such catheters can be utilized for instilling vasodilator drugs directly into ventricles to combat postoperative clinical vasospasm.

- *Shunt system malfunction or infection:* Acts to tide over the time of active infection.
- *Others:* Tumor, meningitis, ischemic stroke, instillation of dye (for ventriculography) or medications (antibiotics for ventriculitis or fibrinolytics in intraventricular hematoma) inside the ventricles.

CONTRAINDICATION

Certain relative contraindications are as follows:
- Uncontrolled coagulopathy
- Scalp infection at the site of proposed EVD insertion.

APPLIED ANATOMY AND PHYSIOLOGY

Ventricular System Anatomy

The ventricular system in humans consists of four ventricles with interconnecting foramina or ducts. There are two lateral ventricles situated on either side of the midline within the cerebral hemispheres. These lateral ventricles connect into a single midline slit like space, known as the third ventricle via interventricular foramen, also called the foramen of Monro. The third ventricle is situated in the diencephalon. The CSF within third ventricle enters into the fourth ventricle located in the posterior fossa between the cerebellum and the brainstem. The connection between the third and the fourth ventricle is called the aqueduct of Sylvius (Figs 1A and B). The CSF from the fourth ventricle then enters either the central canal of the spinal cord through the obex or the basal subarachnoid space via unpaired midline aperture (foramina of Magendie) or the paired lateral apertures (foramina of Luschka). Capillary action, cerebral pulsations and pulsations of the subarachnoid vessels propel the CSF towards the arachnoid villi abutting the superior sagittal sinus (SSS). The arachnoid villi, though which CSF is absorbed into the venous system, are outpouching of the arachnoid mater into the interior of SSS. It is important to remember that CSF passes into venous system in an unidirectional fashion i.e., in venous hypertension, CSF cannot be absorbed into the SSS however, there is no way, blood can make its way into the subarachnoid space from the SSS.

Flow of Cerebrospinal Fluid

The function of CSF is to provide buoyancy to the brain/spinal cord and along with nerve roots, denticulate ligaments and filum terminale, provide structural support to them. It is a modified form of plasma consisting of water, glucose, protein, minerals and a few lymphocytes. CSF is continuously secreted by the choroids plexus of the two lateral ventricles (located at the atrium) at a rate of approximately 20–25 mL/hour in an adult (or 500 mL/day). At any given point of time, approximately 100–150 mL of CSF is contained within the cerebral ventricles and the spinal subarachnoid space (roughly 75 mL each). In health, the rate of reabsorption equals the rate of secretion. Obstructive hydrocephalus results from mechanical obstruction of CSF flow anywhere within the ventricular system until the foramina of Luschka and Magendie. On the other hand, if the obstruction is extraventricular and subarachnoid in location or if there is defective absorption of CSF at the level of arachnoid villi the resultant condition becomes known as communicating or nonobstructive hydrocephalus.

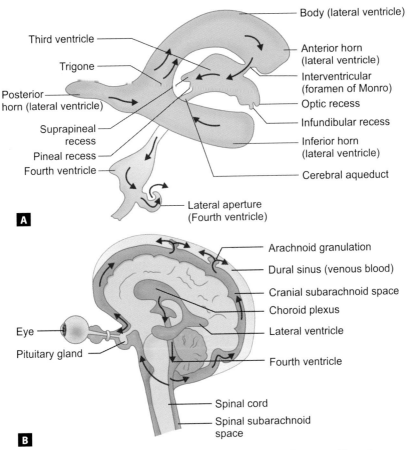

Figs 1A and B Ventricular system of the brain and the direction of flow of CSF under normal circumstances

Effects of Cerebrospinal Fluid on Intracranial Pressure

The Monro-Kellie doctrine states that in a rigid compartment like the skull containing compressible substances like brain, blood and CSF, an increase in volume of one component shall lead to increase of overall pressure inside the skull unless another component decrease in volume reciprocally. Hence, increase in volume of CSF leads to increase in intracranial pressure (ICP). *Such increase in volume may be due to:*

- Increased CSF production (e.g. choroid plexus neoplasm)
- Mechanical obstruction to CSF flow within or outside ventricles (tumors)
- Defective absorption (e.g. after meningitis)

Abnormalities associated with any of the above three processes result in increased ICP and require placement of EVD for CSF drainage. In Figure 2, graph describes the relationship between pressure and volume within the skull (the volume pressure curve, Monro-Kellie doctrine). As can be seen a reasonable increase in volume (irrespective of whether this is edema, mass, blood or CSF) will be tolerated prior to evident changes in the ICP (compensated stage). The key

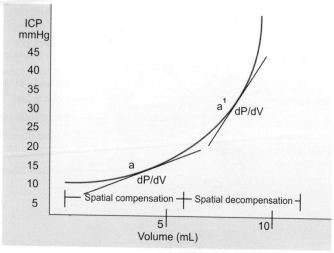

Fig. 2 The volume—pressure curve

is to intervene prior to reaching the critical point after which ICP rises sharply. Clinically, this is associated with bradycardia, hypertension and pupil changes. This is a preterminal event.

Normal ranges/reportable limits: Intracranial pressure is the pressure exerted by the CSF, which circulates from the ventricles around the brain and spinal cord. The normal range of ICP is 0–15 mm Hg; increased ICP is usually referred to as values exceeding the upper permissible limit, i.e. above 15 mm Hg.

Cerebral perfusion pressure (CPP = Mean arterial pressure – ICP) is also measured in patients whilst admitted to ICU with an ICP monitor. Adequate CPP is required to ensure that the brain remains well-perfused (dangerous limit <60 mm Hg). Inadequate CPP may be due to elevated ICP, low blood pressure (BP) or a combination of both and should be managed according to the underlying problem. *The normal range of ICP is shown below:*

- *Neonate:* > 30 mm Hg
- *1-6 months:* > 35 mm Hg
- *6-11 months:* > 40 mm Hg
- *1-4 years:* > 45 mm Hg
- *5-9 years:* > 50 mm Hg.

Symptoms and Signs of Raised Intracranial Pressure

Infants: Irritability, vomiting, full bulging fontanelle, neurological symptoms—decrease in GCS, cranial nerve palsy, sunsetting eyes (eyes unable to look up), irregular respirations and apneic periods, splaying of cranial sutures, a big head—measure head circumference regularly, tachycardia/hypertension/bradycardia, pupil changes (fixed pupils, irregularly shaped pupils or dilated pupils all worrying).

Older children/adults: Headache, nausea, vomiting, lethargy, irritability, worsening concentration, decreased GCS, sixth nerve palsy, other abnormalities—seen at neurologic examination, tachycardia/hypertension/bradycardia, pupil changes (fixed pupils, irregularly shaped pupils or dilated pupils all worrying).

Note: The combination of bradycardia, hypertension and irregular respiration in a neurological patient is a preterminal event. Inform neurosurgeon/neurophysician immediately.

TECHNIQUE AND BASIC PRINCIPLES

First performed by Claude-Nicholas Le Cat in 1744 using a specially invented cannula to treat hydrocephalus in a newborn, EVD remains one of the most common neurosurgical emergency procedures across the world. Subsequently, William Williams Keen first reported the technique and outcome following EVD. Since then, EVD, as a procedure, has seen a sea of change as far as technique, materials and indications for its placement are concerned. In the last century, many improvements were made in the technique along with method of CSF drainage and collection.

External Ventricular Drainage Placement Procedure

Placement of EVD is one of the most important and fundamental skill acquired by a neurosurgeon during his/her training. The usual bony landmarks chosen for EVD placements are Kocher's point (frontal), Keen's point (parieto-occipital), Dandy point, double Dandy point (occipital) and modified Paine's point (intraoperative, perisylvian) (Figs 3 to 7). Usually the Kocher's point is the most common site of putting surgical EVD.

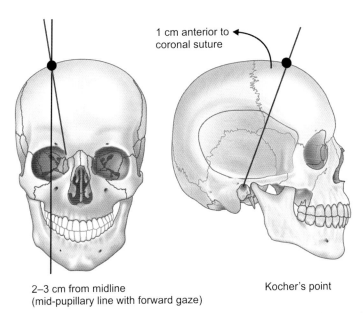

1 cm anterior to coronal suture

2–3 cm from midline
(mid-pupillary line with forward gaze)

Kocher's point

Fig. 3 Kocher's point located 1 cm anterior to coronal suture, 3 cm lateral to midline on the right side. Look at the direction of entry into the ventricles, which is medially and pointing toward external auditory meatus

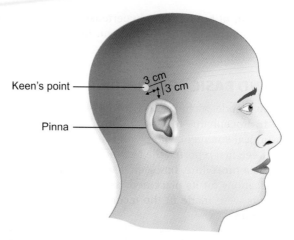

Fig. 4 Keen's point located 3 cm above and behind top of pinna

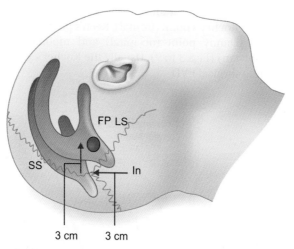

Fig. 5 Dandy point located 3 cm above and 2 cm lateral to inion
(In, inion; SS, sagittal; LS, lambdoid sutures; FP, frontoparietal)

Catheters: External drainage and monitoring system catheters are either translucent or fabricated of radiopaque (barium impregnated) silicone tubing. They feature larger diameter flow holes and larger inside diameter to minimize possible obstruction. Antibiotic impregnated catheters are also available in market.

Several features aid the surgeon during the process of catheter placement:
- Numerical length markers at each centimeter
- Radiopaque stripe down the length of the catheter body for X-ray recognition
- Soft, pliable silicone to minimize trauma to the brain matter
- Large flow holes to reduce potential of clogging.

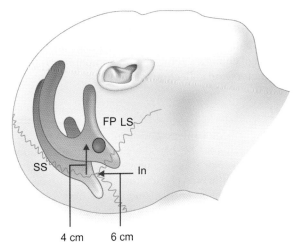

Fig. 6 Double Dandy point, 6 cm above and 4 cm lateral to inion. This point is also known as the Frazier's point (In, inion; SS, sagittal; LS, lambdoid sutures; FP, frontoparietal)

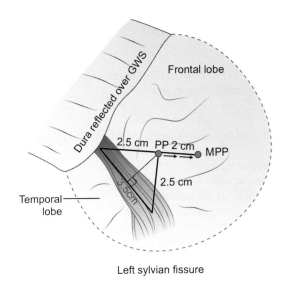

Left sylvian fissure

Fig. 7 Modified Paine's point and its modification. Paine's point is found at the superior apex of the isosceles triangle, whose base of approximately 3.5 cm length rests along the Sylvian veins emanating from under the dura reflected over the greater wing of sphenoid (GWS). Each of the other two limbs of this triangle is 2.5 cm in length. Hyun et al.[1] modified this point of intraoperative ventricular cannulation to avoid trajectory misadventures which are common with Paine's point and described modified Paine's point (MPP). This point lies 2 cm posterosuperior to the original Paine's point

Drainage and collecting system: Once the EVD has been inserted, the surgeon attaches an external drainage and monitoring system. This is a completely closed system for drainage of CSF from the lateral ventricles. This drainage is gravity dependent, unlike shunt tubes, which are provided with pressure valve in the tube system. The drainage system is attached to an IV stand at the head of the bed.

The system comprises a measuring chamber, which is connected to a drainage bag, with a sampling port and stopcock between them. All the connections are "Luer Locked" for safety. A drainage pressure scale (in 1 cm increments) is adjacent to the drainage chamber. A number of companies (Integra, Medtronic, Codman) supply catheters and collection systems.

PREPARATION

- Informed signed consent (unless emergent or no family available) and prepare requisition form for CSF/blood collection, investigations
- Perform baseline neurological assessment and record vitals
- The prophylactic antibiotic is so chosen that the common causes of infection like *Staphylococcus aureus* and *Acinetobacter* are covered. Usually a combination of 3rd generation cephalosporin and an aminoglycoside suffices. We recommend repeating antibiotics if the procedure takes longer than one hour from the time of making the incision.
- Inspection of radiographic images (CT brain) to plan the site and side of ventriculostomy
- Removal of hair is not mandatory. Cleansing with antiseptic solutions and separating them away from the proposed incision site is acceptable.
- *Landmarks (frontal horn placement)*
  - Midline
  - Coronal suture
  - Kocher's point (3 cm from midline/1 cm anterior to coronal suture)
- *Landmarks (occipital horn placement)*
  - Midline
  - Inion
  - Dandy's or double Dandy's point (2 or 4 cm from midline/ 6 or 8 cm above inion)
- *Head position (frontal insertion)*
  - Head looking straight ahead—no rotation
  - Head flat or slightly above heart
  - If required, secure position with tape
  - Appropriate sedation/analgesia as needed
- *Sterile field*
  - Prepare skin with chlorhexidine or betadine paint—let it dry for at least 1 minute before draping
  - Attention to details to prevent contamination of sterile field and hardware
  - Minimize touching the skin with gloved hands
  - Use cranioplasty drape to completely drape the patient and bed
  - Use full barrier precautions (cap, mask, gown, gloves)

PROCEDURE

Frontal Insertion

- Local anesthesia at site of incision and planned exit site of the tube (this ensures that the initial few centimeters of the catheter remains subcutaneously. It goes a long way in preventing catheter infection, hence ventriculitis).

- *Scalp incision*
  - 2–3 cm long, parallel to midline
  - Centered around the proposed entry site (the Kocher's point).
- *Drill (and catheter) trajectory:* Calvarium is drilled with twist drill perpendicular to the brain surface, aiming for ipsilateral medial canthus and EAM (external auditory meatus). Skull may misdirect catheter during the pass if the drill hole is placed in an improper plane.
  - Drill away the entire inner table of bone before violating dura
  - Open dura with back-and-forth action in a controlled fashion.
- *Ventricular catheter placement*
  - Use antibiotic-impregnated ventricular catheter if available (however, these are costly).
  - Insertion length—no more than 6 cm from outer table of skull surface
  - Danger comes from passing too deep or too lateral—if second pass required, direct path more medially, and no deeper.
  - Maximum of three attempts—if unsuccessful, leave catheter in place
- *Once good CSF flow is obtained*
  - Minimize initial CSF drainage
  - Bring catheter externally through skin via a separate stab incision 2–3 cm away from initial incision, by tunneling catheter medially and/or posteriorly without crossing midline
- *Closure*
  - Use 2-0 nylon (monofilament) suture
  - Single layer vertical mattress closure of initial incision, carefully avoiding catheter
  - Tie a purse string around the exit site
  - Simple interrupted sutures to secure the ventriculostomy to the skin (no staples)
  - Make a circle with the catheter after it exits from the stab wound and secure it at multiple points, to reduce chances that it will pull out
- *Connection to drainage system and monitor*
  - Flush the distal system with sterile saline including both the transducer and the drainage tubing
  - Attach the drainage system and the transducer on the sterile field to the ventricular catheter within the sterile field (physicians only)
  - Place a silk tie (braided suture, not monofilament) around the connector that inserts into the ventriculostomy catheter
  - Confirm good waveform
- Dress wound with 2 × 2 sterile gauze and Tegaderm; repeat/change gauze dressing every 24–48 hours while catheter in place
- *CSF studies (collected at insertion):* Gram stain, culture, glucose, protein, cell count, lactate (send on ice)
- Figure 8 shows right frontal EVD (put through the Kocher's point), the tubing and collection bag.

POST-PROCEDURE CARE

- *Dressing:* Initial dressing to remain in place for the first 24–48 hours unless soiled or wet daily maintenance (dressing changes). Thereafter it can be changed on 4th and 7th postoperative day till sutures are removed.

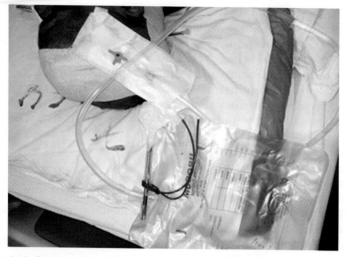

Fig. 8 Right frontal EVD (put through the Kocher's point), the tubing and collection bag

The catheter emanating from the scalp till the three way valve needs to be painted with betadine daily. Then it should be wrapped in sterile gauge. The three way valve should also be covered completely only leaving some area to collect CSF from the side opening and tri way directors.

- *Imaging:* Patient should undergo noncontrast CT scan after the procedure to verify the tip of ventricular catheter and serve as a radiological baseline.
- *Procedure documentation* is very important. Time of changing the catheter should be documented daily and CSF drained over last 24 hours should be clearly documented.
- Documentation of any medications to be administered
- Keeping the collection bag at the level of the external auditory meatus in supine position ensures that it is at the level of foramen of monro. Hence, one can avoid overdrainage of CSF. If the patient position changes, the system has to be repositioned again. Utilize 'lock out' on the bed controls to avoid inadvertent bed position changes. Placing signage *"Do Not Adjust Bed"* at bedside can be useful.
- ICP monitoring, if being done, can be connected at this point of time.
- Patient monitoring includes assessment of GCS, pupillary size and reaction, vitals,CSF volume collected, watching out for soakage at drain site, etc.
- Antibiotic impregnated catheters can be kept for prolonged time (3 weeks or so), however, non antibiotic coated catheters are better changed every 5–7 days. It is important to administer antibiotics during the period of drainage.
- During patient position change and transportation, the triway should be adjusted in such a way that CSF drainage stops. This will ensure not only unwanted leakage of CSF but also sucking in of air inside the ventricles. It is very important to re-open the stop thereafter. The later situation is pretty common in even neurosurgical settings. It goes without saying how dangerous such a thing can turn out to be.
- We recommend sending CSF for biochemical and microbiological analysis daily. The CSF should always be collected from the side opening and never from the collection bag.

- The collection bag has to be changed everyday and a practice of emptying the bag and continuing with the older one is absolutely unacceptable. It goes without saying the importance of maintain asepsis during such changes.
- The EVD catheter needs to be changed every 5–7 days unless one has installed a drug impregnated catheter. Changing catheter requires adherence to all aseptic and antiseptic measures like the first procedure. All one needs is to gently pull out the existing catheter and push in the new catheter through the tract that has already formed. Thereafter, the catheter needs to be secured with a stay suture using 2-0 nylon and rest of the assembly needs to be connected (all new, previous one not to be used under any circumstances).
- *Removal of catheter:* It depends on the indications for which it was put. The basic idea is to tide over the crisis and remove it as soon as one can. On occasions, it may not be possible to do away with CSF diversion. In such cases, conversion to formal shunting can be done. The prerequisite of shunting is absence of biochemical/microbiological absence of infection in the CSF for 3 days prior to the shunt procedure. Otherwise, we keep the EVD closed for about 6 hours and look for clinical deterioration, in the event of which, we repeat CT scan to see increasing hydrocephalus. These patients require permanent shunting or endoscopic third ventriculostomy. In those patients who tolerate clamping of the catheter, for more than 6 hours, the EVD can be removed.

COMPLICATION/PROBLEM

- *Infection:* Infection is a common occurrence. Literature (of indwelling shunts) suggests a 0–28% infection rate per procedure with mean of 8.8%.[2] Inoculation of skin commensals during EVD insertion and colonization of the drainage system during postoperative period with subsequent retrograde infections are the leading causes of EVD related infections.[3] Inoculation related infection is attributed to maintenance of aseptic and antiseptic precautions during the insertion procedure. For obvious reasons, repeated revisions due to some reason or the other heighten the likelihood of further infections. On the other hand, colonization and contamination of the drainage system is directly related to the manipulation of the system, strict adherence to EVD maintenance protocol, and most importantly, the proper technique of EVD insertion.[4] Coagulase negative *Staphylococcus* remains the most common cause of EVD related infection (incidence as high as 47%).[5] Other organisms that have been consistently isolated from infected EVD are *Enterococcus, Enterobacter* and *Staphylococcus aureus.* Tunneling the catheter as far from insertion site as possible is preferred to reduce infection.[6] Antibiotic-impregnated catheters have shown promise in reducing infection rates, as well as a newly designed flexible metallic catheters.[5] Overall, meticulous technique upon insertion, careful wound care, and aseptic technique during CSF sampling are paramount to reduce infection rates. If EVD colonization or meningitis diagnosis is made, then consider strongly for administering intraventricular antibiotics prior to catheter removal as per culture and sensitivity.
- *Hemorrhage:* May occur during placement of EVD from injury to traversing brain tissue or with impact upon the choroids plexus or the deep veins

(periventricular). Irrigation may be needed to wash out the blood and prevent future obstruction. Location of the ventricular catheter tip affects functioning of the EVD and it is recommended that the tip should avoid the choroids plexus if possible to prevent obstruction as well as hemorrhage.

- *Excess drainage:* Excessive drainage of EVD beyond the recommended rate (i.e. > 20 mL/hour for adults, 10–15 mL/hour for pediatrics), there are chances of subdural hematoma formation apart from severe bifrontal headache due to brain sagging, also known as intracranial hypotension. Rarely, EVD placement may lead to remote cerebellar hemorrhage.[7] The thumb rule is, if the patient does not have improvement after EVD and shows some focal neurological signs, one should repeat CT head urgently.
- Catheter pull-out or breakage
- Catheter obstruction or malfunction
- *Fluid and electrolytes imbalance:* Daily serum electrolytes should be monitored for early detection of electrolyte imbalance in patients on EVD. The best available replacement fluid is the normal saline, which closely resembles the composition of CSF. The cause of electrolyte imbalance post EVD placement is continuous loss of CSF that the body normally reabsorbs.

REFERENCES

1. Hyun SJ, Suk JS, Kwon JT, Kim YB. Novel entry point for intraoperative ventricular puncture during the transsylvian approach. Acta Neurochir (Wien). 2007;149:1049-51.
2. Lozier AP, Sciacca RR, Romagnoli MF, Connolly ES Jr. Ventriculostomy-related infections: a critical review of the literature. Neurosurgery. 2008;62:688-700.
3. Lo CH, Spelman D, Bailey M, Cooper DJ, Rosenfeld JV, Brecknell JE. External ventricular drain infections are independent of drain duration: an argument against elective revision. J Neurosurg. 2007;106:378-83.
4. Hetem DJ, Woerdeman PA, Bonten MJ, Ekkelenkamp MB. Relationship between bacterial colonization of external cerebrospinal fluid drains and secondary meningitis: a retrospective analysis of an 8-year period. J Neurosurg. 2010;113:1309-13.
5. Zabramski, JM, Whiting, D, Darouiche, RO, Horner, TG, Olson, J, Robertson, C, et al. Efficacy of antimicrobial-impregnated external ventricular drain catheters: a prospective, randomized, controlled trial. J Neurosurg. 2003;98:725-30.
6. Friedman, WA, Vries, JK. Percutaneous tunnel ventriculostomy. Summary of 100 procedures. J Neurosurg. 1980;53:662-5.
7. Das KK, Nair P, Mehrotra A, Sardhara J, Sahu RN, Jaiswal AK, Kumar R. Remote cerebellar hemorrhage: Report of 2 cases and review of literature. Asian J Neurosurg. 2014;9:161-4.

37
Intracranial Pressure Monitoring

Hemanshu Prabhakar

INTRODUCTION

Intracranial pressure (ICP) is the pressure within cranial cavity relative to the atmospheric pressure. ICP wave is made up of following three components— arterial vascular component, cerebrospinal fluid (CSF) circulatory component and cerebral venous outflow component. The normal ICP wave has three peaks: percussion (P1), tidal (P2) and dicrotic (P3) (Fig. 1).

The normal ranges of ICP vary with age: in adults and older children, it is in the range of 10-15 mm Hg or less. It is 3-7 mm Hg in young children and 1.5-6 mm Hg in term infants. The values may differ in supine and standing positions and also under various physiological conditions such as coughing and Valsalva maneuvers as in defecation and parturition. A sustained elevation of ICP of more than 15 mm Hg in supine position is considered intracranial hypertension.

INDICATION

Though, the indications of ICP monitoring vary from center to center. *Some of the common situations where ICP monitoring is indicated are as follows:*
- Head injury
- Intracerebral hemorrhage
- Subarachnoid hemorrhage
- Hydrocephalus
- Ischemic stroke
- Hypoxic brain injury with cerebral edema
- Meningitis or encephalitis

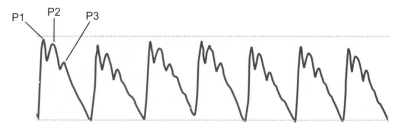

Fig. 1 Waveform during ICP monitoring. Three peaks of normal ICP wave: P1, percussion; P2, tidal; P3, dicrotic

- Hepatic encephalopathy
- Midline shift of more than 5 mm on computed tomography (CT) of head
- Papilledema
- Severe vomiting
- Severe headache
- Transient blindness.

The ICP monitoring of head injured patients with Glasgow Coma Score (GCS) of 8 or less and presence of CT abnormalities, such as brain contusion, swelling, hematoma, compressed basal cisterns or brain herniation, has been recommended by the Brain Trauma Foundation. Those with a normal CT scan but GCS of 8 or less should also receive ICP monitoring if the age is more than 40, and motor posturing (unilateral or bilateral), or systolic blood pressure of less than 90 mm Hg.

CONTRAINDICATION

There are no absolute contraindications for invasive ICP monitoring. However, awake patients and coagulation abnormalities may be considered as relative contraindications.

APPLIED ANATOMY AND PHYSIOLOGY

The brain along with its fluid components, the CSF and blood (arterial and venous), is enclosed in a rigid skull. Whereas the brain occupies nearly 83% of the intracranial compartment, the CSF and blood volume occupies 11% and 6%, respectively. The "Monro-Kellie doctrine" establishes a relationship between the brain, blood, CSF, ICP and cerebral perfusion pressure (CPP). According to the "Monro-Kellie doctrine", the volume of the intracranial compartment must always remain constant to maintain a constant ICP as the skull cannot expand and the brain parenchyma cannot be compressed. ICP may then be defined as "pressure exerted by the blood (arterial and venous) and the CSF on the brain tissue". Normal ICP waves cannot be routinely monitored for the reason that ICP monitoring is not indicated in patients with normal ICP. It has been observed that normally small pulsation waves are observed secondary to the effects of systemic blood pressure, which may be superimposed on slower respiratory variations. In 1960, Lundberg described the three classical ICP waves seen under pathological conditions. The characteristics of these waves are tabulated (Table 1).

Table 1 Characteristics of the Lundberg waves

Wave type	Features	Duration
A-wave (Plateau wave)	Amplitude 20 mm Hg	↑ ICP for 5–20 min
B-wave (Pressure pulses)	Amplitude 10–20 mm Hg 0.5–2/min	30 secs–2 min
C-wave (Traube-Hering-Mayer wave)	Low amplitude 4–8/min	

Abbreviation: ICP, intracranial pressure.

TECHNIQUE AND EQUIPMENT

The continuous measurement of ICP is an important neuromonitor but requires an invasive approach. ICP can be measured in several anatomic spaces (Fig. 2).

- Intraventricular
- Intraparenchymal
- Subdural
- Subarachnoid
- Epidural.

The various advantages and disadvantages related to each location are tabulated (Table 2).

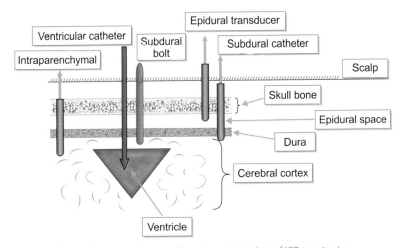

Fig. 2 Schematic diagram showing various sites of ICP monitoring

Table 2 Different techniques of ICP monitoring

Technique	Advantages	Disadvantages
Intraventricular	Accurate	Difficult placement in small ventricles
	Gold standard	Risk of infection
	Allows CSF drain	Risk of bleeding
	Measures IC compliance	
	Repeat calibrations possible	
Intraparenchymal	Low infection rate	Tendency to drift with time
	Reliable	CSF drain not possible
		Recalibration impossible
Subdural	Low infection rate	Easily blocked
	Easy to place	CSF drain not possible
Subarachnoid	Low infection rate	Easily blocked
	Easy to place	
Epidural	Less invasive	Not precise

Abbreviations: CSF, cerebrospinal fluid; IC, intracranial.

Intraventricular or fluid-filled system: This is the most precise method of ICP measurement and is the gold standard against which other methods are measured. The fluid-filled intraventricular catheter is connected to transducer. Additional advantages of this system are that it can be used to measure the intracranial compliance, allows CSF drainage to treat intracranial hypertension and allows periodic recalibration. But sometimes it is difficult or even impossible to insert the catheter when the ventricular size is reduced as in cases of extreme brain swelling. The main disadvantages of intraventricular measurement of ICP are the risks of infection and bleeding.

Transducer-tipped systems: Current transducer systems (ventricular, intra-parenchymal or subdural) reduce the rate of infection. The Codman microsensor transducer system (Fig. 3) consists of minute strain gauge transducer. This transducer is placed on a titanium case at the tip of a flexible nylon tube, 100 cm in length. The microsensor monitors ICP at the source—intraparenchymal, intraventricular or subdural. Information is relayed electronically rather than through hydrostatic system or fiber optics. The main advantage of the microsensor system is that it is position independent, there is no fluid line, it is less invasive, less chance of infection and low drift.

One of the most common methods of ICP monitoring in modern intensive care units (ICUs) is the fiber-optic or "bolt" ICP monitor (Figs 4A and B). This method is advantageous because of its ease of placement, less chance of infection and facility to add other monitoring devices like thermal probes, oximeters, etc. One disadvantage is inability to do therapeutic CSF drainage.

Intraparenchymal system measures localized ICP which may not reflect true ICP (i.e. ventricular CSF pressure).

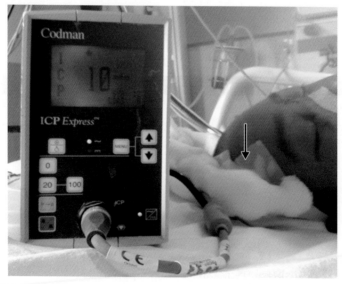

Fig. 3 Codman ICP monitoring system [bold arrow showing location of the catheter (not visible due to surgical dressing)]

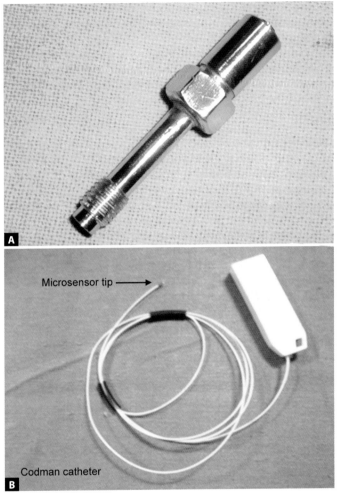

Figs 4A and B (A) Intracranial pressure bolt; (B) Codman catheter showing microsensor tip

A zero drift occurs in microtransducers on long term use and this cannot be recalibrated. Fiber-optic transducers cannot be recalibrated externally; however, their accuracy in practice has proved excellent.

PREPARATION

- Informed consent to be taken
- Measures of sterility to be taken such as washing of hands, sterile gloves and gown, and sterile drapes
- Head should be shaved completely or may be restricted to the surgical site
- A sterile surgical trolley containing the equipment of burr hole, sterile towels/ sheets, sterile bowls for povidone-iodine or any other antiseptic, and 5 cm^3 syringe for local anesthetic
- Catheter set for ICP monitoring

- Routine monitoring of the patient during the procedure should include the heart rate, invasive and non-invasive BP, 5-lead electrocardiogram (ECG) and pulse oximetry
- For apprehensive or uncooperative patients, sedatives such as midazolam 1–2 mg with fentanyl 1–2 µg/kg may be needed (use of sedative in nonintubated patients warrants close monitoring of the respiratory rate and pattern).

PROCEDURE

- The patient lies supine with head in neutral position. Tilting of head is avoided to prevent compression of neck veins that may possibly aggravate ICP.
- Clean the scalp with antiseptic solution and put sterile drapes, usually over the nondominant side of the brain in the frontal lobe.
- The skin of the surgical site is infiltrated with local anesthetic such as lignocaine with adrenalin or bupivacaine.
- The point chosen is in the mid pupillary line, about 1–2 cm anterior to coronal suture, also known as Kocher's point.
- Skin incision is made down to the skull bone.
- A burr hole is made using a twist drill (see Chapter on "Cranial Burr Hole").
- The dura is then opened with the help of blade.
- A ventricular catheter is then passed through the dura, perpendicular to the brain and into the ventricles, approximately 5–7 cm in adults, toward the ipsilateral foramen of Monro. This coincides with the junction of the lines passing from incision point to inner canthus of ipsilateral eye and from tragus of the ear to the incision point.
- Free flow of CSF confirms the position of the catheter. For fiber-optic catheters, a CT scan may be used to confirm the correct placement.
- Catheter should then be fixed with surgical sutures to the scalp using the tunneling method.
- The catheter may then be attached to a pressure transducer for monitoring of ICP waves.
- The transducer should preferably be placed at the tragus or mastoid process which corresponds to the level of foramen of Monro, which is based on the institutional practice. An important fact is to use the same landmark each time the ICP transducer is zeroed.
- Pressure monitoring should preferably be done in supine position.

Note: No more than three attempts should be made to place the catheter, failing to which, decision to place the subarachnoid bolt or intraparenchymal catheter should be taken.

POST-PROCEDURE CARE

- Sterile dressing of the surgical wound should be done. Sterility should be maintained each time the catheter is handled or dressings changed.
- Anticoagulated patient can have their catheters/ICP monitor removed only if their coagulation profile is normal.
- There are no recommendations on the number of days a catheter can be kept in place for ICP monitoring. Most centers prefer keeping the catheter for 5–10 days.

COMPLICATION/PROBLEM

The complications may be related to the type of monitoring site used. These are shown in Table 2. Care should be taken to avoid kinking of the catheter that may dampen the ICP waveforms or even fail to show the waves. Other causes of blocked catheter leading to absence of waves may be air bubble, debris, blood clot or even equipment malfunction.

SUGGESTED READING

1. Cottrell JE, Yound WL (Eds). Neuroanesthesia, 5th edition. Philadelphia: Mosby-Elsevier. 2010.
2. Cucchiara RF, Black S, Michenfelder JD (Eds). Clinical Neuroanesthesia, 2nd edition. US: Churchill Livingstone Inc. 1998.
3. Greenberg MS (Ed). Handbook of Neurosurgery, 7th edition. Thieme Publishers. 2010.
4. Matta BF, Menon DK, Smith M (Eds). Core Topics in Neuroanaesthesia and Neurointensive Care. New York: Cambridge University Press. 2011.
5. Stone DJ, Sperry RJ, Johnson JO, Spiekermann BF, Yemen TA (Eds). The Neuroanesthesia Handbook. US: Mosby Inc. 1996.

38

Nerve and Muscle Biopsy

Sanjeev K Bhoi, Jayantee Kalita, Usha K Misra

INTRODUCTION

Nerve and muscle biopsy involves the process of removing peripheral nerve or muscle for pathological examination. This procedure, considered as "minor surgery", is often used in the diagnosis of neuromuscular disorders. There are limited role of nerve or muscle biopsy in intensive care unit (ICU). It should be considered in selective cases where it will influence the management.

INDICATION

Nerve Biopsy

The important indications of nerve biopsy are in diagnosis, classifications and prognosis of peripheral neuropathy. It is the final step in the evaluation of peripheral neuropathy.
- *Diagnostic:* Vasculitis, amyloidosis, sarcoidosis, Hansen's disease, giant axonal neuropathy, polyglucosan disease.
- *Suggestive abnormality:* Hereditary neuropathy of demyelinating types, chronic inflammatory demyelinating polyradiculoneuropathy (CIDP), paraproteinemic neuropathy.

Muscle Biopsy

- Inflammatory myopathy
- Muscular dystrophies in which genetic testing is not widely available
- Mitochondrial cytopathies
- Metabolic myopathies.

CONTRAINDICATION

Nerve Biopsy

- Should not be done before proper and adequate clinical, laboratory and electrodiagnostic investigations.

Muscle Biopsy

- Bleeding disorder
- Infection at the planned biopsy site.

TECHNIQUE AND BASIC PRINCIPLES

Nerve Biopsy

The commonly biopsied nerves are:
- Sural nerve below lateral malleolus
- Superficial peroneal nerve at the shin
- Intermediate cutaneous nerve of thigh
- Superficial cutaneous branch of radial nerve at the wrist
- Dorsal cutaneous branch of ulnar nerve at wrist

Selection of Nerve

- Ideally the nerve biopsy should be done from a sensory nerve supplying least area of skin.
- Easily identifiable superficial nerves which are not vulnerable to compression or injury are preferred.
- The nerves which can be studied by nerve conduction study are preferred as functionally abnormal nerves are more likely to reveal abnormality.

Muscle Biopsy

Usefulness of muscle biopsy depends on the following considerations: appropriate indication, choice of muscle, biopsy technique and array of histopathology performed.

The biopsy may be punch or open biopsy. The advantage of punch biopsy is quick, cosmetic and less invasive; while disadvantages are poorer yield due to patchy changes in inflammatory myopathy.

Choice of Muscle

- Biceps brachii and vastus lateralis are usually preferred. Muscle should be slightly weak [British Medical Research Council Scale (MRC) III-IV], because more weaker and end stage muscles are fibrous and pathology may be obscured.
- Muscle site should be free of trauma, infections, electromyography (EMG) study and prior biopsy.
- If EMG done on right sided muscle of the body, biopsy should be done on left side muscle.
- Distal muscles such as tibialis anterior and extensor digitorum brevis should be avoided.
- CT, MR may help in choosing the affected muscles.

Note: Combined nerve and muscle biopsy may be more informative.

PREPARATION

- Explain the procedure and obtain written consent.
- *Instruments needed:* Artery forceps, scalpel, forceps, needle holder (Fig. 1).
- Provide relevant details to the pathologist, including nerve conduction findings, creatine kinase (CK) level, EMG findings of previous biopsy, family history and drug history.
- Should be done in clean aseptic condition.

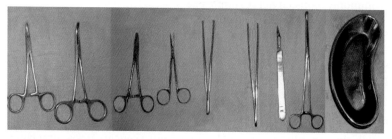

Fig. 1 Instruments required for nerve and muscle biopsy

PROCEDURE

Nerve Biopsy

Methods of sural nerve biopsy is described as prototype:
- Palpate the sural nerve below the lateral malleolus at the midpoint between lateral malleolus and calcaneum and mark the location of nerve (Fig. 2).
- Prepare the skin by povidone iodine and spirit.
- Infiltrate the skin and subcutaneous tissue by 10 mL of 0.5% lidocaine below the lateral malleolus (perform skin sensitivity of lidocaine before).

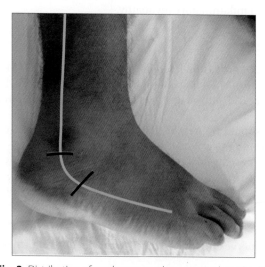

Fig. 2 Distribution of sural nerve on the posterior lateral ankle

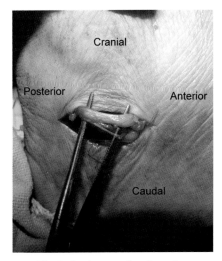

Fig. 3 Sural nerve after dissection

- Place the incision along the course of short saphenous vein, which becomes prominent and visible by compressing the calf by tourniquet.
- Divide Scarpa's fascia and trace the saphenous vein; sural nerve lies medial to saphenous vein.
- After securing bleeders, secure the most proximal portion of exposed nerve and infiltrate it by 0.2 mL of lidocaine.
- Then do dissection of surrounding tissue to make nerve free. Avoid stretching, rubbing or blunt dissection of nerve (Fig. 3).
- Ligate the nerve distal to infiltration site and cut distal to it.
- 3–4 cm of nerve sample is obtained.
- After homeostasis the skin is sutured.

Muscle Biopsy

- Mark the site of biopsy from the belly of muscle. Prepare the skin by povidone iodine and spirit.
- Infiltrate the skin and subcutaneous tissue by 10 mL of 0.5% lidocaine below the lateral malleolus (perform skin sensitivity of lidocaine before).
- Skin incision of 2–3 cm in length is made over the demarcated site (Fig. 4).
- Fatty tissue is gently teased till fascia is exposed (Fig. 5).
- Fascia is incised longitudinally till the muscle belly is exposed (Fig. 6).
- Obtain two intact pieces of muscle, each approximately 1-2 cm in length and 0.5-0.8 cm in thickness.
- Hemostasis is done and fascia is sutured before stitching the skin.

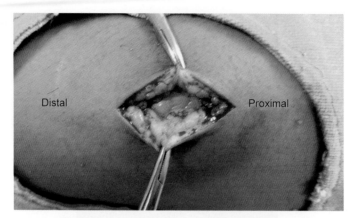

Fig. 4 Skin and soft tissue incision for muscle biopsy

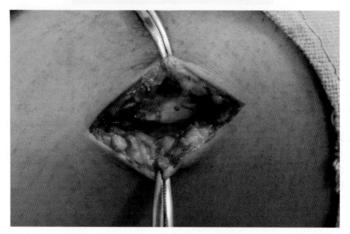

Fig. 5 Muscle belly with glistening overlying fascia

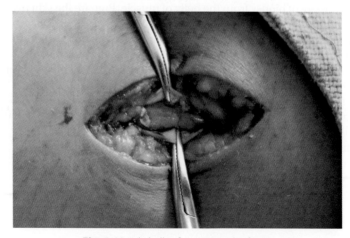

Fig. 6 Muscle belly after cutting the fascia

POST-PROCEDURE CARE

Nerve Biopsy Sample Handling

- Wrap the biopsy specimen in a saline mounted gauge to send to local pathology laboratory.
- If the nerve has to be transported to far off laboratory, the biopsy specimen is placed in 2.5% glutaraldehyde and 1/3 of biopsy piece is placed in formalin.

Muscle Biopsy Sample Handling

- For histochemistry and biochemical studies, muscle samples are immediately frozen.
- For electron microscopy, specimen is preserved in glutaraldehyde.
- For routine neuropathological evaluation, hematoxylin and eosin staining is done in formaldehyde preserved specimens.

COMPLICATION/PROBLEM

There is no major complication. Minor complications are:
- Allergy to local anesthesia
- Bleeding
- Wound infection and dehiscence
- Post biopsy paresthesia and sensory loss
- Stump neuromas.

SUGGESTED READING

1. Dubowitz V. Muscle biopsy—technical and diagnostic aspects. Ann Clin Res. 1974;6(2): 69-79.
2. Dyck PJ, Thomas PK. Peripheral Neuropathy, 4th edition. Philadelphia: Elsevier. 2005. pp. 733-7.
3. Graham DI, Lantos PL (Eds). Greenfield's Neuropathology, 7th edition. Oxford University Press, New York.
4. Hall G. Muscle biopsy. Pract Neurol. 2001;1:113-8.
5. Jaradeh SS, Ho H. Muscle, nerve, and skin biopsy. Neurol Clin. 2004;22(3):539-61.
6. Medline Plus. Muscle biopsy. [Online] Available from http://www.nlm.nih.gov/medlineplus/ency/article/003924.htm. [Accessed March 2015].
7. Nowak L, Reyes PF. Muscle biopsy: a diagnostic tool in muscle diseases. J Histotechnol. 2008;31:101-8.
8. Sommer C, Brandner S, Dyck PJ, Magy L, Mellgren SI, Morbin M, et al. 147th ENMC international workshop: guideline on processing and evaluation of sural nerve biopsies, 15-17 December 2006, Naarden, The Netherlands. Neuromuscul Disord. 2008;18(1):90-6.

39

Spine Immobilization in Trauma Patient

Sandeep Sahu, Indu Lata

INTRODUCTION

The initial and acute management of spinal cord injury (SCI) is very demanding and challenging. The outcome of a patient with SCI depends upon the integrated emergency department and prehospital management. Better resuscitation and rehabilitation depend on trauma system that includes continuum of care in prehospital, trauma unit or centers and SCI centers or rehabilitation unit. The aim is to prevent any type of secondary injury and complications, by proper resuscitation and immobilization, during transfer to hospital or within hospital and proper evaluation integrated trauma system approach.[1] Any trauma patient with or without spine injury may require transport from scene to primary or definitive care hospital or transfer in between hospitals (Fig. 1).

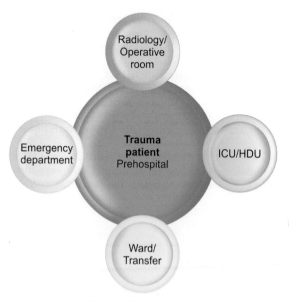

Fig. 1 Patient may have possible transfers that can aggravate unstable spine injury

Abbreviations: ICU, intensive care unit; HDU, high dependency unit.

There is possibility that approximately 30% of patients may have neurological deterioration while undergoing initial management. So, one should be careful with standard precautions in managing unstable spine patient with prevention of any type of secondary injury and complications.[2] There is also possibility that about 5% patients of spine injury may have another nonadjacent fracture elsewhere in the spine.[3]

INDICATION[3,4]

Whenever there is history, sign and symptoms or clinical concern of SCI, spine immobilization should be considered:
- Neurological deficit (e.g. focal deficit, tingling, reduced strength, numbness in an extremity)
- Significant traumatic mechanism and extremes of age
- Intoxication or mental impairment
- Distracting painful injury—other than spine injuries
- Spinal exam reveals point tenderness or pain to range of motion to spinal process at various levels. Any neck pain with or without movement
- Suspected cervical-spine injury: complaining of neck pain or tenderness or limitation of movement.

CONTRAINDICATION OF SPINE IMMOBILIZATION[3,4]

There are no absolute contraindications for spine immobilization in trauma patients. But there may be relative contraindications in conditions in which spine or neck immobilization can lead to: problem in airway and increase chances of aspiration, pain and cutaneous pressure ulcers and increases the intracranial pressure (ICP) and increased difficulty in patient handling, combativeness/resistance.

Spinal immobilization may not be done to the patients with rheumatoid arthritis (especially cervical spine), osteoporosis, presence of hypermobility, muscle spasm, presence of bony bloc, presence of malignancy, fresh/healing fractures, caution in application for pregnant women, hiatus hernia.

APPLIED SPINE ANATOMY

Figures 2A and B explain spinal cord anatomy with dermatome and myotome and, effects of motor and sensory injury in respect to level of spine injury. There are 33 vertebrae: seven cervical, twelve thoracic, five lumbar, five sacral (fused together) and four coccygeal (fused together) vertebrae. The spinal cord segment levels are identified by their nerve roots that may different from corresponding vertebra.

Relevance of Normal Spine Curvature

Remembering that the spinal column is an "S" shape, the lumbar spine is the bottom of the "S". Cervical spine's shape has a lordotic curve. The lordotic shape is like a backward "C". Lumbar spine is similar to the cervical section in that it

Spinal cord and level of injury

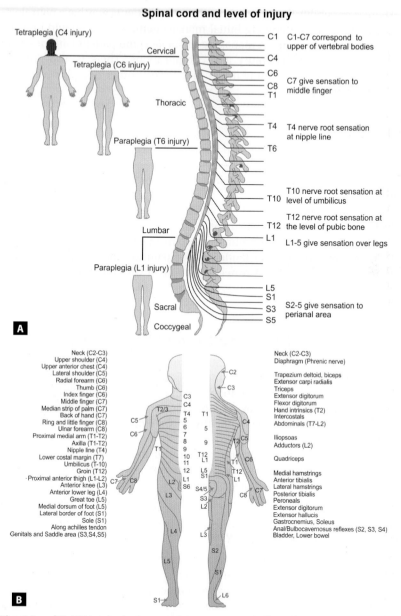

Figs 2A and B (A) Vertebral column with nerve roots and effect of level of spine injury on extent of paralysis; (B) Sensory (dermatomes) and motor (myotomes) distribution of body

has a lordotic curve (a backward "C"). This lordotic curve is due to the result of adaptation of walking and standing erect so also called secondary curvature. The thoracic and sacral spine has kyphotic (S) curve these are same as fetal so these are also primary curvature.

Applied Anatomy in Relation to Common Spine Injury (Area/Part Prone for Injury, etc.)

The level of common spine injury may be one or multiple, depends on mechanism or mode of primary injury and after effect of injury that mean patient fall or thrown and subsequent secondary injuries. But due to anatomical variations in spine one can predict the most common site, if the impact is localized. The most common site for the cervical spine injuries are at level of C4/5. The most common level of thoracic spine injury is at T11/12.

TECHNIQUE AND EQUIPMENT

A patient either having blunt or penetrating spine trauma should receive prehospital spine immobilization as a standard of care. Here, regardless of clinical sign and symptoms, whole spinal column should be immobilized. That meaning application of hard cervical collar with head stabilizer and patient body is fixed on hard backboard.[5-7] The fact that spine immobilization in field during prehospital care of either blunt or penetrating trauma had positive effect on neurological outcomes.[8] But some studies also show that it may cause harm in some selected group of patients.[9,10] The scope of this discussion is out of scope of this chapter.

Precautionary Immobilization

There are always a selected subset of patients who do not required spine immobilization while undergoing prehospital care. But it is shown that about 5 million patients who do not have significant complain or injury gets immobilized during prehospital care/year in US alone.[11,12] This kind of over precautionary practice is called precautionary immobilization.

Recent Techniques[13,14]

The American College of Surgeons course, Advance Trauma Life Support (ATLS') guidelines is widely practiced for neck and spine stabilization worldwide. But still other methods are also have been utilized that have some deviations from ATLS so that better spine immobilization can be achieved, if we had all possible resources. The following methods are being used for shifting or transferring the spine injured patient.[3,4]

- The logroll method/maneuver (Figs 3A to F)
- The straddle lift and slide method/maneuver (Fig. 4)
- The six plus lift and slide method/maneuver (Figs 5A to F)
- The scoop stretcher method/maneuver (Figs 6A and B)

In all the above methods, the person at the patient's head leads and coordinates the team.

Straddle Lift and Slide Method/Maneuver

Five persons are needed for this maneuver. Details of performing this maneuver sequence wise are shown in Figure 4. One rescuer is for providing manual in-line stabilization (MILS) of cervical spine and the second for positioning of the spine

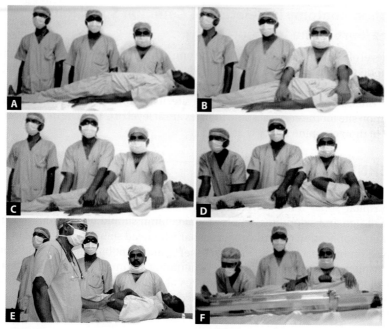

Figs 3A to F Logrolling technique in unstable spine patient, with position of person and hand position. (A) At least four persons needed for it, leader is at head end with manual in-line stabilization and cervical collar, order for movement as a unit; (B) Second person hold torso and pelvis; (C) Third person hold pelvis and another grasp the ankle; (D) Fourth person hold both legs; (E) Fifth person can flex hand and put on chest prior to logroll; (F) All four persons turn patient as a unit with precaution of no movement of the spine

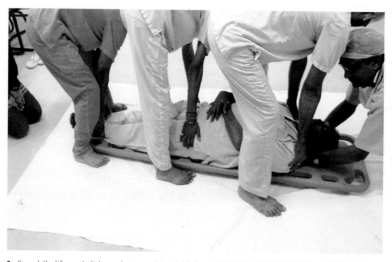

Fig. 4 *Straddle lift and slide technique:* Needed 5 persons, one remains at head end for manual in-line stabilization, 2nd–4th person come across patient torso and 5th person remains at legend

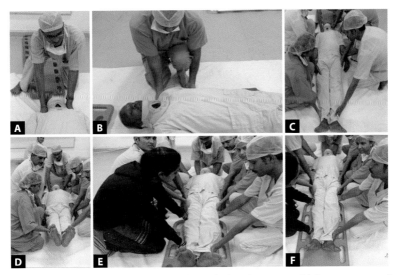

Figs 5A to F Six plus lift and slide method, needed eight person. (A) One person performs manual in-line stabilization; (B) Second person push spine board when other six lift it as unit; (C to F) Six additional rescuers are placed in pairs across from one another at the chest, pelvis, and lower extremities to perform the lift

board. The third, fourth and fifth rescuers straddle the body at the level of the chest, pelvis and lower extremities to perform the lift. The patient is lifted 10–20 cm off the ground, and then the board is slid beneath the patient, from the feet toward the head. The patient is then carefully lowered onto the board.[15]

Six Plus Lift and Slide Method/Maneuver

Eight persons are required during the six plus lift and slide maneuver. Details of performing this maneuver in sequence wise are shown in Figures 5A to F. First and second as above and six additional rescuers are placed in pairs across from one another at the chest, pelvis and lower extremities to perform the lift. Rest of sequence is same as above.[16]

Scoop Stretcher Method/Maneuver

Four persons are required for this transfer. First and second as above, third is located at shoulder level on either side of the patient and the fourth is located at the feet. The two longitudinal halves of the scoop stretcher are separated and then positioned on either side of the patient. Each half of the scoop stretcher is carefully wedged beneath the patient until both ends are securely locked into place (Figs 6A and B).[17]

Manual In-Line Stabilization of Cervical Spine

This is done with the aim to provide immediate temporary stabilization of the cervical spine. *Possible hazards and precautions while doing this maneuver are:*
- If the patient's teeth are clamped closed while performing MILS, the airway may be compromised, if the patient vomits

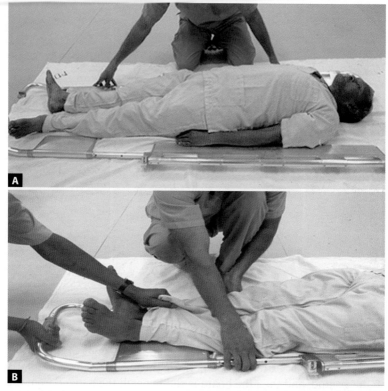

Figs 6A and B Use of Scoop stretcher. (A) Separated longitudinal halves of scoop stretcher along the patient; (B) Once both longitudinal halves of the scoop stretcher are placed beneath the patient, then foot end of scoop stretcher is locked with the remaining part

- Neck pressure increases ICP, so avoid placing hands on the patient's neck
- Do not place traction to the patient's head; it is dangerous in the prehospital setting
- The patient's head must be immobilizes to their chest to prevent neck movement. Failure to do this makes the neck becomes the pivoting point.

Spinal Board

This is patient-transfer device used in transfer of patient in prehospital, inter- and intrahospital transfer of spine injured patient. It provides rigid support to spine during transfer and board immobilization. It is also called as backboard, long spine board, longboard and long backboard (Figs 7C and 8).[18]

PREPARATION

- Equipment or things needed: Hard cervical collar, long spine board or scoop stretcher (Figs 7A and B), team of trained persons, tape, foam blocks and towels, padding, shifting stretcher, straps for binding, blocks to put onside of neck, gurney to shift the patient.

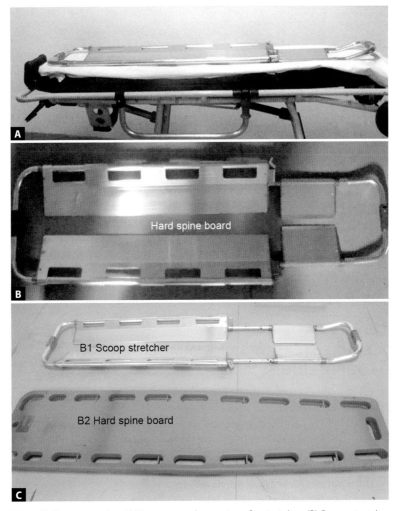

Figs 7A to C Scoop stretcher. (A) Scoop stretcher on transfer stretcher; (B) Scoop stretcher with hard spine board; (C) Scoop stretcher and hard spine board

- *Primary survey and resuscitation:* Follow the principles of ATLS (ABCDE sequence) during assessment and resuscitation of a trauma care and identify life-threatening condition by following the sequence as:
  – A is airway and cervical spine control
  – B is breathing and ventilation
  – C is circulation and hemorrhage control
  – D is to assess neurological disability and
  – E is exposures with environmental control.
- Always try to maintain patient in supine with neutral position with proper techniques of immobilization. Priority is always assessing the airway while maintaining the cervical spine.[19]

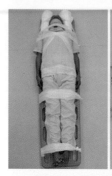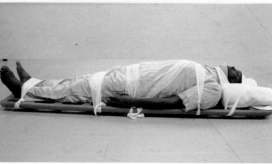

Fig. 8 Spine board stabilization

- *Secondary survey:* To do detailed evaluation from head to toe after primary survey is complete and patient is stabilized. This includes physical examination and complete neurological examination: consciousness, pupil, glasgow coma scale (GCS) score and examination of spinal cord to know level of injury (best motor examination to determine level of quadriplegia and paraplegia, sensory examination by assessing the dermatome as shown in Figure 2B and deep tendon reflexes).[20]

PROCEDURE STEPS OF SPINE IMMOBILIZATION AND LOGROLLING[19]

- There needed at least four–five persons for spine immobilization and logrolling (Figs 3A to F).
  - Team leader can be at head end or aside of all and he directs the procedure and every movement during transfer, person at head end is the most important person to do MILS.
  - Second person to stabilize the torso (pelvis and hips)
  - Third person for holding pelvis and leg
  - Fourth person to move spine board
- First place the long spine board with straps or tape to be across thorax, just above iliac crests, across thighs and just above the ankles of the patient.
- *Cervical spine immobilization/MILS:* Most essential priority is MILS of head and neck with application of semi-rigid cervical collar. This person while do immobilization will further give direction to others to move patient as a unit. Aim is to prevent segmental rotation, lateral bending or sagging of chest or abdomen, any flexion and extension during transfer. Always place padding and blocks on both side of patient head and neck and firmly secure the head and collar with strap/bandages to the board (Figs 9A to D).
- Now, straighten the patients hand with palm in next to torso and leg is straightened in neutral position.
- Logroll the patient as unit toward the two assistants (2 and 3) on the same side of patient torso.
- Second person holds patient opposite shoulder and pelvis (Fig. 3B).

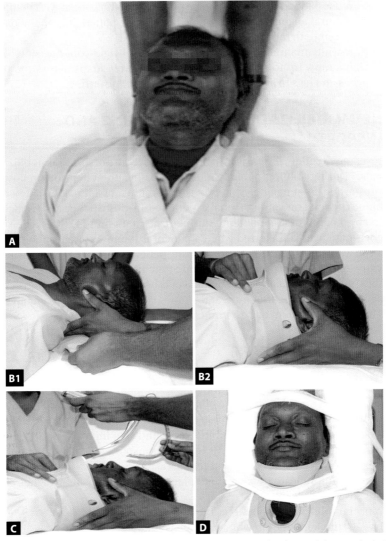

Figs 9A to D Stabilization of unstable cervical spine. (A) Manual in-line stabilization by holding neck and cervical spine; (B1 and B2) Semi-rigid cervical collar in place with manual in-line stabilization and cricoid pressure; (C) Intubation in unstable cervical spine, One person giving manual in-line stabilization with semi-rigid cervical collar, second person is giving cricoid pressure and third person doing oral intubation with all precaution to avoid any possible neck movement; (D) Method of neck stabilization on spine board, by putting roll of cloth on both side of neck to prevent side to side neck movement with double step fixation on spine board

- Third person reaches across and grasp the hip just distal to wrist with one hand and with another hand firmly grasps the ankles together (Fig. 3C).
- The fourth person is responsible for moving the legs together with the upper two people while logrolling as unit (Fig. 3D).

- Now use padded spine board to be put beneath the patient with maintaining neutral alignment of the whole body of the patient logroll the patient in one smooth movement onto the spine board.
- Now while maintaining MILS even after semi-rigid collar or side blocks with straps, try to put and tighten all the given straps across the torso, pelvis and legs to avoid any movement while transferring.

SPINE IMMOBILIZATION DURING IMAGING AND TRANSPORT[21]

Whatever the situation, the basic principle and procedure of spine immobilization are same. During shifting patient from another health system or prehospital, or transporting for imaging, you can choose either of four above described techniques depend on your personal experience, institute policy and availability of persons. Logroll preferably done during resuscitation in ED/ICU. The scoop stretcher maneuver is preferred when a patient is found on prehospital settings when you want little movement during taking patient on stretcher with advantage you can separate the two arms of scoop stretcher. The straddle lift and slide methods and six plus lift and slide maneuver is best for intrahospital transfer and during imaging because literature and studies shows that these two maneuvers leads minimal movement or best immobilization as a unit.[15-17]

POST-PROCEDURE CARE

Always manage the life-threatening injuries first (threat to ABC of life, as given sequence and preference) with minimal movement of the spine. SCIs can be complete, incomplete and it may at any level of spinal column. As soon as resuscitation and survey get completed, one should always try to remove the spine board to avoid possible decubitus ulcer and skin injury in trauma victim. When any patient with unstable spine injury is transported, patient's condition is sufficiently stabilized by following basic rules as:[20]

- Always communicate in advance to place of transfer/hospital/higher center with advance directives
- Spine immobilization should be adequate and secured
- Oxygen supplementation with adequate ventilation
- Secure two large bore intravenous lines and keep it patent
- Airway is patent and anticipatory secure the airway prior to transfer, if needed
- Intercostal drainage of chest tube should be done for suspected of any pneumothorax or hemothorax
- Patient should have multipara monitor for hemodynamic monitoring with battery backup
- When needed nasogastric tube and indwelling urinary catheter is in situ and draining freely
- Skin should be protected from injury due to excessive pressure with proper padding and care
- All the imaging and other treatment records, investigations must accompany the patient

- Always quote in patient records hemodynamic parameter and, clinical and neurological examination as per International Standards Neurological Classification of SCI, prior to transferring the patient.

How to Remove Spine Board[19,20]

In any patient with unstable spine injury, spine protection should be maintained until proven otherwise. For spine injury to be ruled out clinically and radiologically (X-ray of cervical spine AP, lateral and odontoid views and pelvis), X-rays are done on spine board to prevent movements during it. We should consider to remove the long spine board as early as possible, to prevent its complications. Best possible time to remove board while logrolling to examine the back. Patient should be shifted from long spine board to firm, well-padded gurney as soon as possible safely with following all possible guidelines to maintain anatomic alignment of spine by avoiding any movement. While doing this, we should follow modified logroll technique described above with four persons in reversed to remove the patient from spine board (Figs 10A and B). One can use scoop stretcher with firm support under it to safely transfer patient from spine board to gurney. After transfer, the scoop stretcher should be removed and now immobile the patient on gurney also until proven otherwise the stability of spine.[21] It had been proven that lift and slide technique provides least movement as compared to other methods and maneuvers for removal of spine board in a patient with a spine injury.

Maintain and establish proper immobilization of patient's spine until vertebral column and SCIs had been ruled out clinically and radiologically. Obtain early neurosurgeon and/or orthopedician consultation in suspected and detected cases at definitive care center.[21] Untrained or less trained personal can aggravate cervical or whole spine injury while logrolling or transferring the patient. Documentation of neurologic status before and after the procedure and frequently thereafter is advisable.[22]

COMPLICATION/PROBLEM

Patient remained prolong unattained on spine board while resuscitation or transfer for more than 2 hours or on unpadded board may have pressure sores on occiput, scapulae, sacrum and heals areas. So, always remember to remove the spine board after initial resuscitation and stabilization or as soon as possible.[22,23]

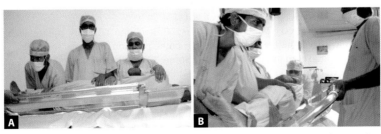

Figs 10A and B Logrolling of patient with spine board application and removal.
(A) Four persons logrolling and application of spine board; (B) Removal of spine board

ACKNOWLEDGMENT

Mr Anil Kumar, chief artist, SGPGIMS for helping in Figures 2, 3 and all the anesthesia technicians of department of anesthesiology, SGPGIMS for supporting in descriptions of procedures as shown in figures.

REFERENCES

1. Tator CH, Hashimoto R, Raich A, Norvell D, Fehlings MG, Harrop JS, et al. Translational potential of preclinical trials of neuroprotection through pharmacotherapy for spinal cord injury. J Neurosurg Spine. 2012;17(1 Suppl):157-229.
2. Conrad BP, Rossi GD, Horodyski MB, Prasarn ML, Alemi Y, Rechtine GR. Eliminating log rolling as a spine trauma order. Surg Neurol Int. 2012;3:188-97.
3. Ahn H, Singh J, Nathens A, MacDonald RD, Travers A, Tallon J, et al. Pre-hospital care management of a potential spinal cord injured patient: a systematic review of the literature and evidence-based guidelines. J Neurotrauma. 2011;28(8):1341-61.
4. Clinical Practice Guidelines for cervical spine assessment of the Royal Children's Hospital Melbourne. [Online] Available from www.rch.org.au [Accessed on 1 March, 2015].
5. Hauswald M, Ong G, Tandberg D, Omar Z. Out-of-hospital spinal immobilization: its effect on neurologic injury. Acad Emerg Med. 1998;5(3):214-9.
6. Baez AA, Schiebel N. Evidence-based emergency medicine/systematic review abstract. Is routine spinal immobilization an effective intervention for trauma patients? Ann Emerg Med. 2006;47(1):110-2.
7. Kwan I, Bunn F. Effects of prehospital spinal immobilization: a systematic review of randomized trials on healthy subjects. Prehosp Disaster Med. 2005;20(1):47-53.
8. Haut ER, Kalish BT, Efron DT, Haider AH, Stevens KA, Kieninger AN, et al. Spine immobilization in penetrating trauma: more harm than good? J Trauma. 2010;68(1):115-20.
9. Brown JB, Bankey PE, Sangosanya AT, Cheng JD, Stassen NA, Gestring ML, et al. Prehospital spinal immobilization does not appear to be beneficial and may complicate care following gunshot injury to the torso. J Trauma. 2009;67(4):774-8.
10. Smith JP, Bodai BI, Hill AS, Fry CF. Prehospital stabilization of critically injured patients: a failed concept. J Trauma. 1985;25(1):65-70.
11. Kwan I, Bunn F, Roberts I. Spinal immobilisation for trauma patients. Cochrane Database Syst Rev. 2001;(2):CD002803.
12. McHugh TP, Taylor JP. Unnecessary out-of-hospital use of full spinal immobilization. Acad Emerg Med. 1998;5(3):278-80.
13. A photographic guide to prehospital spinal care. Emergency Technologies, 5th edition. 2004. Retrieved from www.emergencytechnologies.com.au/psm.htm (Assessed October 2014).
14. Guideline on moving and handling patients with acute or suspected spinal cord injury (SCI), by the Spinal Cord Injury Centres of the United Kingdom and Ireland. Initiated by Multidisciplinary Association of Spinal Cord Injury Professionals: pp. 1-26. available at www.mascip.co.uk (Assessed March 2015).
15. Conrad BP, Horodyski M, Wright J, Ruetz P, Rechtine GR. Log-rolling technique producing unacceptable motion during body position changes in patients with traumatic spinal cord injury. J Neurosurg Spine. 2007;6(6):540-3.
16. Del Rossi G, Horodyski MB, Conrad BP, Di Paola CP, Di Paola MJ, Rechtine GR. The 6-plus-person lift transfer technique compared with other methods of spine boarding. J Athl Train. 2008;43(1):6-13.
17. Del Rossi G, Rechtine GR, Conrad BP, Horodyski M. Are scoop stretchers suitable for use on spine-injured patients? Am J Emerg Med. 2010;28(7):751-6.

18. Vickery D. The use of the spinal board after the pre-hospital phase of trauma management. Emerg Med J. 2001;18(1):51-4.
19. American College of Surgeons. Advanced trauma life support course for physicians. Committee on Trauma. 9th edition. Chicago: American College of Surgeons. 2012.
20. Wing PC. Early acute management in adults with spinal cord injury: a clinical practice guideline for health-care professionals. J Spinal Cord Med. 2008;31(4):360.
21. Schmidt OI, Gahr RH, Gosse A, Heyde CE. ATLS (R) and damage control in spine trauma. World J Emerg Surg. 2009;4:9.
22. Theodore N, Aarabi B, Dhall SS, Gelb DE, Hurlbert RJ, Rozzelle CJ, et al. Transportation of patients with acute traumatic cervical spine injuries. Neurosurgery. 2013;72(Supp 2): 35-9.
23. Muzin S, Isaac Z, Walker J, Abd OE, Baima J. When should a cervical collar be used to treat neck pain? Curr Rev Musculoskelet Med. 2008;1(2):114-9.

40
Nasogastric Tube Placement

Bhuwan Chand Panday

INTRODUCTION

Nasogastric tube (NGT) placement is one of the most commonly performed procedures in a clinical setting for providing enteral nutrition. The tube is placed from one of the nostrils to the stomach for diagnostic or therapeutic purpose. Provision of nutrition through enteral and parenteral route in critically ill patients has been practiced for many centuries (3500 BC).[1,2] This therapy has been described in an ancient Indian, Chinese and Egyptian way of medical treatment.[1] Capivacceus placed the first tube for enteral nutrition in 16th century. Most of the progress in the development of NGT had been done during 17th–19th century.[1]

INDICATION

- *Diagnostic*
  - Evaluation of radiographic material for computed tomography based diagnosis
  - Assessment of gastric pH
  - Gastric bleeding
  - Gastric lavage
- *Therapeutic*
  - Enteral feeding
  - Administration of medicine
- *Preventive measures:* To avoid
  - Nausea, vomiting
  - Gastric distension.

CONTRAINDICATION

- *Absolute*
  - Severe facial trauma
  - Recent nasal surgery
  - Suspected basal skull fracture
- *Relative*
  - Anticoagulant/coagulopathy
  - Esophageal varices
  - Post-bariatric surgery

- Esophageal stricture
- Recent esophageal surgery
- Nasopharyngeal tumor.

APPLIED ANATOMY

The NGT is placed through the nostril to the stomach (Fig. 1). There are two nostrils separated by columella cartilage. Superior boundary of nasal cavity is bounded by sinuses, laterally with the Eustachian tubes, anteroinferiorly with hard palate and posteroinferiorly with soft palate. This passage extends to the oropharynx which is further extended to the upper esophageal sphincter, opening into the long and tubular conduit of esophagus. This tubular passage, i.e. esophagus ends at the lower esophageal sphincter which opens into the stomach. The entire passage from nose to stomach is lined with mucosa. Nasopharynx is unique as it has enlarged or constricted mucosal surface which may lead to unwanted results during NGT placement.

TECHNIQUE AND EQUIPMENT

Nasogastric tube is a flexible medical device with atraumatic blind end and few lateral eyes to decompress the stomach and provide nutrition and medication to the critically ill patients. It is made up of plastic tubing with lumen inside and has a radiopaque lining throughout the length. There are markings at fixed distances on the outer surface of the tube (from blunt tip end) to measure inserted length of the tube. These tubes are made up of different materials, e.g. polyvinyl chloride (PVC), polyurethane or silicone and available in different sizes. Polyurethane tube stays longer than the PVC tube.[3] The distal opening is modified for drain tube and syringe connection (Figs 2A to D).

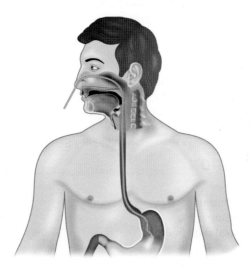

Fig. 1 Route of the nasogastric tube

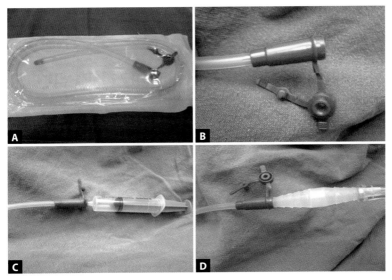

Figs 2A to D (A) Commonly available nasogastric tube; (B) Modified opening of the tube; (C) Modified opening connected to syringe; (D) Modified opening connected to suction tube

Selection of Tube

Selection of the tube plays an important role and is based on its indication (e.g. short/long duration, decompression/nutrition therapy). Numerous types of NGT are available. Medical practitioner can decide about the type, diameter and material, according to the patient requirements (Table 1).

- *Large diameter tube:* It has an advantage of easier aspiration and irrigation with less chance of blockage. However, large size may result in discomfort and irritation. Salem-sump™ is a large diameter double-lumen tube where one lumen is used for aspiration and irrigation and the other lumen is kept open to room air (it equalizes the pressure inside the stomach and atmosphere, when there is no gastric content).
- *Small diameter tube:* Advantages of using fine bore feeding tube are better comfort, less interference with eating and drinking, decreased risk of reflux, early return of swallowing mechanism. The disadvantage, being high chances of obstruction; therefore regular irrigation is mandatory. Soft, flexible, light and small feeding tubes are preferred for administration of nutrition or giving medication.
- *Assessment of adequate NGT length:* Length of the tube is important as neither long nor short length will serve the purpose; rather it may harm the patient. There are many methods to assess the appropriate length of the tube, e.g. nose tip-ear-umbilicus, nose tip-umbilicus and sternal notch to xiphisternum and body length. Most commonly used method is from the tip of the nose to ear tip and then to the xiphisternum (Fig. 3).[2]

Table 1 Different types of tubes[2]

Tube type	Size (Fr)	Length (cm)	Lumen	Function	Material	Comments
Salem-sump tube	6–18	60–122	Double	Gastric decompression Medication delivery Enteral feeding	PVC	Second lumen vents to atmosphere, it prevents suctioning of tube to gastric mucosa. Radiopaque line along its whole length
Levin tube	8–20	122	Single	Gastric decompression Medication delivery Enteral feeding	PVC	Markings at 45, 55, 65 and 75 cm. Radiopaque line along its entire length
Ryle's tube	8–20	105	Single	Gastric aspiration Enteral feeding	PVC	Markings at 50, 60 and 70 cm. Radiopaque line along its full length. Weighted end
Enteral feeding tubes (e.g. Abbot nutrition enteral feeding tube; Cook endoscopy NJFT; Corpak® medical systems CORFLO® tubes; Covidien tubes; teleflex medical tubes)	3.5–12	31–240	Single to triple	Enteral feeding	Polyurethane, silicone and PVC	*Various features may present in the tubes:* Stylet used for less than 12 Fr tubes to stiffen the tube for easy insertion and confirm placement radiographically. Radiopaque markers in every cm length. Weighted tip to allow propulsion into duodenum by peristalsis. Magnets to facilitate jejunal placement. Suture loops to allow endoscopic placement.

Abbreviations: NJFT, nasojejunal feeding tubes; PVC, polyvinyl chloride.

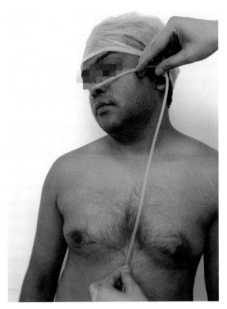

Fig. 3 Measurements for insertion of appropriate length of nasogastric tube

PREPARATION

- Explain the patient about the whole procedure in detail to alleviate anxiety, and to make the patient cooperative and comfortable
- Written informed consent (as per the hospital policy)
- *Adjunct equipment required:* Lubricant jelly, topical local anesthesia, sterile gloves, eye protector, laryngoscope, Magill forceps, syringes, sterile water/saline with bowel, sticking tape
- Suitable size NGT.

PROCEDURE

Selection of Nostril

- Most patent nostril (left/right)—instruct the patient to expire and inspire forcefully through one nostril keeping the other nostril blocked
- Pre-treatment with oxymetazoline or phenylephrine decreases the risk of epistaxis[4]
- Local anesthesia spray/nebulization 5 minutes before procedure will increases the patient comfort.[5]

Awake Patient

- Keep the patient in sitting position with neck gently flexed to align the esophagus and ease the tube insertion
- Prefer to choose lesser diameter NGT to make it less irritating, decreasing risk of reflux and early return of swallowing mechanism[6]

- Insert the tube gently through the selected nostril. As the tube reaches the nasopharynx, the patient might have "gag reflex". He is then advised to swallow the tube
- In case of respiratory distress, coughing or choking withdraw the tube as it is a sign of tracheal irritation. Try again. If the measured length is reached smoothly, the tube has reached the esophagus and then stomach.

Unconscious/Anesthetized/Intubated Patient

- These patients are in supine position but the head-neck position remains the same as that of the awake patient.
- Clean the nostril, if there is debris or mucus plug.
- Apply adequate lubricant.
- The blind end of NGT is passed through one of the nostril and generally reaches the oropharynx uneventfully. Occassionally, resistance may be felt at nasopharynx; at this point do not use any force; withdraw the tube and manipulate it again gently. If still not able to pass the tube, try the other nostril. Once into oropharynx, it can either proceed smoothly through the esophagus to reach the stomach or it can go to trachea. Confirm the tube position (laryngoscopy, end-tidal carbon-dioxide) and then proceed.
    - The most common site of obstruction while insertion is arytenoids.
- Nasogastric tube insertion in unconscious patients is preferably instrument (laryngoscopy, fiberscope, fiberoptic bronchoscopy) guided. There are many techniques described to facilitate the smooth and uneventful insertion of NGT. *These are as follows:*
    - Neck flexion, lateral neck pressure[7]
    - Oral cavity finger manipulation of NGT
    - Ureteric catheter guidewire to guide the NGT[8]
    - Neck flexion and angiography catheter guided cricoids manipulation[9]
    - Rush intubating stylet guided[10]
    - Reverse Sellick's maneuver[11]
    - Glidescope assisted NGT placement.[12]

Confirmation of NGT[13]

There are several methods to confirm the appropriate position of NGT:
- Testing the pH of aspirated liquid—pH of less than 5.5 is confirmatory
- Radiographic imaging—confirming the NGT tip below the left diaphragm
- Aspiration of bile from the tube, but appearance will not confirm the gastric or intestinal placement (Gastric aspirate will show pH <5.0 and bilirubin <5 mg/dL)[13]
- "Whoosh test", auscultation of bubbling sound just below xiphisternum while blowing air into the tube
- Confirmation of the NGT with the magnet tracking device is also a new noninvasive technique to diagnose the correct placement[14]
- Capnography and colorimetric capnometry can also be used to confirm the tube.[13]

Best way to confirm NGT in stomach is with pH (1–5.5) followed by radiographic images.[13,15] Differentiation between the gastric and the intestinal placement of the tube can be done with pH (<5.0) and bilirubin (<5 mg/dL) check.[13]

POST-PROCEDURE CARE

Fixation of Tube

Nasogastric tube placement and confirmation is followed by its fixation. It should be properly fixed with the nose. Fixation with nares may lead to ulceration and necrosis.[16] Various tapes are available to fix the tube (pink tape, butterfly, etc.); securing tube with pink tape has an advantage over others.[17] Suturing may be required for tube fixation in few patients with major gastrosurgical procedure. Nasal bridle can be used as an alternative for suturing. Nasal septal loop is also used in noncooperative patients for short duration.[18] Though different studies have been done for various fixation tools, type of tape and bridle but there is no technique or tool which has proven its efficacy over the other.[18] None has proven its efficacy over the other.[19]

Documentation

Documentation should include time and date of insertion, reason of placement of tube, type and size of tube, length of tube, nostril (right/left), attempts required, aid used to facilitate the smooth insertion, method of confirmation, complications (if any).

Tube Care

- *Maintain patency of the lumen:* Nasogastric and nasoenteric tubes should be routinely checked and flushed 4–8 hourly.[2] It should always be irrigated with saline before and after feeding to avoid blocking.[2]
- *Rechecking of tube position:* Confirm the position before every feed/after shifting or mobilization of patient/patient complaining of discomfort.
- *Routine change of tube:* Follow the manufacturing company instructions.
- *Tube removal:* Gently remove the tape, pinch the tube (to avoid any spill over of the fluid present inside the tubing) and then ask the patient to take deep expiration and removal to be done during expiration.

COMPLICATION/PROBLEM

Error in Diagnosis of Correct Placement[20]

- Untrained personnel
- Wrong interpretation of chest radiograph
- Change in pH due to drugs (H_2 blocker, proton pump inhibitor—increases pH, mixture of lubricating gel and water—decrease in pH)[21]
- Doubtful position, not double checked.

Procedure Related

- *Hemodynamics changes during NGT placement:* NGT placement with the direct laryngoscopy may lead to changes in heart rate, blood pressure and dysrhythmias which come to baseline within a few minutes.[22]

- *Innumerous complications are described in the literature. They are as follows:* Throat (mild irritation, trauma, bleeding); esophageal injury; intrathoracic[23] placement of NGT; intracranial placement[24,25] in head injury/major facial injury.
- Feeding in an unconfirmed tube may lead to tracheobronchial aspiration which increases morbidity and mortality of the patient.[26]
- Rate of accidental removal of NGT is high in critical care, but it can be decreased significantly by educating medical personnel.[27]
- Medicine (pills) and thick feeding may obstruct the tube, instilling the saline without much force may open the tube but if it could not be opened, no need to apply too much pressure, it should be removed and a new tube should be placed.
- In patient with suspected tube migration, confirm the tube position and then feed.
- Tube kept for long duration needs special care as it can lead to nasal ala ulcer, pharyngitis, sinusitis, etc.
- Broken tube can be either removed with the help of forceps, if it is present in the throat; or with the endoscopy guided, in case it is present in the esophagus/gastric lumen.

REFERENCES

1. Vassilyadi F, Panteliadou AK, Panteliadis C. Hallmarks in the history of enteral and parenteral nutrition: from antiquity to the 20th Century. Nutr Clin Pract. 2013;28(2): 209-17.
2. Holdin RA, Bordeianou L. Nasogastric and nasoenteric tubes.Uptodate 2013. (http://www.uptodate.com/contents/nasogastric-and-nasoenteric-tubes).
3. Silk DB, Rees RG, Keohane PP, Attrill H. Clinical efficacy and design changes of "fine bore" nasogastric feeding tubes: a seven-year experience involving 809 intubations in 403 patients. J Parenter and Enteral Nutr. 1987;11(4):378-83.
4. Thomsen TW, Shaffer RW, Setnik GS. Videos in clinical medicine: Nasogastric intubation. N Engl J Med. 2006;354(17):e16.
5. Cullen L, Taylor D, Taylor S, Chu K. Nebulized lidocaine decreases the discomfort of nasogastric tube insertion: a randomized, double-blind trial. Ann Emerg Med. 2004;44(2):131-7.
6. East Cheshire NHS Trust CNSG 007 Guidelines for Insertion and Management of Nasogastric Tubes Created by Maggie Allen. October 2010. Updated August 2012.
7. Mahajan R, Gupta R. Another method to assist nasogastric tube insertion. Can J Anesth. 2005;52:652-3.
8. Appukutty J, Shroff PP. Nasogastric tube insertion using different techniques in anesthetized patients: a prospective, randomized study. Anesth Analg. 2009;109:832-5.
9. Ghatak T, Samanta S, Baronia AK. A new technique to insert Nasogastric tube in an unconscious intubated patient. N Am J Med Sci. 2013;5(1):68-70.
10. Tsai YF, Luo CF, Illias A, Lin CC, Yu HP. Nasogastric tube insertion in anesthetized and intubated patients: a new and reliable method. BMC Gastroenterol. 2012;12:99.
11. Parris WC. Reverse sellick maneuver (letter). Anesth Analg. 1989;68(3):423.
12. Moharari RS, Fallah AH, Khajavi MR, Khashayar P, Lakeh MM, Najafi A. The GlideScope facilitates nasogastric tube insertion: a randomized clinical trial. Anesth Analg. 2010;110(1):115-8.
13. Methods for determining the correct nasogastric tube placement after insertion in adults. Best Practice: evidence-based information sheets for health professionals. 2010;14(1):1-4.

14. Bercik P, Schlageter V, Mauro M, Rawlinson J, Kucera P, Armstrong D. Non-invasive verification of nasogastric tube placement using a magnet-tracking system. JPEN J Parenter Enteral Nutr. 2005;29(4):305-10.

15. NHS Direct. 2011. Reducing the harm caused by misplaced nasogastric feeding tubes in adults, children and infants. [Online] Available from http://www.nrls.npsa.nhs.uk/resources/type/alerts/?entryid45=129640 [Accessed March, 2012].

16. Banerjee TS, Schneider HJ. Recommended method of attachment of nasogastric tubes. Ann R Coll Surg Engl. 2007;89(5):529-30.

17. Burns SM, Martin M, Robbins V, Friday T, Coffindaffer M, Burns SC, et al. Comparison of nasogastric tube securing methods and tube types in medical intensive care patients. Am J Crit Care. 1995;4(3):198-203.

18. Della Faille D, Schmelzer B, Hartoko T, Vandenbroucke M, Brands C, De Deyn PP. Securing nasogastric tubes in non-cooperative patients. Acta Otorhinolaryngol Belg. 1996;50(1):195-7.

19. Brugnolli A, Ambrosi E, Canzan F, Saiani L, Naso-gastric Tube Group. Securing of naso-gastric tubes in adult patients: a review. Int J Nurs Stud. 2014;51(6):943-50. http://www.journalofnursingstudies.com/article/S0020-7489(13)00370-2/abstract

20. Nasogastric tube errors. United Kingdom casebook. 2012;20(3):10-2. (http://www.medicalprotection.org/uk/casebook/casebook-september-2012/nasogastric-tubeerrors).

21. NPSA, Harm from Flushing of Nasogastric Tubes Before Confirmation of Placement. [Online] Available from www.nrls.npsa.nhs.uk/resources/type/alerts/?entryid45=133441. [Accessed March, 2012].

22. Fassolaki A, Athanassiou E. Cardiovascular responses to the insertion of nasogastric tube during general anaesthesia. Can Anesth Soc J. 1985;32(6):651-3.

23. Jain BP, Vegasb A, Bristera S. Thoracic complications of nasogastric tube: review of safe practice. Interact Cardiovasc and Thorac Surg. 2005;4:429-33.

24. Ferreras J, Junquera LM, García-Consuegra L. Intracranial placement of a nasogastric tube after severe craniofacial trauma. Oral Surg Oral Med Oral Pathol Oral Radiol Endod. 2000;90(5):564-6.

25. Başkaya MK. Inadvertent intracranial placement of a nasogastric tube in patients with head injuries. Surg Neurol. 1999;52(4):426-7.

26. Lemyze M. Tracheobronchial aspiration is a potentially life-threatening complication of enteral feeding. CMAJ. 2010;182(8):802.

27. Carrión MI, Ayuso D, Marcos M, Paz Robles M, de la Cal MA, Alía I, et al. Accidental removal of endotracheal and nasogastric tubes and intravascular catheters. Crit Care Med. 2000;28(1):63-6.

41
Nasojejunal Tube Placement

Zafar Neyaz, Praveer Rai, Hira Lal

INTRODUCTION

Nasojejunal tube (NJT) placement is defined as insertion of a long tube through the nostril into the proximal jejunum.[1] The NJT provides a safe access to the gastrointestinal tract for administration of fluids, nutrients and drugs. In critically ill patients, there is slow gastric emptying, while small bowel motility is usually preserved. Therefore, placing a NJT beyond the ligament of Treitz has been shown to reduce gastroesophageal reflux which resulting in lesser incidence of pulmonary aspiration.

INDICATION

- Patients at high risk of aspiration
- Delayed gastric emptying
- Acute pancreatitis
- Chemotherapy-induced nausea
- Hyperemesis gravidarum
- Postoperative paralytic ileus
- Obstructive lesions high in the gastrointestinal tract
- Partial gastric outlet obstruction
- Gastric or duodenal fistula
- As part of barium, computed tomography (CT) or magnetic resonance (MR) enteroclysis.

CONTRAINDICATION

There is no absolute contraindication; the relative contraindications are as following:
- Skull fractures
- Maxillofacial disorders or surgery
- Laryngectomy
- Oropharyngeal tumors or oropharyngeal surgery
- Deranged coagulation profile
- Unstable cervical spinal injuries.

APPLIED ANATOMY

Both nostrils communicate with the respective nasal cavities. Nasal cavities have turbinates and opening of paranasal sinuses laterally, and medially the nasal septum. Roof of nasal cavity is formed by the skull base. Posteriorly, both nasal cavities open into nasopharynx, which opens inferiorly into the oropharynx (Fig. 1). Anteriorly, the oropharynx communicates with the oral cavity. Oropharynx opens inferiorly into the hypopharynx. Anteriorly, the hypopharynx communicates with the laryngeal opening. Opening of the larynx is covered by epiglottis during swallowing. Hypopharynx opens into the esophagus at the level of C5/6 vertebra. Esophagus courses behind the trachea and enters the thoracic cavity. Inside the thorax, esophagus lies anterior to vertebral bodies and inferiorly it joins the stomach at the gastroesophageal junction. Stomach is divided into fundus, body and antropyloric region. Through the pyloric canal, it opens into the duodenal cap (first part of duodenum). The second part of duodenum courses posteriorly and inferiorly, and lies along side of vertebra. The third part of duodenum horizontally crosses the midline toward the left side. Then a short fourth part of duodenum joins jejunum at duodenojejunal flexure.

TECHNIQUE AND EQUIPMENT

Postpyloric enteral feeding has a long history and was first described in 1858.[2] Methods used for NJT placement include blind bedside placement, endoscopic and fluoroscopic placement. Recently an electromagnetic sensing device has been developed for guiding the bedside placement of NJT (Cortrak System, CORPAK MedSystems, Buffalo Grove, USA).[3]

Bedside procedures have success rates ranging from 15% to 95%, and the procedure is usually difficult and requires a skilled operator. In contrast, endoscopic and fluoroscopic-guided NJT placements have success rates more than 90%, and both can be safely and accurately performed in seriously ill patients.[4] Both the fluoroscopic or endoscopic methods are used commonly. Sometimes, the endoscopic technique is combined with the fluoroscopy as well.

Equipment

- Various types of NJT have been developed depending on the indication (feeding or decompression) and mode of placement.[5]
  - *Freka Endolumina (Fresenius Kabi, Germany):* It is an 8 Fr tube and it is placed through the biopsy channel of the endoscope.

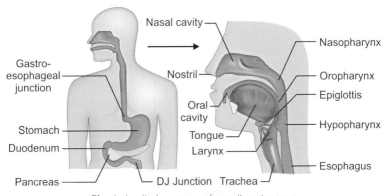

Fig. 1 Applied anatomy of aerodigestive tract

- *CORFLO (CORPAK MedSystems, Buffalo Grove, IL, USA):* It is a 10–12 Fr tube, placed over a guidewire and it does not go through the biopsy channel of endoscope (Fig. 2A). It can be used with CORTRAK enteral access system.
- *Flocare Bengmark nasointestinal tube (Nutricia, Netherlands):* It is inserted nonendoscopically using normal peristalsis.
- *Jejunal feeding tube (Devon Innovation Pvt. Ltd., Bengaluru, India):* It is a non-end-hole NJT and it is usually inserted under fluoroscopic guidance or with the help of endoscopic snare. This tube is 150 cm long, made up of PVC plastic and has 5–6 side-holes near the tip. At the tip, two metallic pellets are embedded in the tube for easy visibility on radiographs (Fig. 2B). A plastic-coated metallic stiffener is used to provide strength for pushing the tube and for manipulations. Generally, 10–14 Fr tubes are used. For feeding smaller gauge tubes are generally sufficient.

PREPARATION

- The patient should give an informed, written consent.
- The procedure is explained to patient.
- Patient should be fasting for 4–6 hours prior to procedure.
- The patient should have patent intravenous 18–20 G cannula.
- *Emergency equipment:* Including oxygen, suction and resuscitation trolley along with availability of adequate skilled staff.
- If endoscopic placement is to be done, the patient should be prepared as for an upper gastrointestinal endoscopy.
- The patient's vitals should be monitored throughout the procedure including pulse oximetry.
- *Following things are generally required for NJT placement:* NJT tube of appropriate size, stiffener (for non-end-hole NJT), guidewire (if Seldinger technique to be used), sterile tray, pad/gauze pieces, sterile gloves, sterile water, tape or other securing device, water-soluble anesthetic jelly, sterile syringes and needles, connector (to connect NJT with syringe), contrast medium, clean endoscope/fluoroscopy unit or both.

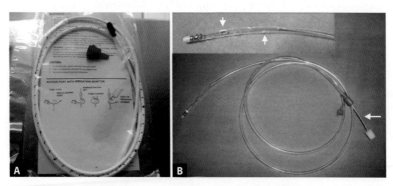

Figs 2A and B (A) CORFLO (CORPAK MedSystems) 12 Fr nasojejunal tube. (B) Jejunal feeding tube (Devon Innovation) with stiffener inside (arrow). Magnified image of tip of NJT showing metallic pellet embedded in tip. Side-holes are located in the proximal part of tube (arrowheads)

PROCEDURE

Fluoroscopic Technique

- Fluoroscopic technique described below is for a non-end-hole tube.[6] Assist patient to sit in a supported upright position. If unconscious, patient is positioned lying on his side. To estimate the length of tube required for reaching stomach, the distance on the tube from the patient's ear lobe to the tip of the nose to the xiphisternum is measured.
- Lumen of NJT is prelubricated for easy manipulation of stiffener (usually with oil recommended by manufacturer). The tube is introduced with stiffener inside (5–10 cm away from tip to keep the tip of NJT flexible). The stiffener tip should never come out of the side holes.
- Patency of nasal passage is checked. Anesthetic gel (preferably 2% xylocaine) is applied inside the patient's nostril and on tip of the NJT.
- The tube is introduced into the nostril and directed posteriorly and inferiorly (Fig. 3A). If there is any difficulty, the patient's head should be extended until the tip of catheter reaches the oropharynx.
- The NJT is then advanced further and swallowed by the patient. Flexing the patient's neck prevents the tip of NJT going into trachea (Fig. 3B). The NJT is then advanced through esophagus into the stomach (Fig. 3C). If the patient starts coughing or NJT comes in oral cavity, withdraw the NJT into the nasopharynx and then reattempt passage. Brief fluoroscopy can be done for negotiating the NJT across the epiglottic region.
- After this, the patient is placed supine on the fluoroscopy table and position of the NJT is checked. The flexible tip of NJT is advanced toward the pylorus and is gently pushed through the pyloric sphincter into the duodenum. The operator rotates the tip of tube toward pylorus by applying torque on the tube near the patient's nostril (Figs 4A to C).
- Across the pylorus the NJT is pushed slowly while the stiffener is withdrawn gradually so that stiffener remains proximal to pyloric sphincter (Figs 5A to C). Pulling out the stiffener may be difficult after it extends into duodenum. The NJT is advanced through the duodenum until its tip is positioned beyond the duodenojejunal flexure.
- Sometimes, on frontal view it is difficult to ascertain whether tube is going into duodenum or coiling back into the stomach. Lateral fluoroscopy may

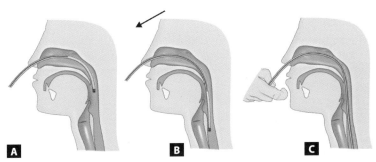

Figs 3A to C Technique of NJT placement in upper aerodigestive tract. (A) NJT insertion through nasal cavity till oropharynx; (B) Flexion of neck (arrow) during advancing tube across epiglottic region; (C) Advancing tube into the esophagus

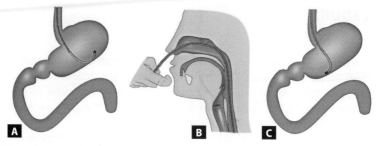

Figs 4A to C Technique of rotating the tip of NJT toward pylorus by applying torque (axial rotation) near nostril

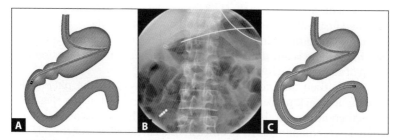

Figs 5A to C Technique of advancing NJT into duodenum across pyloric canal

be helpful in knowing the progress of NJT into duodenum, as it is located posterior to antrum and overlaps the vertebral bodies (Figs 6A to D).

- Sometimes, there may be problem in advancing the NJT through the stomach. NJT may pass up to the greater curve and coil in fundus rather than going toward the pylorus (Fig. 7A). Various maneuvers have been described to direct NJT toward the pylorus.
- Simply applying torque near nostril and gentle pushing may direct the tip toward pylorus (Fig. 7B).
- Double back maneuver may also be used in such cases (Figs 8A to C). In this, the NJT is pushed further till it forms an extra loop with apex directed toward pylorus. The stiffener or guidewire is now advanced as far as the apex of curve. The stiffener or guidewire is now slowly advanced while the NJT is slowly withdrawn, maintaining the stiff end of tube pointed toward pylorus. This technique usually brings the tip of tube from fundus to the antrum region.
- In another maneuver, the NJT is pulled out leaving only small part in stomach, and then patient is put in right decubitus position and tube is readvanced. In right decubitus position, the tip of NJT tends to move toward pylorus due to effect of gravity.
- If NJT coils in antrum and fails to pass into duodenum (Fig. 9A), the NJT is withdrawn a little and stiffener is advanced to uncoil it. While keeping the tip toward pylorus the patient is positioned on their left side to allow air to collect into antrum and duodenal bulb. Small amount of air may be injected at this stage to outline duodenal bulb. Now NJT is advanced slowly toward duodenum.
- Reducing the size of stomach by aspirating gastric content and air with a syringe may help guiding the NJT in desired direction (Fig. 9B). Reducing the

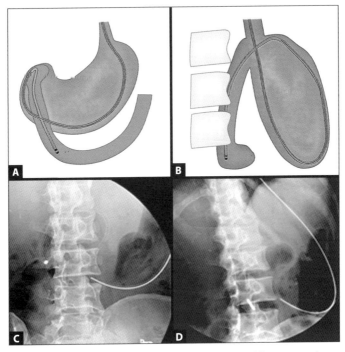

Figs 6A to D Illustration and radiographs showing use of lateral fluoroscopy for confirming location of NJT into duodenum

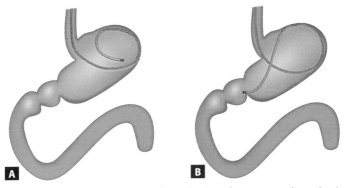

Figs 7A and B (A) NJT coiling in fundus; (B) Application of torque may direct the tip out of fundus toward pylorus

stomach size reduces the tendency of NJT coiling. Applying upward pressure on greater curve of distal antrum by lead-gloved hand may also direct the tip toward duodenum (Fig. 9C).

- Small amount of contrast medium may be injected to outline anatomy in difficult cases.
- Finally the stiffener is withdrawn completely leaving the NJT is position.
- Radiation dose should be kept at minimum by low fluoroscopy current, good collimation, short periods of intermittent fluoroscopy and using last image hold up feature. The average radiation dose is equivalent to 10 chest X-rays (0.21 mSv).[7]

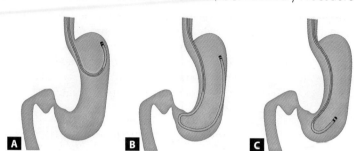

Figs 8A to C Double back maneuver

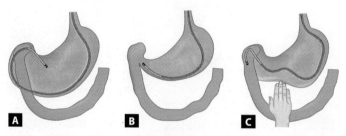

Figs 9A to C (A) NJT is coiling in antrum rather than going into duodenum; (B) Aspirating stomach content and air may reduce tendency of tube to coil in antrum; (C) Upward pressure over greater curvature helps in directing NJT toward pyloric canal

Endoscopic Seldinger (Over Guidewire) Insertion of Nasojejunal Tube

- For this technique, a NJT having an end-hole is needed.[1,5] Patient is positioned left lateral and head is supported with pillow.
- An endoscope is inserted till the third portion of duodenum/duodenojejunal flexure (Figs 10A to C).
- A guidewire is inserted through the endoscope into the jejunum and the endoscope is withdrawn gradually without pulling the guidewire (Figs 10D to H).
- A nasogastric (NG) tube/re-routing catheter is inserted into the clearest nostril and made to slide backward and inward along the floor of the nose to the nasopharynx.
- As the NG tube/re-routing catheter passes down into the nasopharynx, it is visualized at the back of the throat and pulled out through the mouth with the help of a Magill's forceps (a laryngoscope may be needed sometimes).
- Once placed as above, the guided wire is fed into the NG tube/re-routing catheter and the guidewire comes out through the nose (Fig. 10I). The NG tube/re-routing catheter is then removed, leaving the guidewire in place (Fig. 10J).
- The lumen of NJT is flushed with about 20–30 mL of sterile water and outer aspect of proximal tube is lubricated with sterile water.
- NJT is pushed over the guidewire and advanced slowly with gentle pressure until the NJT reaches the jejunum (Fig. 10K). The guidewire is now withdrawn slowly, leaving the NJT in position. NJT position is confirmed by fluoroscopy.

- In another variation of this technique, the NJT is fed over the guidewire through the mouth and after placing tube into jejunum, and the guidewire is removed. A NG tube/re-routing catheter is inserted through the nostril and taken out from mouth. Finally, the NJT is re-routed through it.
- The main disadvantage of this technique is that the oro-nasal transfer of guidewire/NJT may be difficult and uncomfortable for patient.

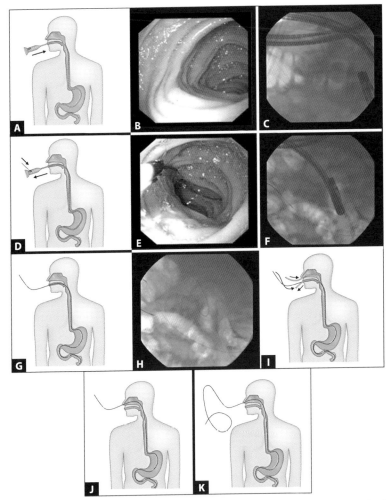

Figs 10A to K Endoscopic (Seldinger) method. (A) Endoscope is inserted till third part duodenum/DJ flexure; (B) Video-endoscopic image; (C) Fluoroscopic image; (D) Guidewire inserted through endoscope; (E) Video-endoscopic image; (F) Fluoroscopic image of the same; (G) Endoscope is removed leaving the guidewire; (H) Fluoroscopic image of the same; (I) Oro-nasal transfer of guidewire; (J) Now guidewire is coursing from nasal cavity to jejunum; (K) NJT placed over the guidewire

Endoscopic Insertion of Nasojejunal Tube Using Endoscopic Snare

- NJT is inserted into stomach as described in fluoroscopic technique.
- Patient is positioned left lateral and head is supported with pillow.
- An endoscope is inserted till the jejunum for inspection, and then it is pulled back into stomach.
- An endoscopic snare is passed through the endoscope and end of NJT is caught with it (Fig. 11).
- The endoscope and snared NJT are advanced till the duodenojejunal flexure.
- After reaching the jejunum, the endoscope and snare are withdrawn, leaving the NJT in position. In this technique, the disadvantage is that, while withdrawing the endoscope, sometimes NJT also comes out.

POST-PROCEDURE CARE

- The tip of NJT is positioned in proximal jejunum. It may be confirmed by injecting small amount of contrast medium either using fluoroscopy or abdominal X-ray (Fig. 12). If NJT is placed as part of CT enteroclysis, positive contrast medium should not be used to check NJT position. Instead of that small amount of air is injected with a 50 cc syringe, and air is seen outlining jejunal loop on fluoroscopy. NJT is fixed to the bridge of nose or upper lip with tape and looped over the ear.
- Abdomen X-ray should be done before starting feeding to confirm the position of the NJT. NJT should be straight without loops formation and tip should be positioned distal to the duodenojejunal flexure.
- NJT should be flushed with 30 mL of cool boiled water before and after the feed or at least once a day.
- Any change in the length of the external portion of tube should be observed.
- NJT can remain in position for up to 4 weeks if the tube and the nose are carefully cared for. If enteral feeding is needed for prolong period then, a percutaneous gastrojejunostomy is recommended.

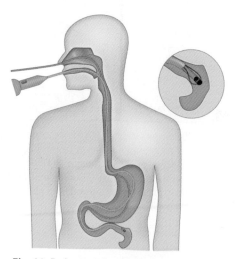

Fig. 11 Endoscopic insertion of NJT with snare

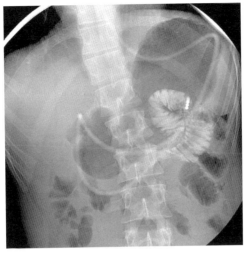

Fig. 12 Confirmation of NJT position by injection of contrast medium

COMPLICATION/PROBLEM

Complications related with fluoroscopic or endoscopic placement of NJT are few as compared with the blind placement.[8,9] Operator's skill not only reduces complications but also makes the procedure less uncomfortable.

- *Traumatic complication*: Although nasal intubation is uncomfortable, traumatic complications are uncommon with the use of fine bore NJT.
  - Perforation of a pharyngeal or esophageal pouch and intracranial insertion of feeding tubes have been reported. Although esophageal, gastric or small bowel perforations are unusual, they have been reported (Fig. 13A).
  - Mild bleeding may take place if there is mucosal injury to nasal, esophageal or gastric mucosa. NJT insertion should probably be avoided for 3 days after acute variceal bleeding. Severe mucosal injury or even perforation may occur if a stiffener is reinserted and accidentally exits via a side-hole (Fig. 13B).
- *Tracheobronchial misplacement*: Accidental bronchial insertion is relatively common with blind placement especially in patients with reduced levels of consciousness or with impaired gag/swallowing reflexes. However, in fluoroscopic or endoscopic placement it is immediately detected and corrected. So, during the NJT insertion, if the patient shows any evidence of respiratory distress, the tube should be withdrawn immediately.
- *Kink*: Sometimes NJT may develop kink near the tip (Figs 13C and D). It is associated with increased resistance while pushing feed into the tube. In such cases, tube should be pulled back till the kink disappears and again pushed over the stiffener or guidewire. A case report of duodenal perforation has been described due to a kink in a nasojejunal feeding tube in a patient with severe acute pancreatitis.[10] Knot formation in feeding tubes has also been reported.
- *NJT displacement back into stomach*: Fine bore NJT may form coil in stomach and tip may be displaced back into stomach spontaneously (Fig. 13E).

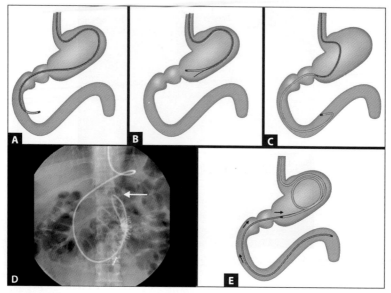

Figs 13A to E Complications and problems with NJT placement. (A) Small bowel perforation; (B) Stiffener exiting from side-hole; (C and D) Kink; (E) Displacement back into stomach

REFERENCES

1. University Hospitals of Leicester NHS Trust (2013). Policy for the insertion and postinsertion management of nasojejunal tubes in the adult patient for registered practitioners. [online] Available from http://www.library.leicestershospitals.nhs.uk. [Accessed July, 2013].
2. Rafferty GP, Tham TC. Endoscopic placement of enteral feeding tubes. World J Gastrointest Endosc. 2010;2(5):155-64.
3. Sinead Duggan (2013). Naso-jejunal feeding: indications and methods of tube insertion. [online] Available from http://www.corpakmedsystems.com/Supplement_Material/SupplementDownloads/Cortrak/Sinead_Duggan_article%20June_2011.pdf. [Accessed July, 2013].
4. Ott DJ, Mattox HE, Gelfand DW, Chen MY, Wu WC. Enteral feeding tubes: placement by using fluoroscopy and endoscopy. AJR Am J Roentgenol. 1991;157(4):769-71.
5. Gastroenterology Training & Education (2013). NJ Tube placement. [online] Available from http://gastrotraining.com/. [Accessed July, 2013].
6. DJ Nolan. Small intestine. In: Whitehouse GH, Worthington BS (Eds). Techniques in Diagnostic Imaging, 3rd edition. London: Blackwell Science Publishing. 1996.
7. Puustinen L, Numminen K, Uusi-Simola J, Sipponen T. Radiation exposure during nasojejunal intubation for MRI enteroclysis. Scand J Gastroenterol. 2012;47(6):658-61.
8. Stroud M, Duncan H, Nightingale J. British Society of Gastroenterology. Guidelines for enteral feeding in adult hospital patients. Gut. 2003;52(Suppl 7):vii1-vii12.
9. Prabhakaran S, Doraiswamy VA, Nagaraja V, Cipolla J, Ofurum U, Evans DC, et al. Nasoenteric tube complications. Scand J Surg. 2012;101(3):147-55.
10. Tong Z, Li W, Wang X, Ye X, Li N, Li J. Duodenal perforation due to a kink in a nasojejunal feeding tube in a patient with severe acute pancreatitis: a case report. J Med Case Rep. 2010;4:162.

42
Percutaneous Endoscopic Gastrostomy

Samir Mohindra, Kundan Kumar

INTRODUCTION

Percutaneous endoscopic gastrostomy (PEG) is an endoscopic guided procedure in which a tube, PEG tube, is inserted into the stomach through the anterior abdominal wall, in patients having poor oral intake and if there is anticipated need of enteral nutritional support for more than 4 weeks required. This procedure provides long-term nutrition through enteral route utilizing natural process of digestion. Placement of PEG tube bypasses the oropharynx and esophagus, and allows nutrients and medications to be delivered directly into the stomach. PEG placement is an excellent alternative to surgical gastrostomy, does not require anesthesia, thus avoiding associated complications. Moreover, by extending the PEG tube into the jejunum using jejunal extension tube, as percutaneous endoscopic jejunostomy (PEG-J) can be achieved. PEG tube insertion is occasionally indicated for decompression of stomach. The technical success of the procedure is high (>95%). The advantage of PEG placement includes utilization of enteral route, avoidance of invasive surgical enterostomy and potential complications related to parenteral nutrition.

INDICATION

Though enteral nutrition is the preferred method of feeding in clinical practice, there are situations where there is hindrance to delivery of nutrients through oral route. In such situations, alternative methods of nutrient delivery, like PEG, are considered. A gastrostomy is generally considered when intermediate (> 4 weeks) or long-term enteral feeding access is needed. Nasogastric or nasojejunal tubes are preferred for short-term feeding.

- *Impaired swallowing:* Most common indications for PEG placement are situations characterized by inability to take sufficient amount of nutrients through the enteral route. *Such clinical situations are:*
  - Neurological events (e.g. Guillain–Barrè syndrome, cerebrovascular accidents, etc.)
  - Anatomical (upper aerodigestive malignancies, head and neck surgeries and radiation, severe facial trauma, facial defects like cleft palate, etc.)
  - Poor volitional intake due to underlying comorbidities.

- *Supplemental feedings:* Usually in high catabolic states like burns, polytrauma, pediatric Crohn's disease, cystic fibrosis (with failure to thrive).
- *Gastric decompression:* "Venting PEG"—marked or prolonged gastric atony, recurrent large volume aspiration of intestinal contents, intestinal pseudo-obstruction (on total parenteral nutrition; TPN), terminal or severely debilitating diseases (intra-abdominal malignancies).
- *Nonalimentation indications:* Prolonged enteral administration of unpalatable medications or diets, fixation of the stomach in patients with recurrent gastric volvulus, bile replacement in patients of external biliary fistula, nonsurgical treatment of the gas-bloat syndrome (post-Nissen fundoplication) and dilation and stenting of obstructing esophageal neoplasms.

CONTRAINDICATION

Various absolute and relative contraindications for the procedure have been identified.[1]

Absolute

- Inability to perform esophagogastroduodenoscopy
- Uncorrectable coagulopathy
- Peritonitis (diffuse)
- Obstruction of bowel (However, could be used for decompression in this situation)
- Rapidly progressive or incurable disease (expected survival of few weeks—terminal disease, advanced dementia).

Relative

- Gross ascites.
- *Gastric mucosal lesions:* Large gastric varices, severe portal hypertensive gastropathy (PHG), severe diffuse gastric antral vascular ectasia (GAVE), etc.
- Past upper abdominal surgery (increases risk of injury to organs interpositioned between stomach and anterior abdominal wall).
- *Morbid obesity:* Difficulty in digital indentation and transillumination of the stomach wall.
- Gastric wall tumors.
- Infection of anterior abdominal wall (increases risk of PEG site infection).
- Intra-abdominal malignancies with peritoneal involvement.

TECHNIQUE AND EQUIPMENT

Percutaneous feeding tube placement can be done by endoscopic, fluoroscopic or surgical methods. Ponsky and Gauderer first described placement of PEG tubes in 1980.[2] *There are three techniques for performing PEG:*
1. Ponsky pull technique
2. Push technique (Sachs Vine)
3. Russell introducer technique.

Except for a postulated higher rate of peristomal infections in pull technique, there are no specific advantages and disadvantages of pull technique over the introducer technique.[3,4] The preferred technique depends on the ease and familiarity of the endoscopist with the specific technique. Success and failure rates are also not different between the technique.[5]

Equipment

- Esophagogastroduodenoscope
- *PEG set (Fig. 1):* Consisting of PEG tube, scalpel, trocar, guidewire, clamp, adaptor.

Size of PEG tube: The size of the tube depends on the planned nutrient to be used for feeding. Commercially available nutrient solutions are of low viscosity and can be easily fed using 15 Fr PEG tube. For feeding homemade cooked food (adequately blended and diluted), 18 or 20 Fr PEG tube should be the preferred size as narrower tubes have risk of getting clogged early.

PREPARATION

- *Informed consent* must be taken before the procedure and relatives need to be explained about the procedure, indication, outcome and possible complications of the procedure.
- *Laboratory workup:* PEG is a high bleeding risk procedure as per American Society of Gastrointestinal Endoscopy (ASGE) guidelines. Therefore, it is imperative to follow strict procedure protocol of testing for platelets and coagulation parameters. Usually platelets more than $50,000/mm^3$ and international normalized ratio up to 1.4 are considered acceptable. Antiplatelet drugs should be withdrawn 5–7 days prior to the procedure. Similarly, warfarin should be discontinued for at least 3–5 days and patient can be put on low molecular weight heparin till 8–12 hours before the procedure.

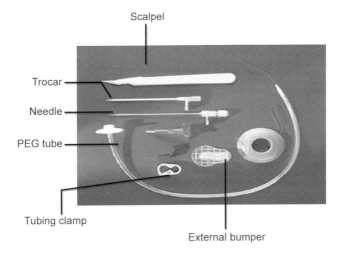

Fig. 1 Components of a PEG set

- *Patient preparation*
  - 8–12 hours nil per os (NPO) is required for the procedure so as to avoid esophageal reflux and aspiration.
  - Shaving of anterior abdominal wall
  - Intravenous access to be secured
  - Rinsing and gargling of mouth with povidone-iodine
  - Local pharyngeal anesthesia (1% lidocaine).
- *Prophylactic antibiotics* are recommended due to risk of infection of the gastrocutaneous tract, by oropharyngeal and cutaneous flora. A single intravenous dose of broad-spectrum antibiotic (amoxicillin plus clavulanic acid or a third generation cephalosporin), is administered approximately 30 minutes prior to the procedure so as to reduce the risk of wound infection and other septic complications.[6]
- *Others:* Lidocaine 1–2% for local anesthesia of the skin and abdominal wall, antiseptic preparation solution such as povidone-iodine or chlorhexidine.
- The procedure is performed using conscious sedation.

PROCEDURE

Pull Technique (Figs 2A to D)

The most common method used for PEG placement is "Ponsky pull technique". Ideally at least two expert individuals (two physicians or a physician and an expert assistant) are required to perform the procedure. Strict attention must be paid to maintain asepsis during the procedure. Procedure is preferably done in supine position. It can be done in left lateral position if patient's condition does not allow a supine position.

- Routine gastroscopy done with standard endoscope for a thorough evaluation of esophagus, stomach and duodenum (up to D2).
- Patient is moved to supine position, air insufflated in stomach for adequate distension, room is darkened (to assess transillumination across stomach/anterior abdominal wall).
- The tip of endoscope is directed toward the anterior abdominal wall and the anterior abdominal wall is observed for transillumination.
- The assistant indents the anterior gastric wall with finger, which is observed by the endoscopist.
- The assistant marks the point on anterior abdominal wall as a site for puncture.
- After applying disinfectant, local anesthetic agent (1% lidocaine) is injected (up to subcutaneous tissue).
- A small (5–10 mm) vertical incision is given on anterior abdominal wall with a scalpel blade (cutting subcutaneous fat and muscle).
- An 18-gauge needle catheter is inserted through the anterior abdominal wall, aspiration done till needle is seen by endoscopist inside the stomach.
- The endoscopist maintains gastric distension with continuous air insufflation.
- The endoscopist puts a snare through the biopsy channel of endoscope and holds the guidewire inserted through the needle catheter.

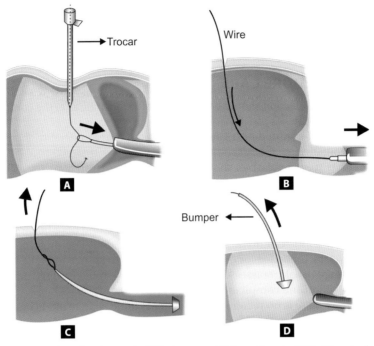

Figs 2A to D Ponsky pull technique for PEG placement. (A) Grasp the wire; (B) Pull the wire through the mouth; (C) Pull the PEG tube down the esophagus; (D) Pull the bumper to gastric wall

- The endoscope along with the snare holding the guidewire is withdrawn through the mouth making sure that adequate guidewire remains outside the anterior abdominal wall.
- The wire loop coming out of the mouth is then connected to the PEG tube by tying figure of "8" knot which is subsequently pulled down through esophagus with pulling of the guidewire coming out on anterior abdominal wall side.
- Too much pulling of the thread should be avoided. There should be adequate "play" at the gastric wall between the internal bumper and stomach wall.
- The external tube is shortened and position secured with external bumper. The external bumper should be placed approximately 1 cm or more from the abdominal wall with the dressing placed under the bumper.
- The endoscope is reinserted after PEG placement, which allows careful examination of the upper digestive tract for any mucosal trauma as well as confirmation of appropriate placement of the internal bolster adjacent to the anterior wall of stomach.

Push Technique[7]

In this technique, guidewire is drawn out through the mouth. Thereafter PEG tube is pushed into position over the guidewire, which extends from stoma site to mouth. Subsequently guidewire is removed.

Russell Introducer Technique[8]

Using Seldinger method, guidewire is placed in gastric lumen. Thereafter size of gastrostomy is increased using serial dilators (Figs 3A to D).

POST-PROCEDURE CARE

- Adequate disinfection should be achieved at the local site after the completion of the procedure.
- Feeding can be started next day, first with plain water preferably, if patient is asymptomatic.
- Patient as well as relatives should be given clear instructions regarding the care of PEG tube.
- Peritubal skin should be cleaned with mild soap and water and thoroughly dried. Use of strong chemicals should be avoided as their use may cause tissue damage, which may lead to leakage around the tube and poor healing.
- Use of antibiotic ointment/solution is to be avoided. Dry dressing of tube insertion site is needed for the first few days after the procedure.
- Patients are usually reassessed after 2–3 weeks for stoma healing, peristomal leak/infection and compliance of feeding advice.
- Currently, there is no recommendation for routine change of PEG tube. PEG tubes are only changed if they are blocked or nonfunctioning.

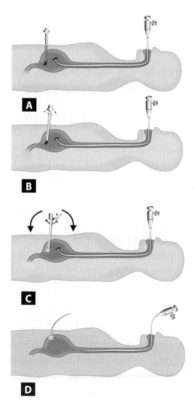

Figs 3A to D Russell introducer technique. (A) Needle puncture under endoscopic vision; (B) Insertion of trocar; (C) Pulling up of bumper; (D) Final position of bumper

Removal of PEG Tubes

Following are the indications for removal of PEG tube:
- Recovery to a state of adequate oral intake (Recovery of swallow after stroke or surgery for head and neck cancer or from brain trauma).
- Persistent PEG site infection
- Ineffective PEG, damaged/broken tubing
- Buried bumper syndrome.

Techniques of PEG Tube Removal (Figs 4A to D)

Percutaneous endoscopic gastrostomy (PEG) tube with rigid bumper is removed endoscopically. PEG tube is pushed into stomach so that tube behind the bumper becomes visible. A snare is passed through the endoscope and part of the tube behind the bumper is held. Thereafter part of the tube on anterior abdominal wall is cut and remaining tube pulled inside stomach and pulled out through the mouth. Alternative method is to cut the external tube and subsequently bumper passes with feces, but there is risk of bowel obstruction with this second method. However, recently published reports describe uneventful passing of the Freka internal bumper with feces.[9] PEG tubes with a collapsible or deflatable bumper can be removed using traction (simply by pulling the PEG tube out through the abdominal wall).

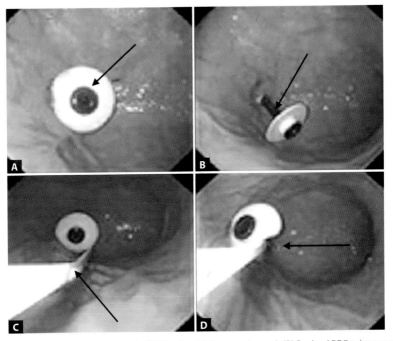

Figs 4A to D Endoscopic removal of PEG tube. (A) Bumper (arrow); (B) Pushed PEG tube to make tube visible behind the bumper (arrow); (C) PEG tube grasped using a snare; (D) PEG tube is being pulled using the snare (arrow)

COMPLICATION/PROBLEM

Major complications occur in approximately 3% and minor complications occur in up to 20% patients, and are possibly related to factors like advanced age, diabetes mellitus, severe cardiorespiratory comorbidities. Procedure-related mortality is approximately 0–2%. As these patients are frequently debilitated, 30-day mortality varies from 6–26%.[10] Various complications reported with PEG placement are:

- Infection may be minor, such as local cellulitis around the exit site of the tube or serious like necrotizing fasciitis of the abdominal wall. Usually occurs if the skin incision is small or if the PEG tube is pulled too tight against the gastric wall. Careful preparation of abdominal wall, swabbing of oral cavity with antiseptic solution, maintenance of asepsis at local site and use of prophylactic antibiotic reduces the incidence of infectious complications.
- Hemorrhage, usually minor.
- Gastric ulcer either at the site of the button or on the opposite wall of the stomach ("kissing ulcer").
- Bowel perforation (usually transverse colon) often resulting in peritonitis.
- Injury to liver capsule, usually in left lobe.
- *Gastrocolic fistula:* Usually present as diarrhea on initiation of feeding. In these cases, the feed goes direct from stomach to colon (usually transverse colon). Diagnosis is made with water-soluble contrast study through the gastrostomy tube; opacification of the colon at fluoroscopy confirms the existence of the fistula. In most instances, this complication is easily managed by removing the gastrostomy tube and allowing the tract and fistula to close. In general, surgical repair is rarely needed.
- *Tube migration into the abdominal wall (Buried bumper syndrome):* Usually occurs due to excessive traction on the tube leading to ischemia and necrosis of the intervening tissue. Present as abdominal pain, resistance to flow of feeds and peritubal leak.
- *Rare complications* like implantation metastases at the gastrostomy tube (may be related to the passage of the gastrostomy tube across obstructive malignant tumors in the upper aerodigestive tract), small bowel fistula, duodenal and colonic obstruction and acute gastric dilatation.

ACKNOWLEDGMENT

Isha Dubey (Pan-Africa e-network, TCIL, School of Telemedicine and Biomedical Informatics, SGPGIMS, Lucknow) for sketching of Figures 2 and 3.

REFERENCES

1. American Society for Gastrointestinal Endoscopy, Bosco JJ, Barkun AN, Isenberg GA, Nguyen CC, Petersen BT, et al. Endoscopic enteral nutritional access devices. Gastrointest Endosc. 2002;56:796-802.
2. Ponsky JL, Gauderer MW. Percutaneous endoscopic gastrostomy: a nonoperative technique for feeding gastrostomy. Gastrointest Endosc. 1981;27:9-11.
3. Deitel M, Bendago M, Spratt EH, Burul CJ, To TB. Percutaneous endoscopic gastrostomy by the "pull" and "introducer" methods. Can J Surg. 1988;31(2):102-4.

4. Maetani I, Tada T, Ukita T, Inoue H, Sakai Y, Yoshikawa M. PEG with introducer or pull method: a prospective randomized comparison. Gastrointest Endosc. 2003;57(7): 837-41.
5. Taylor CA, Larson DE, Ballard DJ, Bergstrom LR, Silverstein MD, Zinsmeister AR, et al. Predictors of outcome after percutaneous endoscopic gastrostomy: a community-based study. Mayo Clin Proc. 1992;67(11):1042-9.
6. Jafri NS, Mahid SS, Minor KS, Idstein SR, Hornung CA, Galandiuk S. Meta-analysis: antibiotic prophylaxis to prevent peristomal infection following percutaneous endoscopic gastrostomy. Aliment Pharmacol Ther. 2007;25:647-56.
7. Sacks BA, Vine HS, Palestrant AM, Ellison HP, Shropshire D, Lowe R. A nonoperative technique for establishment of a gastrostomy in the dog. Invest Radiol. 1983;18(5): 485-7.
8. Russell TR, Brotman M, Norris F. Percutaneous gastrostomy. A new simplified and cost-effective technique. Am J Surg. 1984;148(1):132-7.
9. Kejariwal D, Bromley D, Miao Y. The "cut and push" method of percutaneous endoscopic gastrostomy tube removal in adult patients: the Ipswich experience. Nutr Clin Pract. 2009;24:281-3.
10. Lynch CR, Fang JC. Prevention and management of complications of percutaneous endoscopic gastrostomy tubes. Pract Gastroenterol. 2004;28:66-76.

43
Balloon Tamponade in Upper GI Bleed

Praveer Rai

INTRODUCTION

Balloon tamponade is done to temporarily control life-threatening hemorrhage from gastroesophageal varices. It is only a temporizing measure before definitive therapy like endoscopy, transjugular intrahepatic portosystemic shunt or surgery is done. This tamponade is most commonly done with a Sengstaken-Blakemore tube. The other tubes used for tamponade include Minnesota, Linton-Nachlas tube.

INDICATION

- Balloon tamponade provides temporary control of massive bleed caused by esophageal or gastric varices which results from portal hypertension.
- It may simultaneously be used for drainage and decompression of the stomach.

CONTRAINDICATION

The tube is contraindicated in patients with recent esophageal surgery or esophageal stricture.

TECHNIQUE AND EQUIPMENT

Balloon tamponade was first described by Westphal in 1930.[1] In 1947, Rowntree et al. described the attachment of an inflatable latex bag to the end of Miller-Abbott tube to successfully control variceal bleed.[2] It was known that low pressure (20–30 mm Hg) is needed to collapse veins in the coronary—esophageal collateral circuit and applying traction upon a nasogastric tube with an inflated balloon in the stomach would stop bleed due to esophageal varices. The balloon makes contact with and compresses the coronary veins at their junction with the esophageal veins, and prevents the portal blood flow through this collateral circuit. Constant tension on a nasogastric tube with an inflated balloon at the lower end of the esophagus exerts pressure upon the entire nasoesophageal tract and an upward pull on the stomach. This leads to reflexes, which result in contractions of the stomach and esophagus. As contractions become exaggerated, retching with convulsive attempts at regurgitation supervene.

To abolish regurgitation reflexes and effect tolerance to traction upon a nasogastric tube Sengstaken and Blakemore felt the need of an esophageal balloon which when placed correctly in the esophagus and inflated, it will not go deep into the stomach and thus create a drag upon the nasogastric tube. Thereafter Sengstaken and Blakemore first described the technique of double-balloon tamponade to control variceal bleed.[3] The tube had three channels one for esophageal balloon inflation, one for gastric balloon inflation and one for gastric aspiration. Linton introduced a single balloon tube in 1953.[4] This tube consisted of a gastric balloon and a channel for gastric aspiration. The Linton tube was designed to determine if the source of bleed was above or below the cardia, however, because of coronary vein compression it was also effective to control variceal bleed. The modification of Linton tube was introduced by Nachlas in 1955 and consisted of a third channel to aspirate secretions above the gastric balloon.[5] Linton-Nachlas tube (Fig. 1) is most effective at terminating bleeding from gastric varices. In 1968 the modification of Sengstaken-Blakemore tube, the Minnesota was introduced by Edlich et al.[6] The Minnesota tube had an additional channel for aspiration of esophageal secretions above the balloon and is the most commonly used tube for control of variceal bleed.

Equipment

- *Modified Sengstaken-Blakemore tube (Fig. 2):* It is made of red rubber tube, which is about 85 cm in length and available in different sizes of 12 Fr, 14 Fr, 16 Fr, 18 Fr and 20 Fr. It has two balloons made up of latex, esophageal balloon about 14 cm in length and gastric balloon about 6 cm in length (sizes varies according to manufacturer). It has four ports: one each for esophageal and gastric balloon inflation and one each for esophageal and gastric contents aspiration.
- Syringe (50 mL with catheter tip)
- Hemostat clamp for rubber tubing
- Water-soluble lubricant
- Scissors (for emergency deflation).

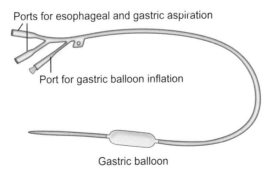

Ports for esophageal and gastric aspiration

Port for gastric balloon inflation

Gastric balloon

Fig. 1 Linton-Nachlas tube

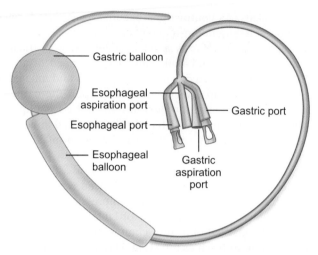

Fig. 2 Modified Sengstaken-Blakemore tube and its parts

PREPARATION

- *Airway prevention:* Endotracheal intubation is preferred in patients with hemodynamic compromise, encephalopathy, or both. The incidence of pulmonary complications is significantly lower when endotracheal intubation is routinely used.[7]
- *Volume correction:* Fluid resuscitation should be undertaken with crystalloids and colloids. A central venous catheter is required especially in patients with decompensated cirrhosis, advanced age or underlying cardiac and pulmonary disease. Coagulopathy should be treated with fresh-frozen plasma and platelets.
- All lumen should be patent, and the balloons should be pre-checked for leaks by inflation with air.

PROCEDURE

- Patient is positioned supine with head of the bed at approximately 30°.
- The tube should be generously lubricated with lidocaine jelly.
- Tube can be inserted through the nose or mouth, but the nasal route is not recommended in patients with coagulopathy.
- The patient is asked to flex neck and tube is gently inserted into a patent naris. Tube is advanced into pharynx, aiming posteriorly and asking the patient to swallow if possible.
- Once the tube is swallowed, confirm that the patient can speak clearly and breathe without difficulty (if not intubated), and gently advance tube to approximately 45 cm into the stomach.
- In patient having endotracheal tube, insertion of Sengstaken-Blakemore tube could be easily done with the help of laryngoscope and Magill's forceps.
- Auscultation in the epigastrium while air is injected through the gastric lumen verifies the tube position, but the position of the gastric balloon must be

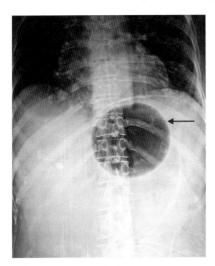

Fig. 3 Gastric balloon (arrow) seen below the gastroesophageal junction

confirmed radiologically at this time. The gastric balloon is inflated with no more than 50 mL of air.

- When the position of gastric balloon is confirmed to be below the diaphragm (Fig. 3), it should be further inflated with air to a volume of 250–300 mL.[8] The gastric balloon of the Minnesota tube can be inflated to 450 mL. Pull the tube backward gently until resistance is felt as the gastric balloon meets the gastroesophageal junction.
- Tube balloon inlets should be clamped with hemostats after insufflation. Hemorrhage is frequently controlled with insufflation of the gastric balloon alone without applying traction, but in patients with torrential hemorrhage, it is necessary to apply traction.[9]
- If the bleeding continues, the esophageal balloon should be inflated to a pressure of approximately 45 mm Hg (bedside manometer). This pressure should be monitored and maintained (Fig. 4).
- Anchor the tube to the patient's nose under minimal tension with padding to prevent damage to the nasal cartilage as shown in the Figure 5.

POST-PROCEDURE CARE

- Intermittent aspiration is done through gastric lumen.
- In Minnesota tube intermittent suction of esophageal lumen is done.
- Inflation of balloons should be checked after insertion and periodically.
- The tube should be left in place for a minimum of 24 hours. The gastric balloon tamponade can be maintained continuously up to 48 hours. The esophageal balloon, however, must be deflated for 30 minutes every 8 hours.
- The position of the tube should be monitored radiologically every 24 hours or sooner if there is any indication of tube displacement.
- A pair of scissors should be at the bedside in case the balloon ports need to be cut for rapid decompression, because the balloon can migrate and acutely obstruct the airway.

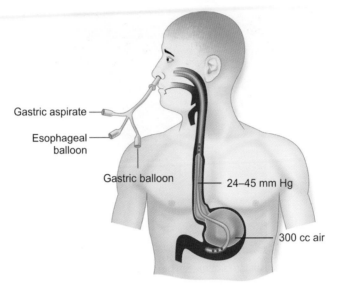

Gastric aspirate

Esophageal balloon

Gastric balloon

24–45 mm Hg

300 cc air

Fig. 4 Correct position of the Sengstaken-Blakemore tube

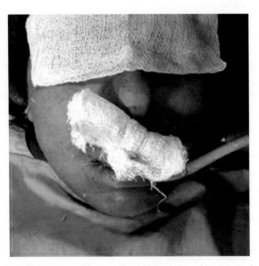

Fig. 5 Fixation of Sengstaken-Blakemore tube at nostril

COMPLICATION/PROBLEM

- Aspiration pneumonia is the most common complication of balloon tamponade. The severity and fatality rate is related to the presence of impaired mental status and encephalopathy in patients with poor control of the airway. The incidence ranges from 0% to 12%.
- Acute laryngeal obstruction and tracheal rupture are the most severe of all complications and the worst examples of tube migration. Migration of the tube occurs when the gastric balloon is not inflated properly after adequate

positioning in the stomach or when excessive traction (greater than 1.5 kg) is used, causing migration to the esophagus or hypopharynx.

- Mucosal ulceration of the gastroesophageal junction is common and is directly related to prolonged traction time (greater than 36 hours). Perforation of the esophagus is reported as a result of misplacing the gastric balloon above the diaphragm so position should be confirmed radiologically before fully inflating the gastric balloon. Rupture of the esophagus carries a high mortality.
- Unusual complications, such as impaction, result from obstruction of the balloon ports making it impossible to deflate the balloon. Occasionally, surgery is required to remove the tube.
- Necrosis of the nostrils and nasopharyngeal bleeding.

REFERENCES

1. Westphal K. Uber Eine Kompressions Behandlung Der Blutungen Aus Esophagus Varizen. Deutsche Med. Wchnschr. 1930;56:1135-6.
2. Rowntree LG, Zimmerman EF, Todd MH, AJAC J. Intraesophageal venous tamponage; its use in case of variceal hemorrhage from the esophagus. J Am Med Assoc. 1947;135(10):630.
3. Sengstaken RW, Blakemore AH. Balloon tamponade for control of hemorrhage from esophageal varices. Ann Surg. 1950;131(5):781-9.
4. Linton RR. The emergency and definitive treatment of bleeding esophageal varices. Gastroenterology. 1953;24(1):1-9.
5. Nachlas MM. A new triple-lumen tube for diagnosis and treatment of upper gastrointestinal hemorrhage. N Engl J Med. 1955;252(17):720-1.
6. Edlich RF, Lande AJ, Goodale RL, Wangensteen OH. Prevention of aspiration pneumonia by continuous esophageal aspiration during esophagogastric tamponade and gastric cooling. Surgery. 1968;64(2):405-8.
7. Cello JP, Crass RA, Grendell JH, Trunkey DD. Management of the patient with hemorrhaging esophageal varices. JAMA. 1986;256(11):1480-4.
8. Duarte B. Technique for the placement of the Sengstaken-Blakemore tube. Surg Gynecol Obstet. 1989;168(5):449-50.
9. Pinto Correia J, Martins Alves M, Alexandrino P, Silveira J. Controlled trial of vasopressin and balloon tamponade in bleeding esophageal varices. Hepatology. 1984;4(5):885-8.

44

Gastric Lavage

Manish Gupta, Nitin Garg

INTRODUCTION

Gastric lavage, which is variously known as *gastric irrigation or stomach pumping*, as the name suggests, is a technique of cleaning out the contents of the stomach. Traditionally, it has been the cornerstone in the management of patients with ingested poison or drug overdose. The value, safety and efficacy of this procedure have been questioned in several clinical studies and its routine use in modern medical practice has been abandoned. However, its use in India and developing nations is still fairly prevalent among healthcare professionals as it is an inexpensive and easily available option for gastrointestinal decontamination.

Gastric lavage should be performed by a trained and experienced healthcare professional and it involves the insertion of a large bore orogastric or nasogastric tube followed by repetitive or sequential instillation and aspiration of small amounts of fluid with the goal of removing or facilitating the recovery of particulate gastric content. It has been mainly recommended for patients who have ingested a life-threatening amount of a toxic substance and present to the hospital within 1 hour of ingestion. Use of gastric lavage in patients who have ingested nontoxic doses of a toxic substance or a nontoxic substance has no clinical benefits. It should also never be used as a deterrent to subsequent ingestion of toxic substance, such an approach is barbaric besides being incorrect.

INDICATION

The American Association of Poison Control Centers (AAPCC) and the European Association of Poison Centres and Clinical Toxicologists (EAPCCT) have released a joint statement discouraging the routine use of gastric lavage in the management of poisoned patients. However, in patients with recent and potentially lethal ingestion of poison, this procedure may be considered after weighing the risk-benefit ratio. *The main indications for a gastric lavage are:*
- To remove or aspirate the unabsorbed fractions of toxins and drug, it is most effective, if done within 60 min of ingestion
- To diagnose and control gastric bleed
- As a cooling technique in hypothermia
- To cleanse stomach before a diagnostic endoscopic procedures.

CONTRAINDICATION

Absolute

- Patients with depressed level of consciousness and unsecured airway
- Ingestion of corrosive agents (acid/alkali) or hydrocarbons/petroleum distillate
- Ingestion of sharp objects
- Ingestion of anticonvulsants or central nervous system depressants
- Patients who have sustained head injury
- Patients with marked hypothermia
- Prior significant vomiting.

Relative

- Patient refusing or resisting the procedure
- Patients with upper airway or GI tract anatomical deformity
- Patients in advanced stage of pregnancy
- Patients who have undergone a recent surgery
- Patients suffering from hemorrhagic diathesis
- Patients with esophageal varices
- If there is a delay in the time of ingestion of toxin and arrival at healthcare facility
- Patients who have ingested poison with effective antidote.

TECHNIQUE

Gastric lavage was one of the major medical advances of the 19th century. In the 1966, it became a standard of treatment for all forms of gastric irritation. There are two chief methods of gastric lavage and some alternative methods as well.

1. *Closed system irrigation*: Connect the bag or bottle of lavage fluid (normal saline/plain water) to orogastric/nasogastric tube with a Y-connector and connect the other end of the Y-connector to the suction tube (Fig. 1). Aspirate the stomach content followed by clamping of the suction tube and then allow 50–200 mL of the lavage fluid to run into stomach by gravity. When the required amount of solution has been instilled, it is drained by gravity or removed by suctioning. Repeat this procedure till the desired results are obtained, that means no further clots are retrieved or the efferent solution returns clear Estimation of gastric output is important to assess the fluid balance and it can be measured by subtracting the irrigant fluid from the total amount of drained fluid. The closed system helps in minimizing the contact risk with body fluid for the healthcare professionals.

2. *Intermittent open system irrigation*: After taking complete personal protective measures as necessary (gown and face protection), empty the gastric content with the help of suction or 50 mL catheter tip syringe. Draw up approximately 50 mL of irrigational solution through the syringe and instill it using gentle pressure. After aspiration of irrigation fluid, discard the solution into measuring container. Continue this procedure until the clear irrigant has been obtained.

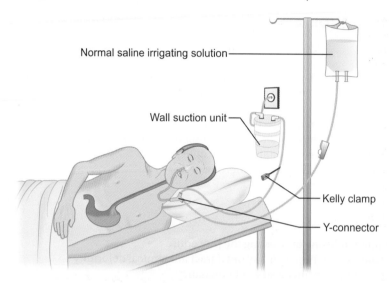

Normal saline irrigating solution

Wall suction unit

Kelly clamp

Y-connector

Fig. 1 Closed irrigation

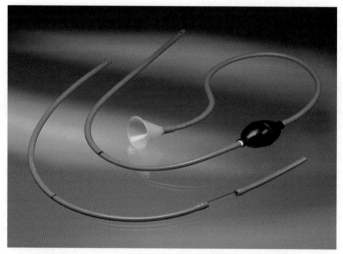

Fig. 2 Funnel-shaped stomach tube
Source: CR Bard Inc.; © 2013

- *Gastric lavage with funnel tube*: If the gastric lavage is made with the tube having funnel (Fig. 2), it is necessary to sink the funnel up to the elbow of the patient sitting on the chair, funnel is then filled with water and gradually lifted above the head, letting 500-600 mL of water enter into the stomach. It is necessary to follow carefully so that not all water from the funnel reaches the stomach because water cannot be removed from stomach again. When there is small amount of water left in the funnel, it must be brought down again to the level of the elbows of the patient and lavage of water with mucus and with oddments of nutrition will be removed from the stomach. The amount of gastric lavage output should be equal to the irrigation/instilled fluid.

- *Tubeless method*: In this method, patient is asked to drink 2-3 glassful of mineral water or light pink solution of potassium permanganate. After that, forced vomiting is done by placing the index and the middle finger of one hand on the root of the tongue.

PREPARATION

- Assessment and documentation of the vital signs, abdominal inspection, abdominal girth measurement and bowel sound auscultation should be done before performing this procedure.
- *Investigations:* Routine investigations such as hemogram and coagulation profile are required before inserting gastric tube.
- *List of equipment:* All the required equipment should be readily available before placement of gastric tube such as orogastric tube sizes (36–40 Fr for adults and 24–32 Fr for children) (Fig. 3), fluid, suction devices, catheter tip syringes, xylocaine spray, adhesive tapes, specimen container, kidney tray, measuring jar, protective shield, IV cannula, IV fluid and crash tray for resuscitation.
- *Medication:* IV fluids, xylocaine spray, activated charcoal and all emergency cardiac medicine
- *Monitoring devices:* Cardiac monitor, pulse oximetry, thermometer, abdominal girth measurement.

PROCEDURE

- In a conscious and alert patient, procedure should be explained and informed procedural consent should be obtained from the patient or the attendants

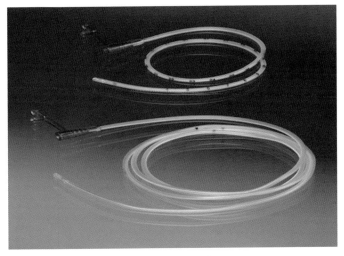

Fig. 3 Stomach tube
Source: CR Bard Inc.; © 2013

in cases of patients with obtunded sensorium. Patient should be instructed in advance to report of any pain, breathing difficulty or any other problem during the procedure.

- Apply the cardiac monitor, secure an intravenous access, and protect the airway by elective endotracheal intubation in patients with poor GCS.
- *Positioning:* Place the patient in Fowler's or semi-Fowler position (Fig. 4) (semi-recumbent 40–60° head up). If elevation of head is not tolerated by the patient because of hypotension, place in left lateral position with 20° head down tilt. This kind of positioning minimizes the risk of aspiration.
- Inspect both the nasal cavity and the oral cavity of patient; remove any loose denture.
- Lavage should be performed with a large bore orogastric tube, ideally, it is Lavacuator (clean plastic gastric hose) but in Indian scenario, an Ewald tube is also used. The size of the tube should be of 36–40 Fr inner diameter for an adult and 24–28 Fr for a child. The tube should be sufficiently pliable not to cause tissue injury, yet firm enough to pass into the stomach.
- Measure the length of the tube so that it should be at the stomach, if tube is too far in stomach it may cause gastric erosion and hemorrhage, and if tube is in esophagus then patient may have blenching or may aspirate during the lavage. The tube length to be inserted can be measured by placing the tube from bridge of the nose to the earlobe to the xiphoid of the sternum. Mark the tube at this point, which usually comes around the 50 cm mark for an adult and the 25 cm for children.
- Lubricate the tube with hydroxyethyl cellulose jelly, place a bite block or mouth gag before inserting the tube to prevent tube bite.
- The operator, standing in front of the patient, passes it gently from nostril, over the base of the tongue into the esophagus, the patient is asked to do swallowing movement (Fig. 5). It may then be further pushed on into the stomach. The mark on the tube will show when it has been introduced far enough.

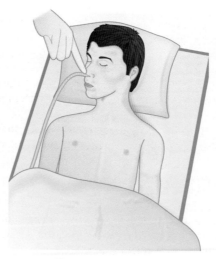

Fig. 4 Fowler's position

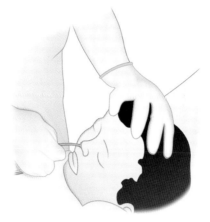

Fig. 5 Insertion of tube

The first introduction of the stomach tube, and sometimes the second, will often cause nausea and retching, but these effects will immediately pass off.

- Correct position of the tube can be confirmed by auscultation at the epigastric area of the insufflated air with 20 mL air filled syringe (Fig. 6), or by testing the pH of the aspirate. Always do X-ray or ultrasonography of stomach to confirm the placement of the tube.
- Aspirate about 30–60 mL of gastric content for specimen analysis (Fig. 7).
- After confirmation of the tube placement lavage is initiated with small (200–300 mL) amounts of warm normal saline or water for adults. In pediatric patients, use 10–15 mL/kg of lavage fluid.
- In certain specific types of poisoning, defined substances have been used, for e.g. paraquat poisoning, Fuller's earth is the adsorbent of choice.
- *Duration and termination of gastric lavage:*
  - Lavage should be given till no particulate matter is visible in aspirated gastric content and the efferent solution is clear.
  - Monitor the vital signs and clinical condition of the patient. The patient may be unstable and may require continuous re-evaluation. Gastric lavage may cause hypothermia; therefore, monitor temperature and look for signs of hypothermia, such as lethargy and changes in heart rate and rhythm.
  - The procedure may be terminated, if the aspirate does not clear after 20–30 minutes of lavage, or if the patient is unable to tolerate the procedure.

POST-PROCEDURE CARE

- After completion of lavage, vital signs and abdominal status should be monitored. Document the amount and type of irrigant fluid used and gastric output during the procedure. The aspirated specimen should be labeled and sent to the laboratory for chemical analysis.
- Most importantly keep a watch on the sensorium and vitals all throughout, pre-, intra- and post-procedure period

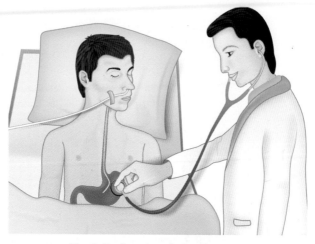

Fig. 6 Confirmation of tube placement

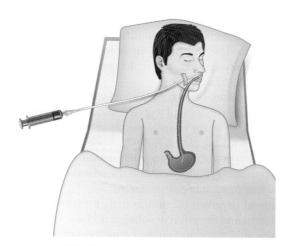

Fig. 7 Aspiration of gastric contents

- In case of any of the problems such as—pain in neck, chest and upper back, blood-stained vomitus, fever, shortness of breath, cough, pain in abdomen immediate note should be made and procedure should be abandoned.

COMPLICATION/PROBLEM

Reported rate of complications is in around 3% of the cases. *The associated complications are:*
- Most common complication is trivial injury of the mucosa, which can occasionally lead to a bleed.
- Improper or unrecognized placement of the orogastric tube.
- *Aspiration pneumonia:* This can take place due to accidental entry of the gastric aspirate, lavage fluid or toxins like hydrocarbon (which carry high-risk

of aspiration) into the respiratory track. Symptomatically, patient may have a sudden difficulty in breathing with fall in saturation. It can be prevented by proper preparation and positioning of the patient.

- *Dyselectrolytemia or fluid imbalance:* Most common of them is hyponatremia with water intoxication. This complication is mainly seen in pediatric patients with the use of disproportionate amount of normal saline or plain water. Patient can go into a state of confusion during the procedure secondary to hyponatremia.
- *Cardiac arrhythmias or ECG changes:* Dyselectrolytemia along with mechanical pressure of the lavage fluid can lead to ECG changes like ST elevation or sinus bradycardia. Vagal stimulation can also at times lead to sinus bradycardia.
- Perforation of viscous like esophagus (which can lead to mediastinitis), stomach or small bowel, when procedure is done unknowingly in poisoning with corrosive agents.
- *Hypothermia:* Due to use of large amount of cold lavage fluid, commonly seen in children
- *Laryngospasm:* Due to upper airway irritation and vagal stimulation
- Hypoxia/Hypercapnia.

SUGGESTED READING

1. Hendrickson RG, Kusin S. Gastrointestinal decontamination of poisoned adults. UpToDate®. *www.uptodate.com* (Assessed April 2015).
2. Krenzelok EP, Vale JA. Gastrointestinal decontamination. In: Brent J, Wallace KL, Burkhart KK, et al (Eds). Critical Care Toxicology: Diagnosis and Management of the Critically Poisoned Patient. Philadelphia: Mosby. 2005. pp. 53-60.
3. Christophersen ABJ, Hoegberg LCG. Techniques used to prevent gastrointestinal absorption. In: Flomenbaum NE, Goldfrank LR, Hoffman RS, et al (Eds). Goldfrank's Toxicologic Emergencies, 8th edition. New York: McGraw Hill, Medical Publishing Division. 2006.
4. Naderi S, Sud P, Acerra J, Pardo S, D'amore JZ, Ward MF, et al. The use of gastric lavage in india for poisoned patients. J Clinic Toxicol. 2012;118(2):2.
5. Proudfoot AT. Abandon gastric lavage in the accident and emergency department? Arch Emerg Med. 1984;1:65-71.
6. Tucker JR. Indications for techniques of, complications of, and efficacy of gastric lavage in the treatment of the poisoned child. Curr Opin Pediatr. 2000;12:163-5.
7. Vale JA, Kulig K. American Academy of Clinical Toxicology; European Association of Poisons Centres and Clinical Toxicologists. Position paper: gastric lavage. J Toxicol Clin Toxicol. 2004;42:933-43.

45

Intra-abdominal Pressure Monitoring

RK Singh

INTRODUCTION

Intra-abdominal pressure (IAP) is the steady state pressure concealed within the abdominal cavity.[1] When this pressure equals or exceeds 12 mm Hg, it is termed as intra-abdominal hypertension (IAH). IAH is further classified into: Grade I (IAP 12–15 mm Hg); Grade II (IAP 16–20 mm Hg); Grade III (IAP 21–25 mm Hg); Grade IV (IAP >25 mm Hg).[1] When IAP exceeds 20 mm Hg and is associated with a new organ dysfunction with or without an abdominal perfusion pressure (APP) below 60 mm Hg, it is termed as abdominal compartment syndrome (ACS). Difference between mean arterial pressure and IAP is the APP. IAP and APP are inversely related and in fact APP (≥60 mm Hg) is considered a better predictor of outcome than arterial pH, base deficit, arterial lactate and hourly urinary output.[2-4] Based on the rapidity of its onset, IAP is often categorized into hyperacute (lasting for seconds, e.g. laughing, coughing, sneezing, etc.), acute (over hours, e.g. trauma or intra-abdominal hemorrhage), subacute (over days, e.g. in medical patients) and chronic (over months, e.g. morbid obese, pregnancy). Most studies evaluating the incidence of ACS are from trauma patients, with incidence varying from 1–14%. However, despite this variability, incidence of ACS is highest among the most critically ill patients.[5] Suboptimal clinical sensitivity warrants measurement of IAP to document its existence and to further categorize it as IAH or ACS.[6]

INDICATION

- Postoperative abdominal surgery
- Patients who have sustained open or blunt abdominal trauma
- *Distended abdomen and clinical assessment consistent with ACS*
  - Oliguria
  - Hypoxia
  - Increased peak end expiratory pressures
  - Hypotension
  - Change in neurological examination results.

CONTRAINDICATION

Any patient requiring Foley's catheter for intravesicular drainage can have IAP measured and monitored. There are only relative contraindications and no absolute contraindication.

- Prostate and lower urologic surgery
- Medical history of bladder pathology
- Bladder and pelvic trauma
- Neurogenic bladder
- Postirradiation of bladder
- Hematuria.

APPLIED PATHOPHYSIOLOGY

Pathophysiological sequelae of raised IAP are as depicted in Figure 1.

TECHNIQUE

There are both direct (intraperitoneal) and indirect (intravesicular, intragastric, intracolonic and intrauterine pressure) methods of IAP estimation. However, being lesser invasive in nature the indirect methods are preferred.

Direct Technique

In this technique, a metallic cannula or a wide bore needle or catheter is inserted directly into the peritoneal cavity. This is then further connected to the pressure transducer. Real-time direct IAP measurement currently is only done during laparoscopic surgery and has been used sparingly since mid-1980s.

Indirect Technique

Intra-abdominal pressure can be indirectly measured by estimating pressure within the gastric, rectum, uterus and inferior vena cava. However, intravesical pressure is the most universally accepted surrogate of IAP. Accuracy and repro-ducibility of IAP measurements are essential to the management of IAH and ACS.

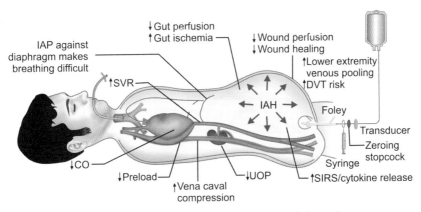

Fig. 1 Pathophysiological consequences of raised intra-abdominal pressure, with intra-abdominal pressure monitoring device *in situ*

PREPARATION

Equipment Required for Intravesicle IAP Measurement

- Appropriate size Foley's urinary catheter
- Urine bag for drainage of urine
- Two-three ways taps
- Luer-Lock connectors
- Pressure transducer kit and tubing
- A 50 mL Luer-Lock syringe
- Sterile 0.9% sodium chloride
- Clamp.

PROCEDURE

Setting up the Intravesicle IAP Monitoring Equipment

- Maintain strict asepsis throughout the procedure
- Ensure that the entire tubing is free of kinks and air bubbles
- Connect the catheter to the drainage bag with connector and three ways taps
- Attach the transducer set to the three ways tap
- Ensure that all connections are Leur locked to prevent frequent disconnections
- Unnecessary clamping and turning off stopcocks can be avoided by the use of an auto-valve of a commercially available IAP monitoring device (Fig. 2).

Estimating the Intra-abdominal Pressure

- The patient is first placed in the supine position
- The transducer is zeroed at the level of the midaxillary line at the iliac crest (Figs 3 and 4).

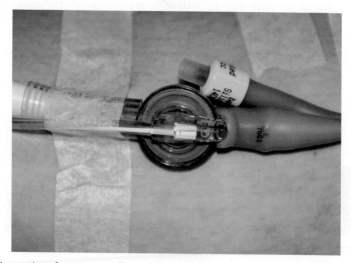

Fig. 2 Auto-valve of a commercially available intra-abdominal pressure monitoring system to help prevent clamping and turning of stopcocks during intra-abdominal pressure measurement

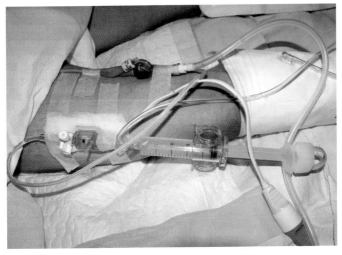

Fig. 3 Transducer fixed at the phlebostatic axis of a supine patient

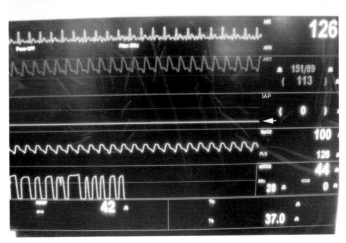

Fig. 4 Intensive care unit monitor showing intra-abdominal pressure tracing (arrow) and intra-abdominal pressure reading of zero after zeroing the transducer

- Intra-abdominal pressure (expressed in mm Hg) is measured at the end of expiration
- Inadvertent contraction of the detrusor muscles of bladder can elevate the IAP. This is prevented by use of optimum sedation[7]
- Spontaneous breathing efforts can alter the IAP readings; hence in a majority of patients IAP readings are estimated during mechanical ventilation
- Using a syringe, the bladder is instilled with a constant volume of 25 mL (in pediatrics 1 mL/kg) of 0.9% normal saline (normal temperature) each time before IAP measurement (Figs 5 and 6). Remember to discard this volume from the daily urine output estimations

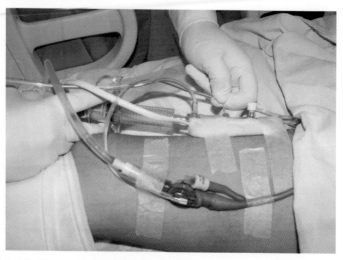

Fig. 5 Prefilled 20 mL syringe of saline bolus for pushing through the transducer channel

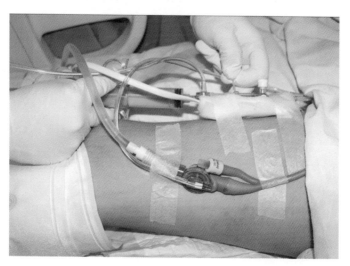

Fig. 6 Empty syringe after pushing the saline bolus

- Close the stopcock of the syringe and allow 30–60 seconds for equilibrium to occur. Obtain the mean pressure reading at the end expiration (this minimizes the effects of pulmonary pressures) (Fig. 7)
- To check correct setting up of the system, pressure on the abdomen should produce fluctuations in the IAP waveform
- Avoid kinking of tubes and presence of air bubbles as it can dampen the waveform
- All transducer monitoring lines should be clearly labeled

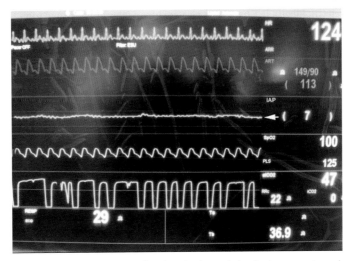

Fig. 7 Intensive care unit monitor showing the intra-abdominal pressure trace (arrow) and the intra-abdominal pressure measurement of 7 mm Hg

POST-PROCEDURE CARE

- Transducer set should preferably be changed every 72 hours
- Discontinuing monitoring: When the patient is clinically improving and successive IAP measurements are below 12 mm Hg for several hours, IAP measurements can be stopped. Using aseptic precautions, remove transducer and IAP assembly kit from the Foley's catheter. Then, re-connect urinary bag to the Foley's catheter. However, continue the clinical observation for any further deterioration and requirement of IAP measurement.

COMPLICATION/PROBLEM

- Air bubbles in the system
- Kinking of the tubing
- Wrong transducer positioning
- Patient not fully supine during IAP measurement
- Urosepsis is a complication of this procedure. Strict aseptic technique during initiation, maintenance and removal of the IAP monitoring device is mandatory to prevent infection and sepsis.

REFERENCES

1. Malbrain ML, Cheatham ML, Kirkpatrick A, Sugrue M, Parr M, De Waele J, et al. Results from the International Conference of Experts on Intra-abdominal Hypertension and Abdominal Compartment Syndrome. I. Definitions. Intensive Care Med. 2006;32(11):1722-32.
2. Diebel LN, Dulchavsky SA, Wilson RF. Effect of increased intra-abdominal pressure on mesenteric arterial and intestinal mucosal blood flow. J Trauma. 1992;33(1):48-9.
3. Schein M, Ivatury R. Intra-abdominal hypertension and the abdominal compartment syndrome. Br J Surg. 1998;85(1):1027-8.

4. Caldwell CB, Ricotta JJ. Changes in visceral blood flow with elevated intra-abdominal pressure. J Surg Res. 1987;43(1):14-20.
5. Malbrain ML, Chiumello D, Pelosi P, Wilmer A, Brienza N, Malcangi V, et al. Prevalence of intra-abdominal hypertension in critically ill patients: a multicentre epidemiological study. Intensive Care Med. 2004;30(5):822-9.
6. Wilson A, Longhi J, Goldman C, McNatt S. Intra-abdominal pressure and the morbidly obese patients: the effect of body mass index. J Trauma. 2010;69(1):78-83.
7. Sessler CN, Gosnell MS, Grap MJ, Brophy GM, O'Neal PV, Keane KA, et al. The Richmond Agitation-Sedation Scale: validity and reliability in adult intensive care unit patients. Am J Respir Crit Care Med. 2002;166(10):1338-44.

46
Paracentesis

Prasad Rajhans, Divyesh Patel

INTRODUCTION

Paracentesis is a procedure to remove fluid from the peritoneal cavity, better described as peritoneocentesis ("cent" meaning to pierce). Needle is inserted in peritoneal cavity to drain peritoneal fluid. It is done basically for two purposes: diagnostic and therapeutic.

INDICATION

- *Therapeutic paracentesis*
  - Therapeutic paracentesis to relieve symptoms due to increased intra-abdominal pressure like dyspnea, poor appetite and declining urine output
  - Percutaneous decompression of resuscitation induced abdominal compartment syndrome related to development of acute tense ascites.[1]
- *Diagnostic paracentesis*
  - New onset ascites to establish cause
  - To diagnose a metastatic cancer (may require recurrent tapping in case of malignant ascites)
  - To diagnose hemoperitoneum in cases of trauma
  - Patient with pre-existing ascites now deteriorating with fever, abdominal pain and tenderness, hepatic encephalopathy and increasing white blood cells (WBC) count and deteriorating urine output.

CONTRAINDICATION

- Acute abdomen that requires surgery is an absolute contraindication.
- Avoid paracentesis in patient with disseminated intravascular coagulation and fibrinolysis and clinically apparent oozing from needle sticks until coagulopathy is corrected.
- Majority of patients who require paracentesis have underlying baseline liver disease and, thereby associated coagulopathy and thrombocytopenia. However, clinically important bleeding events are less in these patient groups, hence routine use of blood products is usually not required.[2,3] There are no specific guidelines for transfusion in such patients. However, if international normalized ratio (INR) is higher than 2 or platelet is lower than 20,000/dL,

then fresh frozen plasma or platelet concentrates should be considered respectively despite scanty evidence, to support safety of patient.
• Relative contraindications include pregnancy, distended bladder and massive ileus with bowel distension, intra-abdominal adhesions or abdominal wall cellulitis.

APPLIED ANATOMY

Understanding certain facts of anatomy is essential to performing the procedure safely. The inferior epigastric artery runs along the rectus abdominis muscle, hence needle insertion site should always be selected lateral to rectus abdominis muscle. Left lower quadrant is better preferred over right lower quadrant as critically ill patients tend to have distended cecum. In practice, preferred needle insertion site is 2–4 cm medially and cephalic to anterior superior iliac spine along the midclavicular line (Fig. 1). Another needle insertion site may be along the midline, 2 cm below the umbilicus. This is along the linea alba (an avascular structure) and hence, chances of vessel injury are not there. However, the left lower quadrant is considerably thinner and has good depth of ascitic fluid than the midline infraumbilical position.[4] This is especially helpful in obese patients and hence, left quadrant is preferred site. In patients with liver disease, there are significant collaterals on anterior abdominal wall. Avoid such highly congested sites. In case of loculated ascites, ultrasound-guided tapping should be done.

TECHNIQUE

There is no definite evidence as to which technique is better than other. *Paracentesis can be basically performed by three techniques:*
1. *Needle technique:* This technique is employed frequently when only small amount of ascitic fluid needs to be removed, that is, in diagnostic paracentesis. Usually, a 20 gauge and 1.5-inch needle is sufficient in thin and lean patients.

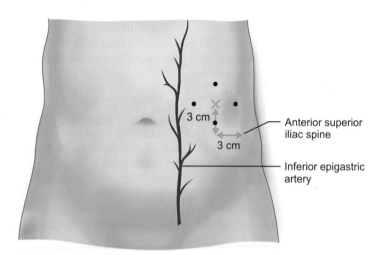

Fig. 1 Preferred site of abdominal paracentesis avoiding the inferior epigastric vessels

In obese patients or patients with thick abdominal wall, an 18–20 gauge lumbar puncture needle shall serve the purpose.

2. *Catheter technique:* In cases where larger amount of fluid is to be removed, that is, in therapeutic paracentesis, catheter technique is recommended as it is associated with lesser complications. A 16–18 gauge angiocath with catheter over needle can be used. Disadvantage with angiocath is that sometimes the plastic catheter may fray or break during insertion or removal and may require unnecessary surgery. Alternatively, a safer option is using a single lumen central venous catheter which can be inserted by Seldinger technique.

3. *Ultrasound guidance technique:* Ultrasound-guided puncture shall particularly be helpful in conjunction with needle or catheter technique especially in patients with intra-abdominal wall adhesions, loculated ascites and patients with deranged bleeding and coagulation parameters. It reduces the complications associated with blind insertion of needles such as perforation of bowel and bleeding.

PREPARATION

- *Laboratory check:* Prothrombin time/international normalized ratio (PT/ INR), activated partial thromboplastin time (aPTT), platelet count and hematocrit.
- *Monitoring:* During procedure at least blood pressure monitoring should be available, preferably electrocardiography (ECG) monitoring also, if done in indoor set-up.
- Always secure a good intravenous access before embarking on procedure.
- *Medications:* An emergency medication trolley should always be by the bedside.
- *Equipment*
    - Sterile gloves, gown, mask and cap.
    - Two percent chlorhexidine for skin preparation.
    - Sterile drapes and sterile gauze pieces.
    - Local anesthetic (2% xylocaine).
    - 10 cc syringe for infiltration of local anesthetic and 50 cc syringe for drawing samples.
    - *Needles*
        - 24 gauge and 1.5-inch needle for local infiltration.
        - 18–20 gauge and 1.5-inch needle for diagnostic tap in thin and lean patients.
        - 18–20 gauge lumbar puncture needle for diagnostic tap in obese patients.
        - 16–18 gauge angiocath or a single lumen central venous catheter for therapeutic tapping.
    - Intravenous set or a noncollapsible tubing for drainage.
    - Drainage bottles (either vacuum or simple bottle).
    - Sample tubes and bottles for hematology, chemistry, microbiology, cytology and cultures.

- *Patient preparation*
  - Written and informed consent should be obtained from patient and if patient is not able to give consent then form the closest caregiver.
  - Ensure the patient has an empty bladder prior to procedure to avoid inadvertent injury.
  - Make the patient lie in bed and make sure head end of bed is raised by 30–45 degree in head up position. This allows the gas filled bowel to ascend and fluid to gravitate at the lower dependent regions where we are intending puncture.
  - Adjust the height of bed so that the operator is comfortable at that level.
  - If available, ultrasound should preferably be obtained prior to going ahead with procedure. This shall help in documenting the exact point of puncture, depth of fluid from skin and depth of bowel from skin and also help to identify any loculation. If ultrasound is not available then on percussion, point of maximum dullness should be found and accordingly puncture site should be selected. Mark the selected site.
  - After proper hand wash and scrub and wearing sterile gown and gloves, paint the selected site and surrounding area with 2% chlorhexidine (Fig. 2) and then cover the area with sterile fenestrated drape (Fig. 3).
  - Anesthetize the skin, subcutaneous tissue and deeper tissue up to parietal peritoneum at the selected site with 2% xylocaine with a 24 gauge and 1.5-inch needle (Fig. 4). Always aspirate before injecting local anesthetic agent.

PROCEDURE

Needle Technique

- Use a 18–20 gauge, and 1.5-inch needle for thin and lean patients or lumbar puncture needle with similar gauge for obese patients or patients with thick abdominal wall.
- *Z-track technique (Figs 5 and 6):* Pull the skin at puncture site taut inferiorly. While tension is maintained on skin inferiorly, prick the skin and then enter

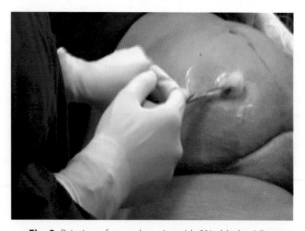

Fig. 2 Painting of procedure site with 2% chlorhexidine

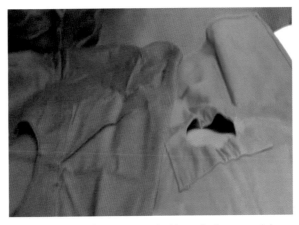

Fig. 3 Painted sterile area covered with sterile fenestrated drapes

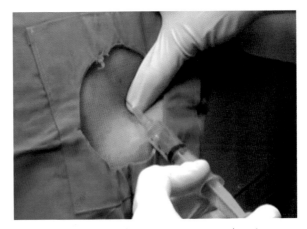

Fig. 4 Local anesthetic injection at procedure site

the abdominal wall fascia and peritoneum perpendicularly. This ensures that the site of entry of skin and peritoneum are at different locations and, thus minimizes the chances of ascitic fluid leak postprocedure.

- As needle is introduced, gentle aspiration should be done intermittently. Continuous aspiration may pull bowel or omentum onto the needle tip, occluding the tip. This may give the false impression that there is no fluid. If bowel or omentum is pulled to the needle tip, releasing the suction on the syringe plunger may allow the bowel or omentum to float away and permit aspiration with free flow of fluid into the needle and syringe. Aspiration of fluid suggests that peritoneal cavity has been entered (Fig. 7).
- Now stabilize the needle with one hand and change the syringe to a 50 cc syringe to collect samples for investigation.
- In case needle technique is used for therapeutic drainage then, you may then connect the needle to an intravenous set or rigid tubing which is then connected to a simple bottle and allowed to drain with gravity or one may also use a vacuum container.

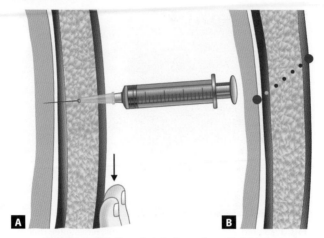

Figs 5A and B Z-track technique of needle insertion

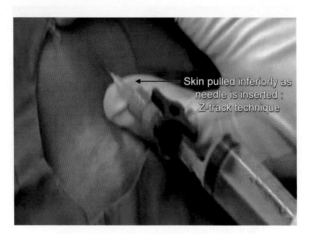

Fig. 6 Z-track technique of needle insertion

Catheter Technique

- If the patient is thin and lean then a 18–20 gauge angiocath can be used as a catheter over needle assembly. In case of obese patients and thick abdominal wall patients a single lumen central venous catheter can be inserted using Seldinger technique.
- The peritoneal cavity is entered with angiocath using similar Z-track technique, while, continuously aspirating as we enter. As soon as ascitic fluid is aspirated the catheter is advanced and needle withdrawn. Now, the catheter is connected to intravenous set or rigid tubing and fluid is allowed to drain with gravity.
- When Seldinger technique is used in patients with large abdominal wall, initial access to peritoneal cavity is obtained with the help of 18 gauge needle with similar Z-track technique. Once the peritoneal cavity is accessed, then a

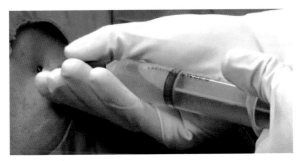

Fig. 7 Aspiration of ascitic fluid on entry into peritoneal cavity

guidewire is inserted through the needle and gradually the needle is removed. Subsequently, single lumen central venous catheter is guided over the wire.

- Then after removing guidewire, the catheter is connected to a draining bottle with the help of intravenous set or rigid tubing.
- It is very important to use Z-track technique for Seldinger technique or else there can be high possibility of post-procedure leak from the puncture site.

Ultrasound-guided Technique

- Under select circumstances as mentioned earlier paracentesis may be done using ultrasound guidance. Needle technique or catheter technique is used in conjunction with ultrasound to accurately localize the fluid in peritoneal cavity.

Collection of Fluid for Laboratory Testing

- Once fluid is aspirated in syringe, we change over to a 50 cc syringe and aspirate the ascitic fluid. This syringe is then handed over to an assistant who is wearing nonsterile gloves. A new 22 gauge needle is then attached to the syringe with sample. 1–2 mL of sample of fluid is the collected in tube with anticoagulant (this tube usually has purple cap) and 1–2 mL of fluid is collected in a plain tube (this tube usually has red cap).
- If cultures are needed then blood culture bottles are used for inoculation of ascitic fluid. It is important to use blood culture bottles because spontaneous bacterial peritonitis (SBP) is an infection which usually has low colony count, just like bacteremia. If a tube or syringe is used for sending ascitic fluid cultures, then sensitivity for detecting SBP is dramatically decreased.[5,6] The assistant wipes the culture bottle cap with alcohol swab and then connects the needle with syringe with culture bottle. Approximately 10 mL of ascitic fluid is used to inoculate blood culture bottle.
- For cytology we collect the whole drained ascitic fluid specimen in a nonsterile glass bottle and send for cytospin. However, some laboratories require fluid for cytology delivered in a syringe or sterile container. Hence, exact sample requirements, including those for unusual tests, should always be coordinated with local laboratory.

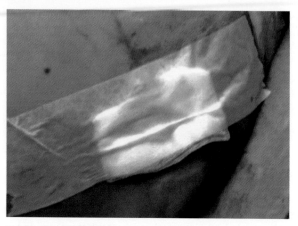

Fig. 8 Dressing at post-procedure site

POST-PROCEDURE CARE

Post-procedure once the needle or catheter is removed, apply a sterile gauze dressing over the puncture site (Fig. 8) and watch for any leak from the site.

Patients with suspected secondary bacterial peritonitis should be investigated with emergent radiograph of abdomen in upright position and if needed a computed tomographic scan of the abdomen. Patient should be taken up for emergency laparotomy, if free air or a surgically-treatable source of infection is documented.[7]

Interpretation of Fluid Analysis

Majority of times ascitic fluid analysis is done to rule out infection and presence of portal hypertension. To determine this, basic fluid tests that need to be done include: assessment of appearance, total count and differential count on ascitic fluid, total protein concentration and serum-to-ascitic albumin gradient (SAAG).

- *Appearance:* Uncomplicated ascites in background of chronic liver disease would give clear ascitic fluid. Turbid fluid would suggest infection or bowel perforation. Milky fluid is suggestive of chylous ascites and bloody fluid may suggest either traumatic tap or malignant ascites.
- *Total leukocyte count and differential leukocyte count:* SBP is diagnosed with absolute polymorphonuclear count more than or equal to 250 cells/mm³ in ascitic fluid and positive culture of ascitic fluid. The total leukocyte count and neutrophil counts need to be corrected in patients with bloody samples. One white blood cell should be subtracted from the ascitic fluid leukocyte count per every 750 RBC to yield the "corrected total count", and one neutrophil be subtracted from absolute polymorphonuclear count per every 250 RBC to yield the "corrected neutrophil count".[8]
- *Serum to ascites albumin gradient:* It is more useful than the conventional exudates/transudate concept and helps identify portal hypertension in such patients.[9] Ascitic fluid albumin value subtracted from the serum albumin value gives SAAG. SAAG more than or equal to 1.1 gm/dL suggests patient has

portal hypertension.[9] However, SAAG will be elevated with any disorder due to portal hypertension.

- *Ascitic fluid protein concentration:* Traditionally ascitic fluid can be classified as an exudate if total protein is more than or equal to 2.5–3.0 gm/dL in ascitic fluid and a transudate if it is below this cut-off. However, this system of classification into transudate and exudates has been replaced by the SAAG, which is a more useful measure.

The total protein concentration may help to differentiate uncomplicated ascites due to liver cirrhosis from cardiac causes, both of which have SAAG more than or equal to 1.1g/dL. In cirrhotic ascites, total protein concentration is usually less than 2.5 g/dL. In ascites due to cardiac causes total protein concentration is usually more than or equal to 2.5 g/dL. In nephrotic ascites, the total protein in ascites is usually less than 2.5 g/dL and SAAG is more than 1.1 g/dL.

- *Additional tests:* Few additional tests may be performed with the initial tests, if there is clinical suspicion for a particular disorder or they may be performed later based on the results of initial testing.
  - Glucose concentration, lactate dehydrogenase concentration, gram stain and culture (infection, bowel perforation)
  - Zn-stain, adenosine deaminase activity and tuberculosis culture (tuberculous peritonitis)
  - Cytology and carcinoembryonic antigen level (malignancy)
  - Triglyceride concentration (chylous ascites)
  - Amylase concentration (pancreatic ascites or bowel perforation)
  - Bilirubin concentration (bowel or biliary perforation).

COMPLICATION/PROBLEM

- *Hypotension:* This usually occurs in large volume paracentesis (defined as >5 L fluid removed at one sitting), where rapid mobilization of fluids from vascular space to third space occurs and thus results in paracentesis induced circulatory dysfunction. Administer a bolus of intravenous fluids. If hypotension is persistent then, consider starting a vasopressor infusion. The American Association for study of liver disease practice guidelines suggest, large volume paracentesis should only be done for refractory ascites.[10] If large volume paracentesis is planned then, it may be done under cover of intravenous albumin infusion of 6–8 gm/L of ascitic fluid to prevent such complication.[10,11] Albumin infusion may be withheld for paracentesis volume less than 5 L. If hypotension is not responding then one must consider a possibility of intraperitoneal bleed and obtain an urgent ultrasound.
- *Persistent leak of ascitic fluid:* Usually occurrence is rare. Treatment usually involves giving 5 minutes pressure over the puncture site and then apply a pressure bandage. If still persistent, then one may consider a purse string suture to close the entry site.
- *Intraperitoneal hemorrhage:* Usually suspected when the returning fluid is persistently bloody and patient is going into hypotension and tachycardia. Correct coagulation abnormalities, if any. If still worsening, then seek a surgical opinion.
- *Bowel perforation and peritonitis:* Infection is usually rare unless bowel is punctured by paracentesis needle. If initial aspirate is fecal then one may

consider this possibility. Patients usually develop abdominal pain and signs of peritonitis. Usually these perforations are small and get walled off by omentum and pain gradually subsides. However, if there is a persistent or worsening sign of peritonitis then plan for an upright X-ray of abdomen to look for gas under diaphragm or CT-abdomen with oral contrast to look for extravasations. Obtain a surgical consult.

REFERENCES

1. Parra MW, Al-Khayat H, Smith HG, Cheatham ML. Paracentesis for resuscitation-induced abdominal compartment syndrome: an alternative to decompressive laparotomy in the burn patient. J Trauma. 2006;60(5):1119-21.
2. Grabau CM, Crago SF, Hoff LK, Simon JA, Melton CA, Ott BJ, et al. Performance standards for therapeutic abdominal paracentesis. Hepatology. 2004;40(2):484-8.
3. McVay PA, Toy PT. Lack of increased bleeding after paracentesis and thoracentesis in patients with mild coagulation abnormalities. Transfusion. 1991;31(2):164-71.
4. Sakai H, Sheer TA, Mendler MH, Runyon BA. Choosing the location for non-image guided abdominal paracentesis. Liver Int. 2005;25(5):984-6.
5. Runyon BA, Canawati HN, Akriviadis EA. Optimization of ascitic fluid culture technique. Gastroenterology. 1988;95:1351-5.
6. Wong CL, Holroyd-Leduc J, Thorpe KE, Straus SE. Does this patient have bacterial peritonitis or portal hypertension? How do I perform a paracentesis and analyze the results? JAMA. 2008;299(10):1166-78.
7. Akriviadis EA, Runyon BA. Utility of an algorithm in differentiating spontaneous from secondary bacterial peritonitis. Gastroenterology. 1990;98(1):127-33.
8. Runyon BA, Antillon MR. Ascitic fluid pH and lactate: insensitive and nonspecific tests in detecting ascitic fluid infection. Hepatology. 1991;13(5):929-35.
9. Runyon BA, Montano AA, Akriviadis EA, Antillon MR, Irving MA, McHutchison JG. The serum-ascites albumin gradient is superior to the exudate-transudate concept in the differential diagnosis of ascites. Ann Intern Med. 1992;117(3):215-20.
10. Runyon B. Management of adult patient of ascites with cirrhosis: an update. Hepatology. AASLD Practice Guidelines Committee. 2009;49(6):2087-107.
11. Sola-Vera J, Minana J, Ricart E, Planella M, González B, Torras X, et al. Randomized trial comparing albumin and saline in the prevention of paracentesis-induced circulatory dysfunction in cirrhotic patients with ascites. Hepatology. 2003;37(5):1147-53.

47
Percutaneous Abdominal Drain

Hira Lal, Rajanikant R Yadav, Zafar Neyaz

INTRODUCTION

Intra-abdominal infections are an important cause of morbidity and mortality in the intensive care unit (ICU). Approximately 30% mortality rates have been reported in ICU patients with intra-abdominal infections.[1] Image-guided percutaneous catheter drainage (PCD) is now treatment of choice for management of abdominal abscesses and the fluid collections. The procedure involves percutaneous placement of a catheter into an abdominal collection or abscess with the help of imaging guidance. The catheter serves to drain the abdominal abscess/fluid collection to the exterior. PCD for abdominal abscesses and fluid collections is associated with lesser morbidity and mortality, lesser hospital cost and lesser length of hospital stay as compared to surgery.[2]

INDICATION[2]

- Infected abdominal collection/abscess.
- Abdominal fluid collection with suspected fistulous communication to hollow viscus.
- Symptomatic abdominal fluid collection (whether infected or not infected), e.g. pancreatic pseudocyst producing bowel or biliary obstruction.

CONTRAINDICATION[2]

There is no absolute contraindication. *However, relative contraindications are:*
- Uncorrectable coagulopathy.
- Hemodynamic instability.
- Unsafe route to abdominal fluid collection (e.g. bowel, vital solid organ or blood vessel in the path between skin and abdominal collection).
- Multiloculated abscesses, hematoma, and infected tumor—PCD may only be partially successful.
- Uncooperative patient.

APPLIED ANATOMY

A good knowledge of the regional imaging anatomy is necessary.

TECHNIQUE AND EQUIPMENT

There are two imaging-guided techniques for placing a PCD catheter into an abdominal abscess or fluid collection:[3,4]

1. *Seldinger technique*: This technique involves imaging-guided percutaneous needle puncture of the abdominal collection/abscess. A guidewire is passed through the needle into the collection/abscess over which the needle is removed and dilatation of the tract and placement of PCD catheter into the collection/abscess is done.

   Advantage

   A PCD catheter can be precisely deployed into the desired location due to the ability to direct the guidewire into that location. This is particularly helpful in large collections, e.g. large psoas abscess and also in deep-seated collections with safe but narrow percutaneous access routes, e.g. subdiaphragmatic collections.

   Disadvantages
   - Multiple serial dilatations over the guidewire may be required.
   - Buckling or kinking of the wire can occur during CT-guided PCD during the process of dilatation over the guidewire, which can lead to failure of PCD procedure.
   - Leakage of contents of the abscess/fluid collection can occur during removal of the needle and during dilatation over the guidewire. This may cause difficulty in placement of the PCD catheter into small abscesses/ fluid collections due to reduced operating space. It may also lead to spread of infectious contents into the abdominal cavity/adjacent organs.
   - The dilator and catheter may not penetrate the wall of the abscess/fluid collection due to high tissue elasticity leading to failure of PCD procedure.

2. *Trocar technique:* This technique involves image-guided direct placement of a catheter mounted on a sharp metal trocar into the abdominal abscess/ collection.

   Advantages
   - PCD catheter can be rapidly deployed.
   - This technique is preferable for large and superficial abdominal collections/abscesses and where there are no important intervening structures (e.g. bowel) between the skin and the abdominal abscess/ collection.

   Disadvantage
   Difficulty in repositioning suboptimally deployed catheters.[3]

Image Guidance Modalities for Percutaneous Drainage

Computed tomography and ultrasound are commonly used modalities for image guidance for PCD. The choice of modality depends on the Interventional Radiologist's preference, location and relationship of the collection with adjacent structures and visualization of the collection with different imaging modalities. Ultrasound is the most commonly used modality, as it is portable, easily available and free of radiation risk. Ultrasound provides real time visualization of needle,

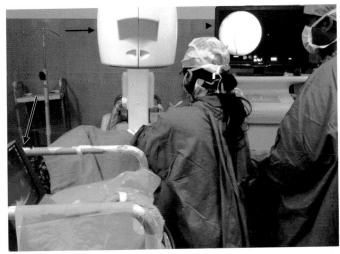

Fig. 1 Interventional radiology room equipped with C-arm fluoroscopy (straight horizontal arrow and arrowhead) and ultrasound machines (slanting black arrow)

guidewire and catheter path. Vascular structures in the needle path can be avoided by using Doppler ultrasound. Ultrasound is preferred for drainage of large and superficial collections. It can also provide access to pelvic collections by transvaginal or transrectal routes. Ultrasound can be used in concert with fluoroscopy if needed. The disadvantage of ultrasound is its inability to penetrate bone and air. It is not suited for drainage of gas-filled collections or drainage of collections deep to the bowel, e.g. pancreatic collections. CT is preferred over ultrasound for identifying the extent of the collection and for planning the access route to the collection. CT with intravenous and oral contrast helps distinguish collection from adjacent normal structures and bowel. CT is preferred for drainage of small and deep collections, air-containing collections, difficult to access collections (e.g. transgluteal route for drainage of pelvic collections). CT fluoroscopy helps precise catheter deployment and decreases procedure time.[3,5]

In the ICU setup, ultrasound is the preferred modality for image-guided PCD as it is portable and the procedure can be done at bedside. When the collection is not visualized or difficult to access by ultrasound, the patient may have to be shifted to the CT room for PCD under CT guidance. In situations where there is requirement of fluoroscopy in addition to ultrasound [e.g. in percutaneous nephrostomy (PCN) or percutaneous transhepatic biliary drainage (PTBD)], the patient may have to be shifted to the interventional radiology suite (Fig. 1).

Drainage Catheters

Most drainage catheters have an inner retention mechanism to hold the catheter within the collection/abscess. *The most commonly used percutaneous drainage catheters are the following:*

Malecot catheter: It is a radiopaque catheter with a flower at its tip. The flower has 2–4 wings, which promote catheter retention and provide enhanced drainage (Fig. 2A).

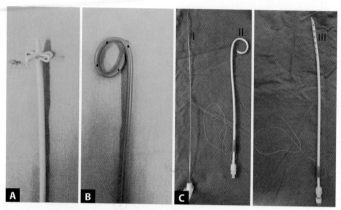

Figs 2A to C Types of percutaneous drainage catheters. (A) Malecot catheter with flower at its tip to promote enhanced drainage and catheter retention; (B) Pigtail catheter with a curled end having few side holes to promote retention; (C) (i) Straightener of Cope-loop pigtail catheter, (ii) Cope-loop pigtail catheter with a string attached to the tip of the catheter, which can be pulled and fixed at the hub end of the catheter to lock the diameter of the curled loop, (iii) Straightened out Cope-loop pigtail catheter with few side holes near its tip

Pigtail catheter: It is a radiopaque catheter with a curled end having few side holes. The curled end is deployed into the abdominal collection or abscess and serves as a self-retaining device (Fig. 2B). Pigtail catheters with locking loop mechanism are called Cope-loop pigtail catheters (Fig. 2C). A small string runs through the center of the catheter and is fixed to the distal curved end. The other end of the string exits just below the hub of the catheter. The curl on the catheter is straightened out by its inner plastic or metal stiffener or as it is advanced over a guidewire. After the stiffener and guidewire are removed, the string is pulled and tied below the hub of the catheter, which causes the distal end of the catheter to curl and lock. The fixed diameter of the locked curl prevents migration. Before removing the catheter, the hub and string are cut releasing the distal lock.

The catheter size to be used is determined by the type and character of the fluid to be drained. Air and thin fluids are drained with 8 and 10 Fr catheters. Larger diameter catheters are required for drainage of viscous fluid or fluid collections with debris. 10–14 Fr catheters may be required for complex abscesses and 24–30 Fr catheters are recommended for drainage of pancreatic and peripancreatic collections in necrotizing pancreatitis.[6,7]

PREPARATION[3,5]

- *Investigations*:
  - *Imaging*: CT, MRI and ultrasound of the patient should be obtained and reviewed to assess the route and appropriate modality to be used (Ultrasound/CT) for percutaneous drainage.
  - Recent coagulation studies—prothrombin time (PT), international normalized ratio (INR), activated partial thromboplastin time (APTT) and platelet count must be done for all patients. PT should be less than 15 sec and INR less than 1.5. Platelet count should be more than 50,000 mm³. Anticoagulant and antiplatelet medications are to be stopped. In the

presence of deranged coagulation parameters, the coagulopathy should be corrected with blood/fresh frozen plasma/platelet transfusion as required.

- Serum creatinine should be within normal limits (< 1.5 mg/dL) if drainage is to be performed under contrast-enhanced CT guidance.

- The patient should be nil per oral for 6–8 hours. Necessary medications as advised by the treating physician should be taken as usual with only a sip of water for oral medications. The dose of insulin or oral hypoglycemic agents should be adjusted as advised by the treating physician.

- Procedure details should be explained to the patient and written informed consent must be obtained.

- Intravenous access of 20 gauge or larger must be obtained.

- Preprocedure dose of suitable intravenous antibiotic should be administered.

- The procedure should preferably be performed under conscious sedation with monitoring of blood pressure, pulse and oxygen saturation.

- General anesthesia/intravenous anesthesia should be administered in children and uncooperative patients.

- Anesthesia equipment for administering local, IV and general anesthesia should be available.

- *Equipment for procedure (Figs 3A to H, 4A to C and 5A to C)*
  - 18 gauge puncture needle
  - 0.035″ or 0.38″ guidewire
  - Serial fascial dilators/Tapered dilator
  - Drainage catheters: Malecot or pigtail catheters with their plastic straighteners when using Seldinger's technique or pigtail catheter with metal trocar when using trocar method.
  - Drainage bag with markings in milliliter, e.g. Urobag, suction drainage device, underwater seal drainage bag/set.
  - Others: Povidone-iodine, sterile drapes including cut sheet, sterile gloves, No. 11 blade, silk suture, needle holder, sterile dressings, syringes, etc.

PROCEDURE

The site where the PCD catheter is to be placed is localized using Ultrasound/CT (Fig. 6A) and the overlying skin is cleaned with povidone-iodine and sterile drapes with cut hole applied at the procedure site (Fig. 6B). Local anesthesia is administered (Fig. 6C). There are two techniques for introducing a catheter into an abdominal abscess or fluid collection.[3,4]

Seldinger Technique (Figs 6A to O)

- An 18 gauge beveled needle with its stilette is inserted into an appropriate position into the abdominal collection/abscess under ultrasound guidance (Figs 6D and E).

- The stilette is removed and a sample of the draining fluid is obtained for the purpose of microbiology, culture and sensitivity.

- A J-tip/curved tip 0.035 or 0.038-inch metallic guidewire is then passed via the hub of the needle into the collection/abscess and the needle angulated so that a suitable position of the wire is achieved (Figs 6F and G).

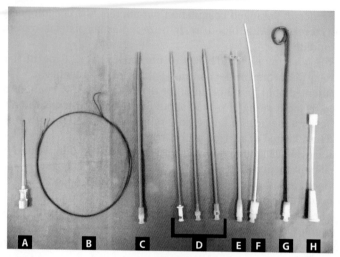

Figs 3A to H Equipment needed for PCD. (A) 18 gauge puncture needle with stilette; (B) Metallic guidewire with curved tip, e.g. Amplatz Ultra Stiff guidewire; (C) Tapered dilator; (D) Serial fascial dilators (8 F, 10 F, 12 F, etc.); (E) Malecot catheter; (F) Stiffener/Straightener of malecots catheter; (G) Pigtail catheter; (H) Connector of catheter

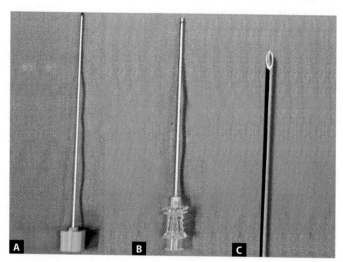

Figs 4A to C Puncture needle. (A) Cannula of puncture needle; (B) Stilette of puncture needle; (C) Close-up view showing sharp bevel of puncture needle cannula

- A small skin incision is made alongside the needle with a No. 11 surgical blade (Fig. 6H).
- The needle is removed keeping the wire *in situ*.
- A tapered dilator is passed over the guidewire into the collection/abscess under ultrasound visualization (Figs 6I and J). Alternately serial dilatation with fascial dilators can be done up to the desired size.
- The dilator is then removed, keeping the guidewire in situ. A suitable catheter (malecot/pigtail) with its straightener is then passed over the guidewire

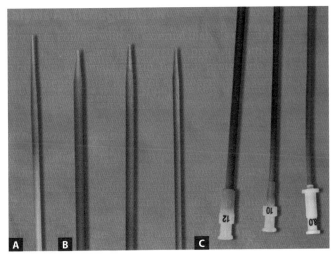

Figs 5A to C Close-up view of various dilators. (A) Leading end of tapered dilator; (B) Leading ends of serial fascial dilators showing their short taper; (C) Hub of serial fascial dilators

under ultrasound guidance into the collection/abscess cavity until the tip of the catheter has reached the desired position (Figs 6K and N). Alternately, fluoroscopy guidance can be used for final positioning of the catheter over the guidewire (Fig. 6L). Additional side holes if desired can be made in the catheter using the No. 11 surgical blade prior to deployment depending upon the length of the abdominal collection. It should be ensured that no catheter side holes are left outside the collection/abscess.

- The straightener of the catheter and guidewire is removed and the catheter is secured to the skin using nonabsorbable silk sutures (Fig. 6M).
- Dressings are applied and the drainage catheter is connected to a drainage bag (Fig. 6O).

Trocar Technique

This technique involves image-guided direct placement of a PCD catheter loaded onto a sharp metal trocar into the abdominal abscess/collection.

- A small incision is made in the skin using a No. 11 blade. The catheter mounted on the trocar is then advanced through the incision site in the abdominal collection/abscess under ultrasound guidance to an adequate position within the collection/abscess cavity.
- Alternately, initially an 18 gauge needle is positioned into the collection/ abscess under ultrasound guidance. A small incision is made in the skin alongside the needle using a No. 11 blade. The catheter loaded on the trocar is advanced parallel to the needle to a predefined location within the collection. This is called tandem trocar technique.
- The trocar is removed when an adequate position as assessed by ultrasound is reached.
- The catheter is then secured to the skin using nonabsorbable silk sutures and connected to a drainage bag.

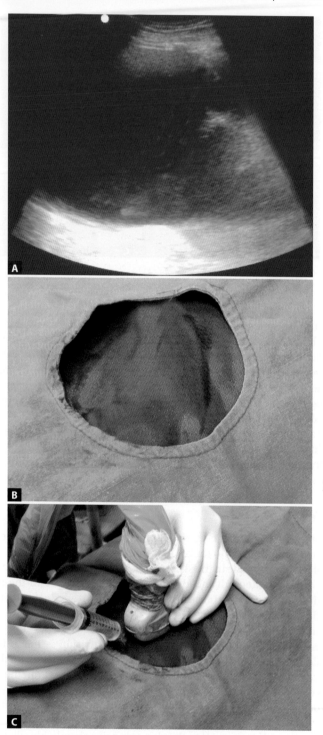

Figs 6A to C (A) Ultrasound image of an abdominal collection; (B) Access site cleaned and cut hole drape applied; (C) Administration of local anesthesia

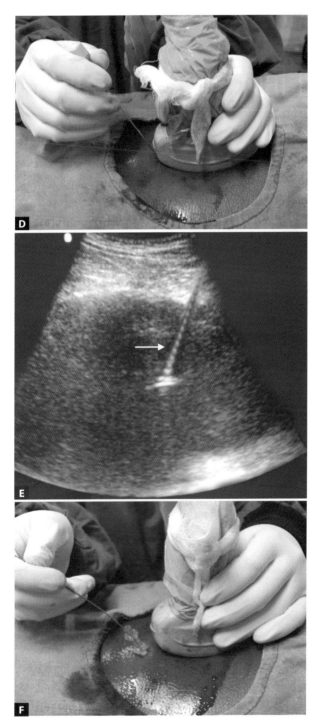

Figs 6D to F (D) Access site puncture with beveled edge needle; (E) Ultrasound image of needle tip and shaft in the collection; (F) Guidewire passed through puncture needle cannula hub after removing its stilette

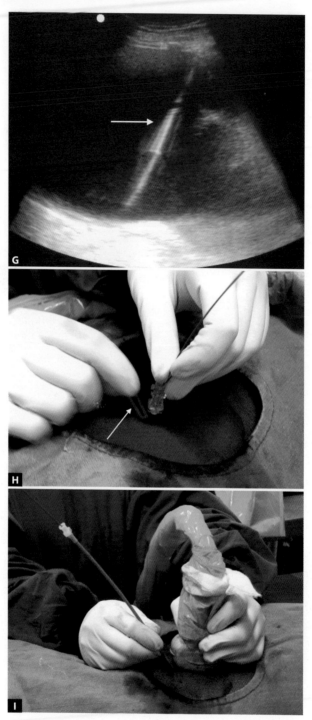

Figs 6G to I (G) Ultrasound image of guidewire passed through needle into the collection; (H) No. 11 blade used to create a small incision around cannula of needle; (I) Tapered dilator passed over the guidewire into the collection after removing the puncture needle over the guidewire

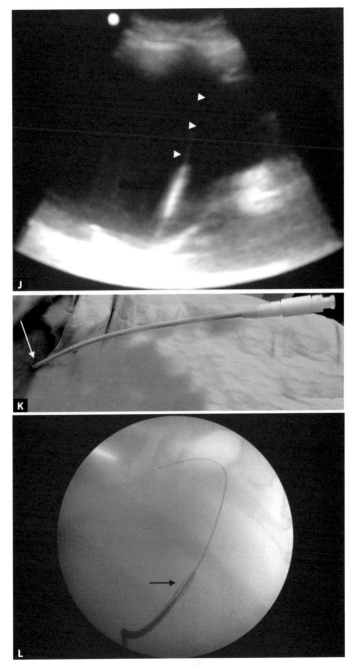

Figs 6J to L (J) Ultrasound image showing change in echogenicity of wire in the region where the dilator has passed over it; (K) Malecot catheter with its stiffener passed over the guidewire after removing the dilator; (L) Fluoroscopic image showing advancement of malecot catheter with its stiffener over guidewire into the collection

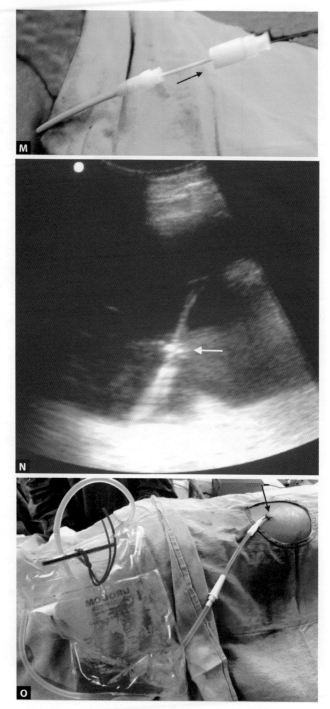

Figs 6M to O (M) Stiffener of malecot catheter detached; (N) Ultrasound image showing malecot catheter flower in the distal part of the collection after detaching stiffener; (O) Hub of malecot catheter attached to connector and connector attached to drainage bag

POST-PROCEDURE CARE[3,5]

- The patient is advised bed rest for 6 hours postprocedure with monitoring of vitals (pulse, blood pressure) and inquired regarding abdominal pain. Daily clinical rounds are taken by the interventional radiologist up to the point of catheter removal and following parameters assessed:
  - 24 hours catheter output
  - Skin access site for leakage or infection
  - Clinical signs (e.g. fever, pain) and laboratory markers (total leukocyte count) of complications or failure of PCD. Persistent fever and leukocytosis after 1–2 days of percutaneous drainage often indicates undrained pus and repeat ultrasonography/cross sectional imaging should be obtained to look for persistence of collection or other undrained collections.
- *Assessment of catheter function*
  - Normal catheter function is indicated by a gradual tapering of fluid output on a daily basis.
  - A gradual decrease in daily fluid output indicates normal catheter function. If the catheter output has markedly decreased over the last 24 hours period, flushing of the catheter with 3–5 mL of sterile normal saline should be done to ensure that it has not clogged. Further imaging may be required to look for resolution/persistence of collection and to assess catheter position/dislodgement.
  - Persistence of fluid collection may require catheter exchange, flushing or upsizing. Kinks in drainage catheter causing its obstruction may require catheter exchange. Viscous collections require more aggressive flushing and catheter diameter may have to be upsized. Multiple catheters may be required.
  - Complex multiseptated collections may respond to intracavitary instillation of thrombolytic agents (streptokinase, urokinase, tissue plasminogen activator). Thrombolytics disrupt fibrin strands in the septations and help drainage of the collection.
  - Catheter dislodgement usually requires a new percutaneous drain. Catheter repositioning may be required if an inadequately draining catheter does not extend across the maximum length of the collection.
- *Catheter removal*: May be considered when the following conditions are met:
  - Obvious clinical improvement
  - Gradual decrease in PCD catheter output to lesser than 10 mL per 24 hours
  - Normalization of leukocyte counts
  - Repeat USG/Cross-sectional imaging suggests significant resolution of collection/abscess cavity.

COMPLICATION/PROBLEM[3,5]

- *Infection:* This may be of following types.
  - Spread of abscess content to the adjacent spaces or organs.
  - *Bacteremia and sepsis*: Transient bacteremia is seen in 5% cases. It occurs due to spill of infected material into the blood and presents with fever with chills and rigor. Cardiopulmonary collapse may occur rarely. Only a few deaths have been reported.

- *Local infection at the skin access*: Occurs with prolonged catheter drainage. It is managed with antibiotics based on culture and sensitivity, antiseptic dressings (iodoform gauze) and catheter change/removal or a new PCD catheter from a different site. In patients with severe infection, surgical management may be required.

Prevention

- Supportive measures such as cardiopulmonary resuscitation equipment, intravenous antibiotics, and pethidine (for management of rigors) should be readily available and administered immediately when required.
- Contrast injection into the abscess cavity/collection should not be done as far as possible as it may cause over-distention of the cavity leading to spillage of infected contents into blood or adjacent spaces with resultant bacteremia or peritonitis. It should only be done in difficult situations to guide catheter placement or rarely to confirm access into abscess cavity/collection.
- Potentially infectious routes (e.g. transvaginal or transrectal routes for drainage of pelvic collections) should be avoided if possible.
- New sterile equipment should be used for drainage of each collection in cases with multiple fluid collections to prevent cross-contamination.

- *Fistulous communication to bowel, biliary tree or urinary system*: A fistulous connection may be present prior to PCD or may occur during PCD due to traversal of the catheter through bowel. This is indicated by persistent output of large volume of fluid from the PCD catheter, which may contain enteric/tube feed/fecal contents, bile or urine. An "abscessogram/cavitogram" under fluoroscopy can be done to confirm the fistulous communication.

- *Non-target catheterization or puncture*: Inadvertent PCD catheter traversal through the intestine, liver, spleen and stomach has been reported. PCD catheter traversal through small bowel presents with high output of bowel contents from the catheter or bowel obstruction and may not have serious consequences but catheter traversal through the colon may lead to life-threatening peritonitis and sepsis. In all cases of bowel traversal, a surgical consultation should be obtained. If peritoneal signs and sepsis are not present, the patient can be managed with bowel rest and antibiotics. Withdrawal of the catheter can be done when a mature tract has formed. This can be confirmed with an "over-the-wire tractogram" done with contrast injection under fluoroscopy. Slow withdrawal of the catheter can be done over days to weeks to allow time for the enterocutaneous tract to close.

  Catheter traversal through solid parenchymal organs may result in parenchymal, subcapsular or peritoneal bleeding. Patients who do not present with significant bleeding can be managed with catheter removal following adequate tract formation or catheter removal with embolization of the tract with gelfoam pledgets. Patients who present with significant bleed due to pseudoaneurysm and arteriovenous fistula formation require transarterial embolization or surgery.

  Prevention: Administration of contrast via the mouth, rectum or stoma prior to CT-guided drainage decreases the risk of PCD catheter traversal through the bowel.

- *Bleeding*: Injury to adjacent vessels can occur during PCD. Vessel injury is suggested by sudden onset of bloody output via the catheter or pericatheter.

Temporary capping, upsizing, or repositioning of the catheter may tamponade acute bleeding. Intravenous fluids and blood transfusion should be started when indicated. Imaging should be obtained in cases of persistent bleeding. Bleeding from small vessel lacerations, pseudoaneurysms and arteriovenous fistulae require endovascular transcatheter embolization. In cases with large vessel injury, a surgical consultation should be obtained. The catheter should not be prematurely removed as it may result in catastrophic bleeding.

Prevention

- Doppler ultrasound should be used to avoid vascular structures during ultrasound-guided drainage procedures.
- Seldinger technique should be preferred in cases where the risk of bleeding is high. Narrow bore puncture needles and drainage catheters (6–8 Fr) can be used for initial drainage. Catheters can be upsized at a later date.

REFERENCES

1. Marshall JC, Innes M. Intensive care unit management of intra-abdominal infection. Crit Care Med. 2003;31(8):2228-37.
2. Wallace MJ, Chin KW, Fletcher TB, Bakal CW, Cardella JF, Grassi CJ, et al. Quality improvement guidelines for percutaneous drainage/aspiration of abscess and fluid collections. J Vasc Interv Radiol. 2010;21(4):431-5.
3. Thabet A, Arellano RS. Catheter drainage of abdominal abscesses and fluid collections. In: Kandarpa K, Machan L (Eds). Handbook of Interventional Radiologic Procedures, 4th edition. Philadelphia: Lippincott Williams & Wilkins. 2011. pp. 527-34.
4. Gervais DA, Brown SD, Connolly SA, Brec SL, Harisinghani MG, Mueller PR. Percutaneous imaging-guided abdominal and pelvic abscess drainage in children. Radiographics. 2004;24(3):737-54.
5. Lorenz J, Thomas JL. Complications of percutaneous fluid drainage. Semin Intervent Radiol. 2006;23(2):194-204.
6. Nair AV, D'Agostino HR. Transcatheter fluid drainage. In: Valji K (Ed). The Practice of Interventional Radiology with Online Cases and Videos, 1st edition. Philadelphia, Pa: Elsevier Saunders. 2012. pp. 106-25.
7. Shenoy-Bhangle AS, Gervais DA. Use of fibrinolytics in abdominal and pleural collections. Semin Intervent Radiol. 2012;29(4):264-9.

48

Bedside Laparoscopy

Biju Pottakkat

INTRODUCTION

Acute abdominal conditions like acute pancreatitis, acute cholecystitis, mesenteric ischemia, hollow viscous perforation, diverticulitis, post-traumatic bleeding, intra-abdominal abscess, etc. are frequently encountered in patients admitted in critical care units. The interpretation of standard bedside modalities like clinical examination and ultrasonography in diagnosing suspected abdominal conditions in critically ill patients is challenging due to factors like low level of consciousness, high threshold for stimulus, absence of reflexes, abdominal wall edema, effects of medications, presence of transudative fluid in the peritoneal cavity, bowel distention, dyselectrolytemia and postoperative status. Usage of computed tomography (CT) or magnetic resonance imaging are sometimes limited by risk related to the transport of critically ill patient to radiology suite, time taken for the examination, renal failure risking contrast nephropathy and the inability to introduce adequate oral contrast agents due to paralytic ileus and delayed gastric emptying. Diagnostic peritoneal lavage has limited specificity in critically ill patients with suspected intra-abdominal conditions as presence of blood cells, bacteria or amylase in the peritoneal fluid may not prompt a laparotomy. The maximally invasive approach like diagnostic and therapeutic laparotomy cause major stress in an already physiologically compromised patient. Direct visualization of the peritoneal cavity and intra-abdominal organs through small incisions using telescopes (laparoscopy) can be utilized as a diagnostic and therapeutic tool and is already well established in various acute and chronic abdominal conditions. An abdominal condition which can make the patient critically ill will be usually evident on laparoscopy. Considering all these factors, the role of bedside laparoscopy (BSL) is becoming relevant.

Bedside laparoscopy is a modality in which the abdominal cavity with intra-abdominal organs is inspected through sub-centimeter incisions using telescopes and therapeutic procedures are executed in specific feasible circumstances through laparoscopic techniques on bedside.

INDICATION

Major trauma, systemic sepsis of suspected abdominal source and post-cardiac operation status constitute the majority of patients undergoing BSL. A patient based multifactorial decision making process has to be followed before selecting patients for BSL. Bedside diagnostic laparoscopy could be considered if clinical signs and/or laboratory and/or imaging findings were suggestive, but not conclusive, for intra-abdominal cause. BSL is employed in the following situations in an ICU patient.

Diagnostic

- Suspected bowel gangrene
- Re-look laparoscopy after laparotomy for suspected bowel ischemia.
- Suspected hollow viscous perforation
- Suspicion of acute pancreatitis despite negative findings on imaging.
- Suspected slippage of percutaneous gastrostomy or jejunostomy tubes.
- Re-look laparoscopy after temporary tamponade for bleeding in trauma.

Therapeutic

- To drain localized collections
- Insertion of peritoneal drains
- To take tissue samples for biopsy, e.g., liver biopsy along with diagnostic laparoscopy.

  With the availability of better helical CT which can help in virtual visualization of intra-abdominal viscera, BSL cannot be considered as an alternative tool if CT can be performed.

CONTRAINDICATION

- Patient with very high ventilatory support who may deteriorate after pneumo-peritoneum.
- High intra-abdominal pressure (above 15 mm Hg) measured by intravesical pressure measurement.
- Uncorrected coagulopathy
- Significant bowel distention which prevents port placement.

PREPARATION

- Informed consent
- Measure intravesical pressure
- Correct coagulopathy
- Maintain blood pressure adequately with optimum inotropes.
- Check availability of bottles for collecting fluid and specimens.
- *Staff*: One surgeon and one assistant surgeon, one anesthetist, two nurses.

TECHNIQUE AND EQUIPMENT

An experienced surgeon who is well familiar with the expected finding in acute abdominal conditions is required to perform the BSL quickly and effectively in an already sick patient. Some of the conditions can be spot diagnostic. General anesthesia is to be achieved by standard induction, maintenance and neuromuscular blockade. Patient has to be restrained to the bed. Trendelenburg or anti-Trendelenburg position is used as required. Unlike operation table, as side tilt of the bed is not possible usually and hence pillows for side elevation can be used instead. The entire diagnostic BSL procedure usually takes less than 40 minutes.

A decision can be expected in 70% of patients. The requirement for open surgery depends on the suspected intra-abdominal condition and open diagnostic laparotomy can be avoided in up to two-thirds of patients in whom laparotomy is planned. Those who undergo open operation are mainly patients with mesenteric ischemia.

Equipment required include direct vision ports, optical trocars of 5 mm and 10 mm, zero and 30 degree 10 mm and 5 mm telescopes, camera, monitor, insufflator, basic laparoscopy instruments like dissector, grasper, bowel holding forceps, suction irrigation cannula, electrocoagulator, basic open surgical instruments, suture materials and light.

PROCEDURE

After putting the patient on full general anesthesia, abdomen is cleaned and draped with povidone-iodine 3%. Small subumbilical incision is made and umbilical port is inserted under direct vision. Veress needle is not advised as it may puncture a distended bowel. In patients with previous laparotomy, introduce blind tipped trocar through the incision. Introduce the pneumoperitoneum with carbon dioxide very slowly after watching the effects of abdominal distention on the blood pressure. Keep the intra-abdominal pressure below 15 mm Hg.

Introduce the laparoscope and look for findings. Always put additional ports for introducing instruments for retraction and visualization. Always take sample of peritoneal fluid for bacterial culture and amylase estimation. Proceed visualization from superior to inferior as the Trendelenburg position at the end of examination may help both in inspection of the pelvis as well as to prevent further drop in blood pressure.

Following findings needs to be observed.
- Look for free fluid and its nature. Always expect some amount of peritoneal fluid in critically ill patients. Bile may suggest a gallbladder perforation, enteric content is suggestive of hollow viscous perforation.
- Saponification of omental fat suggests acute pancreatitis.
- Look liver to see congestion which may suggest hepatitis. Nodular liver suggests cirrhosis.
- Look for infected collections in subphrenic, perihepatic, perisplenic, pelvic and paracolic spaces.
- Retrogastric phlegmon suggests acute pancreatitis.
- Look for color of the jejunal and ileal loops to rule out mesenteric ischemia.
- Look for the gallbladder for inflammation or perforation, pericholecystic fluid and spilled stones.
- Look first part of duodenum and distal ileum to rule out perforation, appendix for acute appendicitis and sigmoid colon for diverticulitis.
- Look ovaries for ruptured ectopic pregnancy.
- Look spleen for bleeding lesions and lacerations.

Therapeutic BSL can be used for drainage of infected collections, introduce peritoneal drains and for peritoneal lavage. Therapeutic surgical procedures like appendectomy or cholecystectomy is better avoided in a non-operation theater environment.

At the end of laparoscopic examination, wash the peritoneal cavity thoroughly and suck out all fluid if an additional port is already inserted. If a surgically correctable pathology is diagnosed on laparoscopy, shift the patient to operation room as soon as possible for the definite procedure.

POST-PROCEDURE CARE

Watch for port site bleeding and bleeding through drains if inserted.

COMPLICATION/PROBLEM

The complication rate is less than 10%.
- Patients with cardiac diseases constitute a risk group for post BSL complications.
- Ventilatory support and inotropic support may increase after BSL.
- Port site infection can occur. Intra-abdominal and port site bleeding may happen in patients with coagulopathy.
- Ascites leakage through peri-drain area and ports can be a complication which can delay healing.

SUGGESTED READING

1. Bender JS, Talamini MA. Diagnostic laparoscopy in critically ill intensive-care-unit patients. Surg Endosc. 1992;6(6):302-4.
2. Ceribelli C, Adami EA, Mattia S, Benini B. Bedside diagnostic laparoscopy for critically ill patients: a retrospective study of 62 patients. Surg Endosc. 2012;26(12):3612-5.
3. Jaramillo EJ, Treviño JM, Berghoff KR, Franklin ME Jr. Bedside diagnostic laparoscopy in the intensive care unit: a 13-year experience. JSLS. 2006;10(2):155-9.
4. Karasakalides A, Triantafillidou S, Anthimidis G, Ganas E, Mihalopoulou E, Lagonidis D, et al. The use of bedside diagnostic laparoscopy in the intensive care unit. J Laparoendosc Adv Surg Tech A. 2009;19(3):333-8.
5. Kelly JJ, Puyana JC, Callery MP, Yood SM, Sandor A, Litwin DE. The feasibility and accuracy of diagnostic laparoscopy in the septic ICU patient. Surg Endosc. 2000;14(7):617-21.
6. Peris A, Matano S, Manca G, Zagli G, Bonizzoli M, Cianchi G, et al. Bedside diagnostic laparoscopy to diagnose intra-abdominal pathology in the intensive care unit. Crit Care. 2009;13(1):R25.
7. Walsh RM, Popovich MJ, Hoadley J. Bedside diagnostic laparoscopy and peritoneal lavage in the intensive care unit. Surg Endosc. 1998;12(12):1405-9.

49

Dynamic Abdominal Wall Closure for Open Abdomen

Fahri Yetisir, A Ebru Salman, Oskay Kaya

INTRODUCTION

If abdominal closure takes more than 7 days for any reason, risks of serious complications (such as large abdominal wall defects, fistula, giant ventral hernias) and mortality rates increase.[1,2] Temporary abdominal closure (TAC) system is very important in the management of open abdomen. Several TAC systems have been proven to decrease mortality and early postoperative complications and increase the chance of definitive closure of open abdomen.[2,3] There are lots of advantages and disadvantage of TAC systems, which are listed in Table 1. The dynamic wound closure for open abdomen systems [Abdominal reapproximation anchor system (ABRA)® Canica, Almonte, Ontario, Canada] provides dynamic reduction of retracted abdominal defects with the goal of maintaining or restoring the definitive primary closure option by transfacial elastomers.[4,5] The dynamic wound closure system has three different types of product named as Surgical Skin Closure, Adhesive Skin Closure and Abdominal Wall Closure system for different type of wound.

ABRA and VAC (vacuum-assisted closure) therapy can be used together so that dynamic traction was provided by ABRA, and drainage of abdominal exudate and reduction of edema were ensured by VAC dressing. This combination of ABRA with VAC therapy is the most ideal. TAC method for open abdomen management according to recent literature (Table 1).[6,7]

INDICATION

Abdominal reapproximation anchor system is designed for the delayed definitive closure of almost all open abdomens. It is based on continuous dynamic tension to achieve reapproximation of the fascia edges of the abdominal wall by adjustable transfacial elastomers.[4]

CONTRAINDICATION

There is no known contraindication of ABRA during management of open abdomen. We can use ABRA for reapproximation of all the retracted open abdomen. However, the important point is timing and duration of application.

Table 1 Advantages and disadvantages of temporary abdominal closure methods

No:\nYes:+	1\nEvacuation of exudates	2\nReduction of edema	3\nCheap	4\nMinimizing heat and fluid loss	5\nReducing the risk of evisceration	6\nMaintenance of abdominal domain	7\nEasy to apply	8\nKeeping the patient dry	9\nReducing the incidence of ACS	10\nAllowing multiple abdominal re-explorations	11\nDynamic (It can change according to abdominal pressure)	12\nUsing successfully in the presence of infection	13\nReducing the damage to the skin or fascia	14\nReducing development of giant hernia	Total number of yes
Skin approximation	–	–	+	–	–	–	+	+	–	+	–	–	–	–	4
Bogota bag	–	–	+	–	–	–	+	–	+	+	–	–	–	–	4
Absorbable mesh	–	–	–	–	+	+	–	–	–	–	–	–	–	+	3
Marlex with zipper	–	–	–	–	+	+	–	–	–	+	–	–	–	+	4
Wittman patch	–	–	–	–	+	+	–	–	–	+	–	–	–	+	4
Retension suture	–	–	+	–	–	+	+	–	–	–	–	+	–	–	4
Ramirez compartment separation technique	–	–	+	+	+	+	–	+	–	–	–	–	–	–	5
ABRA	–	–	–	–	+	+	+	–	+	+	+	+	+	+	9
VAC therapy	+	+	–	+	–	–	+	+	+	+	+	+	+	–	10
ABRA and VAC therapy	+	+	–	+	+	+	+	+	+	+	+	+	+	+	13

The earlier we can start application of ABRA, the more we can increase the chance of treatment success by shortening the duration of the treatment. Furthermore, this system should be used by a qualified surgical practitioner.

TECHNIQUE

There are many TAC techniques for management of open abdomen. Most famous TAC systems, which are skin approximation, Bogota bag, absorbable mesh, Marlex with zipper, Wittman patch, retention suture and Ramirez compartment separation technique have been used. Due to their limitations and disadvantages, success rates of these TAC techniques are not very high (Table 1).

For management of open abdomen, an ideal TAC technique must prevent evisceration and loss of domain, preserve fascia and skin and minimize damage to the viscera. It can be used successfully in the presence of infection, by evacuating exudates, lowering bacterial counts, reducing edema and inflammation and minimizing heat and fluid loss. It should keep the patient dry and intact. It must be dynamic, cheap and easy to apply. It should offer the advantage of reducing the incidence of abdominal compartment syndrome (ACS), development of giant hernia.[6-9] In our previous studies combination of ABRA with VAC therapy seem to be the most suitable TAC technique providing all these requirements.[6,7] The combination of both techniques has been successful in providing 13 of 14 requirement of ideal TAC (Table 1).

Abdominal reapproximation anchor system has two main parts; anchors and elastomers. During application, cannulator and lancet are used. Elastomers pass through full thickness of abdominal wall (skin, adipose tissue and fascia) minimum 5 cm lateral from wound margin. Abdominal content is covered with silicon sheet. Abdominal domain is maintained and wound edge is drawn toward midline in a constantly dynamic way by elastomer (Fig. 1).

PREPARATION

Abdominal reapproximation anchor system should be applied in operating room in complete sterile condition under general anesthesia. The entire abdomen,

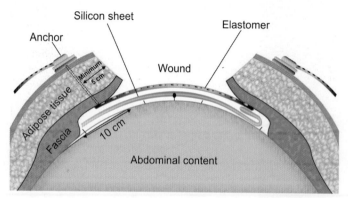

Fig 1 Schematic illustration of ABRA application to open abdomen

extending 20–25 cm from each wound margin should be shaved and cleaned. All necrotic tissue, adhesions between abdominal content and wall should be excised to create clean, mobile abdominal wall wound margins. The whole abdominal content including the all recesses should be washed with warm normal saline and cleaned (Fig. 2).

PROCEDURE

- With a skin marker, draw placement margins at 5 cm from the wound edge and 3–5 cm intervals starting from the upper aspect of the wound to lower aspect (Fig. 2).
- Following the marks on the layout, make 3 mm holes in the skin by using electrocautery.
- The fat and muscle tissues and the fascia are divided by the help of the cannulator. Elastomers are passed through full thickness of the abdominal wall at both sides by the help of cannulator (Fig. 3).
- Anchors are installed to each end of the elastomers at both sides.
- In order to protect abdominal content is covered with the silicone viscera protector sheet. To prevent adhesions, the silicone sheet must extend beyond the elastomer entry points.
- Elastomers are stretched up to 1.5–2 times of their nontensioned length (Fig. 4). The black bars on the elastomer provide a visual indication of elastomer tension. It is critical to set and maintain appropriate elastomer tensions at all times. Failure to maintain correct elastomer tensions will reduce system effectiveness. Tension of all elastomers is controlled. We try to make around 2 times tension at the center of wound and 1.5 times tension at the lateral sides. After that, VAC therapy is applied over the ABRA (Figs 5 and 6).

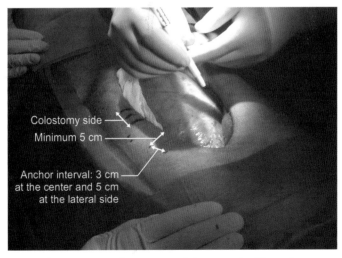

Fig. 2 Drawing of entry point of elastomers by skin marker

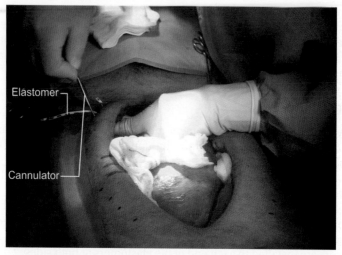

Fig. 3 Passing of elastomers through full thickness of abdominal wall by the help of cannula

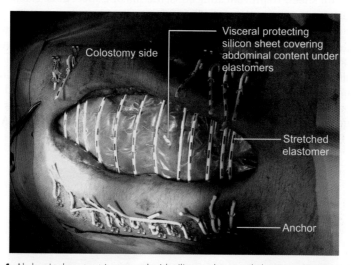

Fig. 4 Abdominal content is covered with silicone sheet and elastomers are stretched

POST-PROCEDURE CARE

Patient's general conditions, wound status, working of applied systems (ABRA and VAC therapy) whether proper or not are controlled every day. VAC dressing is changed every 2–4 days and at the same time the tension of elastomer is readjusted. When two edge of wound come across fascia is closed completely by polydioxanone suture (PDS) 1/0 suture firstly, 2 days later, if there is no problem; skin is also closed. One week after skin closure, anchors of ABRA are removed (Fig. 7).

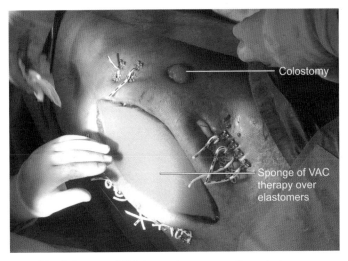

Fig. 5 Sponge of VAC therapy is seen over silicon elastomers

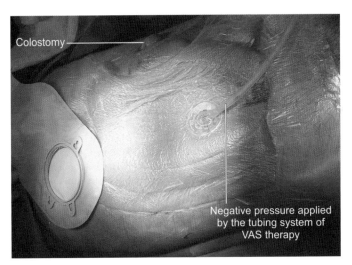

Fig. 6 Application of VAC therapy over ABRA was complete

COMPLICATION/PROBLEM

If it is a long-term treatment, serious pressure sores on the edges of the wound may occur, depending on compression of the anchors. Tension of elastomer should be controlled and readjusted if needed. It is very important to prevent the development of pressure sores, otherwise management of these sores and related infections can be very difficult.

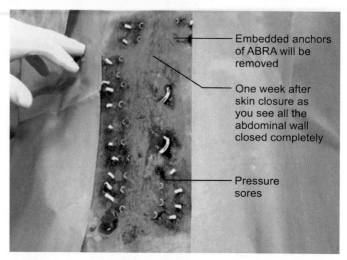

Embedded anchors of ABRA will be removed

One week after skin closure as you see all the abdominal wall closed completely

Pressure sores

Fig. 7 One week after skin closure anchors of ABRA will be removed

REFERENCES

1. Regner JL, Kobayashi L, Coimbra R. Surgical strategies for management of the abdomen. World J Surg. 2012;36:497-510.
2. Cano-Lopez M, Armengol-Carrasco M. Use of vacuum-assisted closure in open incisional hernia repair: a novel approach to prevent seroma formation. Hernia. 2013;17(1):129-31.
3. Björck M, D'Amours SK, Hamilton AE. Closure of open abdomen. Am Surg. 2011;77(1):S58–61.
4. Reimer MV, Yelle JD, Reitsma B, Doumit G, Allen MA, Bell MS. Management of open abdominal wounds with a dynamic fascial closure system. Can J Surg. 2008;51:209-14.
5. Urbaniak RM, Khuthaila DK, Khalil AJ, Hammond DC. Closure of massive abdominal wall defects: a case report using the abdominal reapproximation anchor (ABRA) system. Ann Plast Surg. 2006;57:573-7.
6. Salman AE, Yetisir F, Aksoy M, Tokac M, Yildirim MB, Kilic M. Use of dynamic wound closure system in conjunction with vacuum-assisted closure therapy in delayed closure of open abdomen. Hernia. 2014;18(1):99-104.
7. Yetisir F, Salman AE, Özdemir F, Durak D, Özlü O, KılıçM. Modified application of dynamic wound closure system in the management of septic open abdomen. World J Trauma and Crit Care Med. 2013;1:1-8.
8. Kaplan M, Banwell P, Orgill DP, Ivatury RR, Demetriades D, Moore FA, et al. Guidelines for the management of the open abdomen. Supplement to wounds: 2005;17(Suppl 1): 1-24.
9. Losanoff JE, Richman BW, Jones JW. Temporary abdominal coverage and reclosure of the open abdomen: frequently asked questions. J Am Coll Surg. 2002;195:105-15.

50

Urethral Catheterization

Vijai Datta Upadhyaya, Eti Sthapak

INTRODUCTION

Urinary catheterization involves insertion of hollow tubular instrument into urinary bladder via urethra through urinary meatus. Few indwelling catheters can be secured in bladder by inflating the balloon. In males, catheterization is found to be more difficult because of natural curvature, narrow (anatomical) sites and its long length compared to females. One should be very cautious while putting urinary catheter in an individual with urethral stricture or suspected urethral injury to avoid false passage.

INDICATION

- Acute urinary retention
- Chronic urinary retention if associated with symptoms or have back pressure changes
- Monitoring of renal function
- Postoperative period
- To bypass any obstruction
- To collect sterile urine specimen.

CONTRAINDICATION

Absolute

Suspected traumatic injury to lower urinary tract, which may be indicated by history of pelvic or straddle type injury. The signs of suspicious injury are high ridding or boggy prostrate, perineal hematoma or blood at the external urinary meatus.

Relative

- Urethral stricture
- Recent urethral or bladder surgery
- Uncooperative patient.

APPLIED ANATOMY

The urethra in males is relatively fixed at the level of the urogenital diaphragm and pubic symphysis. Downward traction on the penis promote urethral folding making it difficult to catheterize at the level of the suspensory ligament (Fig. 1). Usual length of the male urethra is around 20 cm. The male urethra is divided into three part, namely—penile urethra (largest part), membranous urethra (around 4 cm) and prostatic urethra (3.5 cm).

TECHNIQUE AND EQUIPMENT

The word "catheter" originated from Greek word, which means "to let or send down". From way back 3000 BC for relieving pain from retained urine, during that period straw, rolled up palm leaves and hollow tops of onions are used as a catheter. In 11th century, malleable catheters were developed and in 18th century rubber catheters were introduced. The revolutionary change in catheter system came in 1953 when Dr Frederic EB Foley introduced latex balloon catheter, which now properly called as Foley catheter.

Duration of catheterization: When catheterization is required for less than 2 weeks is termed as short-term catheterization, when it is required for 2–5 weeks it is termed as intermediate-term catheterization. When it is necessary to keep catheter for more than 6 weeks it is termed as long-term catheterization. The catheter material will determine the duration of catheter stay (see here).

Catheters

Type

- *Foley catheter:* This is an indwelling urinary catheter, which prevent the tube from sliding out because of balloon at the tip, which can be inflated with sterile water (Fig. 2).

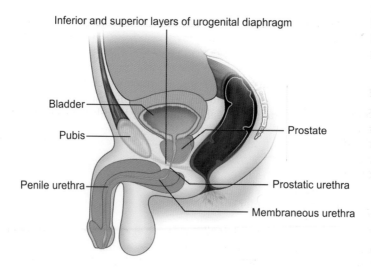

Fig. 1 The anatomy of the male urethra

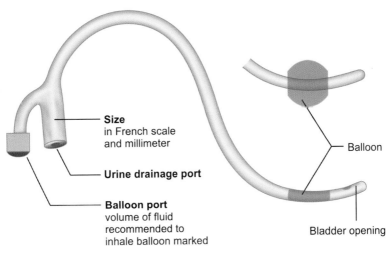

Fig. 2 The parts of Foley catheter

- *Robinson catheter*: These are catheter usually used for short term or as intermittent catheterization.
- *Coudé catheter*: This catheter is designed for the cases where negotiation of catheter is difficult in prostatic urethra (swollen prostrate); the upward curvature of the tip of the catheter facilitates the passage through the natural curvature of prostatic urethra.
- *Hematuria catheter*: This is a triple or double-lumen catheter used for post TURP patients to control hemostasis. This is a variant of Foley catheter.

Size and Length

- Catheter diameter is measured in French (Fr or Ch) units. In diameter it ranges from 6 Fr to 22 Fr. Color coding at the funnel end help in easy identification of different size of Foley catheter.
- Foley catheter available in 6–12 inches length. The catheter with length of 12 inches (about 40 cm) is used for adult male and shorter length catheters (20–40 cm) are used in children and females.

Tips

- *Straight tip*: This type of Foley catheter is used for normal catheterization, the tip is tapered to pass smoothly through the urethra.
- *Coudé tip*: This is type of Foley catheter, which has curved tip and used for cases with enlarged prostrate or narrow urethra.
- *Olive tip*: Used in females.

Material

- Urethral catheters were originally made of natural latex rubber, and were prone to infection, toxicity and hypersensitivity. PTFE (polytetrafluoroethylene) provides no advantage over latex catheter. Both, PTFE and latex catheter could be used for short to intermediate-term catheterization.

- Polyvinyl chloride and polyethylene catheters are recommended for short-term postoperative period because of wide lumen, which facilitates rapid flow of urine.
- For long-term catheterization silicone catheters should be used. These catheters usually have wider lumen. It also reduces the urethritis and decreases the chances of urethral stricture in long term.

Catheter selection: The catheter should be selected on the basis of need of catheterization, duration of catheter needed and tip design. Whistle tip enable larger drainage area hence are appropriate for cases where debris or clot is suspected and Roberts's catheter facilitates drainage of residual urine.

- *Size selection as per age*
  Less than 6 months: Feeding tube (5 Fr)
  6 months – 2 years: 8 Fr
  3 years – 7 years: 10 Fr
  8 years – 12 years: 12 Fr
  12 years and adults: Foley (straight tip) catheter (16–18 Fr)
      Children (how to decide the size of Foley); Divide the age (in years) of child by 2 and then add 8 to get the exact size of catheter in children.
- *Other special condition*
  - *Adult males with obstruction of prostatic urethra:* Coudé tip (18 Fr)
  - *Gross hematuria:* Foley catheter (20–24 Fr) or 3-way irrigation catheter (20–30 Fr)

PREPARATION

- Consent (as per hospital policy)
- *Equipment needed:* appropriate size urethral catheter, disposable sterile towel and drapes, sterile gauze pieces, two pair of sterile gloves, sterile lubricating (water soluble) jelly, cleansing solution (antiseptic solution), sterile water, syringe and needle, closed urinary drainage system including urinometer.

PROCEDURE (IN MALE PATIENT)

- Steps should be explained to the patient at the beginning (explaining the steps and what we want from patient will relax the patient and avoid the anxiety of the patients).
- Ask the patient to lie on his back with leg should be open (this maneuver will relax the bladder and urethra). Proper position for catheterization is supine with frog-leg position, with knees flexed. It is difficult to insert catheter in tense urethra and may cause complication (opening the leg will ensure the penis is accessible).
- Wash hand properly and put on the gloves (gloves are important part of personal protective equipment of health care worker and it make the procedure sterile and minimize the risk of infection).
- Open the appropriate size Foley catheter in sterile manner and make all other arrangements ready, like, sterile syringe, Urobag, sterile water and cleansing solution and drapes. Choose correct size of catheter. If contaminated urine is expected than the accepted size is 16 Fr but if gross contamination or

hematuria is likely than 18 Fr catheter size will be more appropriate.[1-3] It is also important to check the competency of the balloon and the patency of the catheter before insertion.

- Paint the genital area with cleansing solution, lift the penis, paint it, clean the foreskin and then retract the foreskin; if foreskin is present for proper exposure of glans by using gauze swab. It should be kept in mind that cleansing should be done from inside to outside not in reverse manner (Fig. 3).
- Drape should be placed properly in sterile manner (the genital should be exposed properly for inserting the catheter but meanwhile other area should be covered to maintain the sterility). By lifting the penis, penile urethra can be made straightens which facilitates the catheterization (Fig. 4).[4,5]
- Apply lubricant to the distal part of the catheter with balloon deflated, insert 10–15 mL of local anesthetic gel in the urethra slowly (Fig. 5), after inserting gel penis should be held properly to close external urethral meatus between the thumb and finger (Fig. 6) to avoid leakage of gel.[2,6] It is mandatory to wait for 2 to 4 minutes after putting lidocaine jelly in urethra.[2,4,5] This will minimize the discomfort to the patient by pain relief and will also reduce the friction of catheter to mucosal surface, which will facilitate smooth insertion while catheterization.
- The gloves should be replaced with new sterile gloves after this stage and place new sterile drape around the penis (this will prepare sterile filed for catheterization).
- Hold the penis in one hand and insert the catheter into the urethral meatus with other hand taking care of sterility (Fig. 7). The catheter should be advance in the urethra gently (2–3 cm at a time)[1] and once urine flow begins continue to push the catheter into the bladder another 2 inches to ensure that it has reached the bladder[6] preferably insert the catheter up to bifurcation mark (Fig. 8) and palpate the catheter against bladder neck. Always ensure that urine is flowing from the catheter (Fig. 9). In case there is no flow of urine even

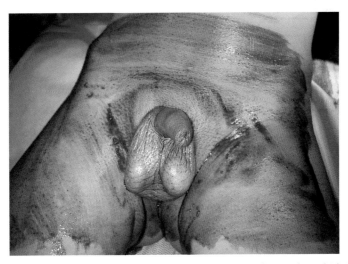

Fig. 3 Proper painting area for urethral catheterization using povidone-iodine which includes the genital, thigh and lower abdomen

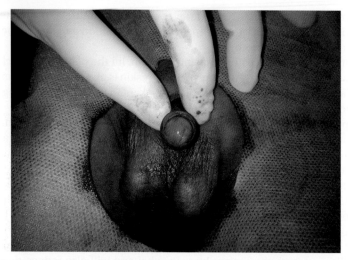

Fig. 4 Properly drape the area with sterile sheet and retract the prepuce to open the glans for clear visualization of urinary meatus

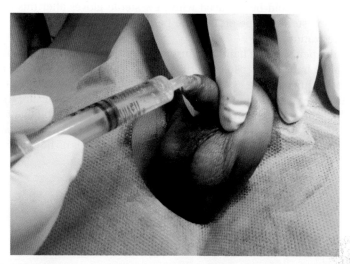

Fig. 5 Installation of the local anesthetic (lignocaine jelly) with the help of syringe

after pushing whole of the catheter, a gentle pressure should be applied over the pubic symphysis area.[7,8] Also ensure that lumen is not kinked/blocked which usually occur in smaller size catheter. Do not inflate the balloon unless the urine flow is seen.

- Inflate the balloon with appropriate volume of sterile water (Fig. 10) as indicated on the catheter.[8,9] The volume of the balloon varies according to the size of Foley catheter like it is 5 mL for pediatric Foley and it ranged from 10 mL to 30 mL depending on the size and type of Foley, but care should be taken that amount installed in balloon should not exceed the upper limit

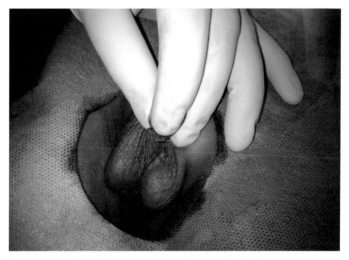

Fig. 6 Closing the tip of the penis with thumb after installing the local anesthetic or one can hold the penis between two fingers

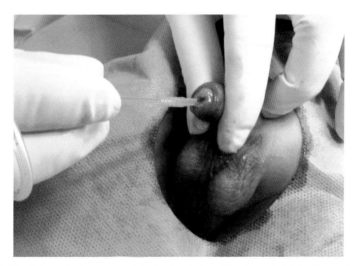

Fig. 7 Gently introducing appropriate sized catheter with adequate lubrication and slowly progress it into the bladder

as mentioned on the Foley.[1] The following substance should be avoided for filling the balloon—air, nonsterile water and normal saline.

- Withdraw the catheter slightly to place it in the dependable position and attach the drainage bag (Fig. 11) (withdrawing the catheter will ensure proper placement of catheter at bladder base for optimal drainage of urine). On desire of patient catheter may be secured taking care that the catheter is not taut.
- Clean the glans after the procedure. It is very important to reposit the foreskin (retraction of the prepuce) to avoid paraphimosis after catheterization.[6]

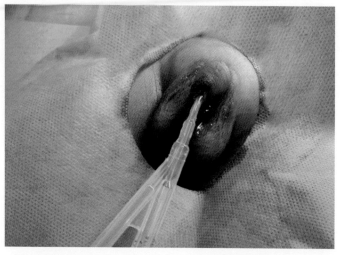

Fig. 8 Introducing the Foley catheter till its bifurcation

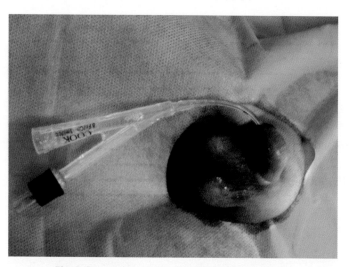

Fig. 9 Ensure that urine is draining from the catheter

- Amount of the urine should be measured after catheterization and it is better to collect the specimen of urine for laboratory examination.
- Record the information relevant document like reason for catheterization, residual volume, date and time of catheterization, catheter type and size, amount of water instilled into the balloon and any problem during negotiation of catheter (to provide point of reference or comparison in event of later queries).

Clinical Pearl

- Always retract the foreskin in uncircumcised males and hold it in place with a piece of gauze.

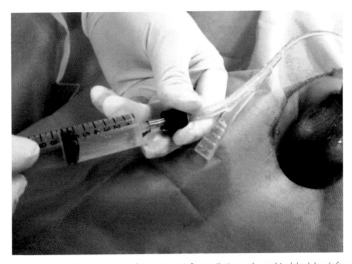

Fig. 10 Inflating the balloon once catheter is satisfactorily introduced in bladder (after ensuing that urine is draining form the catheter)

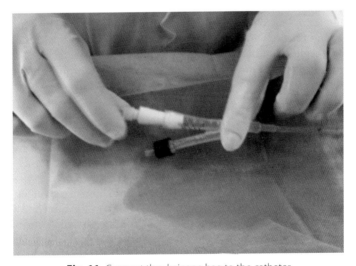

Fig. 11 Connect the drainage bag to the catheter

- Use your nondominant hand to achieve adequate meatal exposure.
- Always advance the catheter fully in male patients.
- If patient feels pain while inflating the balloon, immediately deflate the balloon because catheter might be lying in the urethra.

Difficulty in Catheterization

- In case of difficult catheterization it is advisable to insert little extra gel, it will help in lubricating the urethra as well as will dilate the urethra for smooth passage of catheter.

- If resistance is felt at external urinary sphincter, traction of penis, gentle pressure on catheter and asking patient to strain (as if passing urine) will help in negotiating the catheter
- Sometime tip of the catheter is caught between the urogenital diaphragm and urethra. Negotiation of catheter into the bladder in such situation can be facilitated by upward pressure on the perineum
- Kinking of the catheter can be overcome by slightly bigger size catheter.

POST-PROCEDURE CARE

- *Fixation of catheter*
  - *In adult:* It is preferable to secure the catheter to the thigh, ensure there is no tension in the tubing. Securing the catheter will minimize the bladder irritation during mobilization.
  - *In children:* It is preferable to secure the catheter to lower anterior abdominal wall in young children.
- *Position of Urobag:* The Urobag should always be kept lower than your bladder. This keeps urine from flowing back into your bladder. Take care that bag should not touch the floor.
- *Dressing/Cleaning:* Hygiene of hand[10] should be kept in mind while handling the catheter or bag to maintain sterility. The patients should be counseled for higher fluid intake.[11] Ensure regular cleaning of the meatus with sterile water but avoid regular bladder washout to maintain the sterility.[12]
- *Routine changing of catheter:* The data is very scanty for routine change of the catheter but most widely it is accepted that catheter may be changed every 2–3 weeks if prolonged catheterization is needed.
- *Removing a catheter*
  - It is better to remove catheter early in the morning
  - Patients should be counseled that symptoms like frequency and dysuria may occur after removal of the catheter and can persist for 24–48 hours after removing the catheter.
  - Check the volume of water filled in balloon and then use syringes to deflate the balloon. If balloon cannot be deflated—keep the attached syringe to the inflation arm of the Foley at least 30 minutes to deflate the balloon by effect of gravity. Sometime simple procedure like squeezing of the rubber tubing can displace the organized crystal in inflation channel. If all other means of deflating the balloon fails, it is recommended to deflate the balloon by rupturing it under ultrasound guidance.
  - While removing the catheter ask the patient to breathe deeply which relax the pelvic floor muscles.
  - Clean the meatus using gauze with sterile water after removing the catheter.

COMPLICATION/PROBLEM

- Urinary tract infection
- Urethral mucosal trauma—may occur because of incorrect size of catheter or poor technique of insertion.

- Inability to tolerate catheter—may occur due to urethral or bladder mucosal irritation. It can be resolved by strapping of catheter to prevent unnecessary pulling of catheter. Use of 100% silicone catheter if hypersensitivity with latex is suspected or use of anticholinergic medication may resolve the problem.
- Inadequate drainage of urine—may occur due to kinking of drainage of tubing, blocking of tubing with blood clot or debris in infected urine or it may be due to incorrect placement of catheter
- Leakage of urine—may occur because of bladder irritation or due to irritation of balloon of catheter or it may be due to use of incorrect size of catheter.

ACKNOWLEDGMENT

Dr Mangal Singh—for providing the photograph; and Esha Dube—for sketching the figures.

REFERENCES

1. Pomfret I. Catheter care—trouble shooting. J Community Nurs. 1999;13(6):20-4.
2. Carr HA. A short history of the Foley catheter: from handmade instrument to infection-prevention device. J Endourol. 2000;14(1):5-8.
3. McGill S. Catheter management: it's the size that's important. Nurs Mirror. 1982;154(14): 48-9.
4. Bandy JP, Moors J. Urology for Nurses. Oxford: Blackwell Scientific Publication; 1996.
5. Baxter A. Urinary catheterization. In: Mallet J, Dougherty L (Eds). Manual of Clinical Nursing Procedures, 5th edition. Oxford: Blackwell Publishing; 2000. pp. 600-12.
6. Hadfied-Law L. Male catheterization. Accid Emerg Nurs. 2001;9(4):257-63.
7. Lowthian P. The dangers of long-term catheter drainage. Br J Nurs. 1998;7(7):366-8.
8. Trout S, Dattolo J, Hansbrough JF. Catheterization: how far should you go? RN. 1993; 56(8):52-4.
9. Winn C. Complications with urinary catheters. Prof Nurse. 1998;13(5):S7-10.
10. Wilson J. Control and prevention of infection in catheter care. Community Nurse. 1997; 3(5):39-40.
11. Asscher AW, Sussaman M, Waters WE, Davis RH, Chick S. Urine as a medium for bacterial growth. Lancet. 1966;2(7472):1037-41.
12. Simpson L. Improving community catheter management. Prof Nurse. 1999;14(12): 831-4.

51

Suprapubic Cystostomy

Vijai Datta Upadhyaya

INTRODUCTION

Cystostomy is the general term for the surgical creation of an opening into the bladder; it may be a planned component of urologic surgery or an iatrogenic occurrence. The aim of suprapubic catheterization is to provide an emergency, temporary bladder drainage. Urinary bladder lies in the midline of the lower abdomen. When distended, its position can be determined by palpation, percussion or ultrasonography. In cases where urinary bladder is not distended, it can be distended by oral or intravenous hydration. Percutaneous suprapubic cystostomy should not be done when bladder is not distended. In a setting where an individual is unable to empty his or her bladder appropriately and urethral catheterization is either undesirable or impossible, suprapubic cystostomy offers an effective alternative.

INDICATION[1,2]

- Urethral stricture
- Acute retention of urine where urethral catheter cannot be passed
- Acute prostatitis
- Periurethral abscess
- Traumatic urethral disruption
- Requirement of long-term urinary diversion (like in cases of neurogenic bladder)
- Management of complicated lower genitourinary infections.

CONTRAINDICATION

Absolute[3,4]

- Nondistended, nonpalpable bladder
- History of bladder cancer.

Relative[3,4]

- Prior midline infraumbilical incision or recent cystostomy
- Pelvic irradiation
- Placement of orthopedic hardware for pelvic fracture repair

- Coagulopathy
- Gross hematuria (with blood clots in the bladder)
- Pregnancy.

In cases where percutaneous placement is contraindicated, an open surgical approach for suprapubic cystostomy is necessary to provide appropriate dissection through adhesions to avoid bowel injury and to achieve effective hemostasis for proper placement of suprapubic catheter.

APPLIED ANATOMY

The adult bladder is located in the anterior pelvis and is enveloped by extraperitoneal fat and connective tissue. It is separated from the pubic symphysis (Figs 1 and 2) by an anterior prevesical space known as the retropubic space (Cave of Retzius). The dome of the bladder is covered by peritoneum, and the bladder neck is fixed to neighboring structures by reflections of the pelvic fascia and by true ligaments of the pelvis. The body of the bladder receives support from the external urethral sphincter muscle and the perineal membrane inferiorly and the obturator internus muscles laterally.

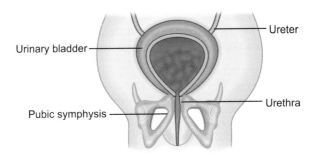

Fig. 1 The anatomical position of urinary bladder in anterior view

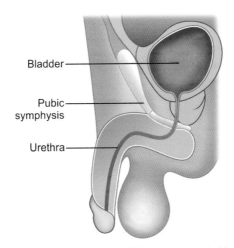

Fig. 2 Anatomical position of urinary bladder with anatomical landmark in lateral view

TECHNIQUE AND EQUIPMENT

The first operation of suprapubic cystostomy was performed in 1474.[5] *Suprapubic cystostomy can be performed in two ways, as follows:*

1. Open approach, in which a small infraumbilical incision is made above the pubic symphysis deep up to the bladder after dissecting all the muscle.
2. Percutaneous approach, in which the catheter is inserted directly through the abdominal wall, above the pubic symphysis, for which different available techniques are:
   - Percutaneous placement of a suprapubic cystostomy using Seldinger technique
   - Percutaneous placement of a suprapubic catheter over or through a sharp trocar
   - Percutaneous placement of a suprapubic cystostomy under direct cystoscopic visualization
   - Percutaneous placement of a suprapubic cystostomy under direct ultrasonographic visualization.

The two important things, which should be kept in mind while planning for suprapubic cystostomy catheters, are:

1. First is, if bladder can be drained by perurethral catheter, uretheral catheterization is better.
2. The second issue is the method that will be used to place the suprapubic cystostomy, either an open approach or a percutaneous approach.

Equipment: The equipment required for the suprapubic cystostomy using trocar cannula methods are (Fig. 3):

- Percutaneous suprapubic catheter set (trocar with cannula and Foley catheter)
- Closed urinary drainage system (sterile tubing and empty bag).

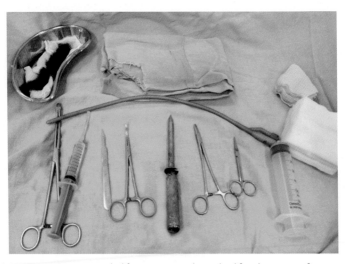

Fig. 3 Necessary equipment needed for trocar cannula method for placement of suprapubic tube

PREPARATION

- *Consent:* Informed valid consent should be taken from the patients or guardian if patient is minor.
- Arrange all the equipment before hand
- Preferably ask patients to take bath
- Distend the urinary bladder.

PROCEDURE

Position: Supine position is appropriate for this procedure though if procedure is done under guidance of cystoscopy lithotomy is a better choice.[6]

Anesthesia: Local anesthesia should be used for a percutaneous suprapubic cystostomy, though sedation may be added in pediatric patients. Appropriate local anesthesia would be a 1:1 formulation of lidocaine 1% 5 mL and bupivacaine 0.25% 5 mL, for a total of 10 mL. Few surgeons may prefer general anesthesia for the procedure, especially in children.

Procedural Steps

- Shave the suprapubic operative field
- Clean the abdominal wall properly with povidone-iodine solution and spirit
- Prepare the site with an antiseptic solution
- Drape the site with sterile towels, ensuring that the pubic symphysis and anterior superior iliac spine can be visualized
- Ensure the fullness of bladder
- Palpate the distended bladder; mark the site with marking pen (Fig. 4), landmark is two fingerbreadths above the pubic symphysis in the midline. Do not place the catheter in natural crease.
- Apply local anesthetic in skin at the marked site (Fig. 5), then infiltrate the anesthetic into the subcutaneous tissue and rectus abdominis muscle fascia, aiming the needle at a 10–20° angle toward the pelvis. Advance the needle in this direction, while aspirating the syringe; and aspiration of urine will confirm the entry into the bladder (Figs 6 and 7). Once the entry in bladder is confirmed mark the distance with hemostat.
- Make a small skin incision of around 1 cm size at the marked site (Fig. 8). Incise the superficial fascia and preferably linea alba and dissect the muscle with hemostat (Fig. 9). After incising fascia/linea alba trocar with cannula is traduced and advance further aiming it at 10–20° angle toward the pelvis (Fig. 10) as soon as trocar will pierce the bladder there will be a feeling of loss of resistance and urine will flow out of the cannula confirming the entry of trocar in bladder.
- Remove the trocar and insert the Foley catheter (Figs 11 and 12) of appropriate size. Advance the catheter more than 4–5 cm beyond, from where bladder fluid is first seen to coming out (Fig. 13). This ensures that the balloon is fully in the bladder (not in the subcutaneous tissue) before inflation.

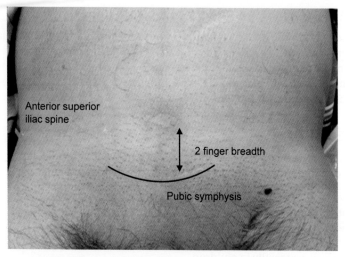

Fig. 4 Marking of the site in relation with anatomical landmark

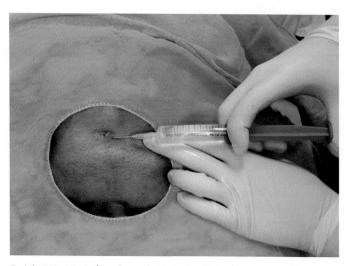

Fig. 5 Administration of local anesthetic in the skin, subcutaneous tissue and fascia

- Using a Baumgartner needle holder, an Adson tissue forceps (Figs 14 and 15), and 3-0 nylon suture on a curved needle, secure the catheter to the skin of the anterior abdominal wall. Place an air knot at the skin, adjacent to the cystostomy site, and then use the two loose ends of the suture to place another knot around the catheter itself.

POST-PROCEDURE CARE

- Dressing should be changed daily
- Clean the area around catheter with mixture of equal volume of water and hydrogen peroxide daily
- Empty the drainage bag timely to avoid leakage

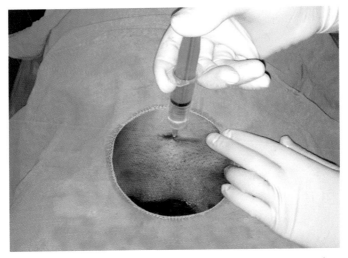

Fig. 6 Syringe advanced in the bladder and confirmed with aspiration of urine

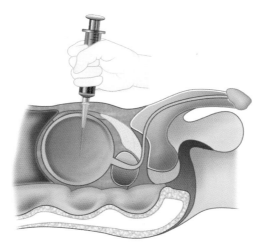

Fig. 7 Schematic diagram showing the position of needle in the urinary bladder

- Skin suture should be removed after 5 days
- Vital signs should be checked, along with serum electrolyte, magnesium, blood urea nitrogen and creatinine concentrations.[1]

Follow-up[2]

- Ideally, all patients with suprapubic tube should be managed with urologist so that correction of underlying disease and care of tube is properly supervised.
- It takes around 4–6 weeks for maturation of tract so first tube change must be done after this period.
- Subsequently catheter can be changed monthly.

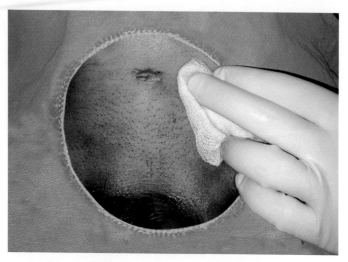

Fig. 8 Skin incision at the marked site

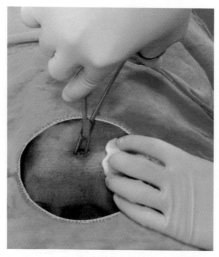

Fig. 9 After skin incision subcutaneous tissue was incised and plane is developed between the muscles up to the fascia

- It is advisable to put catheter of size more than 16 Fr, to avoid frequent blockage.
- Anticholinergic may be added in cases of urethral leakage.
- If suprapubic wound is large, it can be closed with suture.

How to Prevent Complications

- Distend the bladder properly before putting suprapubic cystostomy tube
- If bladder cannot be distended use either cystoscopic or USG guidance for placing percutaneous cystostomy tube.

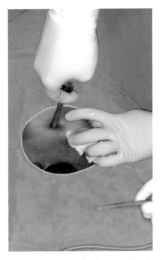

Fig. 10 Trocar with cannula is introduced and advanced in the bladder further aiming it at 10–20° angle toward the pelvis

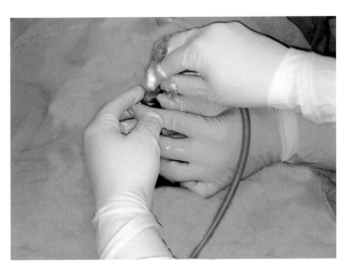

Fig. 11 Foley catheter is introduced into the bladder after removing the trocar and flow of urine was confirmed

- To prevent gram-negative bacteremia, an appropriate preprocedural intravenous gram-negative antibiotic should be administered before instrumentation of the genitourinary tract.

COMPLICATION/PROBLEM

- Immediate complications of suprapubic catheter placement include gross hematuria, which is usually transient, and the possibility of post-obstructive diuresis, in which urine output may be greater than 200 mL/hour.[3,7]

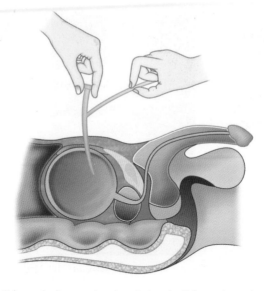

Fig. 12 Schematic diagram showing placing the Foley catheter through the cannula into the bladder

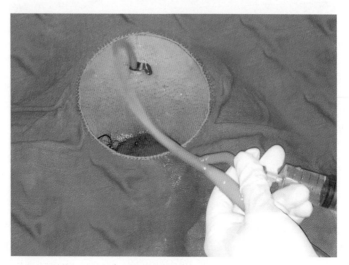

Fig. 13 Cannula is removed after placing the Foley into the bladder

- Serious complications of the procedure include bowel perforation[8] and other intra-abdominal visceral organ injuries and urosepsis, whose manifestations may be delayed.[7]
- A mucous or mucopurulent discharge around the exit site may occur; if present, it can be managed with local hygiene measures alone if there is no cellulitis and no evidence of systemic infection.
- Inadvertent puling of catheter leading to loss of cystostomy tract.

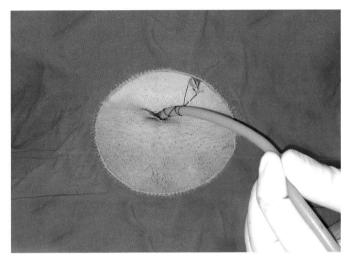

Fig. 14 Foley is properly secured with suture

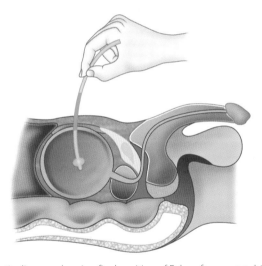

Fig. 15 Schematic diagram showing final position of Foley after suprapubic puncture

- Suprapubic catheter use may be additionally complicated by exit site infections, over granulation of cystostomy site or leakage from cystostomy site.
- Bladder stones developed in 22–45% of patients with long-term suprapubic catheter use.[9]

ACKNOWLEDGMENTS

Dr Abhishek, Department of Urology, SGPGIMS, Lucknow and Isha Sharma, Technician, School of Telemedicine, SGPGIMS, Lucknow for photographs and sketching.

REFERENCES

1. Awojobi OA, Lawani J. Suprapubic cystostomy: indications and complications. Trop Doct. 1984;14(4):162-3.
2. Harrison SC, Lawrence WT, Morley R, Pearce I, Taylor J. British Association of Urological Surgeons' suprapubic catheter practice guidelines. BJU Int. 2011;107(1):77-85.
3. Katsumi HK, Kalisvaart JF, Ronningen LD, et al. Urethral versus suprapubic catheter: choosing the best bladder management for male spinal cord injury patients with indwelling catheters. Spinal Cord. 2010;48:325-9.
4. Patterson BM. Pelvic ring injury and associated urologic trauma: an orthopaedic perspective. Semin Urol. 1995;13(1):25-33.
5. Cumston CG. A short account of early history of suprapubic cystostomy. Boston Med Surg J. 1912;166:516-25.
6. Irby PB 3, Stoller ML. Percutaneous suprapubic cystostomy. J Endourol. 1993;7(2):125-30.
7. Robinson J. Insertion, care and management of suprapubic catheters. Nurs Stand. 2008;23(8):49-56.
8. Ahmed SJ, Mehta A, Rimington P. Delayed bowel perforation following suprapubic catheter insertion. BMC Urol. 2004;4(1):16.
9. Sugimura T, Arnold E, English S, Moore J. Chronic suprapubic catheterization in the management of patients with spinal cord injuries: analysis of upper and lower urinary tract complications. BJU Int. 2008;101(11):1396-400.

52
Peritoneal Dialysis Catheter Placement

Basant Kumar, MS Ansari

INTRODUCTION

Dialysis is a form of treatment that performs many of the kidney's functions. It is often used to treat advanced chronic kidney diseases, where the kidneys have lost most or all of their functions. It excretes toxic wastes from the blood and removes excess water from the body. In the process of peritoneal dialysis, peritoneal membrane acts as a filter and removes not required toxic products from the body. Dialysis cycle (or peritoneal exchange) has three phases; filling by dialysate, dwelling and draining of dialysate with waste products (Figs 1A and B). It is palliative and helps to feel better and live longer, but it does not cure for end-stage renal disease (ESRD). The intraperitoneal administration can be used for blood transfusion, chemotherapy, insulin and nutrition.

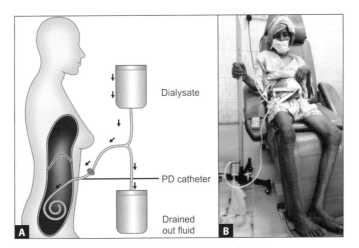

Figs 1A and B Peritoneal dialysis

INDICATION

Strong Indications

- Hemodialysis intolerance
- Failure to vascular access (canulation)
- Congestive cardiac failure/prosthetic valvular disease/poor cardiac function
- Peripheral vascular disease
- Children aged 0–5 years
- Patient preference
- Distance from a hemodialysis center.

Peritoneal Dialysis Preferred in Patients with

- Bleeding diathesis/disorders
- Chronic infections
- Possibility of renal transplantation in the near future
- Children above 5 years and in adolescent
- Multiple myeloma/diabetes mellitus.

Peritoneal Dialysis has been Utilized Infrequently for Non-renal Indications with Variable Benefit in

- Refractory congestive heart failure
- Hepatic failure/pancreatitis
- Hypothermia/hyperthermia
- Hyponatremia
- Dialysis-associated ascites
- Drug poisonings.

CONTRAINDICATION

Absolute

- Loss of peritoneal functions
    - Multiple abdominal adhesions
    - Sclerosis/fibrosis of the peritoneal membrane
    - Documented type II ultrafiltration failure
- Women with third trimester of pregnancy
- Severe/active inflammatory bowel diseases
- Acute diverticulitis/diverticulosis
- Infected abdominal collections or abscess
- Active ischemic bowel disease
- Severe psychotic disorders/significant intellectual disability.

Relative

- Severe malnutrition/hypercatabolism
- Multiple abdominal adhesions/fresh intra-abdominal surgery
- Peritoneal leaks

- Frequent episodes of diverticulitis
- Bowel stoma (ostomy)
- Proteinuria greater than 10 g/day
- Morbid obesity/body size limitations
- Dementia/poor personal hygiene
- Upper limb amputation with homelessness.

Peritoneal Dialysis is not Preferred but is Possible in Selected Circumstances

- Obesity/fatty abdomen
- Multiple hernias including inguinal, incisional, etc.
- Severe backache
- Previous abdominal surgeries
- Poor home hygienic conditions.

APPLIED ANATOMY

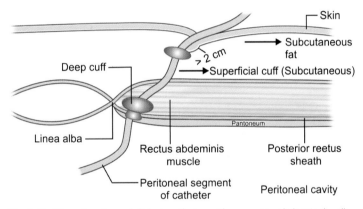

Fig. 2 Position of peritoneal dialysis catheter with respect to abdominal wall

TECHNIQUE AND EQUIPMENT

Peritoneal dialysis (PD) was first used in 1959 by Richard Ruben for the management of ESRD but popularized by Popovich and Moncrief. They developed continuous ambulatory peritoneal dialysis (CAPD) for patients with chronic renal disease. In 1968, Henry Tenckhoff described the technique of placement of the indwelling peritoneal catheter via an open surgical technique. Subsequently, percutaneous and laparoscopic techniques for PD catheter placement have been introduced by Allon M et al. (1988) and Amerling R et al. (1993), respectively.

Peritoneal dialysis has several advantages including:
- Better hemodynamic control
- Biocompatible membrane
- No extracorporal circulation of blood
- Increased mobility and lifestyle
- Less fluid and dietetic restrictions

- Flexible schedule/more autonomy
- Lower prevalence of hepatitis C
- Preservation of residual renal functions.

Surgical or Dissection Technique

This is the most commonly used technique. *Merits of open surgical technique are:*
- Good hemostasis and low risk of bleeding
- Tissue injury or viscous perforation is completely eliminated
- Precise positioning of the inner segment is possible
- All types of catheters can be inserted
- Low risk of dialysate solution leaks.

Demerits of open surgical technique:
- Larger incision may predispose to late hernias
- Immediate use is not recommended due to risk of dialysis solution leak
- High cost of surgical procedure (dependence on surgeon's availability, OT time).

Laparoscopy Technique

- Preferred method
- Visualization of the course of catheter
- Air-filled cavity
- Catheter is placed under direct vision.

Blind or Guidewire Technique

- No direct visualization of peritoneum
- Devices to guide the catheter
- Fluid-filled cavity
- Least preferred in adults
- Can perform at bedside under local anesthesia.

Peritoneoscopy/Y-TEC® Technique

- Air-filled cavity
- Visualization of the course of catheter
- Specialized equipment
- Cost is modest.

Equipment: Peritoneal Dialysis Catheter

- Peritoneal dialysis catheters are manufactured either of silicone rubber or polyurethane with Dacron cuffs. Try to avoid the polyurethane catheters because it may damage by local antibiotics (mupirocin or gentamycin).
- Peritoneal dialysis catheter has a flexible silicon tube and an open end-port with several side holes for proper drainage and absorption of the dialysate. *It has three segments (Fig. 2):*
  1. *External:* It lies outside the skin and visible
  2. *Tunneled:* It lies between peritoneum and below skin
  3. *Intraperitoneal:* It lies within peritoneal cavity.

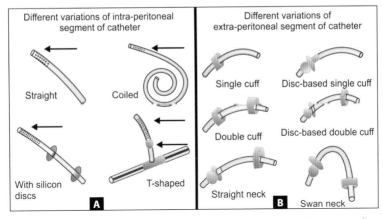

Figs 3A and B Different variations of intra- and extra-peritoneal segment of peritoneal dialysis catheter

Catheters are available in different shapes (straight, curved: swan neck, curled-pigtail), lengths and number of Dacron cuffs (single or double cuffs) (Figs 3A and B). Most of the catheters that are used today have a coiled tip and doubly cuffed.

The catheter holds its position at peritoneal site by the help of proximal cuff while the distal cuff acts as a barrier near subcutaneous plane to prevent infections from the exit wound and skin (Fig. 2).

Types of Catheter (Figs 3 and 4)

- *Intraperitoneal part of catheter has four basic designs*
  1. *Straight Tenckhoff;* with a 100 mm section; containing 1 mm side-holes
  2. *Curled Tenckhoff;* with a coiled 200 mm section; containing 1 mm side-holes
  3. *Straight Tenckhoff;* catheter with perpendicular discs [Toronto-Western design (rarely used)]
  4. *T-fluted catheter;* (investigational) with grooved perpendicular limbs; positioned against the parietal peritoneum
- *Subcutaneous portion (between the peritoneal-entry and skin exit sites) has three basic shapes*
  1. Straight or gently (slight) curved
  2. Arcuate or "swan neck" with 150-degree bending
  3. 90-degree bends (no longer available)
- *Depending on Dacron cuffs, there are three options*
  1. *Single-cuffed catheter;* usually placed in the rectus muscle
  2. *Dual-cuffed catheter;* one in the rectus muscle and other one in subcutaneous tissue
  3. *Disc-shaped deep cuff with a silicone ball within the peritoneum;* with or without a subcutaneous cuff

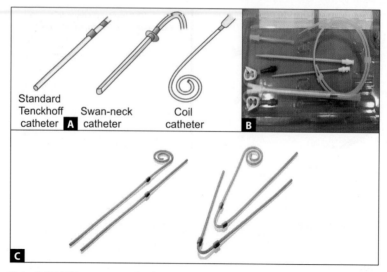

Standard Tenckhoff catheter | A | Swan-neck catheter | Coil catheter | B

C

Figs 4A to C (A) Different types of catheters; (B) Percutaneous catheter with dilator, needle and guidewire; (C) Medcomp® peritoneal dialysis catheter devices: single-cuffed straight and coiled catheter, double-cuffed straight and coiled swan-neck catheter

Source: Fig. 4C: Medical Component, Inc, 1499 Delp Drive, Harleysville, PA 19438. www.medcompnet.com

- Depending on internal diameter (the outer diameter being essentially constant at 5 mm), *there are three choices of catheters:*
  1. 2.6 mm inner diameter; standard Tenckhoff catheter size
  2. 3.1 mm inner diameter; Cruz® catheter
  3. 3.5 mm inner diameter; Flexneck™ catheter

PREPARATION

- All routine investigation required for general anesthesia
- Prophylaxis antibiotics
- Nephrology team should be involved preoperatively
- The patient and his/her family should be counseled about different modalities of therapy (pros and cons) and given full freedom to choose type of therapy
- The patient should be explained about the catheter insertion procedure and informed about complications of the insertion procedure and of the therapy
- Proper consent to be taken
- The patient should be evaluated for any evidence of hernias, diaphragmatic eventration or/and any weakness of the abdominal wall (if any of these are evident; it is advisable to repair these defects during catheter insertion. In such conditions, the peritoneal dialysis should delay for 4 weeks after repair to avoid leakage)
- The abdomen should be marked preoperatively for location of deep cuff, superficial cuff and exit site in relation to abdominal wall (Fig. 5)
- Direction of exit site (downward, lateral or upward) and location of superficial cuff in relation with exit site should be marked preferably in standing position

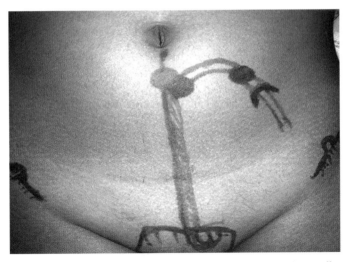

Fig. 5 Preoperative marking of abdomen (red-incision, blue-deep cuff, black-superficial cuff and exit site)

of patient taking into account of patient's beltline and should be placed laterally
- The exit site should be placed; either above or below to the beltline. It should not lie on a scar or within the abdominal folds.

Pre-insertion Patient Assessment and Preparation

Patient should be throughly evaluated for body size, right or left handedness, previous abdominal surgery, ascites, any peritonitis history, constipation, urinary tract obstruction, uncontrolled hypertension/vision, intra-abdominal mass: polycystic kidney disease (PKD), aneurysm, huge myoma, bleeding tendency, drugs (coumadin, antiplatelet drug), arrange a meeting with another patient on peritoneal dialysis (PD) for introduction to PD, demonstrate catheter and transfer set.

Night Before Surgery

Bowel preparations, i.e. ensure regular bowel motions; preferable to give an enema 12 hours before and on the morning of surgery. Keep patient nil per os (NPO) as per anesthetist's instructions. The preparation of the skin should be done properly. If possible, patient should have a bath with chlorhexidine soap on the morning of the surgery. The part should be prepared by shaving the skin hair from xiphisternum to mid-thigh. The abdomen should be cleaned with betadine 12 hours before and on the morning of the surgery.

Day of Catheter Insertion

Ensure empty bladder prior to transfer to theater. Label any limbs with *arteriovenous* (A-V) fistula access, stating normal blood pressures or venipuncture from that limb. Prophylactic antibiotics (first generation cephalosporin, such as cefazolin and an aminoglycoside) are given 1 hour before and for 12 hours postoperative. Vancomycin is generally avoided.

PROCEDURE

Open Surgical Technique

- *Position:* Supine. Under general anesthesia.
- A midline vertical incision about 5 cm is made; starting from 2–3 cm below the umbilicus (Figs 6A and B).
- Subcutaneous layer is dissected up to the anterior rectus sheath.
- Rectus abdominis muscle fibers are bluntly dissected after opening the anterior sheath.
- The entry site of catheter should be paramedian (Figs 7A and B). It should not enter through the linea alba (to minimize leaks).
- Posterior rectus sheath is incised and stay sutures should be taken before abdominal cavity is opened (Figs 8A and B).
- The abdominal wall is carefully inspected for adhesions after lifting the abdominal wall by a retractor.
- Now, the position of patient is changed to Trendelenburg position.
- After placing stylet in the PD catheter; it is advanced into the peritoneal cavity; deep in the pelvis. The landmark that corresponds to a deep pelvic location for the tip of dialysis catheter is the pubic symphysis.
- Tip of catheter should be placed in the deep pelvis for optimal hydraulic functioning and to minimize the chances of omental wrapping around catheter.
- Stylet is removed from catheter. The deep cuff of catheter is placed into the preperitoneal space and anchor with sheath using resorbable suture. The deep cuff should never be placed in the peritoneal cavity (Figs 9A and B).
- The peritoneum, anterior and posterior rectus sheaths are closed carefully with resorbable sutures; ensuring not to obstruct/knick the catheter.

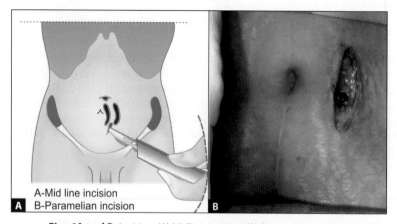

Figs 6A and B Incision. (A) Midline incision; (B) Paramedian incision

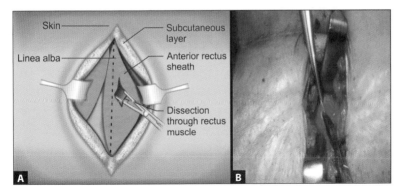

Figs 7A and B Dissection through rectus abdominis muscle

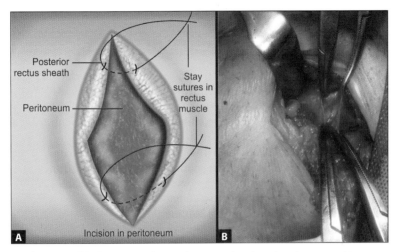

Figs 8A and B Dissection of posterior rectus sheath and peritoneum with stay

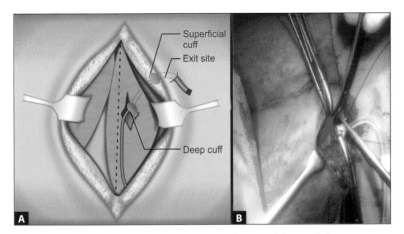

Figs 9A and B Placement of catheter in pelvis and fixation of deep cuff above peritoneum

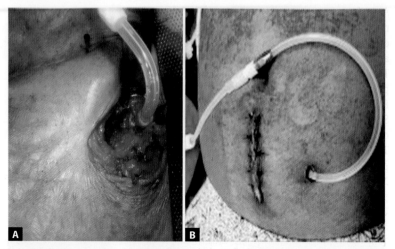

Figs 10A and B Creation of subcutaneous tunnel, fixation of superficial cuff and exit site

- A tunnel is created in subcutaneous plane and the superficial cuff is placed subcutaneously; about 2 cm away from the exit site (it minimizes the extrusion of superficial cuff) (Figs 10A and B).
- The preferred exit site is created at lateral and caudal to the entrance site by using a needle.
- Exit site should be avoided near the patient's belt area, skin creases and abdominal folds, and should be fashioned about 2 cm away from superficial cuff. It should be clearly visible to patient for daily exit-site care.
- Catheter type and exit location must be patient specific:
  Lower abdominal exit site: For high beltline.
  Mid-abdominal exit site: For low beltline or low skinfolds.
  Upper abdominal exit site: For obesity or floppy skinfolds.
  Presternal exit site: For patient with obesity, incontinence or stomas.
- Avoid suturing and stapling near the exit site.
- After securing hemostasis, close the skin incision. It is advisable to avoid fixation of catheter at exit site by suture.
- Patency of catheter should be checked by filling the abdomen with 100 mL saline. Entrance site is looked for leakage and saline is allowed to drain. Inspect the drained fluid for any evidence of hemoperitoneum and fecal contamination.

Laparoscopic Technique

- *Position:* Supine. Under general anesthesia.
- Open technique to create pneumoperitoneum is preferred over use of Veres needle. The abdomen is insufflated with CO_2 gas to create pneumoperitoneum of 12–14 mm Hg after inserting a 5 mm trocar.
- In Trendelenburg position of patient, a 5 mm trocar is placed about 2 cm below the umbilicus; after creating pneumoperitoneum.
- Abdomen is thoroughly inspected (diagnostic laparoscopy) with a 5 mm scope.

- At the planned exit-site position of the PD catheter (i.e. paraumbilical left or right 2–3 cm below the umbilicus); an extra 5 mm trocar is inserted under direct vision. It is important that this trocar is introduced through the anterior and posterior rectus sheaths, but not through the peritoneum.
- Then, a double-cuffed curled-tip PD catheter is introduced via the paraumbilical port, ensuring no torsion or kinking.
- Finally, a stiff stylet is used to introduce the catheter into the peritoneal cavity. Sometimes, an extra 5 mm trocar/port needed for proper positioning of catheter into the deep pelvis.
- The distal cuff should be positioned outside the peritoneum (in the preperitoneal space or between both the rectus muscle sheaths).
- Now, the paraumbilical trocar is removed and the catheter is placed to its planned exit-site position.
- Use needle to create the subcutaneous tunnel on the left or the right side of abdomen. The proximal cuff should be lying in this tunnel.
- The catheter is checked for its patency and then; the abdomen is desufflated, with the camera still in position to check the location of the catheter.
- At end, the trocar is removed and the rectus sheaths and wounds are closed carefully with resorbable sutures.

Percutaneous Technique

- *Position:* Supine
- Under local anesthesia
- Performed using a Seldinger technique
- A small incision is made on the entrance site (usually in the midline) by blunt dissection of the abdominal rectus sheath
- The peritoneal cavity is entered with an 18-gauge needle and the cavity is filled with around 500 cc of saline. The patient should be painless and ensure that there is no resistance, if needle is placed accurately
- A guidewire is directed into the abdomen through needle and needle is removed
- The tract is dilated by the dilators by advancing it over the guidewire into the abdominal cavity
- After desired dilatation of tract, dilators and wires are removed. Now, the PD catheter with preplaced stylet is advanced into abdomen through the sheath. It is advanced into the deep pelvis until the proximal cuff is located in the preperitoneal space
- Finally, the peel-away sheath and stylet are removed and the catheter position is checked
- Subcutaneous tunnel is created up to the planned exit site and distal cuff is placed in tunnel about 2 cm away from the exit site
- The abdomen is filled with 500 cc of saline and drained by gravity to check the patency of catheter.

POST-PROCEDURE CARE

- *Immediate flushing*
  - Flush the catheter with repeated small volumes of saline until the effluent is clear

- Flush the catheter with 500–1000 mL of heparinized (500–1000 u/L) PD solution to check patency of the catheter and to halt the fibrin or blood clot formation
- Once the effluent becomes clear; the catheter can be capped safely
- Before capping the catheter, instill 15,000 units of undiluted heparin into the catheter
- Flushing can be repeated after 7 days
- Vitals monitoring
- Look for bleeding from the exit site
- Nil per os for 6 hours in postoperative period. Then allow sips of water as soon as the bowel sounds heard and then gradual conversion to semisolid diets
- Minimal movement of patient and catheter in postoperative period for first 24 hours
- The surgical dressing should not be changed for 72 hours unless there is obvious soaking of dressing, bleedings or signs of infection
- Frequent dressing changes (in the immediate postimplantation period) are not necessary
- The fewer the dressing changes, the less is the risk of local trauma due to manipulations and less risk of contamination of the exit site
- After 2–3 weeks, frequent dressing changes are indicated when the exit site is colonized with bacteria
- Patients should avoid taking a bath until the exit site has fully healed
- The catheter should be immobilized using a firm dressing or tapes on multiple sites
- Avoiding turning movement and minimizing handling of catheter until exit site/tunnel are completely healed; will reduce the incidence of trauma and will promote the tissue growth
- To avoid cross contamination of wound/exit site; good handwashing practice is essential. Primary aim of long-term exit-site care is to prevent exit-site infections
- Apply local antibacterial at the exit site.

Indication of PD Catheter Removal

Refractory/frequent peritonitis and/or refractory wound (exit site and tunnel) infections.

COMPLICATION/PROBLEM

Early (<30 days) Complications

- Wound/exit-site infections
- Subcutaneous tunnel infections
- Cuff protrusion
- Catheter block/outflow/inflow failure
- Pericatheter dialysate leaks
- Hernias
- Bowel perforation
- Bleeding wound
- Leakage.

Late (> 30 days) Complications

- Infection (exit site/subcutaneous tunnel)
- Outflow/inflow failure (clots or blockage in the catheter/kinking in the subcutaneous tunnel/omental wrap over catheter or bowel adhesions
- Malpositioning or displacement of the catheter into the upper abdomen
- Leakage of dialysate
- Hernias
- Peritonitis.

Other Complication

- Malnutrition
- Catheter migration
- Exit site cuff erosion
- Low backache
- Hydrothorax
- Pain or cramping pain on infusion
- Genital edema
- Sclerosing encapsulating peritonitis.

ACKNOWLEDGMENTS

Professor RK Sharma (Director and Head, Department of Nephrology, Sanjay Gandhi Postgraduate Institute of Medical Sciences (SGPGIMS), Lucknow, Uttar Pradesh and his team for permission of photographs of their patients; Dr Sanjay Surekha and Dr Sharmad Kuchadker, Senior Resident, Urology, SGPGIMS, Lucknow; Miss Isha Dubey, Technician (*PAN Africa e-network*), TCIL, School of Telemedicine and Biomedical Informatics, SGPGIMS, Lucknow, Uttar Pradesh.

SUGGESTED READING

1. Allon M, Soucie JM, Macon EJ. Complications with permanent peritoneal dialysis catheters: experience with 154 percutaneously placed catheters. Nephron. 1988;48(1): 8-11.
2. Blagg CR. The early history of dialysis for chronic renal failure in the United States: a view from Seattle. Am J Kidney Dis. 2007;49(3):482-96.
3. Crabtree JH. Selected best demonstrated practices in peritoneal dialysis access. Kidney Int Suppl. 2006;103:S27-37.
4. Figueiredo A, Goh BL, Jenkins S, Johnson DW, Mactier R, Ramalakshmi S, et al. Clinical practice guidelines for peritoneal access. Perit Dial Int. 2010;30(4):424-9.
5. Li PK, Szeto CC, Piraino B, Bernardini J, Figueiredo AE, Gupta A, et al. Peritoneal dialysis-related infections recommendations: 2010 update. Perit Dial Int. 2010;30(4):393-423.
6. Mehrotra R, Kermah D, Fried L, Kalantar-Zadeh K, Khawar O, Norris K, et al. Chronic peritoneal dialysis in the United States: declining utilization despite improving outcomes. J Am Soc Nephrol. 2007;18(10):2781-8.
7. Peppelenbosch A, van Kuijk WHM, Bouvy ND, van der Sande FM, Tordoir JHM. Peritoneal dialysis catheter placement technique and complications. NDT Plus. 2008;1(Suppl 4):iv23-8.
8. Popovich RP, Moncrief JW, Nolph KD, Ghods AJ, Twardowski ZJ, Pyle WK. Continuous ambulatory peritoneal dialysis. Ann Intern Med. 1978;88(4):449-56.
9. Tenckhoff H, Curtis FK. Experience with maintenance peritoneal dialysis in the home. Trans Am Soc Artif Intern Organs. 1970;16:90-5.

53

Hemodialysis

Harsh Vardhan, Dharmendra Bhadauria

INTRODUCTION

Acute kidney injury (AKI) is a major health problem that affects millions of patients worldwide, leading to increased mortality, and progression to chronic kidney disease in patients who survives. The true incidence of AKI in intensive care unit (ICU) has been difficult to establish due to lack of standardized definition, but it has been estimated that 3–7% of hospitalized patients and 25–30% of patients in the ICU develop AKI, with 5–6% of the ICU population requiring renal replacement therapy (RRT) after developing AKI.[1]

INDICATION

Emergency:
- Pulmonary edema
- Refractory metabolic acidosis
- Refractory hyperkalemia (K >6.5 mEq/L)

Urgent:
- Uremic encephalopathy
- Uremic pericarditis

Planned:
- Oliguria more than 24 hours
- Anuria more than 12 hours
- Creatinine more than 10.0 mg/dL
- Urea more than 200 mg/dL.

HISTORY AND BASIC PRINCIPLE

Historically in 1854, Thomas Graham of Glasgow, presented the principles of solute transport across a semipermeable membrane.[2] Abel, Rountree and Turner in 1913 developed the artificial kidney.[3] Hass in 1924 performed the first hemodialysis in humans[4] and the artificial kidney was developed by Kolff in 1943–1945.[5,6] Alwall in 1946 at Lund University[7,8] modified this kidney inside a stainless steel canister to which negative pressure was applied thus performing the ultrafiltration. In 1962, Scribner started the world's first outpatient dialysis facility, Seattle Artificial Kidney Center.[9] The principle of hemodialysis involves diffusion of solutes across a semipermeable membrane. It utilizes counter current flow with the dialysate and blood flowing in opposite direction in the extracorporeal circuit. Concentration gradient is maintained across the membrane by counter current mechanism increasing the efficiency of the dialysis. Fluid removal (ultrafiltration) is achieved by altering the hydrostatic pressure of the dialysate compartment, causing free water and some dissolved solutes to move across the membrane along a created pressure gradient. Urea and other waste products, potassium and phosphate diffuse into the dialysis solution.

MODALITIES OF RENAL REPLACEMENT THERAPY

Multiple modalities of RRT (Flow chart 1) are available for the management of patients with AKI, including conventional intermittent hemodialysis (IHD), peritoneal dialysis, multiple forms of continuous renal replacement therapy (CRRT) and "hybrid" therapies, such as sustained low-efficiency dialysis (SLED; also known as extended duration dialysis or EDD).

- *Intermittent hemodialysis*: Short-term IHD has been the mainstay of RRT in AKI for more than five decades. Patients typically undergo dialysis treatments for 3–5 hours on a thrice-weekly, alternate-day or daily schedule depending on catabolic demands, electrolyte disturbances and volume status.
- *Continuous renal replacement therapy*: The CRRTs represent a spectrum of treatment modalities. Initially, CRRT was provided using an arteriovenous extracorporeal circuit.[10] Although this approach offered technical simplicity, blood flow was dependent upon the gradient between mean arterial and

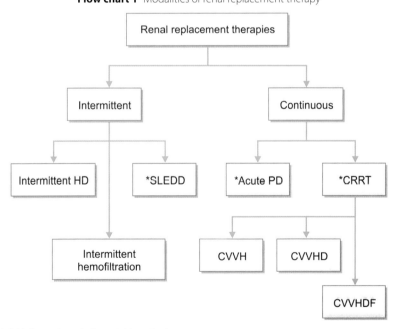

Flow chart 1 Modalities of renal replacement therapy

*Helpful in hemodynamically unstable patients.
Abbreviations: HD, hemodialysis; SLEDD, slow extended daily dialysis; CRRT, continuous renal replacement therapy; CVVH, continuous veno-venous hemofiltration; CVVHD, continuous veno-venous hemodialysis; CVVHDF, continuous veno-venous hemodiafiltration

central venous pressure, and there was an increased risk of complications from prolonged arterial cannulation.[11] As a result, the continuous arteriovenous therapies have largely been supplanted by pump-driven, veno-venous CRRT.[12] The modalities of veno-venous CRRT vary primarily in their mechanism of solute removal, in continuous veno-venous hemofiltration (CVVH), solute transport occurs by convection; in continuous veno-venous hemodialysis (CVVHD), it occurs by diffusion; and in continuous veno-venous hemodiafiltration (CVVHDF), it occurs by a combination of the two.[13] Although, at the same level of urea clearance, convective therapies provide enhanced clearance of higher-molecular-weight solutes than diffusive therapies, no clear clinical benefit has been demonstrated for CVVH or CVVHDF compared with CVVHD.

- *Hybrid therapies*: The hybrid modalities of RRT represent therapies in which conventional hemodialysis equipment is modified to provide extended-duration dialysis using lower blood flow rates and dialysate flow rates.[14] A variety of terms have been used to describe these therapies, including SLED,[15,16] EDD[17] and sustained low-efficiency daily diafiltration (SLEDD-f).[18] Because these therapies extend the duration of the dialysis treatment while providing slower ultrafiltration and solute clearance, they are associated with enhanced hemodynamic tolerability compared with IHD. The degree of metabolic control attained with these treatments is comparable to that observed with CRRT.[19]

Intermediate Versus Continuous

If we compare IHD with continuous therapies, then we will find that IHD is mainly diffusive and is generally done with a low flux membrane while CRRT is mainly convective and is done with a high flux membrane. The dialysate flow rate is more in IHD with high clearance rate as compared with CRRT. CRRT is more labor intensive and it cannot be done without anticoagulation when compared with IHD (Table 1).

Table 1 Blood flow rates in various forms of hemodialysis

Type of therapy	Transport mechanism	Urea clearance (mL/minutes)	Ultrafiltration (L/day)
IHD	Diffusion and convection	200–400	4–6
SLED	Diffusion and convection	150–200	6–8
CAVH	Convection	7–10	0–12
CVVH	Convection	15–17	0–12
CAVHD	Convection and diffusion	16–39	4–12
CVVHD	Convection and diffusion	16–39	4–12
PD	Diffusion and convection	12–17	1–3

Abbreviations: IHD, intermittent hemodialysis; SLED, sustained low-efficiency dialysis; CAVH, continuous arteriovenous hemofiltration; CVVH, continuous veno-venous hemofiltration; CAVHD, continuous arteriovenous hemofiltration with dialysis; CVVHD, continuous veno-venous hemodialysis; PD, peritoneal dialysis.

Choice of Mode of Hemodialysis

The choice of a particular mode of hemodialysis mainly depends on cost and patient characteristics. In patients with hemodynamic instability, CRRT or SLED can be offered to the patient. SLED is preferred in patients with coagulopathy or those having active bleed as it can be done with minimal or no anticoagulation while theoretically, CRRT has the advantage of removal of proinflammatory cytokines [tumor necrosis factor (TNF), interleukin-1 (IL-1) and IL-6] and anti-inflammatory cytokines (IL-10, IL-1 R antagonist) equivalent and is also preferable in patients with cerebral edema. When continous infusion of fluid, blood products and nutrition is required CRRT may be preferable.[19]

Dialysis Apparatus

Hemodialysis apparatus can be broadly divided into a blood circuit and a dialysis solution circuit, which meet at the dialyzer. The blood circuit begins at the vascular access. From there, blood is pumped through an arterial blood line to the dialyzer. Blood is returned from the dialyzer to the patient via a venous blood line (Fig. 1). These terms are used even though often only venous blood is being accessed. Various chambers, side ports and monitors are attached to the inflow and outflow blood lines, and are used to infuse saline or heparin, to measure pressures and to detect any entrance of air. The dialysis solution circuit includes the dialysis solution supply system, which makes dialysis solution online from purified water and concentrate, and then pumps the solution through a different compartment of the dialyzer. The dialysis solution circuit includes various monitors that make sure that the dialysis solution is at the right temperature, has a safe concentration of dissolved salts, and is not being exposed to blood (due to a leak in the dialyzer membrane) (Fig. 2).

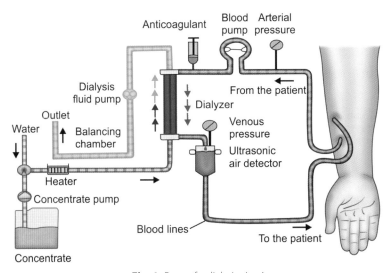

Fig. 1 Parts of a dialysis circuit

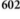

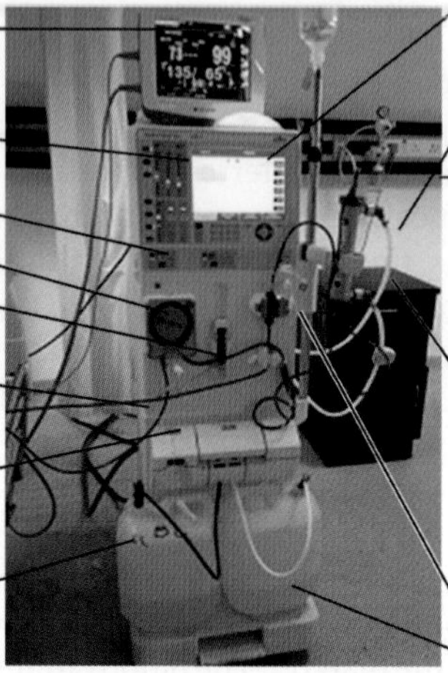

Cardiac monitor

Pressure of blood flow

Blood pump speed

Blood pump

Heparin pump

Blood returning to patient

Blood coming from patient

The source of bicarbonate part (B)

Display showing time left on treatment fluid to be removed and much more

Dialyzer holder

Blood then flow to the kidney where unwanted component are removed by diffusion. Excess fluid removed by pressure

Blood is diffused against the dialysate fluid which is made up of acid and bicarbonate mixed to the correct strength with treated water

Air detector

The source of bicarbonate part (A)

Fig. 2 Parts of dialysis machine

Filters

The filters are cylindrical in shape with clear plastic outside and dialyzer membrane visible inside (looks like thick paper). It is 15–18 inches in length and 2–3 inches in thickness. Connectors are present at the arterial and the venous side. The blood flows into a chamber (header) at one end. Blood then enters thousands of small capillaries tightly bound in a bundle. After the capillaries, the blood collects in a chamber at the other end of the cylindrical shell, the second header, and is then routed back to the patient through the venous tubing and venous access device. In parallel-plate dialyzers, now rarely used in the United States, the blood is routed between sheets of membranes laid on top of one another. The dialyzer is configured so that blood and dialysis solution pass through alternate spaces between the membrane sheets.

Membranes

Four types of membranes are currently used in dialyzers: cellulose, substituted cellulose, cellulosynthetic and synthetic.
1. *Cellulose*: Cellulose is obtained from processed cotton. Cellulose membranes go by various names, such as regenerated cellulose, cuprammonium cellulose (cuprophane), cuprammonium rayon and saponified cellulose ester.
2. *Substituted cellulose*: The cellulose polymer has a large number of free hydroxyl groups at its surface. These free hydroxyl group are responsible for blood cell activation causing bio-incompatibility of the dialyzer. In the cellulose acetate, cellulose diacetate and cellulose triacetate membranes, a substantial number of these groups are chemically bonded to acetate, reducing the free hydroxyl moieties and making membranes more biocompatible.
3. *Cellulosynthetic*: A synthetic material (a tertiary amino compound) is added to liquefied cellulose during formation of the membrane. As a result, the surface of the membrane is altered, and biocompatibility is increased. This membrane goes under the trade names of cellosyn or hemophan.

4. *Synthetics*: These membranes are not cellulose based but are synthetic plastics, and materials used include polyacrylonitrile (PAN), polysulfone, polycarbonate, polyamide and polymethyl methacrylate (PMMA).

Product Water for Hemodialysis

Patients are exposed to 120–200 L of dialysis solution during each dialysis treatment. Any small molecular weight contaminants in the dialysis solution can enter the blood unimpeded and accumulate in the body in the absence of renal excretion. Therefore, the chemical and microbiologic purity of dialysis solution is important, if patient injury is to be avoided. Dialysis solution is prepared from purified water (product water) and concentrates, the latter containing the electrolytes necessary to provide dialysis solution of the prescribed composition. Each dialysis unit has a water purification plant (Fig. 3).

Dialysate Fluid

During hemodialysis, there is countercurrent flow of blood and dialysate. This countercurrent flow optimizes the concentration gradient for solute removal. The dialysate is essentially a physiologic salt solution that creates a gradient for removal of unwanted solutes and maintains a constant physiologic concentration of extracellular electrolytes (Table 2).

Dialysis Access

Hemodialysis requires access to blood vessels capable of providing rapid extracorporeal blood flow. Vascular access can be permanent or temporary.

Permanent Access

It consists of arteriovenous fistula (AVF) or graft. AVFs are the preferred access method. They are created by joining an artery with a vein through an anastomosis.

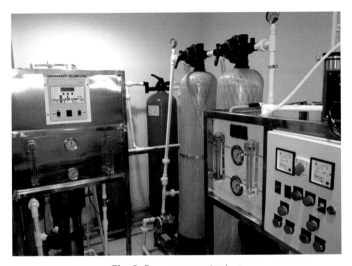

Fig. 3 Reverse osmosis plant

Table 2 Composition of dialysate fluid (units are in mEq/L, except for pH)

Sodium	135–145
Potassium	0–4
Chloride	102–106
Bicarbonate	30–39
Acetate	2–4
Calcium	0–3.5
Magnesium	0.5–1
Dextrose	11
pH	7.1–7.3

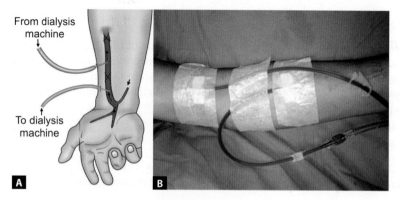

Figs 4A and B Arteriovenous fistula

They are usually created in the nondominant arm. The preferred sites are the anatomical snuffbox, the forearm (usually a radiocephalic fistula or so-called Brescia-Cimino fistula, in which the radial artery is anastomosed to the cephalic vein) or the elbow (usually a brachiocephalic fistula, where the brachial artery is anastomosed to the cephalic vein). Usually, 4–6 weeks are required for its maturation. Two AVF needles are needed for the initiation. The "arterial" needle draws blood from the "upstream" location while the "venous" needle returns blood "downstream" to avoid recycling. AVF is advantageous as it is associated with lower infection rates, higher blood flow rates and a lower incidence of thrombosis (Figs 4A and B).

Arteriovenous Graft

Arteriovenous graft is an artificial vessel, joining the artery and vein. The material used to make a graft is often polytetrafluoroethylene (PTFE), but sometimes sterilized veins from animals are also used. Grafts are used when patient's native vessel's dimension are unsuitable for a fistula creation. They mature faster than an AVF. Arteriovenous grafts have higher risk for thrombosis and infection (Fig. 5).

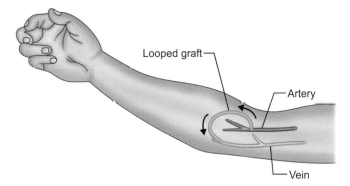

Fig. 5 Arteriovenous grafts

Temporary Access

Non-tunneled Catheters

Non-tunneled hemodialysis catheters are designed for short-term use and are the preferred catheter for immediate hemodialysis vascular access. Many different nontunneled catheters are available and are composed of materials such as polyurethane, polyethylene, polyvinyl chloride and medical grade silicone. The luminal diameter ranges from 1–2 mm and pump flow rates are 300–400 mL/minutes. Most nontunneled dialysis catheters have a conically-pointed tip and are relatively rigid at room temperature to facilitate insertion, but the catheter generally softens at body temperature to minimize the potential for vessel trauma. Because the more rigid material used in nontunneled catheters can perforate through the veins or heart, verification of correct catheter tip positioning is essential. Nontunneled catheters are usually short (9–20 cm) in length to ensure that the catheter tip does not extend into the right atrium.[20] The rigidity of the catheter makes insertion time slightly less by avoiding the use or need for an introducer sheath or possibly a soft tissue dilator, which are associated with an increased risk of blood loss and air embolism. Precurved catheters and curved extensions for nontunneled catheters are available to minimize catheter kinking at the exit site from the skin. The use-life of nontunneled catheters varies with insertion site. Mechanical malfunction and infectious complications are the principle reasons for removing a nontunneled dialysis catheter. In general, internal jugular and subclavian vein catheters are suitable for 2–3 weeks of use although longer periods have been reported[21] (Fig. 6).

Femoral catheters are generally limited to a single dialysis session in ambulatory patients, and 3–7 days in bed-bound patients.[21] Femoral catheters in ambulatory patients are removed after each dialysis session because of the issues of safety and difficulty maintaining the catheters which are prone to malposition and kinking.

Tunneled Catheters

Tunneled dialysis catheters are associated with lower rates of infection compared with nontunneled catheters.[22,23] The larger lumen size of tunneled catheters

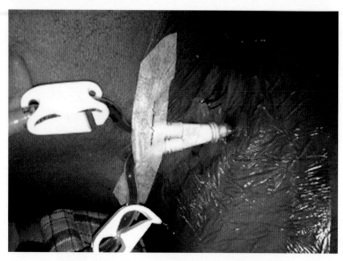

Fig. 6 Right internal jugular venous catheter *in situ*

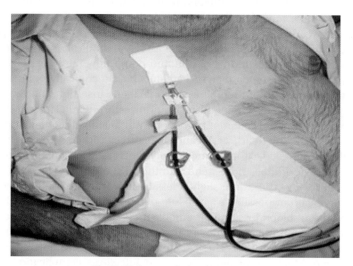

Fig. 7 Right tunneled catheter *in situ*

also allows for greater blood flow rates (> 400 cc/minutes) than nontunneled catheters. Tunneled catheters are primarily used for intermediate or long-term (> 2 weeks) hemodialysis vascular access. Placement of a tunneled catheter rather than a nontunneled catheter may be prudent for ambulatory patients diagnosed with AKI given that the duration of dialysis cannot be predicted.[23] Tunneled dialysis catheters are generally double lumen catheters with a polyester cuff generally positioned at the skin exit site that allows tissue ingrowth, sealing off the catheter tunnel. They are composed of silicone and other soft flexible polymers like thin polyurethane, which are less thrombogenic than the materials used in nontunneled catheters. These catheters are blunt, soft and flexible (Fig. 7).

Hemodialysis Anticoagulation

As blood comes in contact with an external dialysis circuit during hemodialysis, some form of anticoagulation is required to prevent clotting of blood. Strategies include no heparin, minimal heparin, heparin protamine and standard heparin use. In some patients, other forms of anticoagulation such as regional citrate, prostacyclin or citrate as a dialysate is used

No-heparin Hemodialysis

No-heparin hemodialysis is used in patients with at high risk of bleeding.[24] These include active bleed (except menstruation), recent surgery or patients with uremic pericarditis. The protocol requires rinsing both the dialyzer and blood lines with 2,000–5,000 units of heparin contained in a liter of normal saline. The heparinized saline is flushed out from the extracorporeal lines prior to dialysis. Usually, high blood flow rates are maintained with frequent flushing with normal saline to prevent clotting. Extra volume of saline infused should be calculated and later removed with ultrafiltration.

Minimum Dose Heparin

This protocol involves lower heparin doses to reduce bleeding risk (10% versus 19%) with frequent activated clotting time (ACT) monitoring. The dose consists of boluses of 500 units of heparin every 30 minutes or continuous infusion of heparin to keep the ACT above 150 seconds but below 200 seconds.[25-27]

Regional Anticoagulation with Protamine

The method involves infusion of heparin at the arterial end of the dialyzer and reversing this with protamine infusion at the returning end. This is one of the earliest methods used. Whole blood ACT is monitored and maintained at 250 seconds before dialyzer inlet and the predialysis baseline before returning blood to the patient. Protamine dosage is adjusted as per protamine titration test.[27]

Regional Citrate Anticoagulation

This method is based on the principle that calcium depletion with citrate prevents the progression of coagulation cascade. Isosmotic trisodium citrate solution (102 mmol/L) is infused into the arterial side of the dialyzer.[28] The dialyzer removes the citrate-calcium complex. Five percent calcium chloride is infused into the venous return line at a rate of 0.5 mL/minutes. Several modifications of this technique have been described.[28] The citrate infusion rate is adjusted to keep the ACT above 200 seconds in the arterial limb. Calcium level is frequently measured to prevent hypo- or hyperkalemia.

Citrate Dialysate

The use of citric acid as the acid in dialysate concentrates has been described. Citric acid-based dialysates result in reduced clotting in no-heparin dialysis (by lowering serum calcium enough to interfere with the clotting cascade but not enough to cause symptomatic hypokalemia) and increases patient bicarbonate levels (by the conversion of citrate to bicarbonate). The major disadvantage is that, at a citric acid concentration of 2.4 mEq/L, a small but significant change in serum calcium does occur, although usually not enough to cause symptoms. Further studies are needed to delineate the role of citric acid-based dialysates. It is commercially available.

Prostacyclin Regional Anticoagulation

Prostacyclin is a platelet aggregation inhibitor with vasodilatory properties. It is infused into the dialyzer circuit at 4–8 ng/kg/minutes. Its plasma half-life is 3–5 minutes. Headache, lightheadedness facial flushing and hypotension are major side effects which has limited use in present times.[29,30]

PREPARATION

- *Consent*: Before starting dialysis, a written consent needs to be taken from the patient or guardian. Monitoring of vital status.
- *Dialysis order*: A clear and comprehensive order has to be documented for the staff to start the dialysis procedure. It starts with the mode of hemodialysis, the duration and the amount of ultrafiltration, the access and any additional information including the transfusion of blood products.

PROCEDURE

Predialysis

- A dialysis machine is prepared before a patient is connected to it. Plumbing on the machine is set by the technician or the nurse.
- The pump works by applying pressure to the tubing and moving that pressure point around. The tubing is pressed between the disk and enclosure through 270 degrees. It is characteristic of dialysis machines that most of the blood out of the patients' body at any given time is visible. This facilitates troubleshooting, particularly detection of clotting.
- Access is set-up. For patients with a fistula, two large gauge needles are inserted in opposite direction into the fistula. For other patients, access may be via a catheter.
- When access has been set-up, the patient is then connected to the pre-configured plumbing, creating a complete loop through the pump and filter (Figs 8 to 10).

Dialysis

The pump and a timer are started. Hemodialysis is underway (Figs 11A and B).

Blood pressure is checked periodically. In each session, a definite amount of fluid is removed (ultrafiltration) which is practically calculated on the basis of weight gain and the extra fluid which has to be given to the patient as drugs or enteral nutrition or blood product transfusion.

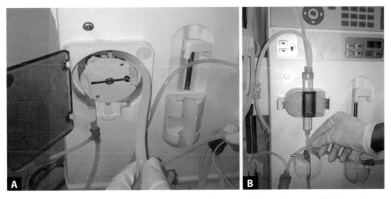

Figs 8A and B Dialysis machine is being set-up. (A) Part of the tubing is rolled over the rotor pump and (B) venous bubble catcher is being set in the holder

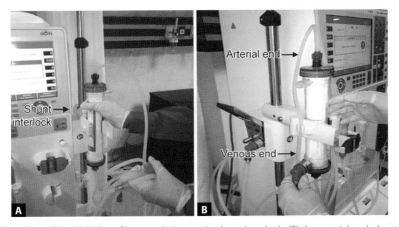

Figs 9A and B (A) Dialysis filters are being set in shunt interlock; (B) the arterial end placed above and venous end placed below

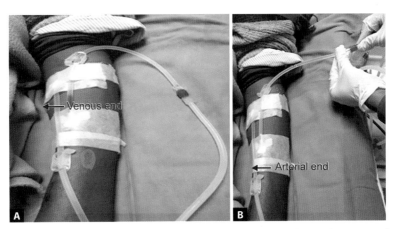

Figs 10A and B Arteriovenous access (fistula) is connected to the dialyzer tubings. Arterial end is punctured away from the heart and venous end towards it with a minimum distance of 5 cm between them to prevent recirculation

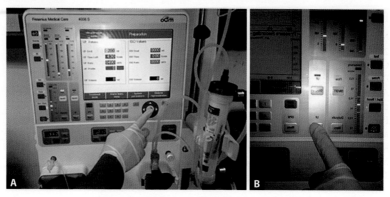

Figs 11A and B Dialysis machine is started

POST-PROCEDURE CARE

Patient is disconnected from the machine. Dialysis filter may be preserved for future reuse.

Needle wounds (in case of fistula) are bandaged with gauze, held for 10–15 minutes with direct pressure to stop bleeding, and then taped in place.

In case of dialysis catheter, maintain utmost sterility and put heparin in the lumen (as per manufacturer advice), after disconnection from the machine.

Blood pressure, weight and temperature are again measured.

COMPLICATION/PROBLEM

Patient Complications

- Hypotension
- Muscle cramps
- Disequilibrium syndrome
- Nausea and vomiting
- Headache
- Chest pain
- Itching
- Fever and chills
- Pyrogen reaction
- Hypertension.

Technical Complications

- Clotting
- Blood leak
- Power failure
- Hemolysis
- Air embolism
- Exsanguination
- Dialyzer reaction.

REFERENCES

1. Nash K, Hafeez A, Hou S. Hospital-acquired renal insufficiency. Am J Kidney Dis. 2002;39(5):930-6.
2. Graham T. The Bakerian lecture: on osmotic force. Philosophical Transactions of the Royal Society in London. 1854. pp. 177-228.
3. Abel JJ, Rowntree LG, Turner BB, et al. The removal of diffusible substances from the circulating blood by means of dialysis. Transfus Sci. 1990;11(2):164-5.
4. Paskalev DN, Haas Georg (1886–1971). The Forgotten Hemodialysis Pioneer, Dialysis and transplantation. 2001;30(12):828-30.
5. Kolff WJ, Berk, HTJ. Artificial kidney, dialyzer with great area. Geneesk Gids. 1944.
6. McKellar S. Gordon Murray and the artificial kidney in Canada. Nephrol Dial Transplant. 1999;14(11):2766-70.
7. Alwall N, Norvitt L. An artificial kidney: clinical experiences of dialytic treatment of uremia. Acta Med Scand. 1948;131:237-50.
8. Shaldon S. Development of Hemodialysis, From Access to Machine, Hypertension, dialysis and clinical nephrology HDCN 2002. [*www.hdcn.com (Accessed on November 2014)*].
9. Blagg CR. The Early Years of Chronic Dialysis: The Seattle Contribution. Am J Nephrol. 1999;19:350-4.
10. Kramer P, Schrader J, Bohnsack W, Grieben G, Gröne HJ, Scheler F. Continuous arteriovenous hemofiltration: a new kidney replacement therapy. Proc Eur Dial Transplant Assoc. 1981;18:743-9.
11. Bellomo R, Parkin G, Love J, Boyce N. A prospective comparative study of continuous arteriovenous hemodiafiltration and continuous venovenous hemodiafiltration in critically ill patients. Am J Kidney Dis. 1993;21(4):400-4.
12. Wendon J, Smithies M, Sheppard M, Bullen K, Tinker J, Bihari D. Continuous high volume venous-venous haemofiltration in acute renal failure. Intensive Care Med. 1989;15(6):358-63.
13. Ronco C, Bellomo R. Basic mechanisms and definitions for continuous renal replacement therapies. Int J Artif Organs. 1996;19(2):95-9.
14. Tolwani AJ, Wheeler TS, Wille KM. Sustained low-efficiency dialysis. Contrib Nephrol. 2007;156:320-4.
15. Marshall MR, Golper TA, Shaver MJ, Alam MG, Chatoth DK. Sustained low-efficiency dialysis for critically ill patients requiring renal replacement therapy. Kidney Int. 2001;60(2):777-85.
16. Marshall MR, Golper TA, Shaver MJ, Alam MG, Chatoth DK. Urea kinetics during sustained low-efficiency dialysis in critically ill patients requiring renal replacement therapy. Am J Kidney Dis. 2002;39(3):556-70.
17. Kumar VA, Craig M, Depner TA, Yeun JY. Extended daily dialysis: a new approach to renal replacement for acute renal failure in the intensive care unit. Am J Kidney Dis. 2000;36(2):294-300.
18. Marshall MR, Ma T, Galler D, Rankin AP, Williams AB. Sustained low-efficiency daily diafiltration (SLEDD-f) for critically ill patients requiring renal replacement therapy: towards an adequate therapy. Nephrol Dial Transplant. 2004;19(4):877-84.
19. Kielstein JT, Kretschmer U, Ernst T, Hafer C, Bahr MJ, Haller H. Efficacy and cardiovascular tolerability of extended dialysis in critically ill patients: a randomized controlled study. Am J Kidney Dis. 2004;43(2):342-9.
20. Ponikvar R, Buturović-Ponikvar J. Temporary hemodialysis catheters as a long-term vascular access in chronic hemodialysis patients. Ther Apher Dial. 2005;9(3):250-3.
21. Cheesbrough JS, Finch RG, Burden RP. A prospective study of the mechanisms of infection associated with hemodialysis catheters. J Infect Dis. 1986;154:579-89.
22. Coryell L, Lott JP, Stavropoulos SW, Stavropoulos SW, Mondschein JI, Patel AA, Kwak A. The case for primary placement of tunneled hemodialysis catheters in acute kidney injury. J Vasc Interv Radiol. 2009;20(12):1578-81.

23. Weijmer MC, Vervloet MG, ter Wee PM. Compared to tunnelled cuffed haemodialysis catheters, temporary untunnelled catheters are associated with more complications already within 2 weeks of use. Nephrol Dial Transplant. 2004;19(3):670-7.
24. Sanders PW, Taylor H, Curtis JJ. Hemodialysis without anticoagulation. Am J Kidney Dis. 1985;5(1):32-5.
25. Stamatiadis DN, Helioti H, Mansour M, Pappas M, Bokos JG, Stathakis CP. Hemodialysis for patients bleeding or at risk for bleeding, can be simple, safe and efficient. Clin Nephrol. 2004;62(1):29-34.
26. Swartz RD, Port FK. Preventing hemorrhage in high-risk hemodialysis: regional versus low-dose heparin. Kidney Int. 1979;16(4):513-8.
27. Pinnick RV, Wiegmann TB, Diederich DA. Regional citrate anticoagulation for hemodialysis in the patient at high risk for bleeding. N Engl J Med. 1983;308(5):258-61.
28. von Brecht JH, Flanigan MJ, Freeman RM, Lim VS. Regional anticoagulation: hemodialysis with hypertonic trisodium citrate. Am J Kidney Dis. 1986;8(3):196-201.
29. Swartz RD, Flamenbaum W, Dubrow A, Hall JC, Crow JW, Cato A. Epoprostenol (PGI2, prostacyclin) during high-risk hemodialysis: preventing further bleeding complications. J Clin Pharmacol. 1988;28(9):818-25.
30. Caruana RJ, Smith MC, Clyne D, Crow JW, Zinn JM, Diehl JH. Controlled study of heparin versus epoprostenol sodium (prostacyclin) as the sole anticoagulant for chronic hemodialysis. Blood Purif. 1991;9(5-6):296-304.

SECTION 5

Miscellaneous

54

Bone Marrow Aspiration and Biopsy

Gaurav Srivastava, Barnali Banik, Narendra Agrawal

INTRODUCTION

Bone marrow aspiration means to withdraw the fluid portion of the marrow and the bone marrow biopsy means to take out a piece of bone core with help of a wide bore needle. Bone marrow aspiration and biopsy are collectively referred to bone marrow examination.

Bone marrow drilling is one from oldest of surgical practices which still have relevance and is most basic and important test in the field of medicine. The currently practiced way of testing bone marrow came into practice since 1905 after a report by "Pianese" of marrow Leishmaniasis. In modern medicine, bone marrow examination is a valuable tool in evaluation of varied diseases.

INDICATION[1]

- Diagnosis, staging and monitoring of therapeutic response in various hematological diseases like:
  - Acute leukemias
  - Lymphoproliferative disorders
  - Myeloproliferative disorders
    Myelodysplastic syndrome
  - Plasma cell disorders (multiple myeloma, primary amyloidosis, etc.)
- To rule out metastasis
- Evaluation of cytopenias, unexplained anemia, leukocytosis, thrombocytosis, erythrocytosis
- Evaluation of iron status
- Pyrexia of unknown origin
- Chronic and disseminated infections and granulomatous diseases like tuberculosis, leishmaniasis, fungal infection, sarcoidosis, HIV specially when associated with cytopenias
- Unexplained splenomegaly
- Storage disorders (Gaucher's disease, etc.)
- Chromosomal disorders in neonates.

CONTRAINDICATION

There is actually no absolute contraindication. All of the mentioned below are relative contraindications.[1,2] It is imperative to ensure hemostasis after the procedure especially in a patient with coagulopathy or thrombocytopenia.

- Hemophilia
- Disseminated intravascular coagulation (DIC) or severe bleeding disorder (coagulopathy)
- Severe thrombocytopenia
- Avoid sternal aspirate in suspected multiple myeloma (high risk of perforation)
- Avoid in bone suspicious of osteomyelitis.

APPLIED ANATOMY

Bone marrow is a spongy tissue which consists of hematopoietic stem cells along with maturing hematopoietic elements, supporting stroma (macro- and microenvironment) and fat. The tissue lies within the hollow center of all the bones. At birth, almost all the marrow spaces are filled with hematopoietic tissue. As age advance, the tissue gets replaced by fat in long bones so in an adolescent and adults, the hematopoietic tissue is chiefly confined to axial skeletal (flat bones). Not only the bone marrow shrink in its extent but also the cellular portion decreases in whatever the bone marrow remains there in adults with advancing age. Whereas a marrow space shows a nearly 100% areas containing cellular components in a new born, the adults have it in range of 30–70% depending upon age.

TECHNIQUE AND EQUIPMENT

Site Selection[1,3]

- Posterior superior iliac spine (PSIS) is the most preferred site due to several reasons. Apart from advantage of having a good amount of marrow tissue in iliac crest, the PSIS is a superficial and fairly immovable landmark which can be palpated and located easily. The thickness of cortical bone is lesser at PSIS as compared to other parts of iliac crest. The thickness of iliac crest blade at or near PSIS is more so that we can get a good length marrow biopsy and the chance of cutting through the bone is less. Moreover, the amount of pain felt is usually lesser than any other site in body.
- Anterior superior iliac spine (ASIS) and area 2.5–5 cm posterior to it can be chosen as second option in a person who is not able to lie on lateral positions or having a disease/deformity affecting PSIS. ASIS can be accessed in supine posture. ASIS is also easily palpable and a relatively fixed landmark. The skin overlying ASIS is not fixed and can slide during the procedure making it difficult to poke the bone at desired site. The thickness of cortical bone is more at this site so, it sometimes becomes difficult to get access to marrow spaces.
- Sternum is last option and should be avoided in routine. Sternal puncture should never be done in patients younger than 12 years. Sternum can be accessible in morbidly obese patients. The preferred site is area close to second or third intercostal space. A bone marrow biopsy should never be attempted and only bone marrow aspiration can be done.

- Tibia contains marrow in infants and can be a good site for bone marrow sampling in infants. Ideal site is medial surface of tibia just below tibial tuberosity. Both marrow aspiration and biopsy can be done from this site.
- Surgical biopsy (open biopsy) or CT-guided biopsy (ribs, vertebrae or greater trochanter) can be done to target the affected sites of bone/bone marrow. Such kind of procedures is useful in diseases with focal bone marrow involvement.

Bone Marrow Aspirate, Smear and Imprints/Touch

Smears are good for morphologic assessment of cells and to get a differential counts (myelogram). If marrow fragments are visible then an idea of cellularity of the marrow can also be taken. Occasionally, the marrow aspirate is diluted with blood and no or only occasional marrow components are visible. In such cases, the diagnosis rests on marrow biopsy. The imprint/touch smears made by putting and rolling of bone marrow biopsy piece on slides can help to get morphologic details of cells in such cases. Apart from routine morphological tests on marrow, the slides can be tested with various cytochemical stains to look for particular type of disease for example, the myeloperoxidase (MPO) stain for acute myeloid leukemia and iron stain to look for iron stores and also to diagnose myelodysplastic syndromes. The aspirated marrow can be taken into heparinized or ethylenediaminetetraacetic acid (EDTA) vials to subject to various molecular/fluorescence in situ hybridization (FISH), cytogenetic studies and flow cytometric immunophenotyping. Other tests which can be performed at aspirated marrow are cultures for mycobacterium, Leishmania, bacteria/fungi, etc. as indicated.

Bone Marrow Biopsy

Biopsy is a long thin piece from core of the bone. We should try to get at least 1.5 cm long piece so that to see at least 10 marrow spaces (intertrabecular spaces) under the microscope to call it an adequate biopsy, otherwise you may get an equivocal report from your pathologist or the pathologist can state that biopsy was inadequate to give a final opinion. Biopsy is good tool to assess cellularity of marrow and arrangement or localization of various cellular components within the marrow spaces. Biopsy is also useful to look for malignant infiltrates like solid tumors, lymphomas. Biopsy from bilateral PSIS or iliac crests is sometimes recommended to more reliably look for lymphoma or solid tumor infiltrates. Nowadays, bilateral biopsies are not routinely recommended and in diseases with known focal marrow involvement, it is preferable to do computed tomography (CT) or positron emission tomography (FDG-PET) guided biopsies.[4] Other tests which can be performed at biopsy tissue are reticulin stain for fibrosis and immunohistochemistry as indicated.

Equipment

- *Bone marrow aspiration needle:* Usually a smaller, 16-gauge needle with a stylet
- *Bone marrow biopsy needle:* A wider bore, usually 11 gauge for adults (some prefer 9-gauge needle) or 13-gauge needle for pediatric age group. Needle is accompanied by a stylet and a "J" shaped device (obturator) for removing the biopsy core from the needle (Fig. 1).

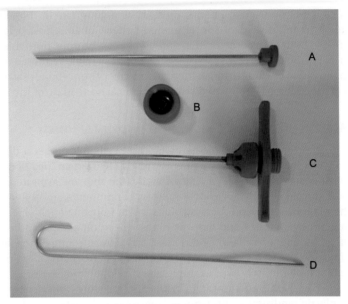

Fig. 1 Jamshidi bone marrow biopsy needle and its parts. (A) Stylet, (B) cap, (C) biopsy needle 11 gauge, (D) obturator

PREPARATION

- Bone marrow aspiration and biopsy should be an absolutely aseptic procedure. Every care should be taken to maintain so, to avoid any chances of infection
- *Consent:* A written informed consent should also be signed, explaining the procedure and the possible risks involved in it. This also leads to allay the apprehension in the patient's mind and make him feel comfortable
- General anesthesia or sedation may be required in pediatric cases or in anxious/non-cooperating adults
- *Monitoring required:* Usually, the vitals and oxygen saturation are checked before starting the procedure. A check is also kept on the oxygen saturation in cases of mild sedation
- *Laboratory work-up:* Generally, coagulation profile and platelet counts are checked before the procedure
- Arrange major equipment (bone marrow aspiration and biopsy needles of appropriate size
- *Arrange adjunct equipment (Fig. 2):*
  - A thin knife (usually size 11) to give a stab at the selected site
  - Five disposable syringes with needles, 5 and 10 cc (to give local anesthesia and then to collect samples)
  - Glass slides (should be a fresh pack or recently opened pack)
  - Glass or plastic container with 10% formalin or B5 solution to put biopsy in it
  - Heparinized/EDTA vials, culture bottles, etc. as per the requirement
  - Cleansing solutions (alcohol and povidone iodine or 2% chlorhexidine), sterile pack containing bowls, drapes, sponge holder, gauge pieces/pads, injectable lidocaine 2% for local anesthesia
- Also, one of the most important is an assistant who is good in making slides.

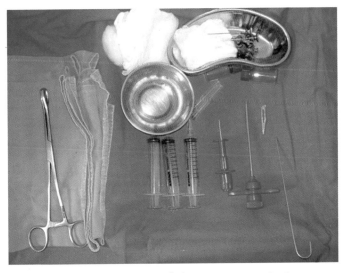

Fig. 2 Adjunct equipment for bone marrow examination

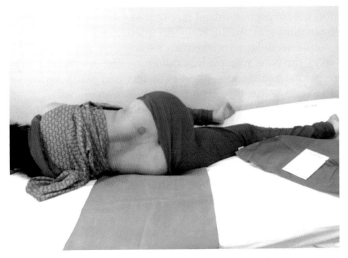

Fig. 3 Ideal position for bone marrow examination for a right handed person

PROCEDURE

For Posterior Iliac Crest Site

- The patient should be placed in lateral decubitus position (if you are a right handed person then left lateral position will be more convenient) with the top leg flexed and the lower leg straight (Fig. 3). Alternatively, prone positioning can be done.
- Examine site for any evidence of infection; palpate and locate the posterior iliac crest and PSIS. ASIS should also be palpated and located, as the needle will be pointed in this direction once the bone has been entered.

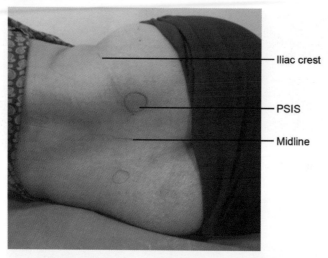

Fig. 4 Important landmarks for bone marrow examination
Abbreviation: PSIS, posterior superior iliac spine.

- Common site for aspiration and biopsy is approximately three finger-widths from the midline and two finger-widths inferior to the iliac crest (Fig. 4).
- Using sterile technique, protective clothing and gloves (and eye wear if necessary), the bone marrow tray should be first opened and organized for easy access to needed items. Needles, stylets, and plastic syringes should be checked to ensure that they are intact and function properly.
- Cleanse the chosen area with povidone-iodine or chlorhexidine solution and drape a sterile field (Fig. 5A).
- Use 1–2% lidocaine solution using a 23-gauge needle to anesthetize the skin, subcutaneous tissue. Infiltrate the periosotium repeatedly by injecting small amounts of lidocaine solution at different points on the surface of the bone with a 21–22-gauge needle. Anesthetize a small area around the target region as aspirate and biopsy should be taken from different sites (Fig. 5B).
- While waiting for the anesthetic to produce its effect, extra syringes for special studies (e.g. flow cytometry, cytogenetics and molecular studies) can be appropriately anticoagulated. Specimens for molecular studies should not contain heparin.
- Once local anesthesia has been achieved, make a small (3 mm) skin incision with a scalpel blade at the site of insertion of the aspiration needle. The incision should be perpendicular to the long axis of body to avoid gaping of wound (Fig. 6).
- Hold the bone marrow needle (with stylet in place) perpendicular to the skin at the previously marked point, and gently advance it to the periosteum. When the needle has reached periosteum, it should be directed toward the ASIS.
- Use twisting motion and do not twist more than 180 degree in either direction to penetrate the periosteum. A steady twisting back and forth motion. When the periosteum is penetrated there is a give way feeling. At this point patient feels deep seated pain. Patient should be alerted of this pain beforehand

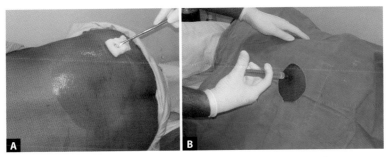

Figs 5A and B (A) Cleaning of area; (B) Draping and local anesthesia

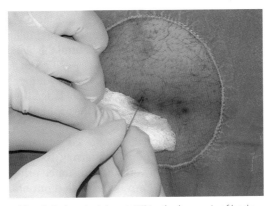

Fig. 6 Stab or incision at 90° to the long axis of body

otherwise he may be taken by surprise. Continue to advance the needle slightly to ensure that it is anchored into the bone.

- Remove the stylet, attach a 2 mL syringe to the aspiration needle, and again advise the patient that the aspiration may cause a brief period of pain (Figs 7A and B).
- Only aspirate 0.2–0.5 mL of bone marrow as excessive drainage may lead to dilution with peripheral blood. This initial specimen should be used for preparing smears.
- The non-anticoagulated specimen should be handed to the assistant, who will assess the quality of the sample (i.e. determine the presence or absence of grossly visible bone spicules) and prepare the various smears. Anti-coagulated specimens should be sent to the laboratory for further preparation and other tests (e.g. cytogenetics, molecular studies, cultures and flow cytometry). The patient should be made aware of the need for multiple specimens at the outset, since each separate aspiration may be painful, despite fully adequate local anesthesia.
- If aspiration attempts are not successful, reinsert the stylet (the needle may be rotated) and advance the needle a short distance; repeat attempts at aspiration with the syringe and suction. If multiple aspiration attempts are unsuccessful, an alternate site (e.g. the other posterior iliac crest) may be approached with the same sterile strategy after the bone marrow biopsy has been obtained.

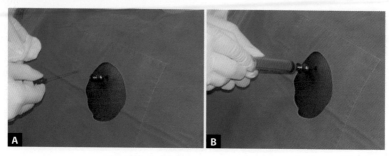

Figs 7A and B Bone marrow aspiration

- Once it has been determined that the aspirate is satisfactory, reinsert the stylet and remove the needle (with stylet in place) by using a similar twisting motion, and apply pressure to the site with small gauze until the bleeding stops.
- If a biopsy is necessary, prepare the Jamshidi™ needle and advance it into the cortical bone, using the same incision but a slightly different point in bone, with a steady twisting movement until it is firmly lodged. This may require a greater amount of pressure than was used for the aspiration. Remove the stylet and with a rotating motion advance the needle for another 15–20 mm (Fig. 8A).
- Redirect the needle tip and rotate it 360 degrees in both directions to separate the biopsy specimen from the surrounding marrow tissue. Following this step, the needle should be advanced a very short distance prior to removal. This step may prevent the specimen from being pulled out of the needle at the biopsy site.
- Remove the needle with a slight twisting motion, place a sterile dressing over the site and apply pressure for several minutes until the bleeding stops. Once hemostasis is achieved, a bandage should be applied, and the patient should be instructed to lie supine for 10 or more minutes. Pressure dressings may be required in thrombocytopenic patients.
- Once the biopsy needle has been removed, the specimen may be extracted from the needle by inserting the obturator (or stylet) through the distal (cutting) end of the needle. The bone marrow biopsy can then be placed on a slide, where imprints (touch prints) are made before the core specimen is further processed for cytologic investigations. This step is especially useful in situations where a bone marrow aspirate could not be obtained (Fig. 8B).
- Examine the biopsy specimen. If the specimen consists mostly of homogeneous, white material (cortical bone) or glistening tissue (cartilage), it may be necessary to attempt a second biopsy for a more satisfactory specimen. This should be done with a new biopsy needle, as the original needle may have been damaged by the process of inserting the obturator or stylet through the distal end of the biopsy needle.

Special Consideration

Precautions to be taken when dealing with a particular disease for example, in patients with multiple myeloma, the bone may be extremely soft and if one applies a normal force, the needle may pierce the entire blade of bone to injure

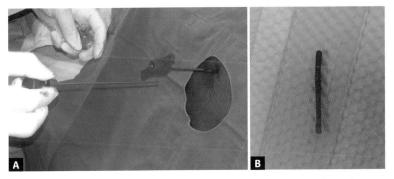

Figs 8A and B Bone marrow biopsy needle in place and a good length bone marrow biopsy piece

underling structures. Also, it is very difficult to get a biopsy from soft and fragile bone. To take a biopsy from such cases, you need to palpate the bone by the needle and chose a firm to hard point on the surface of bone.

Dry tap, where one is unable to get aspirate, is more commonly due to faulty technique but occasionally associated with certain underlying conditions like marrow fibrosis, tumor infiltrates, leukemia and aplastic anemia.

POST-PROCEDURE CARE

- Document vitals during procedure, postprocedure recovery and hemostasis
- If the patient is in pain after the procedure, give him some analgesia (e.g. paracetamol).
- Firm pressure and dressing. Advise patient to rest for at least 30 minutes to be sure about his vitals and also the hemostasis at the biopsy site. Keep the area dry. Bandage can be removed after 24 hours. Wound site should be checked to look for signs of infection or hematoma formation.
- *Preparation of bone marrow slides (Figs 9A to C):* Put few drops of the aspirate on each glass slide and transfer the remaining aspirate into EDTA tubes to prevent clotting. Slides can be prepared by following methods.
  - *Wedge method:* Place few aspirate particles on one slide and use the second slide at an angle of 30 degree to spread it.
  - *Particle crush technique:* This is a better technique but requires practice. Particles are put over the end of the first slide and the second slide is placed parallel to the first one to crush the particles and then run over. This method gives better evaluation of hematopoietic cells and mast cells.
  - *Touch (imprint) smear:* When aspirate is unsatisfactory. Biopsy piece is rolled in between two slides with mild compression making sure not to break the biopsy sample.

COMPLICATION/PROBLEM

Complication rate is reported to be 0.05–0.07% in large studies.[5-7]
- Dizziness and headache under influence of local anesthetic agent
- Local site infection/abscess formation
- Bleeding or oozing from puncture site, hematoma

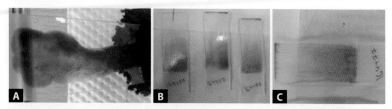

Figs 9A to C Preparation of bone marrow aspiration smears. (A) The aspirated marrow is poured over a slanting slide; (B) The blood slides down while the marrow particles remain on top; (C) Then, these particles are picked up with help of a spreader slide and smeared over glass slides

- Needle breakage
- Sternal perforation
- Deaths reported due to sepsis, laceration of blood vessels and massive hemorrhage[6,7]
- Pain
- Anaphylactic reactions
- Fractures
- Specific complications of sterna puncture are perforation with penetration of underlying structures leading to pulmonary embolism, pneumothorax, cardiac temponade or perforation.

REFERENCES

1. Bain BJ. Bone marrow aspiration. J Clin Pathol. 2001;54(9):657-63.
2. Eikelboom JW. Bone marrow biopsy in thrombocytopenic or anticoagulated patients. Br J Haematol. 2005;129(4):562-3.
3. Malempati S, Joshi S, Lai S, Braner DA, Tegtmeyer K. Videos in clinical medicine. Bone marrow aspiration and biopsy. N Engl J Med. 2009;361(15):e28.
4. Campbell JK, Matthews JP, Seymour JF, Wolf MM, Juneja SK. Australasian Leukaemia Lymphoma Group. Optimum trephine length in the assessment of bone marrow involvement in patients with diffuse large cell lymphoma. Ann Oncol. 2003;14(2): 273-6.
5. Le Dieu R, Luckit J, Sundarasun M. Complications of trephine biopsy. Br J Haematol. 2003;121(6):822.
6. Bain BJ. Morbidity associated with bone marrow aspiration and trephine biopsy—a review of UK data for 2004. Haematologica. 2006;91(9):1293-4.
7. Bain BJ. Bone marrow biopsy morbidity and mortality. Br J Haematol. 2003;121(6): 949-51.

55

Postmortem Organ Needle Biopsy

Rajanikant R Yadav, Namita Mehrotra

INTRODUCTION

Failure to reach antemortem diagnosis is a common problem in medicine. Even with the exclusion of lack of facilities and diagnostic experience, there are other unavoidable factors that include:[1]

- Limited time prior to demise
- Cardiovascular instability of the patient for invasive investigations or exploratory laparotomy
- The presence of coagulopathy
- Limitations of serological or radiological markers in diagnosis.

Hence, there is a need for autopsy that provides answers for the deceased relatives[2] and also provides important information for both research and clinical practice.[1] Unfortunately, the standard autopsy technique is declining due to difficulty in obtaining consent, financial reasons or technical difficulties. Concerns of the next-of-kin, about delaying the rituals and esthetic appearance of the deceased are other major factors that have limited autopsies. Postmortem biopsy sampling of tissues from certain organs can provide "meaningful pathological alterations" that aid in diagnosis of disease.[2] Postmortem needle biopsy is ideal for detecting conditions producing diffuse changes in an organ.

INDICATION

- *To determine the cause of death*
  - When relatives of the deceased have refused to give their consent for a conventional necropsy.
  - When a full necropsy is not justified owing to the risk of infection.[3]
- To improve our understanding of the pathogenesis of diseases which require human samples to be studied.

CONTRAINDICATION

Relatives unwilling to give consent for minimally invasive biopsy.

APPLIED ANATOMY AND TECHNIQUE

Multiple needle biopsy tissue samples of the liver, spleen, heart, kidneys, lungs, muscles, brain are collected in the immediate postmortem period using a Tru-cut biopsy needle. Advantages of bedside postmortem biopsy are: (1) it is less time-consuming and is performed at bedside before decomposition occurs, thereby making it possible to apply a wide range of investigational methods that include microbiological and immunological studies, frozen sections and electron microscopy, (2) acceptance of the "limited postmortem sampling" technique by next of kin is higher than conventional autopsy primarily due to the "nondeforming" nature of needle biopsy.

- *Nonimaging-guided techniques*
  Fouroudi et al. described a nonimaging-guided technique for obtaining samples from viscera.[4]
  - *Liver:* Multiple biopsies from both lobes of the liver at the transabdominal line.
  - *Heart:* Through the left, third and fourth intercostal spaces just lateral to the sternum.
  - *Kidney:* At 1 cm below the twelfth rib and 2 cm lateral to the lateral border of the quadratus lumborum muscle.
  - *Lung and pleura:* Tissue samples can be collected, directly through small incisions (1 cm) from the suspected sites or randomly from the third left and right midaxillary lines.
  - Other sites, e.g. muscle, intestine can be sampled via an open incision, if they have clinical and/or radiological evidence of disease.[1]
- *Imaging-guided techniques*
  Farina J et al. described an ultrasound-guided technique for obtaining postmortem biopsy samples.[5] Ultrasonography is performed to detect any focal lesions using 2–5 MHz convex or sectorial probe to study the liver, kidneys, spleen, pancreas, the gastrointestinal and urogenital tracts, heart, lungs, pleural and peritoneal cavities. The breasts, testes, thyroid gland, other superficial structures and all the organs in children can be studied using a multifrequency 5–7.5 MHz linear probe. Ultrasound examination of the adult brain can be done via a 3 cm window created in the skull or via the foramen magnum and biopsy samples can be obtained under ultrasound guidance. The brain of newborns and infants can be accessed via the fontanelles.[5]

Tru-cut® Biopsy Gun

Spring loaded Tru-cut® biopsy guns from 14–18 gauge with needle shaft lengths of 9–20 cm and sample slot of size 1–2 cm can be used (Figs 1 to 4).

PREPARATION

- *Consent:* The relatives are made aware of the importance of autopsy, which includes the possibility of an infectious process in the deceased, the underlying hereditary or familial factor predisposing to death and the exact causes of death.
- *List of all equipment:* Image-guidance modality (ultrasound machine with 2–5 MHz convex or sectorial probe and 5–7.5 MHz linear probe), povidone

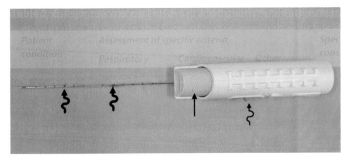

Fig. 1 18 gauge spring loaded biopsy gun with its shaft (thin curved black arrows) having markers at 1 cm distances, cocking mechanism (straight arrow) and trigger (bold curved arrow)

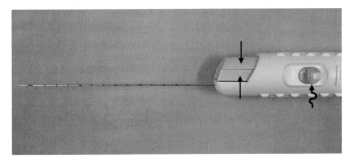

Fig. 2 Side view of biopsy gun showing its two cocking levers (straight arrows) and trigger (bold curved arrow)

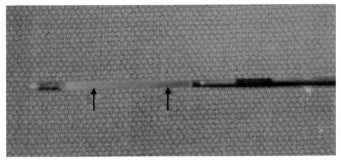

Fig. 3 Partially cocked biopsy gun showing its 2 cm length tissue core sample slot (straight arrows)

iodine, sterile drapes including cut sheet, sterile gloves, blade no. 11, 14–18 gauge Tru-cut biopsy gun, formalin jar, 18 gauge lumbar puncture needle for fluid aspirations, syringes, sutures.

PROCEDURE

- Select the site for biopsy (see above).
- The skin overlying the organ of biopsy is cleaned with povidone iodine and sterile drapes with cut hole applied at the procedure site (Fig. 5).

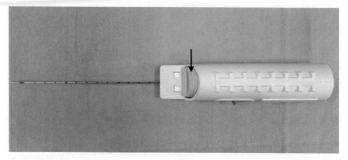

Fig. 4 Fully cocked biopsy gun with retracted cocking levers (straight arrow)

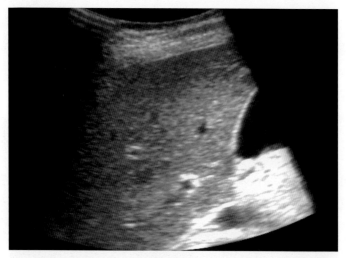

Fig. 5 Ultrasound image of liver using 2–5 MHz convex probe

- Generally five or more samples from lesions or from organs, in which disease had been suspected while the patient was alive, should be considered.
- For liver and kidney biopsies, a draped sterile ultrasound probe is used to focus the organ and guide the direction and depth of the needle insertion (Figs 5 to 8).
- For lung biopsies samples are obtained directly through small incisions (1 cm) from the suspected sites and the wound closed with sutures. Samples can also be obtained randomly from the third left and right midaxillary lines.
- For aspiration of effusions and other fluids a spinal needle (18–20 gauge) connected to a syringe is inserted under sonographic guidance under full aseptic precautions to prevent contamination of samples.
- Whenever possible, blood samples are obtained for laboratory testing.

POST-PROCEDURE CARE AND PROBLEMS

Handling/Storage of Samples

All biopsy samples are immediately placed in a container containing buffered formalin. The patient name, hospital registration number and the organ from

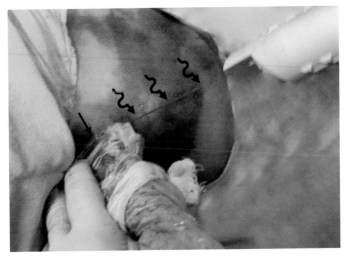

Fig. 6 Alignment of ultrasound probe (straight arrow) and biopsy gun (bold curved arrows) for biopsy

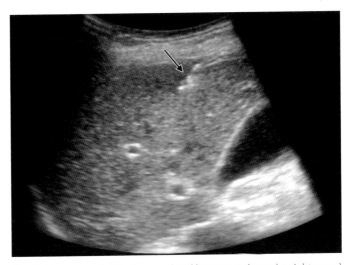

Fig. 7 Biopsy gun shaft in the peripheral liver parenchyma (straight arrow)

which the biopsy sample has been obtained are labeled on the container. The samples obtained for histological analysis are sent for conventional histological analysis and for immunohistochemistry, genetic and other diagnostic techniques. Aspirates from effusions and other fluids are sent for cytological and microbiological studies.

Problems

- *Inadequate and non-representative samples*: The concordance rate between needle autopsy and conventional autopsy regarding the cause of death

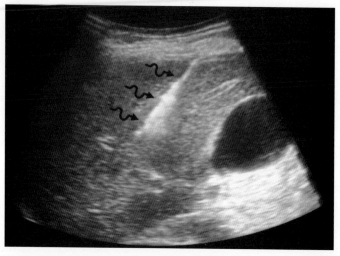

Fig. 8 Complete tract (bold curved arrows) of the biopsy gun shaft in the liver parenchyma after triggering the biopsy gun

and the main pathological findings has been variably reported to range from 60–83%. However, the postmortem needle biopsy technique has not gained popular acceptance due to failure to obtain adequate tissues in the sampled areas and, more importantly for pathologists, it does not provide the macroscopic appearance of organs in situ and might fail to sample focal lesions or small organs (e.g. parathyroid glands) or lesions in the nervous system.

- *Inability to diagnose cause of death in certain cases*: e.g. metabolic causes.

REFERENCES

1. El-Reshaid W, El-Reshaid K, Madda J. Postmortem biopsies: the experience in Kuwait. Med Princ Pract. 2005;14(3):173-6.
2. Rigaud JP, Quenot JP, Borel M, Plu I, Hervé C, Moutel G. Post mortem scientific sampling and the search for causes of death in intensive care: what information should be given and what consent should be obtained? J Med Ethics. 2011;37(3):132-6.
3. Underwood JC, Slater DN, Parsons MA. The needle necropsy. Br Med J (Clin Res Ed). 1983;286:1632-4.
4. Foroudi F, Cheung K, Duflou J. A comparison of the needle biopsy postmortem and the conventional autopsy. Pathology. 1995;27(1):79-82.
5. Farina J, Millana C, Fdez-Acenero MJ, Furio V, Aragoncillo P, Martin VG, et al. Ultrasonographic autopsy (echopsy): a new autopsy technique. Virchows Arch. 2002;440(6):635-9.

56
Managing Pressure Ulcer

Ankur Bhatnagar

INTRODUCTION

Patients in intensive care unit (ICU) settings are considered to be at greatest risk for development of pressure ulcers. They are likely to present with rapid progression of symptoms, may require mechanical ventilation and subsequent administration of sedatives and pharmacological drugs, potentially reducing the peripheral circulation which leads to rapid development of pressure ulcers. The presence of these lesions contributes to overall septic load, and patient thus enters a spiraling downfall of ulcer-related sepsis and multiorgan dysfunction. The most effective treatment of pressure ulcer continue to be its prevention. Every ICU should implement strategies to prevent hospital-acquired Stage III and IV pressure ulcers. However, it is imperative to remember that pressure ulcers are bound to occur in ICU patients in spite of best care. Unlike paraplegics, children, terminally ill and even patients under home care, accurate risk assessment tools for pressure ulcer development are not available for ICU patients.[1] Management of pressure ulcers especially in ICU settings is a complex job requiring close cooperation between various categories of caregivers like intensivist in charge, nursing personnel, wound care specialist, surgeon, plastic and reconstructive surgeon, dermatologist, dietician, occupational therapist.

PATHOPHYSIOLOGY OF PRESSURE ULCER

The primary cause of any pressure ulcer is prolonged ischemia and continuous frictional stress to the tissues. When tissue pressures exceed the normal intracapillary pressures, it produces local capillary occlusion, ischemia and tissue hypoxia, leading to tissue breakdown. Muscles are more prone to develop ischemic changes as compared to the overlying skin when subjected to equal amount of sustained pressure. Unlike other patients, e.g. paraplegics, ICU patients are continuously exposed to multiple risk factors which can lead to the development of pressure ulcers, which are divided into extrinsic and intrinsic causes.[2]

- *Extrinsic factors*: Excessive pressure (infrequent turning), shear and friction force, impact injury (pressure from tubes, catheter, rubbing pulling of patient), heat, moisture, posture, incontinence, length of ICU stay.
- *Intrinsic factors*: Critical illness (hypotension), reduced mobility, age, skin (dry thin papery), body type (obesity), nutrition, sepsis.

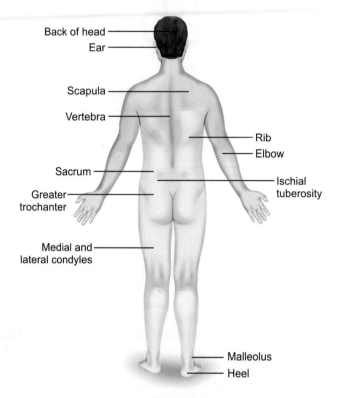

Back of head

Ear

Scapula

Vertebra

Rib

Elbow

Sacrum

Greater trochanter

Ischial tuberosity

Medial and lateral condyles

Malleolus

Heel

Fig. 1 Multiple sites of ulcer

Where it occurs? Figure 1 showing multiple sites of ulcer.

Grades:[3,4] Various stages of pressure ulcer are described in Table 1 and are shown in Figures 2A to D.

PREVENTION

Preventing pressure ulcers is of paramount importance especially in critically ill patients, as definitive treatment for pressure ulcers may not be always possible due to poor general condition. It involves:
- Risk assessment
- Nutritional assessment
- Patient positioning
- Choice of support surface.

Risk assessment: Every ICU should have a protocol to analyze every new admission and to identify at risk individuals. Multiple scoring systems are used but the modified Brendon score is the simplest[1] and the most commonly used. Scoring is done on various risk factors which provide a structured documentation

Table 1 Features of various stages of pressure ulcer

Category	Features
Stage I	Intact, non-blanchable skin
	Pain disproportionate to the ulcer
Stage II	Partial thickness dermal loss
	Presents as a dry, shallow ulcer or a serosanguinous blister with absence of slough
	Often confused with tape burns, incontinence-associated dermatitis, maceration or excoriation
Stage III	Full thickness skin loss with exposed subcutaneous tissue slough present
	Minimal undermining and tunneling present
Stage IV	Full thickness tissue loss with exposed bone, tendon or muscle
	Slough or eschar may be present
	Extensive undermining and tunneling
Unclassified pressure ulcers	Extensive slough and eschar prevent localization of the stage of ulcer. Once debridement is done only then true depth of ulcer is known

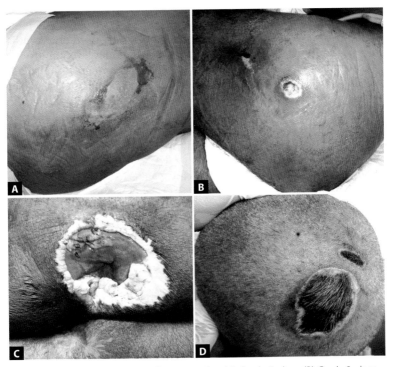

Figs 2A to D Various grades of pressure ulcer (A) Grade 2 ulcer; (B) Grade 3 ulcer; (C) Grade 4 ulcer; (D) Device-related scalp ulcer

of at risk individuals. All individuals who are confined to the bed with no or limited mobility and intact skin with alterations are at high risk of pressure ulcer development. Friction, sensory perception, general health status and body temperature should be an important part of assessment of at risk individuals. Skin inspection should include assessment for localized heat, edema, or indurations (hardness), especially in dark skin individuals.[3]

Nutritional assessment: Serum albumin, hemoglobin and weight are the most important indicators. Each patient is given 30–35 kcal per kg body weight per day, with 1.25–1.5 g/kg/day protein and 1 mL of fluid intake per kcal per day.[5] Oral nutrition (via normal feeding, tube feeding and/or with additional sip feeding) is the preferred route for nutrition, and should be supported whenever possible.[5]

Patient repositioning:[1,6] Repositioning involves moving the patient to prevent prolonged pressure over bony prominences and patient-related devices. The repositioning schedule for every patient should be tailor-made and depends on the inherent mobility, general medical condition, treatment objectives and assessments of the individual's skin condition, and varies between frequent turning every 2–4 hours. Individuals on ventilators or deep sedation with poor cardiovascular status will also require protection against shear stress. Figures 3A and B showing various repositioning figures.

Support surface:[5,6] Currently, there are over 200 of these devices commercially available. Most ICU patients have limited mobility, are hooked onto ventilators, multiple life-support systems, and require head end elevation to prevent ventilator-associated pneumonia (VAP), making frequent turning next to impossible. Precedence of VAP prevention leads to higher shear stress on the coccyx. Support surfaces are of two types: *pressure reducing* and *pressure relieving*. Pressure relieving devices increase the surface contact area to reduce pressure and include foam mattresses and low air loss mattresses. Pressure reducing devices relieve pressure over specific body areas by using timed pressure cycles known as alternating pressure support. However, no device has been proved to be superior and there is no substitute for regular repositioning. The nursing personnel should not be lulled into a false sense of security while using these devices and modify their patient positioning routine.[5] Higher-specification foam mattresses should be used for all individuals assessed as being at risk for pressure ulcer development. Heel-protection devices distribute the weight of the leg along the calf without putting pressure on the Achilles tendon, with knee kept in slight flexion.

General guidelines for prevention of pressure ulcers in ICU patients:[5,6]
- Skin should be checked daily for at risk individuals and documented.
- Skin should be cleaned regularly.
- Hot water and irritating chemical agents should be strictly avoided. Normal saline or lukewarm water is the best.
- The skin should be adequately moisturized after each cleaning using neutral pH soaps.
- Incontinent individuals should be provided with barrier absorbent dressings to keep at risk skin well lubricated and dry.
- Do not use massage or vigorously rub skin but gently dab or pat dry.

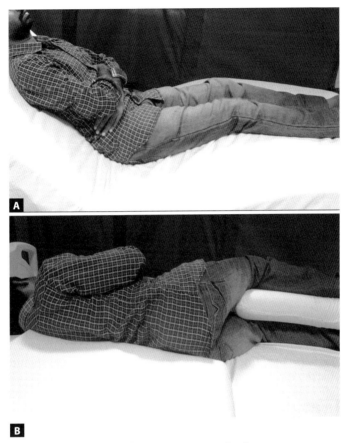

Figs 3A and B Various repositioning figures

- Use of skin emollients prevents dry skin.
- Excessive skin moisture should also be avoided to prevent maceration.
- Use of transfer aids to reduce friction and shear.
- Multiple individuals should position the patient in tandem by lifting and avoid dragging.
- The heels should be always on the surface and support should be applied underneath the calf when lying supine.
- Avoid positioning over medical devices such as tubes and drainage catheters.
- Patient should be nursed in 30° side lying or prone position. Ninety degree lateral and supine position should be avoided.
- Head end elevation beyond 30° should be avoided to prevent slouched position which places excessive pressure and shear over the sacrum and coccyx.
- For ventilated patients the head end elevation should be around 30° so as to prevent VAP while reducing shear stress on the coccyx.
- Minimum amount of linen should be there between the patient and the support surface.

- Use an active support surface (overlay or mattress) for patients where repositioning is not possible.
- Frequent turning and repositioning should continue even in the presence of a support surface.
- Synthetic sheepskin pads, cut out ring, or donut-type devices and water-filled gloves should be avoided.

TREATMENT OF PRESSURE ULCER[7]

The objectives for management of pressure ulcers vary depending on the stage of the wound:
- Recently closed wound, Stage I pressure ulcer, denuded or excoriated skin— require skin protection to avoid further damage.
- Stage II—encourage regeneration of tissue and protect wound surface.
- Stage III/IV—promote granulation and contraction (epithelialization), followed by definitive skin cover if required.

PREPARATION

- *Routine work-up:* Before embarking on wound care of a patient in ICU, following points are to be ascertained: check for vitals, check for bleeding profile, inform the intensivist and the patient attendants, adequate analgesia/ sedation, proper exposure and lighting.
- *Dressing personnel:* Intensive care unit dressing personnel should use cap, mask, barrier disposable Mackintosh at all times. There should be a minimum of two people at time of dressing (one for dressing and other for providing sterile material).
- *Dressing tray (Fig. 4):* Dressing tray with lid and should have: two medium-size sterile sheets (one plain and one cut), two artery forceps (one large and one small), one small bowl, one tissue cutting scissors, one tooth forceps heavy, sterile gauze and cotton pads, scalpel blade no. 4 one, cleansers and antibacterial like povidone-iodine, normal saline, large sterile Gamzee pads (10° × 10°) and rolls (6° × 1 m), sealing sheets of various sizes (e.g. opsite).
- *Assessment of wound:[8]*
  - *Pressure ulcer stage:* All assessments and skin inspection findings should be documented as early as possible after admission. Once layers of tissue and supporting structures are lost, they can only be replaced with granulation tissue. Hence, a Stage IV pressure ulcer becomes a healing Stage IV, once granulation starts. Apart from the stage, the anatomical location, size of ulcer, condition of wound bed along with presence of sinuses and wound discharge should also be documented.
  - *Condition of periwound skin:* Healthy periwound skin reduces chances of wound infection and also helps in applying dressing to the wound. When the surrounding skin is macerated or has significant dermatitis, it becomes difficult to provide good dressing to the ulcer. Once the condition of the wound is documented, a detailed discussion has to be made with treating physician regarding the type of care for the wound.
  - *Wound history:* Previous records of wound care should always be consulted. All previous dressing strategies should be documented after consulting the previous healthcare providers if possible.

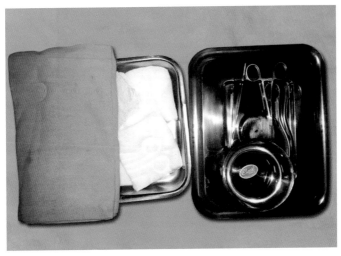

Fig. 4 Dressing kit

- *Etiology:* Pressure ulcers having extensive undermining require packing to fill dead space. In Grade 4 wounds, there may be presence of deep sinuses, which again require packing to obliterate dead space. Hence, for such wounds, cover should be augmented with antibiotic-impregnated gauze packing which helps in reducing wound discharge.
- *Size:* Size and extent of tissue loss is a major determinant of the type of wound dressing. Wound packing may be needed for larger wounds; however, exposed tendons and ligaments will require moist hydrophilic environment to prevent tissue desiccation.
- *Exudates:* Control of wound exudates is essential to manage increased bioburden, protect the periwound skin, control odor and avoid overuse of wound care products. Wounds with copious exudates should have absorbent dressings while low-exudate wounds require skin protection only.
- *Base:* Wound base is an independent determinant of the healing process. Clean healthy granulation signifies a healing wound and hence a moist environment should be maintained to promote healing. Chlorine water and hydrogen peroxide should be avoided in such wounds to prevent granulation tissue damage.
- *Slough:* It is detrimental to wound healing. Debridement is required depending on the amount of slough and patient's general condition. In slight amount, moist wound environment promotes autolysis during dressing change. In moderate amount, chemical or mechanical agents are used while for large amounts, serial sharp debridement along with intermittent chemical or mechanical debridement is required (Fig. 5).
- *Epithelium:* Growing epithelium also signifies healing wound and should be maintained in a moist environment.
- *Odor:* It is a very important part of wound management from the attendant's and nursing staff's point of view. A patient having wounds with malodor is a source of stress and inconvenience to other patients, staff nurses and attendants. Moreover, a malodor wound is a frequent cause of

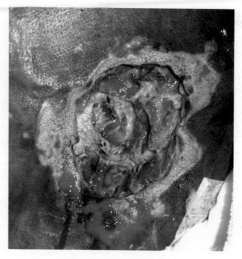

Fig. 5 Slough in wound

dissatisfaction among patient attendants regarding quality of care. Odor is commonly associated with an infected, fungating, necrotic wounds with high bacterial load. Such wounds require frequent dressing change, debridement if possible, and closed bulky dressings.

– *Comorbid conditions:* These patients require frequent wound inspection as chances of complications and failure of dressing protocols are high. Most common are diabetes, obesity, immunosuppression, cardiac failure and shock due to any cause.

• *Dressing material:* An ideal dressing for pressure ulcer should have the following qualities: nonadherent to the wound bed, should confirm to the wound bed shape, obliterates dead space, decreases bacterial load, promotes debridement of necrotic tissue, promotes granulation tissue and wound healing, able to absorb exudates, protects periwound skin, easy to apply and manage, economically viable.

Any dressing for pressure ulcer will have the following layers:

– *Non-adherent layer* resting on the wound bed. This layer prevents the dressing from sticking to the wound thus reducing pain during dressing change. Most commonly, a paraffin gauze is used.

– *Absorbent layer for the exudates* is the most important layer of the entire dressing. If there is excessive bioload as evidenced by large copious exudates or foul smell, this layer may be augmented with antibiotic and bactericidal agents like silver dressings, hydrofera blue, cadexomer iodine, and honey.

– *Superficial barrier layer* to prevent contamination and allow oxygen and water vapor circulation. This layer can be an adhesive layer which allows the dressing to stay in place without damaging the periwound skin.

Some of the commonly used dressing types are[9] (Fig. 6) (Table 2):

– *Gauze:* Most commonly used dressing material. Highly absorptive as packing material, economical but requires frequent changes to prevent

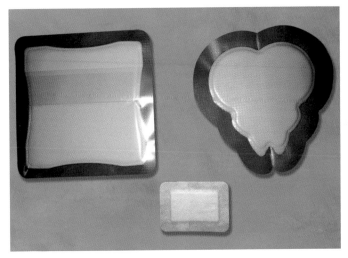

Fig. 6 Various dressing types

drying and desiccation. Unless kept moist, will adhere to the wound, leading to a nonselective debridement. Frequent changes make it unsuitable for use in ICU settings, especially for Grade 3 and 4 ulcers. The wound bed and gauze should always have an intervening layer of paraffin gauze to prevent adherence.

- *Calcium alginates or other fiber gelling dressings:* Obtained from brown seaweed. These are used for packing moderate to heavily exudative wound. The fibers absorb the exudates about 20 times its weight, and turn into a gel, which in turn maintains a moist wound bed.
- *Foam:* Contains an absorptive nonadherent hydrophilic polyurethane film coat layer. It confirms to the wound shape thus reducing dead space. Combined with negative pressure wound therapy (NPWT).
- *Hydrocolloids:* Are gel-forming agents and form an adhesive, impermeable barrier when they come in contact with exudates and are available in variety of shapes. Generally used for partial and full thickness wounds in combination with other dressings. Highly comfortable and can be left in place up to several days.
- *Hydrogel:* Provides moisture to the wound; is nonadherent.
- *Transparent films:* They decrease friction, are permeable to oxygen and water vapor. Not recommended for an infected wound.
- *Wound fillers:* They are used for shallow wounds with mild to moderate exudates with an add-on secondary dressing for retention.
- *Antimicrobials:* They decrease bacterial load (e.g. silver dressings, hydrofera blue, cadexomer iodine, honey).
- *Collagen:* It enhances collagen fiber reorientation thus enhancing wound repair.

Table 2 Commonly used dressing materials

Dressing type	Description	Advantages	Disadvantages	Indication	Brand name
Gauze	Saline/povidone-iodine/antibiotic soaked	Simple and cheap	Labor-intensive, frequent changes, painful dressing change	For packing of sinuses in deep wounds	Plain gauze
Alginate	Fibers from brown seaweed	Highly absorptive, fills dead space, forms gel, hydrates wound, promotes autolytic debridement, easy to apply	May dehydrate wound, not to be applied in superficial wounds	Primary dressing for deep ulcers with sinus and undermining	Algicell, 3M Tegagen, Melgisorb, Kaltostat
Foam	Polyurethane foam made in sheet or pad form	Highly absorptive, can fill dead space	Not able to fill sinuses (gauze packing required)	For moderate exudates, if combined with NPWT can be used for heavy exudates	Allevyn, Biatain, Hydrocell
Hydrocolloid	Occlusive or semiocclusive dressing available as wafers/paste/powder	Impermeable to bacteria, self-adherent, molds well	Does not fill sinuses, not used in heavy exudates (will require supplement with alginate), can damage periwound skin	Used for ulcers with slough and necrosis as it promotes autolytic debridement, for moderate exudates wounds	Comfeel, Duoderm
Hydrogel	Water or glycerin-based amorphous gels, impregnated gauze or sheets	Rehydrates wound, relieves pain, fills dead space and sinuses, easy to apply, promotes autolytic debridement	Not effective in heavy exudates, can dehydrate wounds, difficult to apply	Good for all types of ulcers except Grade 1	AcryDerm, DermaGauze, 3M Tegagel, Aquagauze
Transparent film	Adhesive, semipermeable, polyurethane membrane	Preserves moisture, impermeable to contaminants and bacteria	No absorptive capacity, requires healthy per wound skin for application	For superficial ulcers with low exudates, as secondary dressing to hold other dressings like hydrocolloid, hydrogel in place for exudative wound	Opsite, 3M Tegaderm

Abbreviation: NPWT, negative pressure wound therapy.

PROCEDURE

Cleaning

- Prior to wash the type, amount, color and odor of wound discharge are noted.
- Wash with a thin powerful stream of normal saline. Normal saline is the cleanser of choice; however, lack of preservative allows early bacterial colonization within the saline. Hence, all bottles should be discarded within 24 hours of opening. A 35 mL syringe with 19-gauge angiocatheter creates an 8-psi irrigation pressure stream, which may be used to remove adherent material in the wound bed.[10] This can also be done using a 50 mL/20 mL syringe mounted with an 18G IV cannula.
- Wound is cleaned gently with moist gauze in a circular pattern, starting at the center of the wound and working toward the edge of the wound and surrounding skin.
- Hard pressure and scrubbing should be strictly avoided.
- Never return to the wound center with the same gauze to prevent recontamination.
- In the presence of heavy colonization, topical antimicrobials are indicated (e.g. povidone-iodine, sodium hypochlorite solution, hydrogen peroxide or acetic acid) for a limited period (usually 2 weeks).[9]
- These should be discontinued when a clean wound bed and a reduced volume of exudates is achieved.
- Commercial wound cleansers containing surfactants are used in cases of heavy exudates and adherent material as they help to remove bacterial biofilm.[11]
- High-pressure irrigation can reduce the necrotic tissue needed in the presence of slough and necrotic tissue.
- Once the wound is clean, an assessment of the size, depth is made and then appropriate management strategy is formulated based on the above noted parameters and patient's general condition.[12]
- Treatment goals should be identified and can be curative or palliative.[12]

Debridement

If slough or eschar is present then debridement of the slough is required along with dressing of the wound. Debridement is of two types (Figure 5 showing slough in wound).[13]

- *Non-selective*: Rarely done in ICU. This involves removing the entire, both healthy and unhealthy, tissue till a uniform healthy layer is available which can be provided a graft or flap cover. It is done through major debridement and is performed in OT in hemodynamically stable patients with good general condition, when a definitive skin cover is to be given.
- *Selective*: It involves removal of only the necrotic tissue so as to decrease the bacterial bioload and improve the healing process. This procedure is most commonly done in ICU patients. Various types are:
  - *Autolytic:* Using the body's own immune mechanism to remove necrotic tissue by providing healthy moist wound environment. Avoided in immune-compromised and unstable patients.

- *Chemical/enzymatic:* Using commercially available concentrated enzymes to degrade slough. Ointments require a moist environment and specific pH for optimal action. They do not penetrate an eschar and easily deactivated by wound cleansers and heavy metals.
- *Surgical:* Here, only the dead eschar or slough is removed surgically as a bedside procedure unlike nonselective debridement.
- *Biosurgical:* Use of disinfected maggots to remove dead necrotic tissue. Not commonly used due to lack of availability. The secretions of *Lucilia sericata* or *Phaenicia sericata* also have antimicrobial properties even for methicillin-resistant *Staphylococcus aureus* by promoting human fibroblast activity.[14]
- *Ultrasonic:* Saline mist coupled with ultrasonic waves produces mechanical and thermal effects. However, if the probe comes in contact with the tissue it can lead to nonselective debridement.[15]

Selective debridement goes hand in hand with dressing process and is repeated as and when required. Most ICUs use a combination of various selective procedures to achieve healthy wound environment.

Adjunct Therapies

Apart from debridement and wound dressings, these modalities are used to augment wound healing by increasing epithelialization and granulation tissue formation.

However, these therapies do not work in the presence of infection, heavy wound exudates and necrotic tissue. These therapies are therefore instituted once bacterial bioload has decreased and adequate debridement has been done. Moreover, if during the course of these therapies wound condition deteriorates, these should be immediately discontinued and conventional wound care strategies should be reinstated. They are:

Biophysical Agents

- Electrical stimulation.
- Induced-electrical stimulation.
- *Negative pressure wound therapy (NPWT):*[16] These devices apply negative pressure, or suction to the wound bed. The negative pressure has three main physical effects:
  - Increased tension on tissues that stimulate mitosis
  - Increased local blood flow in the capillary bed
  - Drainage of excess exudates.

  These lead to better exudate control, promote granulation tissue formation and reduce wound periwound edema thereby augmenting wound contraction and epithelialization.[17] It should be applied and monitored by a clinician trained in its indications, contraindications, precautions and different methods of application. NPWT is mostly used for Stage III or IV pressure ulcers that fail to progress healing with conventional dressing and debridement.[18,19] Figure 7 showing NPWT.
- *Hyperbaric oxygen:* It is the application of high pressure oxygen to the host's tissues. Hyperbaric oxygen (HBO) increases oxygen diffusion to the wound

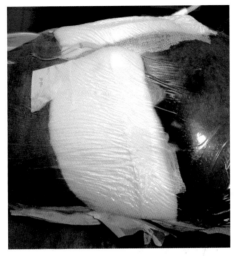

Fig. 7 Negative pressure wound therapy

and the oxygen carrying capacity. It reduces oxygen free radicals, bacterial growth and increases the white blood cell's activity, granulation tissue formation, epithelialization and wound contraction.[20]

- Noncontact, nonthermal ultrasound.
- Phototherapy.

Biological Applications

They donate physiological constituents to the wound bed. These are in the form of gels and sheets, reducing the bacterial bioburden. Various types include platelet gels, platelet-derived growth factor.

Palliative Care[21]

Many a times in acute care settings, patients with pressure ulcers have multiple comorbidities and poor general condition. Many of these patients are on various life-support systems, heparin and inotropic drugs, have unstable parameters with poor long-term prognosis. In such a scenario, definitive and extensive treatment of pressure ulcers including surgical debridement and definitive skin cover of ulcers is not possible, wherein the focus of the intensivist is to maintain the vital parameters of the patient and to control multiorgan dysfunction.

In this setting, we perform what is known as "palliative care" of pressure ulcer. The goal of this care is to prevent further increase in the size and grade of the wound, control wound discharge, wound odor and decrease overall sepsis load. This helps in not only keeping the patient clean but also comforts the patient attendants and care providers.

Palliative wound care has two basic components:[7,21] Firstly, symptom management (elimination or reduction of pain, control of odor and exudates, treatment/ prevention of infection) and secondly, quality of life objectives (restoration of some sense of control, maintenance of function and independence, control of caregiver burden, reduction of distress for patient and family). These are achieved using various forms of dressing and selective debridement. Once the general condition of the patient improves, management can be pursued with a curative intent.

General Guidelines for Pressure Sore Dressings[10,11,14,20]

- Dressing has multiple layers.
- Commercially available dressings have multiple layers incorporated into one.
- The wound environment should be hydrated to prevent tissue desiccation.
- Dressing is not a substitute of regular turning protocols.
- All cavities and sinus tracts should be packed with bactericidal/antibiotic-impregnated gauze at the start of dressing.
- The innermost layer of the dressing should always be a nonadherent layer which should be in touch with wound base, e.g. paraffin gauze.
- If necrotic tissue is present then chemical/enzymatic debridement agents should be added to the wound bed.
- If high bacterial load is suspected, antibiotic ointment should be added to the wound base.
- Absorbent material forms the second layer.
- Type of absorbent depends on the amount of exudates.
- The dressing should confer to the wound shape and eliminate dead space.
- If excessive odor is present then activated charcoal can be added.
- The absorbent material is covered with a transparent film to prevent contamination and allow oxygen and water vapor to circulate.
- The transparent film also has adhesive capacity thus allows the dressing to be kept in place.
- Change of dressing is done depending on the amount of exudates.
- In Grade 1 or very superficial wound, absorbent layer can be eliminated.
- Dressings are changed as soon as there is soakage, pain, signs of local inflammation.

REFERENCES

1. Cox J. Predictors of pressure ulcers in adult critical care patients. Am J Crit Care. 2011;20(5):364-75.
2. Reilly EF, Karakousis GC, Schrag SP, Stawicki SP. Pressure ulcer in the intensive care unit: The 'forgotten' enemy. Scientist. 2007;1(2):17-30.
3. National Pressure Ulcer Advisory Panel. http://www.npuap.org/.
4. Agency for Healthcare Research and Quality. (2012). 3D: The Braden scale for predicting pressure sore risk. [online] Available from http://www.ahrq.gov/research/ltc/pressureulcertoolkit/putool7b.htm.
5. Theaker C. Pressure sore prevention in the critically ill: what you don't know, what you should know and why it's important. Intensive Crit Care Nurs. 2003;19(3):163-8.
6. Ayello EA, Sibbald RG. Preventing ulcers and skin tears. In: Capezuti E, Zwicker D, Mezey M, Fulmer T (Eds). Evidence-based Geriatric Nursing for Best Practice, 3rd edition. New York: Springer Publishing. 2008. pp. 403-29.
7. Perry D, Borchert K, Burke S, Chick K, Johnson K, Kraft W, et al. Institute for Clinical Systems Improvement. Pressure Ulcer Prevention and Treatment Protocol. Updated January 2012.
8. Watret L, Armitage M. Making sense of wound cleaning. J Comm Nurs. 2002;16:27-34.

9. European Wound Management Association (EWMA). Position Document: Identifying criteria for wound infection. London: MEP Ltd. 2005.

10. Sussman C, Bates-Jensen BM. Wound Care: A Collaborative Practice Manual. Lippincott Williams & Wilkins. 2007.

11. White RJ, Cutting K, Kingsley A. Topical antimicrobials in the control of wound bioburden. Ostomy Wound Manage. 2006;52(8):26-58.

12. Price MC, Whitney JD, King CA, Doughty D. Development of a risk assessment tool for intraoperative pressure ulcers. J Wound Ostomy Continence Nurs. 2005;32(1):19-30, quiz 31-2.

13. Stanisic MM, Provo BJ, Larson DL, Kloth LC. Wound debridement with 25 kHz ultrasound. Adv Skin Wound Care. 2005;18(9):484-90.

14. Gray M. Is larval (maggot) debridement effective for removal of necrotic tissue from chronic wounds? J Wound Ostomy Continence Nurs. 2008;35(4):378-84.

15. http://www.fda.gov/MedicalDevices/Safety/AlertsandNotices/ucm244211.htm.

16. Gupta S, Cho T. A literature review of negative pressure wound therapy. Ostomy Wound Manage. 2004;50(11A Suppl):2S-4S.

17. http://www.fda.gov/Safety/MedWatch/SafetyInformation/Safety Alerts for Human Medical Products/ucm190704.htm.

18. Myers B. Wound Management: Principles and Practice, 2nd edition. 2007.

19. Bradley M. When healing is not an option. Palliative care as a primary treatment goal. Adv Nurse Pract. 2004;12(7):50-2, 57.

20. Whitney J, Phillips L, Aslam R, Barbul A, Gottrup F, Gould L, et al. Guidelines for the treatment of pressure ulcers. Wound Repair Regen. 2006;14(6):663-79.

21. Alvarez OM, Kalinski C, Nusbaum J, Hernandez L, Pappous E, Kyriannis C, et al. Incorporating wound healing strategies to improve palliation (symptom management) in patients with chronic wounds. J Palliat Med. 2007;10(5):1161-89.

57

Mobilization of Patient

Abraham Samuel Babu, Vishal Shanbhag, Arun G Maiya

INTRODUCTION

The role of the physiotherapist in the intensive care unit (ICU) has been established in the area of bronchial hygiene and respiratory care. Over the last few decades, the role of the physiotherapist has expanded by providing early mobilization for patients in ICU to facilitate faster weaning and early discharge from the ICU. It is described as the mainstay of treatment to ensure recovery and return to functional status through progressive mobilization.[1] Early mobilization and critical care rehabilitation are an evidence-based treatment that should be delivered through teamwork and be considered in every critically ill patient from the very beginning of admission to the ICU.[2] Physiotherapy utilizing the principle of a "patient-centered rehabilitation manual" has shown significant benefits in a randomized controlled trial.[3] Physical rehabilitation through physiotherapy should start within the ICU and has been shown to be safe even when administered to patients who are still ventilated.[4,5] Early initiation of exercises and mobilization of patients improve the general well-being of the patient and while facilitating faster and better progression of rehabilitation, quicker weaning and extubation.[6]

INDICATION FOR EARLY MOBILIZATION

Any patient admitted to the ICU can be a candidate for mobilization as soon as they are medically stable or if the treating physician and the rehabilitation team decide on initiation of rehabilitation—ideally, it can be initiated as early as within 24 hours.

CONTRAINDICATION FOR EARLY MOBILIZATION

Contraindications need to be assessed prior to mobilization exercises. This is crucial to ensure safe mobilization and optimize maximum benefits from mobilization of ICU patients.

General

- Hemodynamically unstable patients (i.e. hypotension, uncontrolled hypertension, fluctuating BP)
- Uncontrolled arrhythmias

- Acute coronary event or ongoing ischemia
- Decompensated heart failure
- Patients with hypoxemia and severe acute respiratory distress syndrome (ARDS) in first 24 hours
- Partial pressure of oxygen (PaO_2) less than 80 mm Hg [for non-chronic obstructive lung disease (COPD) patients] and PaO_2 less than 70 mm Hg (for COPD patients)
- High positive end expiratory pressure (PEEP) (>8 cm H_2O) and fractional inspired oxygen (FiO_2) (>0.8) to maintain oxygen saturation measured by pulse oximetry (SpO_2) more than 95%
- Untreated deep venous thrombosis
- Unstable spinal injuries
- Raised intracranial pressure
- Acute massive cerebrovascular accident (CVA) in the first 48 hours.

Specific to Various Exercises

Contraindications to various exercises are important for the rehabilitation expert so as he can decide appropriate interventions. Table 1 summarizes the contraindications to specific exercises (viz. passive exercises, active-assisted exercises, active exercises and resisted exercises) being carried out on patients in the ICU.

TECHNIQUE AND BASIC PRINCIPLES OF MOBILIZATION

Mobilization of patients in the ICU was once considered impossible and unsafe for patients in ICU. Patients admitted to ICU suffered from consequences of bed rest which further increased their morbidity and mortality. However, with the growing development of medicine, the rising survival rates of critically ill patients have only strengthened the need for mobilization and rehabilitation of ICU patients. Griffiths et al. in their paper identified profound physical weakness with good recovery among other problems seen in ICU survivors.[7] Critical illness polyneuropathy (CIPN) has been established as a condition seen specifically in ICU patients along with ventilator-induced diaphragmatic dysfunction (VIDD). In very long stay ICU patients, electromyographic evidence of chronic denervation may be detected many years later, but very few have corresponding clinical weakness or important limitation in activities of daily living at that time point.

Table 1 Contraindications to various exercises

Passive	Active-assisted	Active	Resisted
Septic arthritis	Can be performed within limits of pain		Septic arthritis
	Acute demyelination	Acute demyelination	Acute demyelination
Deep venous thrombosis			
Untreated fractures			
Side of hemodialysis port			
Cellulitis*			

*Can be performed, but with caution.

Physiologic Basis for Mobilization

Immobilization coupled with critical illness has deleterious effects on the body. Muscle wasting has been seen to be highest within the first 2–3 weeks of ICU stay. The consequence of ICU stay results in the onset of CIPN, VIDD, increased dependence for activities of daily living and psychological consequences. Thus the need for early mobilization. Mobilization refers to physical activity which is sufficient to elicit acute physiological effects causing a change in ventilation, perfusion, circulation, muscle metabolism and alertness. It also acts as a countermeasure for venous stasis and deep venous thrombosis. Positioning is an important part of the mobilization which can be used to increase gravitational stress and associated fluid shifts through head tilt and other positions that approximate the upright position. The upright position increases lung volumes and gas exchange, stimulates autonomic activity, and can reduce cardiac stress from compression.[8]

Thus, it is clear that exercises and mobilization are essential components of ICU care. Exercises are provided to the patient according to each specific need and aim. Exercises can be classified as passive, active-assisted and active. Passive mobilization requires the movement to be performed by the therapist with no assistance from the patient. This is usually required in patients who have no muscle power and/or are not able to take active participation either due to neurological deficits, sedation or due to neuromuscular blockade. Passive movements help maintain joint range of movement and prevent development of tightness in muscles and ligaments. Active-assisted exercises are for those patients who can initiate movements, but cannot perform the entire range of movement on their own. Hence, they require some assistance. Patients requiring this type of exercises are usually responsive and can follow commands. Active exercises are reserved for those patients who can perform movements on their own without any assistance. Active exercises can be progressed to resisted exercises—depending on the condition of the patient and the specific rehabilitative goal to be achieved. These patients are responsive and able to follow commands. These forms of exercises can be applied to all patients in the ICU provided there are no specific contraindications (Table 1). Active forms of exercises help in improving muscle power, and progression of these exercises can be used to further improve strength or endurance of the muscles as well.

Adjuncts to Mobilization

In instances where mobilization of the patient is difficult, alternate arrangements can be made to help move the patient out of bed. Devices like a tilt table (Fig. 1) and standing wheelchair (Figs 2A and B) can be used to help achieve the erect posture for patients who cannot be made to sit with therapist support. It is important to understand space constraints especially when using tilt tables. Other devices like standing beds can be used; however, the cost of procuring these beds in the Indian context needs to be kept in mind. Apart from these, physiotherapists can also use oxygen therapy and noninvasive ventilation to aid in early mobilization of patients in the ICU. Even though, these have been widely used as part of pulmonary rehabilitation, their role in critical care rehabilitation is yet to be determined.

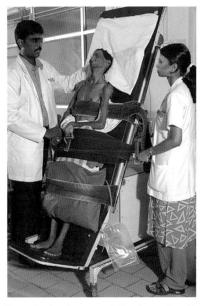

Fig. 1 Patient being mobilized on a tilt table

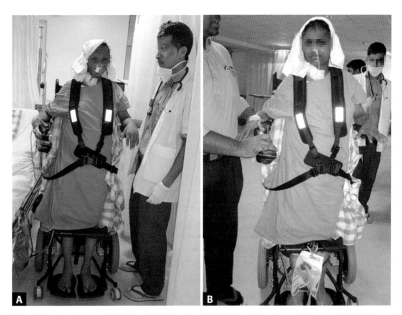

Figs 2A and B (A) Patient made to stand using a standing wheelchair; (B) Patient mobilized using the motorized standing wheelchair

PREPARATION AND ASSESSMENT

Assessment of Patient

The assessment of patients forms a crucial component prior to initiation of mobilization. Detailed evaluation of the patient with emphasis on musculoskeletal and neurological systems, blood and biochemical reports, arterial blood gases (ABGs) and chest X-ray is required. Specific evaluations such as muscle strength, respiratory muscle strength and evaluation of functional performance also need to be performed for all patients prior to mobilization.[2] Discussion with the medical team by the physiotherapist will help in setting realistic goals for the patient to achieve through early mobilization.

Recently, a new scale—the Chelsea Physical Assessment tool, a bedside scoring system, is introduced to grade physical morbidity in the critical care population.[9] This can be used in the ICU to evaluate patients prior to mobilization. However, its applicability and relevance in various ICUs are to be established. Nevertheless, it is still a useful tool in the current scenario.

Endotracheal suctioning is to be performed prior to mobilization so as to prevent the mobilized secretions from affecting the mobilization process. Check the cuff pressure of the advanced airway and ensure the airway is properly secured prior to mobilization.

Based on the general condition, patients can be categorized into three categories as described by Hanekom et al.[10]

- Category A—Unconscious patients
- Category B—Conscious and physiologically stable patients
- Category C—Deconditioned patients.

Table 2 describes the assessment of patients to be considered prior to mobilization. This categorization is useful when stratification of patients is required to help formulate focused rehabilitation interventions for ICU patients.

If the above criteria for a particular category are not met, the patient can be treated as belonging to the previous category. At this point, it is important to re-emphasize the importance of a detailed clinical evaluation to decide the readiness for mobilization. The above mentioned criteria are a guideline and should not serve as hard criteria to prevent mobilization of patients in the ICU.

Monitoring during Mobilization

Monitoring during mobilization is important to ensure safety of the patient during mobilization. If the patient is being made to stand or being ambulated, portable oxygen saturation probes can be used to monitor saturation. It is important to ensure adequate oxygenation during the mobilization. Therefore, it is key to ensure oxygen saturations more than 94% during exercise for those with no lung pathology and more than 90% for those with COPD. FiO_2 can be titrated to maintain this oxygenation status during mobilization. Monitor for signs of increased work of breathing and respiratory distress during mobilization. For patients who are being made to stand or ambulated, the Borg's rating of perceived exertion (RPE) can be used to guide the difficulty the patient has while performing the particular activity. Intensities between 9–11/20 on the RPE are adequate during the initial stages of mobilization in the ICU. Patients with heart failure and acute myocardial infarction requiring cardiac rehabilitation can be mobilized guided symptoms, heart rate and RPE.[10,11]

Table 2 Categorization of patients in ICU and their respective assessment

Patient category	Patient condition	Assessment of specific criteria			Special consideration
		Respiratory	Cardiovascular	Other	
A	Unconscious patients	• SpO$_2$ > 94%	• <20% variability in blood pressure • Low inotrope support*		
B	Conscious and physiologically stable patients	• PaO$_2$/FiO$_2$ > 300 • SpO$_2$ > 94% (<4% variation) • Good respiratory pattern • Adequate respiratory support (FiO$_2$ < 0.6), low dose of catecholamines, less than 20% variability in blood pressure, PEEP < 10 cm H$_2$O, resting heart rate <50%, age predicted maximum	• Normal ECG • Absence of orthostatic hypotension	• Hemoglobin >8.5 g/dL • Platelets	In case the patient does have orthostatic hypotension, the patient can still be gradually mobilized out of bed provided blood pressure and symptoms are monitored
C	Deconditioned patients	• Normal respiratory pattern on stable ventilation or breathing spontaneously • Controlled secretions • SpO$_2$ > 92% with FiO$_2$ < 0.5, PEEP ≤ 5 cm H$_2$O		• No arrhythmia, heart failure, angina • Controlled sepsis	In case of heart failure or acute coronary syndrome, in-hospital cardiac rehabilitation supervised by a physiotherapist trained in cardiac rehabilitation can be initiated[11,12]

*Less than 0.1 µg/kg/min.

Care during Mobilization

It is important to keep the following points in mind while mobilizing patients in the ICU.

• Ensure the advanced airway is secure and no displacement of the tube occurs during mobilization.

- Ensure the intravenous (IV) lines and catheters do not get pulled while mobilizing patients.
- Optimize timing of exercise for those with diabetes receiving insulin to prevent hypoglycemia from occurring during mobilization.
- If the patient is breathing spontaneously but with an advanced airway, ensure the ventilator is on standby for any emergency.

PHYSIOTHERAPY TREATMENT

Once the patient has been categorized, it is appropriate to begin planning the possible interventions that can be performed by the patient. The interventions will be discussed according to each category as described by Hanekom et al. We have also added a note on what alternate interventions could be done.

Category A

- Positioning with head end elevated 30–45°
- Regular position change.

Exercises

- Passive movements to all limbs in the supine position—10 repetitions twice a day (Figs 3A and B)
- Passive stretching to the Achilles tendon, hip adductors, hip internal rotators, long flexors of the upper limb and shoulder adductors—10-second hold, five repetitions twice a day
- Neuromuscular electrical stimulation—Target the large muscle groups of the lower limb (quadriceps and gastrosoleus).

Additional Treatments Possible

- Splinting and positioning of limbs in case of neurological diseases are also important during this time.
- Low level LASER therapy can be used to help promote wound healing and control of infection for bed sores.

Category B

Exercises

- Active exercises to the upper and lower limbs—begin with 3–5 repetitions × 2–3 sets (as tolerated by the patient). Progress repetitions and number of sets as tolerated by the patient.
- Gentle resistance exercises can be initiated during this time.
- Inspiratory muscle training can be initiated during this phase to facilitate faster weaning and in preventing VIDD. This could be done in intubated patients by altering the pressure support and trigger while ensuring the patient inhaled a predetermined tidal volume 5 times for 2–3 sets twice a day. The repetitions and sets can be gradually increased according to the patient's tolerance. It is better to hyperoxygenate the patient during this process.

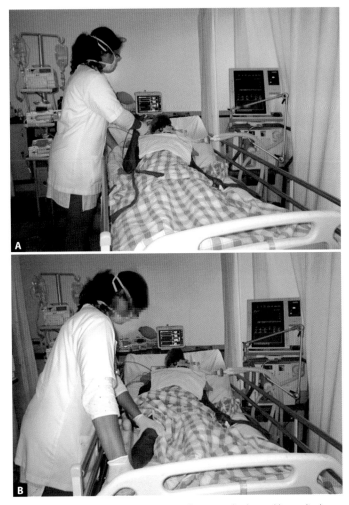

Figs 3A and B Passive exercises to the upper limbs and lower limbs

Other Activities

- *Sitting in bed (Fig. 4):* Balance training in static postures (i.e. sitting) can be initiated to help promote sitting balance.
- Sit to stand activities.
- *Transfer to chair (Fig. 5):* Chair sitting beside the bed while on ventilator support could be performed without any complications. This improves the orientation of the patient and also prevents abnormalities in ventilation perfusion from occurring.
- Walking.

Category C

- Resistance training to upper and lower limbs at an intensity of 11–13 on the RPE.
- Endurance training to the limb and trunk muscles (Fig. 6).

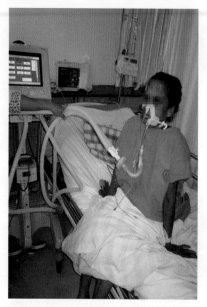

Fig. 4 Patient in high sitting position while on continuous positive airway pressure via endotracheal tube

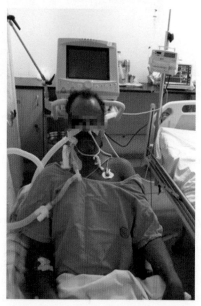

Fig. 5 Patient in chair sitting position while on T-piece via endotracheal tube

- If the patient has lower limb muscle power of more than three with moderate trunk stability, standing with walker and ambulation can be initiated with or without assistance (Figs 7 and 8). Portable oxygen or continuous positive airway pressure (CPAP) may be required during ambulation depending on the oxygenation status and work of breathing.

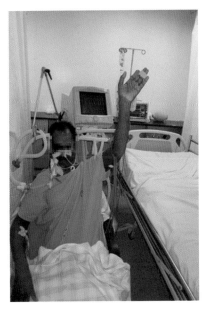

Fig. 6 Patient in chair sitting position while on T-piece doing active upper limb exercises

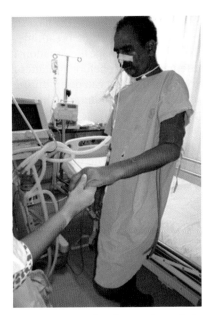

Fig. 7 Patient standing and performing lower limb exercises

POST-PROCEDURE CARE

- Following mobilization, it is important to assess the patient to look for signs of respiratory distress and hemodynamic instability.
- Check the position of the advance airway, IV lines and catheters, following mobilization.

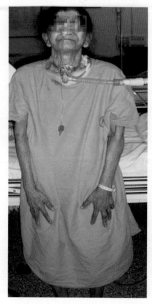

Fig. 8 Patient on bilevel positive airway pressure via tracheostomy being made to stand

- Ensure adequate rest for the patient before the next session of mobilization.
- If a patient develops increased work of breathing, appropriate ventilator strategies can be utilized to help manage the situation. It may also be necessary to hyperoxygenate the patient both before and after mobilization to help in counteracting the oxygen deficit that can occur during mobilization.
- The use of bronchodilators may be required if there is severe bronchospasm, following mobilization.
- Documentation is an important part of any medical record. It is essential to have detailed documentation available for the assessment, goals, mobilization and post-mobilization assessment. The utility of these documents will also help the medical team in assessing the progress of the condition of the patient in the ICU.

COMPLICATION/PROBLEM

All interventions performed in the ICU carry some risk to the patient. However, proper screening and monitoring during exercises ensure that patients are kept safe throughout the process of early mobilization. Nevertheless, some of the commonly seen problems that occur following mobilization according to the category of the patient are given below.

- *Category A:* Hypoxemia, increased work of breathing and tachycardia
- *Category B:* Hypoxemia, increased work of breathing, tachycardia, fatigue, joint pain (if weight bearing is initiated) and muscle soreness
- *Category C:* Fatigue, joint pain and muscle soreness.

Special care should be taken while mobilizing elderly patients with severe osteoporosis and those with metastasis to the bone.

To conclude, early mobilization is an important component of ICU care. Physiotherapists and the intensive care team should work together to initiate critical care rehabilitation as early as possible so as to allow for good functional recovery of the patient.

ACKNOWLEDGMENT

The authors thank the patients for their willingness to participate in adding to the pictorial part of this chapter. We also thank the Medical Superintendent and the ICU staff at Kasturba Hospital, Manipal University, Manipal, for all their support and co-operation.

REFERENCES

1. Stiller K. Physiotherapy in intensive care: an updated systematic review. Chest. 2013;144(3):825-47.
2. Gosselink R, Needham D, Hermans G. ICU-based rehabilitation and its appropriate metrics. Curr Opin Crit Care. 2012;18(5):533-9.
3. Jones C, Skirrow P, Griffiths RD, Humphris GH, Ingleby S, Eddleston J, et al. Rehabilitation after critical illness: a randomized, controlled trial. Crit Care Med. 2003;31(10):2456-61.
4. Bailey P, Thomsen GE, Spuhler VJ, Blair R, Jewkes J, Bezdjian L, et al. Early activity is feasible and safe in respiratory failure patients. Crit Care Med. 2007;35(1):139-45.
5. Schweickert WD, Pohlman MC, Pohlman AS, Nigos C, Pawlik AJ, Esbrook CL, et al. Early physical and occupational therapy in mechanically ventilated, critically ill patients: a randomised controlled trial. Lancet. 2009;373(9678):1874-82.
6. Babu AS. Critical care rehabilitation: a neglected part of ICU care. Oman Med J. 2012;27(4):268.
7. Griffiths RD, Jones C. Seven lessons from 20 years of follow-up of intensive care unit survivors. Curr Opin Crit Care. 2007;13(5):508-13.
8. Gosselink R, Bott J, Johnson M, Dean E, Nava S, Norrenberg M, et al. Physiotherapy for adult patients with critical illness: recommendations of the European Respiratory Society and European Society of Intensive Care Medicine Task Force on Physiotherapy for Critically Ill Patients. Intensive Care Med. 2008;34(7):1188-99.
9. Corner EJ, Wood H, Englebretsen C, Thomas A, Grant RL, Nikoletou D, et al. The Chelsea critical care physical assessment tool (CPAx): validation of an innovative new tool to measure physical morbidity in the general adult critical care population; an observational proof-of-concept pilot study. Physiotherapy. 2013;99(1):33-41.
10. Hanekom S, Gosselink R, Dean E, van Aswegen H, Roos R, Ambrosino N, et al. The development of a clinical management algorithm for early physical activity and mobilization of critically ill patients: synthesis of evidence and expert opinion and its translation into practice. Clin Rehabil. 2011;25(9):771-87.
11. Babu AS, Maiya AG, George MM, Padmakumar R, Guddattu V. Effects of combined early in-patient cardiac rehabilitation and structured home-based program on function among patients with congestive heart failure: A randomized controlled trial. Heart Views. 2011;12(3):99-103.
12. Babu AS, Noone MS, Haneef M, Naryanan SM. Protocol-guided phase-1 cardiac rehabilitation in patients with ST-elevation myocardial infarction in a rural hospital. Heart Views. 2010;11(2):52-6.

58

Surveillance of ICU-acquired Infection

Armin Ahmed, Richa Misra

INTRODUCTION

It is said that what cannot be measured, cannot be improved. Surveillance is the method by which we measure rate of specific events/infection or disease. The collected information is then analyzed, interpreted and disseminated for improving the outcome with one or another interventions. Patients admitted to intensive care unit (ICU) are at higher risk of acquiring nosocomial infection due to intrinsic (e.g. immunosuppression) as well as extrinsic (e.g. invasive procedures) factors. ICUs are priority areas for surveillance because they are the epicenter of antimicrobial resistance in the hospital.

OBJECTIVE

- To monitor the rate and magnitude of infection and to take preventive measures.
- To compare infection rates among various units or ICUs. This will not only ensure the use of best practices for infection control but also assess the effectiveness of infection control strategies employed in a given unit or ICU.
- To develop, implement and evaluate new infection control practices.
- To analyze the local epidemiology with respect to risk factors and the common pathogens associated with ICU-acquired infections.
- To document the antimicrobial resistance rates.

ICU-ACQUIRED INFECTION AND SURVEILLANCE SYSTEM

Health care-associated infections (HAIs) can be broadly classified as two types: (1) Endogenous infections and (2) Exogenous infections.

- *Endogenous infections* are caused by organisms already inhabiting various body sites such as orodigestive tract, skin, vagina, etc. There occurs qualitative as well as quantitative change in the gastrointestinal flora of critically ill patients. Qualitative changes include colonization with abnormal flora, i.e. organisms which are not found in healthy states [e.g. aerobic Gram-negative bacteria (GNB) like *Pseudomonas, Klebsiella, Enterobacter* and methicillin-

resistant *Staphylococcus aureus* (MRSA)]. Along with qualitative changes there occurs quantitative change in the form of gut overgrowth which is defined as more than 10^5 potential pathogens per milliliter of saliva or per gram of feces. Overgrowth of potentially pathogenic organism predisposes for infection.
- *Exogenous infections* are those in which the potential pathogen is not carried at all. Such infections are acquired from healthcare personnel, visitors, equipment, etc.

Definition of intensive care unit-acquired infection: An infection that was "not present or not in incubation at admission to the ICU", but occurs 48 hours after admission and until 48 hours after discharge of the patient. An exception to the 48-hour criterion is made in cases of catheter-related bacteremia when a relation with the origin of infection can be established. In practice, all infections with onset from day 3 onward in the ICU (whereby the day of admission to the ICU is counted as day 1) should be reported.

Device-associated health care-associated infection: A device-associated ICU infection refers to pneumonia (intubation), bloodstream infection (central vascular catheter), or a urinary tract infection (catheter) that occurs in a patient with a device that was used for two or more days before onset of infection.

Health care-associated infection surveillance systems: Several surveillance network systems (Table 1) came in existence worldwide in last one to two decades with aim of standardizing surveillance practice by protocols and training programs. They have shown benefit by providing feedback to the concerned units and allowing corrective action.

Role of on-site microbiology laboratory: It plays a pivotal role in monitoring and controlling HAIs in ICUs since the microbiologist is the Infection Control Officer. *The following are the responsibilities of the microbiology laboratory:*
- Prepare protocol on specimen collection and transport
- Identify common bacterial isolates recovered from clinical specimens to at least species level
- Provide the local antimicrobial susceptibility pattern (antibiogram)
- Identify sources of infection through culture of environment and identify carriers (however, routine microbiological sampling and testing are not recommended)

Table 1 Examples of health care-associated infections surveillance systems

Surveillance network	Country
National Healthcare Safety Network	United States
Improving Patient Safety in Europe	Austria, Spain, France, Belgium, Germany, etc.
International Nosocomial Infection Control Consortium	Latin American Countries
Krankenhaus-Infektions-Surveillance-System	Germany
National Institute for Public Health and the Environment, RIVM	The Netherlands
National Surveillance Study in Intensive Care Units	Spain
Scottish Surveillance of Healthcare-associated Infection Programme	Scotland

- Provide facilities for microbiological testing with techniques of sterilization and disinfection including biological monitoring
- Conduct epidemiological typing of isolates in case of outbreak of infection
- Train and educate infection control personnel.

Surveillance and challenges: The current methods of ICU surveillance are associated with several challenges (Table 2).

METHOD OF SURVEILLANCE: BASIC PRINCIPLES

There are four key stages of surveillance: (1) Data collection; (2) Validation; (3) Analysis; (4) Interpretation. After completing these four steps, the data is reported to those who can take measures to improve outcome.

Data Collection and Validation

- *Defining the event and collecting information:* For doing surveillance, first step is to clearly define the event to be surveyed, for example, if we want to do surveillance for ventilator-associated pneumonia (VAP) in an ICU, criteria for VAP should be clearly established. Once the criteria are made, the definition is applied to all patients who form the study population. Besides this, other relevant information regarding the infection is also noted like patient's unique identification number, demographic details, microorganism causing infection, antimicrobial therapy given, and susceptibility pattern, etc. Generally, such information is collected by person who is dedicated for this work and is called infection control practitioner (ICP). Information collection can be active or passive.
  - Passive method involves asking the physicians or staff nurse to fill the infection control form. Such method is not encouraged because there are high chances of underreporting of the infectious event.
  - Active method involves searching for an infectious event by routinely reviewing the microbiological reports, daily/periodic ward rounds and review of postdischarge follow-up, because some of the infections might be incubating at the time of discharge.

Table 2 Surveillance—problems and solutions

Challenges/disadvantages of surveillance	Solution
Yields excessive data, is labor-intensive as well as time-consuming	Electronic data files can be maintained with software for analysis or data manager can help reduce the workload
Expensive—per annum cost of ICU-acquired infection is 5 times more than cost of routine surveillance	Cost-benefit ratio should be calculated
May miss out on specific pathogens or clusters of infection	Establish microbiology laboratory alerts
Collects only targeted data, limited information about endemic rates in entire hospital	Can be correlated with hospital prevalence surveys and complement it to determine patient groups beyond ICU setting

- *Inclusion criterion of patient*: An ICU-acquired infection is considered when a patient stays for more than 48 hours in the ICU. It is calculated by subtracting the date of admission to the ICU from the date of discharge from the ICU and adding one. The result should be greater than two, i.e.

  Date of discharge from the ICU – Date of admission to the ICU + 1 > 2

  All infections with date of onset after day 2 of admission and later in the ICU should be reported and be regarded as HAIs, even if there are reasons to believe that the infection was acquired in another ward or in the community.
- *Infection data* are collected for each infection episode by type of infection.
  - Date of onset of infection, or date of onset of symptoms, or if unknown, date when treatment was started, or date first diagnostic examination was done.
  - Site of infection [bloodstream infection, pneumonia, urinary tract infection (UTI)].
  - Origin of the bloodstream infection (if a recognized pathogen is recovered from one or more than one percutaneous blood cultures after 48 hours of catheterization, and this pathogen is not related to an infection at another site, or if patient improves after removal of the catheter within 48 hours).
- *Micro-organism and antimicrobial resistance data:*
  - Isolate result
  - Antibiotic with code
  - Final interpretation result of all different susceptibility tests performed as SIR (S = sensitive, I = intermediate, R = resistant)
  - Antimicrobial resistance markers with codes [e.g. *Staphylococcus spp*, methicillin-sensitive *Staphylococcus aureus* (MSSA), methicillin-resistant *Staphylococcus aureus* (MRSA), vancomycin intermediate-resistant *Staphylococcus aureus* (VISA); *Enterococcus spp*, vancomycin-resistant *Enterococcus faecium* (VRE)]
  - Similarly, note resistance to third generation cephalosporins, or to carbapenems in Enterobacteriaceae.
- *Antimicrobial use data* is also collected by episode, for each antimicrobial agent and indication.
  - Antimicrobial start date
  - Antimicrobial end date
  - Indication for antimicrobial use (empiric treatment or documented treatment or selective digestive decontamination or any other).
- *Denominators:* In order to calculate the infection rate, there are various methods used for defining the denominator. One method is to use the total number of patients admitted or discharged. Another method is to add the total number of days for which all the patients remained in the hospital during the surveillance period. In this way, patient day denominators are calculated. However, these include only infected patients and fail to include patients at risk. Recently, computer-based calculations are done by maintaining a record of all patients at risk for the infection. The risk factors are recorded in the computer. Whenever a patient develops infection the information is added. Whatever time period and population ICP selects, rates are thus calculated from the patient information database using summary denominator.

- *Rate calculation:* Rate is calculated to know the probability that a particular event can occur. It is given by the following formula:

  Rate = $k(x/y)$

  Where,

  x = Number of times the event has occurred in a given period

  y = Total number of patients admitted, or number of patient days, or number of patients at risk in a given period

  k = Base (100, 1,000, 10,000 and so on) is selected such that rate is expressed as a convenient whole number.

  There are three types of rates—incidence, prevalence and attack rates. Prevalence represents the number of active cases (both old and new) during a specified period of time in a given population. Incidence represents the number of new cases reported during a specified period of time in a given population. Attack rates are calculated only for epidemics.

Analysis and Interpretation

The tabulated data is analyzed and relationship of its various component parts is studied. Current rates are compared with previous rates to determine the effect of control measures taken. The data is thus interpreted and reported to authorities responsible for taking control measures.

SURVEILLANCE FOR SPECIFIC ICU-ACQUIRED INFECTION

Catheter-associated Urinary Tract Infection

Health care-associated UTIs are frequently associated with catheterization of the urinary tract. It can be associated with complications such as cystitis, prostatitis, pyelonephritis, bacteremia, etc. Rarely, infection can spread to distant sites causing endocarditis, septic arthritis and meningitis.

- *Setting:* Surveillance can be done in any inpatient location where denominator can be calculated, e.g. ICU, high dependency unit (HDU). Surveillance is done for at least one calendar month.
    - *Definition of catheter-associated urinary tract infection:* Urinary tract infections occurring in patient with a urinary catheter in situ for more than 2 days (the criteria also require urinary catheter to be present on the date of the event or the day before).
- *Date of infection:* The date on which patient fulfills all the criteria for UTI.
- *Numerator data:* Information is collected using UTI reporting form which should include following minimum points:
    - Brief instructions regarding data collection and filling of form
    - Demographic information
    - Whether urinary catheter was present or not
    - Additional information like whether patient also developed secondary bacteremia, survivor and non-survivor, organisms isolated, and susceptibility patterns.
- *Denominator data:* Denominators used are device days and patient days. Device days are calculated by counting the number of patients with indwelling urinary catheter per day and then summing the daily counts for 1 month.

- *Data analysis:* The catheter-associated urinary tract infection (CAUTI) standardized infection ratio is obtained by dividing the observed rate of CAUTI by the expected rate of CAUTI.

Surveillance for Central Line-associated Bloodstream Infection

Central line-associated bloodstream infections (CLABSIs) can be prevented by taking due precautions at the time of insertion and maintaining adequate post-insertion catheter care.

- *Settings:* Any inpatient setting where denominator can be calculated is eligible for surveillance. Surveillance should be done for minimum period of 1 month.
- *Definition of central line-associated bloodstream infection:* This is defined as bloodstream infection in a patient who has a central line or umbilical catheter in situ for more than 2 days (the criteria require that catheter should be in situ on the date of the event, or the day before the event).
- *Definition of central line:* This is defined as any catheter which terminates in one of the great vessels or close to the heart, and is used for giving infusions, withdrawing blood, or hemodynamic monitoring. It is important to remember that site of insertion or type of catheter used does not decide whether a line qualifies for central line.
  Following devices are not central lines: Pacemaker wire, femoral artery catheters, intra-aortic balloon pump (IABP) devices, extracorporeal membrane oxygenator (ECMO).
- *Numerator data:* A bloodstream infection form which includes the demographic details, central line was present or not, microbiological details, etc., can be used for data collection.
- *Denominator data:* Most commonly used denominators for CLABSI are device days and patient days. Data should be collected at the same time every day.
- *Data analysis*
  - Central line-associated bloodstream infection standardized infection ratio can be calculated by dividing the observed number of CLABSI with the expected number of CLABSI. The expected number of infections is calculated from a standard population for a baseline time period.
  - Central line-associated bloodstream infection rate per thousand days is obtained by following formula:
    CLABSI rate/1,000 days = (number of CLABSI/number of central line days) × 1,000

Surveillance for Ventilator-associated Event

Ventilator-associated pneumonia is associated with increased risk of death, prolonged ICU stay and increased cost of patient care. All VAP prevention guidelines strongly recommend surveillance in order to know the disease trend and implement control measures. The traditional definition for VAP includes radiographic findings as one of the criteria. However, chest radiograph findings depend on the quality of the film and observer variation. Due to this reason, traditional VAP definition cannot be used for surveillance purpose.

A new approach under the name of ventilator-associated events (VAEs) has been designed by National Healthcare Safety Network (NHSN) to make the surveillance and infection control programs convenient at large scale.

- *Setting:* Surveillance can be done in any inpatient location where denominator can be calculated. This can be done in ICUs, neonatal ICUs, specialty care areas, etc. PNEU (VAP) criteria are used for patients less than 18 years of age. VAE criteria are used for patients more than 18 years of age. This article deals with VAE only.
- *Definition:* Ventilator-associated event includes three categories namely, ventilator-associated condition (VAC), infection-related ventilator-associated complication (IVAC) and possible and probable VAP. The VAE algorithm and definitions are designed for surveillance purpose and should not be used for clinical management of the patient.
  - *Ventilator-associated event* is defined as deterioration in patient's respiratory condition after an initial stabilization or improvement on mechanical ventilation, associated with evidence of infection or inflammation and laboratory features of respiratory tract infection (The criteria require the patient to be present on mechanical ventilation for at least 2 days before the event. It also requires 2-days period of worsening, following initial stabilization or improvement).
    1. *Improvement* on mechanical ventilation is defined as daily decrease in fractional inspired oxygen (FiO_2) and/or the level of positive end-expiratory pressure (PEEP) till the day before on which deterioration in respiratory condition is noted.
    2. *Ventilator-associated condition:* After a period of initial stability or improvement in a patient, who has been on mechanical ventilation for at least two calendar days, develops one or both of the following features of worsening oxygenation:
       - Increase in FiO_2 requirement by more than 20% which is sustained for two or more calendar days
       - Increase in PEEP requirement by three or more centimeters which is sustained for two or more days.
    3. *Infection-related ventilator-associated complication:* A patient of VAC on or after 3 days of mechanical ventilation and within 2 days before or after onset of oxygenation deterioration develops:
       - Temperature more than 38°C or less than 36°C or total leukocyte count (TLC) more than 12,000/mm³ or less than 4,000/mm³
       - A new antimicrobial is started and continued for at least four or more days.
  - *Probable VAP* is defined as a patient who is a case of VAP and IVAC, has one of the following features on or after 3 days of mechanical ventilation and within 2 days before or after onset of oxygenation deterioration develops any one of the criteria:
    - Purulent respiratory secretions
    - Positive culture of sputum or endotracheal aspirate or bronchoalveolar lavage (BAL) or protected specimen brush (PSB) sample.
  - *Possible VAP* is defined as a patient who is a case of VAP and IVAC, has one of the following features on or after 3 days of mechanical ventilation and

within 2 days before or after onset of oxygenation deterioration develops any one of the criteria.

- Purulent respiratory secretions and positive culture or
- *Any of the following:*
    (i) Positive pleural fluid culture
    (ii) Positive lung histopathology
    (iii) Positive laboratory diagnosis of *Legionella*
    (iv) Positive laboratory diagnosis of pathogenic virus such as influenza, respiratory syncytial virus (RSV), adenovirus, parainfluenza, etc.

- *Date of event:* It is the first calendar day on which PEEP or FiO_2 increases above its defined level for VAE.
- *Numerator data:* It is collected via form which has filling instructions, demographic records, indication for mechanical ventilation, days on mechanical ventilation, outcome, etc.
- *Denominator data:* Device days are frequently used as denominator. Ventilator days are calculated by counting the number patients on mechanical ventilation each day and then summing the daily count for the whole month.
- *Data analysis:*
    - Standardized infection ratio is calculated for VAE in the same way, as we calculate the standardized infection ratio for other infections. Expected VAE is statistical prediction done by calculating VAE in a standard population within a baseline period.

    Standardized infection ratio = observed VAE/expected VAE

    - Ventilator-associated event rate per thousand days is obtained by following formula:

    VAE rate/1,000 days = Number of VAE/Number of ventilator days × 1,000

Surveillance for *Clostridium difficile*-associated Diarrhea

Clostridium difficile is a growing cause of diarrhea in hospitalized patients. Presentation of *Clostridium difficile*-associated diarrhea (CDAD) can vary from uncomplicated diarrhea to pseudomembranous colitis and toxic megacolon. CDAD surveillance is important to guide and monitor CDAD control programs. Surveillance for CDAD can be performed in any inpatient location where denominator can be calculated, e.g. ICU, HDU.

- *Definition of a Clostridium difficile-associated diarrhea case (numerator):* It is defined as a case of diarrhea or toxic megacolon along with positive laboratory results of *C. difficile* toxin (A/B or both) or positive finding of pseudomembranous colitis on endoscopic or histopathological examination.
- *Denominator data:* Denominator used is per 10,000 patient days.
- *Rate of Clostridium difficile-associated diarrhea:* Rate of CDAD/10,000 days = (number of cases in the reporting duration/number of inpatients during the reporting period) × 10,000

SUGGESTED READING

1. Bénet T, Allaouchiche B, Argaud L, Vanhems P. Impact of surveillance of hospital-acquired infections on the incidence of ventilator-associated pneumonia in intensive care units: a quasi-experimental study. Crit Care. 2012;16(4):R161.

2. Horan TC, Andrus M, Dudeck MA. CDC/NHSN surveillance definition of health care-associated infection and criteria for specific types of infections in the acute care setting. Am J Infect Control. 2008;36(5):309-32.

3. Suetens C, Morales I, Savey A, Palomar M, Hiesmayr M, Lepape A, et al. European surveillance of ICU-acquired infections (HELICS-ICU): methods and main results. J Hosp Infect. 2007;65(Suppl 2):171-3.

4. Tokars JI, Richards C, Andrus M, Klevens M, Curtis A, Horan T, et al. The changing face of surveillance for health care-associated infections. Clin Infect Dis. 2004;39(9): 1347-52.

5. Website of Centers for Disease Control and Prevention: *http://www.cdc.gov.*

59

Blood and Urine Sampling for Microbiology

Armin Ahmed

INTRODUCTION

Microbiological samples require proper handling from the time of specimen collection to transport, storage and processing. Error at any step from collection to processing can lead to wrong results. Specimen should be collected from anatomic sites, which are likely to give growth of pathogen and contamination with commensal flora is avoided. One should maintain strict asepsis while collecting the sample. Adequate amount of specimen should be collected especially in case of blood, cerebrospinal fluid and urine culture. As a general principle, body fluid or tissue is preferred over swab from any site. A specimen requisition form should be filled and sent with the specimen. The form should include information regarding the patient's working diagnosis; name of the sample, site and method of sample collection, antimicrobial therapy patient is receiving, any specific pathogen being sought or whether suspected pathogen is likely to be hazardous for the laboratory personnel. Transportation of the specimen should be done in sterile containers. Culture specimens should be transported to laboratory as early as possible. If storage is required before processing, refrigeration is used for most specimens as it prevents the growth of contaminants and maintains the viability of pathogens. However, blood culture specimens are not refrigerated. They are stored at 35 °C or in incubator. Specimen for *Neisseria* requires stable temperature, sufficient atmospheric CO_2 and humidity. Improper or unlabeled samples, samples in broken or defective containers and unpreserved samples (collection done more than 12 hours ago) are unfit for processing.[1]

BLOOD SAMPLING

Indication

- Any patient with suspected bacteremia (One should remember that absence of fever or a normal white blood count does not rule out bacteremia).
- Suspected meningitis, arthritis, endocarditis, pneumonia, osteomyelitis and fever of unknown origin.
- Surviving sepsis guidelines recommend two sets of blood culture (*one set means one aerobic and one anaerobic blood culture, therefore two sets means*

total four bottles, two aerobic and two anaerobic, each set from a different puncture site) to be sent before starting antimicrobial therapy in all patients of severe sepsis and septic shock. Blood culture sample collection should not cause delay (> 45 minutes) in initiation of antimicrobial therapy.[2]

Contraindication

There are no contraindications for blood culture. The infected skin should not be used as puncture site.

TECHNIQUE AND BASIC PRINCIPLES (BLOOD SAMPLING)

- *Collection:* Blood cultures require meticulous collection, as they are prone to contamination by the skin flora.
- *Site:* Blood culture samples should be collected via peripheral venipuncture rather than indwelling catheter or venous cannulae as it minimizes the chances of contamination. Samples from indwelling catheters should be taken only when catheter-related infection is suspected. Separate sites should be used for collection of two or more blood cultures. Arterial blood provides no advantage over venous blood.

  When catheter-related bloodstream infection is suspected blood culture is drawn from all invasive lines that are more than 48 hours old. Blood can be drawn from any port. It is preferable not to draw blood culture from the port in which antibiotic was given during last 1 hour.
- *Volume:*[3]
  - Around 20 mL blood (10 mL for aerobic and 10 mL for anaerobic bottle) should be taken from each venipuncture site.
  - At least two sets, each from two different puncture sites (total 40 mL) should be taken during evaluation of each sepsis episode.
  - Using adequate volume of blood for culture ensures that the blood to broth ratios (1:5 to 1:10) well maintained which increases the likelihood of pathogen recovery.[4]
  - For infants and small children the volume drawn should not be more than 1% of the total blood volume.
- *Number:* Two to three sets of blood culture samples will detect most episodes of bacteremia including continuous or intermittent bacteremia. Single blood culture sample should be discouraged, as it will not detect all septic episodes and is difficult to differentiate from normal flora.
- *Timing:*
  - In patients who are severely sick with anticipated continuous bacteremia 2–3 sets of samples can be collected simultaneously as most studies have shown no difference in yield between samples collected simultaneously or at intervals.[5]
  - However, in certain selected cases with suspected intermittent bacteremia multiple samples should be collected 6–36 hours apart.
  - Blood culture should be drawn before initiation of antibiotic therapy, whenever possible.
  - If the patient is already on antibiotic therapy, blood culture should be taken just before the next dose of antibiotic.

Culture Media

Automated aerobic bottles are employed in most hospitals. They are suitable for growth of the common aerobes and facultative anaerobes but obligate anaerobes require separate culture media. Routine use of anaerobic blood culture remains controversial in literature due to decrease in the incidence of anaerobic bacteremia. However, current National Committee for Clinical Laboratory Standard (NCCLS) guidelines recommended both aerobic and anaerobic cultures to be sent with every venipuncture.[3] Anaerobic cultures are more important under specific circumstances like severe immunosuppression, deep-seated abscess or wound infection. Culture bottles for disseminated mycobacterial infections are also available. They are not routinely recommended but should be used when suspecting disseminated infection with *Mycobacteria* (both tubercular and nontubercular). Blood culture media are made in the laboratory as well as commercially available. Soybean casein digest (SCD) is most commonly used media for aerobic cultures while brain heart infusion (BHI) media is used for fastidious organisms. Manual blood culture bottles are incubated for a period of 7 days. Commercially available fully automated microbiology growth and detection systems called as BACTEC blood cultures (Becton Dickinson Microbiology Systems) are frequently used nowadays in many centers. These systems detect the presence of microorganism by monitoring the CO_2 level in the bottle released as a result of consumption of ^{14}C-labeled metabolic precursors present in the broth. These systems are more efficient than manual systems and require incubation for 5 days.[4]

While interpreting the result of blood culture it should be kept in mind that there are some isolates that are nearly always represent true infection (*S. aureus, E. Coli, Pseudomonas aeruginosa, Streptococcus pneumoniae, Candida* spp.) and some organisms most of the times do not represent true bacteremia (*Corynebacterium* spp, *Bacillus* spp and *Propionibacterium).*

PREPARATION AND PROCEDURE (FIGS 1A TO D) (BLOOD SAMPLING)

- Hands are washed with soap and water followed by alcohol rub.
- After verifying patient's identity, the procedure is explained to the patient.
- Procedure tray is placed near the patient zone. It should contain all required equipment (two blood culture bottles set, i.e. two bottles for aerobic and two bottles for anaerobic, sterile gloves, tourniquet and 2% chlorhexidine in 70% alcohol swabs, syringe, needle, commercially available blood collection device, etc).
- Bottle top is disinfected with 2% chlorhexidine in 70% isopropyl alcohol wipe using no touch technique.
- Tourniquet is applied and appropriate vein is identified.
- Hand hygiene is performed again.
- The 3–4 inches area around the puncture site is cleaned with 2% chlorhexidine in 70% isopropyl alcohol with forward and backward strokes (some centers use full draping and maximum barrier precaution for collection of blood culture especially in critically ill, transplant and immunocompromised patients). The skin should remain 'wet' for 30 seconds with alcohol to act and allowed to dry.

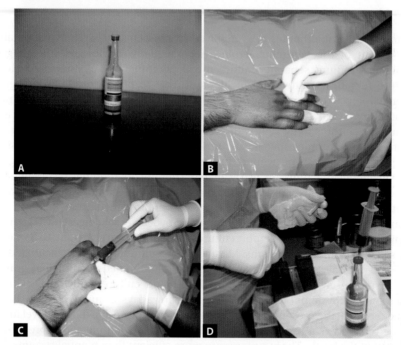

Figs 1A to D (A) Blood culture bottle; (B) Skin preparation with alcohol and chlorhexidine; (C) Sample collection by peripheral venipuncture; (D) Transfer of collected sample into blood culture bottle

- In children less than 2 months of age, chlorhexidine should not be used, only 70% alcohol swabs should be used for skin preparation.
- Sterile gloves should be worn, if vein needs to be palpated after skin preparation.
- Sample is collected via gentle venipuncture. Tourniquet is released during the procedure where appropriate.
- Around 20 mL blood is withdrawn from each site. This amount is equally divided into aerobic and anaerobic bottles. First aerobic bottle is inoculated with 10 mL of blood and then 10 mL is added to anaerobic bottle.
- Cotton ball and pressure is applied at the puncture site.
- Though changing needle between sample collection and transfer to the bottle has shown some reduction in contamination, the risk of needle stick injury outweighs the advantage.
- After adding the blood to culture bottle, it can be gently rotated to mix the contents but vigorous shaking should not be done. Blood culture bottles are kept in upright position.
- While collecting sample for catheter-related bloodstream infections, the hub of the catheter is cleaned with 70% alcohol for 15 seconds and then allowed to air dry. Blood is then drawn from any of the port via a syringe. Blood culture from central line should always be paired with peripheral venipuncture for diagnosis of catheter-related bloodstream infection. Sample collection for blood culture from central line does not require a discard amount while other laboratory tests require a discard amount. Therefore, it is advisable to draw blood culture first and it acts as the discard amount for other tests.

POST-PROCEDURE CARE (BLOOD SAMPLING)

- Blood cultures should be immediately transported to the laboratory.
- If there is any delay in transportation the bottle should be left at room temperature (20–25°C for 4–6 hours) and should not be refrigerated.

URINE SAMPLING

Indication

- Patients with clinical signs and symptoms of urinary tract infection
- Patients of severe sepsis and septic shock in which cause is unknown
- Many ICUs use weekly or biweekly urine culture in all catheterized patients as a part of their surveillance program for nosocomial infections.

Contraindication

There is no contraindication for sending urine culture.

TECHNIQUE AND BASIC PRINCIPLE (URINE SAMPLING)

Collection: Urine should be collected in clean containers free of particles and interfering substances. Microbiological specimen should be collected in sterile container. It should be leak-resistant and secured with lid to prevent specimen loss. Specimen containers should not be reused. The recommended size of the container is one, which can hold 50 mL and has a wide base. The container should be well labeled with patient name, identity number, date and time of collection. The requisition form should be sent along with the specimen. The form should include collection technique (catheter, clean catch or morning specimen), storage technique before transport, time of collection and time of receiving of the sample in the laboratory.

- *Volume:* Around 10 mL should be collected for culture.
- *Timing:* In patients who are not hospitalized, the best time to collect urine sample is on arising because morning urine is concentrated and bacteria get time to multiply in the bladder. Such type of advantage is lost in specimen collection from catheterized patients.

The type of technique used for urine specimen collection depends on the patient profile and the setting in which collection is being done. Adhesive perineal bags are used in children who are not toilet trained but this method has high contamination rate. Urethral catheterization and suprapubic aspiration are preferred due to least chances of contamination but both are invasive procedures.[6]

While interpreting the urine culture report, quantitative value of colony forming units (CFU) per milliliter (mL) of urine is important. A colony count above 10^5 CFU/mL is considered significant bacteriuria.[7] However, in case of symptomatic patients, even lower count (as low as 10^3 CFU/mL) should be taken into account.[7]

PREPARATION AND PROCEDURE (URINE SAMPLING)

Urine specimen can be collected by various methods described here.

Patient Collection

- This is done in cooperative patients after giving them instructions.
- The genitalia are first cleaned with soap and water.[8]
- The foreskin is withdrawn in uncircumcised males.
- Patient is asked to void the initial portion and collect only the mid portion of the urine without contaminating the container (clean catch).
- Rest of the urine is then passed into the bedpan or toilet.

Assisted Collection

Catheter Specimen (Figs 2A to D)

- After verifying the identity of the patient and explaining the procedure, the rubber bung of the urinary catheter is cleaned with alcohol swab and allowed to dry. This is done to prevent contamination of urine sample.
- The catheter can be clamped for some duration before sample collection to allow urine to collect in the tubing.
- A sterile needle with a syringe is then inserted at 45° into the rubber bung and urine sample withdrawn.
- The needle is taken out and the rubber bung again cleaned with alcohol swab. Sample is collected in a sterile container.
- Catheter is unclamped, if it was clamped for sample collection.

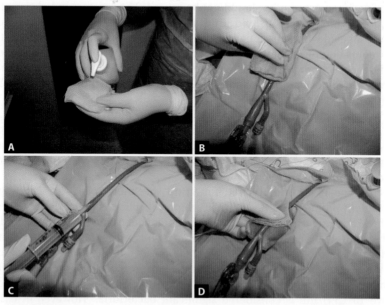

Figs 2A to D (A) Alcohol swab; (B) Cleaning of catheter with alcohol swab; (C) Urine sample collection with a sterile needle; (D) Catheter cleaning with alcohol swab after sample collection

Suprapubic Specimen

In this technique, urine is aspirated from the distended bladder using a needle, which punctures through the anterior abdominal wall using strict aseptic technique. It is useful in infants and small children.

POST-PROCEDURE CARE (URINE SAMPLING)

If the sample is not transported immediately, then any of the following methods can be used for storage.[9]

- The sample can be refrigerated at 2–8 °C for up to 24 hours.
- Bacteriostatic preservative agents (e.g. boric acid) can be added to the specimen after discussions with laboratory. Such samples do not require refrigeration.[10]
- An agar film can be dipped into the urine and container is closed properly. The container is sent to the laboratory where subcultures are done from agar sample.

REFERENCES

1. Wilson ML. General principles of specimen collection and transport. Clin Infect Dis. 1996;22(5):766-77.
2. Dellinger RP, Levy MM, Rhodes A, Annane D, Gerlach H. Surviving Sepsis Campaign Guidelines Committee including the Pediatric Subgroup, et al. Surviving Sepsis Campaign: international guidelines for management of severe sepsis and septic shock, 2012. Intensive Care Med. 2013;39(2):165-228.
3. Clinical and Laboratory Standards Institute. Principles and procedures for blood cultures: Approved guideline M47-A. Clinical and Laboratory Standards Institute, Wayne, PA. 2007.
4. Reimer LG, Wilson ML, Weinstein MP. Update on detection of bacteremia and fungemia. Clin Microbiol Rev. 1997;10:444-65.
5. Li, J, Plorde JJ, Carlson, LG. Effects of volume and periodicity on blood cultures. J Clin Microbiol. 1994;32:2829-31.
6. Karacan C, Erkek N, Senel S, Akin Gunduz S, Catli G, Tavil B. Evaluation of urine collection methods for the diagnosis of urinary tract infection in children. Med Princ Pract. 2010;19(3):188-91.
7. Centers for Disease Control and Prevention. Catheter-associated urinary tract infection (CAUTI) event. [online] Available from *www.cdc.gov/nhsn/pdfs/pscmanual/7psccauticurrent.pdf.* [Accessed July, 2013].
8. Shrestha R, Gyawali N, Gurung R, Amatya R, Bhattacharya SK. Effect of urogenital cleaning with paper soap on bacterial contamination rate while collecting midstream urine specimens. J Lab Physicians. 2013;5(1):17-20.
9. NCCLS. Urinalysis and transportation, and preservation of urine specimens. Approved Guideline. NCCLS Document. GP16-A2 Vol. 21 No. 19. Wayne, PA: NCCLS. 2001.
10. Lum KT, Meers PD. Boric acid converts urine into an effective bacteriostatic transport medium. J Infect. 1989;18(1):51-8.

60

Blood Component Handling at Bedside

Atul Sonker, Anju Dubey

INTRODUCTION

Blood transfusion (BT) is a vital component of the modern healthcare system. If used judiciously, it may be lifesaving. In cases where BT is required, one should weigh the risk of potential adverse reactions and probable transfusion-transmitted infections against the benefits of infusing other pharmacological substitutes (crystalloids or colloids). The appropriate use of blood and blood components implies that blood and/or components should be transfused only to treat a condition leading to significant morbidity or mortality which cannot be prevented or managed effectively by other means.

The term "blood components" refer to various parts separated from whole blood, donated by healthy subjects (blood donors), which are intended for transfusion to different subjects (recipients). Each whole blood donation has potential to be separated into three different types of blood components, i.e. packed red blood cells (PRBC), plasma components (fresh frozen plasma, cryoprecipitate and cryo-poor plasma) and platelet concentrate (random donor platelet). There should be written standard operating procedures (SOPs) for the administration of blood and blood components in every hospital, especially for checking the final identity of the patient, the blood bag, the compatibility label and there should be documentation at each step to prevent the errors.

BLOOD COMPONENTS: BASIC PROPERTIES

Whole Blood

Whole blood is unaltered anticoagulated blood primarily collected from: (a) Volunteer or replacement blood donors for transfusion to the patients (allogeneic transfusions) or (b) Patients donating for transfusion to themselves, later on (autologous transfusions). The whole blood is collected from those donors who have satisfactorily undergone a health assessment which includes a questionnaire on past and present illnesses, and have met standard criteria required for whole blood donation.

Blood Components

Blood components are therapeutic parts of whole blood intended for transfusion, such as PRBCs, platelets and plasma components separated by centrifugation due to their different specific gravities. Table 1 shows the variants of packed red blood cells (PRBC) and their specific features. Table 2 shows various platelet and plasma preparations along with their properties and storage recommendations.

Cellular Components

- Red blood cells (RBC) or packed red blood cells (PRBC)
- Leukocyte depleted PRBC
- Random donor platelet concentrates (RDP)
- Single donor platelet concentrates (SDP)
- Leukocyte depleted platelet concentrates

Plasma Components

- Fresh frozen plasma (FFP)
- Cryoprecipitate
- Cryo-poor plasma (CPP)

Types of PRBCs

- *PRBC with no additive solution:* Red cells in a volume of 150–200 mL (depending on the volume and hematocrit of whole blood collected) from which approximately 80% of the plasma has been removed. Hematocrit is around 65–75%.
- *PRBC suspended in additive solution:* Red cells in a volume of 150–200 mL (depending on the volume and hematocrit of whole blood collected) having minimal residual plasma to which 100 mL of additive solution has been added. Hematocrit is around 50–70%.
- *Advantage of transfusing PRBC over whole blood*
    - PRBCs increase oxygen carrying capacity of recipient's blood without increasing its volume. This component is useful in cases of chronic anemia, congestive heart failure (CHF) and in old, debilitated patients.
    - When plasma is removed from whole blood, quantity of plasma proteins decrease thus leading to lesser chances of allergic or anaphylactic reactions.
- *Advantages of using PRBC suspended in additive solution*
    - Viscosity of PRBC is reduced, which makes the transfusion easy.
    - Shelf life of PRBC is increased from 35–42 days.
    - Increase in post-transfusion viability of red cells.

Storage

Blood bank refrigerator used for storage of PRBC units has feature of maintaining a uniform temperature of 4–6°C. It is equipped with digital thermometer which displays the temperature continuously, continuous temperature recording device and audible alarm system.

Labeling of Blood and Blood Component

The label on blood/blood component bag should contain following information: Type of blood or blood component; name and address of blood bank; license

Table 1 Whole blood and red cell components

Volume of parent whole blood	Approximate volume of usable final product	Physical appearance	Type of bag used	Storage temperature	Shelf life
Packed red blood cell (PRBC) component					
450 mL blood + 63 mL anticoagulant (CPD)	350 +/- 20 mL	Dark red in color	With additive solution	4–6°C in BBR	42 days, if unopened 24 hours, if spiked
350 mL blood + 49 mL anticoagulant (CPD)	300 +/- 20 mL	Dark red in color	With additive solution	4–6°C in BBR	42 days, if unopened 24 hours, if spiked
450 mL blood + 63 mL anticoagulant (CPDA1)	280 +/- 40 mL	Dark red in color	Without additive solution	4–6°C in BBR	35 days, if unopened 24 hours, if spiked
350 mL blood + 49 mL anticoagulant (CPDA1)	230 +/- 40 mL	Dark red in color	Without additive solution	4–6°C in BBR	35 days, if unopened 24 hours, if spiked
Whole blood	350 mL/450 mL whole blood + 49 mL anticoagulant (CPDA1)	Red in color	Single or double blood-bag system	4–6°C in BBR	35 days, if unopened 24 hours, if spiked
Saline washed red blood cells	275–300 mL	Red in color	Red cells in normal saline	4–6°C in BBR	24 hours

Abbreviations: CPD, citrate phosphate dextrose anticoagulant solution; CPDA1, citrate phosphate dextrose adenine anticoagulant solution; BBR, Blood bank refrigerator.

Table 2 Platelet concentrates and plasma components

	Physical appearance	Approx vol (mL)	Storage temperature	Shelf life	ABO compatibility	Rh-compatibility	Post-transfusion effect
Platelet products							
RDP	Liquid, straw colored	50–60 mL	20–24°C	5 days	NR	NR	1 unit ↑ platelet count by ~10 × 10³/µL. (4–6 units can be pooled)
SDP	Liquid, straw colored	200–300 mL	20–24°C	5 days	R	NR	↑ platelet count by 30–50 × 10³/µL.
Plasma products							
FFP	Frozen, clear yellowish	220–250 mL	–18°C or lower	1 year	R	NR	↑ level of clotting factors by 8–10% at a dose of 10–15 mL/kg
Cryoprecipitate	Frozen, cloudy yellowish	10–15 mL	–18°C or lower	1 year	NR	NR	↑ fibrinogen level by 50 mg/dL at a dose of 1 unit/10 kg.

Abbreviations: R = Required; NR = Not required

number of blood bank; unit number of blood/component; blood group (ABO and RhD); date of preparation of blood/blood component; date of expiry; volume of blood or blood component with nature and percentage of anticoagulant; instructions for use; and non-reactive serological status of Transfusion Transmitted Infections such as, antibody of against human immunodeficiency virus (HIV) 1 and 2, antibody against Hepatitis C Virus (HCV), surface antigen of Hepatitis B Virus (HBsAg), Syphilis and Malaria parasite.

Compatibility Labeling on Red Cell Units

Along with above mentioned details, the following additional information should be there on compatibility label (for red cell component only):

- The compatibility label and certificate indicating patient's name, age, gender, hospital's identification number, ward and bed number.
- ABO and RhD type of recipient and donor, type of blood component which is issued.
- Signature of the authorized person from BT service.

BEDSIDE HANDLING OF BLOOD COMPONENTS

General Principles

Informed Consent

There are variations in documentation related to transfusion of blood and blood component, e.g. dedicated transfusion consent form versus documentation in patient's medical records. In cases where patient is unable to give consent to administer blood and blood components either due to medical reasons, e.g. unconsciousness or patient is minor, attempts to seek an alternative person legally entitled to provide consent should be made prior to any BT, unless in an emergency life-threatening situation where transfusion should be given as a part of life-saving treatment.

Requisition Form and Pretransfusion Blood Sampling for Blood and Blood Components

- The requisition form is the means of communication with the transfusion service provider(s), asking them to prepare and issue the blood component for administration to a particular patient.
- After making documentation for transfusion requirement, it is necessary to make positive identification of the patients and labeling the samples at the patient's bedside. If this is not followed, a *wrong blood in tube* (WBIT) event may happen and result in lethal transfusion reaction.
- It is also important to mention history of previous transfusion episode and associated event, if any. The history of adverse event associated with previous transfusion help the BT personnel to perform other reference laboratory test and procedures to prevent recurrence of such event, e.g. recurrent febrile nonhemolytic transfusion reaction, transfusion delayed hemolytic transfusion reaction, etc.

- The request must include the indication for transfusion and whether there is any special blood component requirement for the patient, e.g. saline-washed PRBC in case of IgA deficient patient.

Table 3 addresses various issues related to release of blood components from BT services depending on clinical urgency.

Table 3 Issues related to release of blood from blood transfusion service

Blood component	Clinical situation	Approximate required for release	ABO and Rh(D) group of component	Cross-match
PRBC	Immediate requirement	< 5 min	O Rh(D) Neg	Uncross matched
	urgent requirement	~ 15 min	Blood group matched/ identical	Uncross matched
	Planned	2–3 hours	Blood group matched/ identical/compatible	Cross matched
FFP	Any	45–60 min	Only ABO matching or neutral blood group	Not required
Cryo-poor plasma (CPP)	Any	45–60 min	Only ABO matching or neutral blood group	Not required
Cryoprecipitate	Any	45–60 min	Any blood group	Not required
Platelets	Any	15–30 min	ABO identical is preferred else random group can be given in case of adult. ABO identical is must in case of neonate < 4 months	Not required

Requisition in Emergency

- If a patient is in critical condition and there is no time of blood sample collection for pre-transfusion testing, then the doctor in emergency can request for O negative (preferred) or O positive blood (if O negative is not available).
- In no condition, the patient having anti-D (unexpected red cell antibody) and RhD negative women of child-bearing age should be transfused with RhD positive blood unless there is no other choice available in a life-threatening situation.
- Blood sample of the patient should be sent to blood bank as soon as sampling becomes possible. All documentary formalities should be completed once the emergency is over.

Blood Component Bag Identification Check

- The most important step before actual administration of blood components is proper recipient identification and ensuring the compatibility of the component. When blood is issued from a blood bank, a manual or computer print document (compatibility form) is sent along with the blood/blood component bag.

- This compatibility form contains information pertaining to the recipient such as:
  - ABO and Rh(D) group
  - Unit number and
  - Information identifying the intended recipient (name, registration number, blood group, ward and bed number).
- There should not be any discrepancy between the ABO, Rh(D) group and donation number on blood bag and that on compatibility label.

Inspection of blood component bag: Following point need to be checked:
- Integrity of the bag
- If there are any large or small visible clots
- If there is any evidence of hemolysis in the plasma or at the interface between red cells and plasma.
- Discoloration or any signs of leakage which may warn that the blood has been contaminated by bacteria and may lead to severe or fatal reaction when transfused.
- The blood bag which appear abnormal or damaged or which has remained out of the refrigerator for more than 30 minutes should never be transfused.
- Checking must take place at the bedside of the patient.

Bedside re-checking of blood component bag: Following point need to be ensured
- *First step*
  - Ask the patient (conscious) to tell his or her name, age and hospital registration number.
  - If the patient is confused or unconscious a responsible relative or another member of staff who knows the patient can be asked to verify the patient's identity.
- *Second step:* Check the patient's name and ID against compatibility form and label of the blood component.
- *Third step*
  - Now check the ABO group and Rh(D) status of the blood component unit and match them with those recorded on the compatibility label on blood component. The blood groups should be compatible.
  - On the blood bag label, check the expiry date.
  - Finally, ask a second personnel to repeat checking process at the bedside.

Blood Transfusion Set

- All blood components (PRBCs, platelets, FFP and cryoprecipitate) must be given through standard BT set to remove fibrin clots or other particulate debris.
- Standard BT set have pore size of 170 microns, capable of removing macroaggregates.
- Take aseptic precaution, including cleaning of port of blood component bag before spiking with BT set.
- In order to reduce the risk of bacterial growth, the blood administration set must be changed with completion of each transfusion or every 12 hours, if the transfusion is going on.
- To assist transfusion of large volumes of red cells in the setting of critical bleeding, external pressure devices (bags) and rapid infusion devices are

used. The pressure in the device should never exceed 300 mm Hg to avoid hemolysis in blood unit.

- When blood components need to be administered through a multi-lumen venous access device, other lumens should not be used concurrently for infusing medications and fluids.

Monitoring during Transfusion of Blood and Blood Component

Closely observe, monitor and document patient's vitals: every 5 minutes for first 15 minutes; every 15 minutes for next half hour; every half hour for next 1 hour; and every hour till the end of transfusion; 30 minutes post-transfusion.

Documentation

Following points should be documented in patient's records after blood and blood component transfusion: Type of component, volume transfused; unit ID number of blood component; blood group of blood component unit transfused; time of start and completion of transfusion; signature of person administering the blood.

Blood and Blood Components Specific Issues

Whole Blood

- *Indications*
  - Transfusion therapy in massively bleeding patient
  - Exchange transfusion
- *Dosage:* One unit of whole blood increases hemoglobin approximately by 1.0 gm/dL and hematocrit by 3% (in case of adult)
- *Administration*
  - Must be ABO and Rh(D) compatible with patient's blood
  - Must be through standard BT set
  - Pre-transfusion warming is never recommended in routine transfusions; however in cases of massive transfusion, blood warming is done using standard warmer.
  - Never add any medicines to the blood unit
  - Complete transfusion within 4 hours of initiation.

Packed Red Blood Cell

- *Indications*
  - In cases of acute or chronic normovolemic anemia, for restoration of oxygen carrying capacity.
  - In case of acute blood loss, use with crystalloid replacement fluid or colloid solution.
- *Non-indications*
  - Deficiency anemia that is pharmacologically treatable
  - Known deficiency of coagulation factors
  - Decrease in platelet count
  - Only for volume replacement

- To enhance healing of wound
- For general *well-being* improvement
- Substitute to a hematinic.

- *Dosage effects*
    - Adults who is not bleeding actively, an unit of RBC increases:
        - Hemoglobin by 0.75–1 gm%
        - Hematocrit by 2.5–3%
    - Children who are not bleeding actively, a dose of 8 mL/kg body weight of whole blood or RBC prepared from it, increases:
        - Hemoglobin by 0.75–1 gm%
        - Hematocrit by 2.5–3%
    - Infants who are not bleeding actively, a dose of 3 mL/kg body weight of whole blood or RBC prepared from it, increases:
        - Hemoglobin by 0.75–1 gm%
        - Hematocrit by 2.5–3%
- *Administrations*
    - Must be ABO and Rh(D) compatible with recipient's blood type
    - No medication should be added to the unit of blood
    - Transfusion should be completed within 4 hours of commencement
    - Pre-transfusion warming is never recommended in routine transfusions; however, in cases of massive transfusion, blood warming is done using standard warmer.

Fresh Frozen Plasma

- *Indications*
    - For patients who have undiagnosed coagulopathy and multiple coagulation factor deficiencies.
    - Liver diseases
    - Warfarin (anticoagulant) reversal
    - Disseminated intravascular coagulation (DIC)
    - Replacement of coagulation factors in patients who receive large volume transfusions such as massively transfused cases.
- *Non-indications*
    - Should not be used as a source of albumin or as a volume expander
- *Dosage:* 10–15 mL/kg
- *Administration*
    - ABO blood group compatible
    - No cross-matching required
    - FFP should be thawed in blood bank in thawing bath at temperatures between 30°C and 37°C, before use.
    - FFP should be administered soon after thawing and within 24 hours, if kept at 2–6°C.
    - Transfuse FFP using standard BT set as soon as possible after thawing.

Cryoprecipitate

- *Indications*
    - *Fibrinogen replacement:* Fibrinogen consumption (e.g. DIC) or loss (e.g. massive hemorrhage), or both

- In the treatment of inherited deficiencies of (as an alternative to factor VIII concentrate):
  - von Willebrand factor (von Willebrand disease)
  - Factor VIII (hemophilia A)
  - Factor XIII
- *Dosage*
  - 2 units/10 kg weight.
  - One bag contains more than 80 units of factor VIII and more than 150 mg of fibrinogen.
  - Plasma level of factor VIII is increased by 2% from each unit of factor VIII per kg.
- *Administration*
  - Before transfusion, it should be thawed in blood bank in thawing bath between 30°C and 37°C.
  - It should be transfused immediately after thawing.
  - If not transfused immediately, cryoprecipitate should not be stored later than 4 hours at 2–6°C.

Cryo-poor Plasma

- *Indications:* Thrombotic thrombocytopenic purpura (TTP)
- *Dosage:* 10–15 mL/kg
- *Administration*
  - Should be ABO compatible
  - Cross-matching is not required
  - Should be thawed in blood bank in thawing bath between 30°C and 37°C before use.
  - Transfuse as soon as possible through standard BT set after thawing.

Platelet Components

Random donor platelet (RDP) or single donor platelet (SDP)
- *Indications:* Treatment of bleeding due to:
  - Thrombocytopenia due to any disease
  - Platelet function defects
  - To prevent bleeding due to thrombocytopenia such as in bone marrow failure.
- *Contraindications*
  - As prophylaxis of bleeding for surgical patients unless preoperative platelet count is low
  - Idiopathic autoimmune thrombocytopenic purpura (ITP) except in life-saving conditions.
  - Thrombotic thrombocytopenic purpura
  - Thrombocytopenia associated with septicemia until treatment has been initiated.
  - Heparin-induced thrombocytopenia, unless there is life-threatening hemorrhage.
- *Dosage*
  - *For RDP:* 1 unit of RDP unit/10 kg of body weight/dose for adult
  - *For SDP:* 1 unit of SDP/dose for adult

- *Administration*
  - ABO compatible (preferred but not a mandate)
  - Check that the platelet bag do not show clumping or appear unusually cloudy, which may be a sign of bacterial contamination.
  - Transfused through standard BT set
  - Should be transfused immediately once received in the ward.
  - If not transfused, the platelet product should be sent back to the blood bank for appropriate storage in agitator with incubator.

Table 4 shows issues pertaining to transfusion of various blood and blood components.

Table 4 Issues related to transfusion of blood and blood components

Component type	Start administration	Complete transfusion
Packed red cell	≤ 30 minutes of issue	Within 4 hours
Random platelet unit/apheresis platelet concentrate	≤ 30 minutes of issue	Within 4 hours
Fresh frozen plasma (FFP)/cryoprecipitate	< 30 minutes of issue	< 6 hours

ADVERSE REACTION DUE TO BLOOD COMPONENTS

The healthcare personnel who are involved administering transfusions must be trained so as to recognize a transfusion reaction and take appropriate actions promptly. If a reaction occurs, the critical event is to stop the transfusion immediately, maintain the patency of intravenous line with saline and evaluate the clinical situation. Patient's vital signs should always be measured immediately if a reaction occurs. Table 5 shows classification and features of various transfusion reactions.

Adverse Transfusion Reaction

1. *Acute transfusion reaction*: Occurs within 24 hours of transfusion
2. *Delayed transfusion reaction*: Signs appear 5–10 days after transfusion

Acute Transfusion Reaction

- *Febrile nonhemolytic transfusion reaction:* ≥ 1°C rise in temperature associated with transfusion and without other cause for fever. Patient has muscle cramps, nausea, headache, flushing of the skin, tachycardia, chills and rigors. Transfusion should be stopped immediately. Vital signs of the patient and urine output should be monitored.
  Treatment: Acetaminophen, meperidine for chills.
  Prevention: Use of leukoreduced blood for transfusion
- *Urticaria:* Pruritus, flushing, rash. Use antihistamine. May restart transfusion slowly, if symptoms resolve.
- *Acute intravascular hemolysis of transfused red cells due to incompatible transfusion:* This occurs soon after transfusion is started. Patient complains of pain at infusion site, back and flank pain, shortness of breath, fever, rigors. There is hypotension, bleeding from wounds or venipuncture sites,

Table 5 Adverse reaction due to transfusion of blood and blood components

Categories of transfusion reaction	Severity	Signs	Symptoms	Possible causes
I	Mild	*Localized cutaneous reactions:* • Urticaria • Rash	Pruritus (itching)	Hypersensitivity (mild) to plasma proteins
II	Moderate	• Flushing • Urticaria • Rigors • Fever • Restlessness • Tachycardia	Anxiety Pruritus (itching) Palpitations Mild dyspnea Headache	Hypersensitivity (moderate-to-severe) Febrile nonhemolytic transfusion reactions (FNHTR) due to antibodies to WBC &/cytokines Possible contamination with pyrogens and bacteria
III	Severe	Rigors Fever Restlessness Hypotension (fall of 20% in systolic BP) Tachycardia (rise of 20% in heart rate) Hemoglobinuria Unexplained Bleeding [disseminated intravascular coagulation (DIC)]	Anxiety Chest pain Pain near infusion site Respiratory distress/ shortness of breath Loin/back pain Headache Dyspnea	Acute intravascular hemolysis Bacterial contamination and septic shock Fluid overload Anaphylaxis Transfusion associated lung injury (TRALI)

hemoglobinuria in unconscious patients. Transfusion should be discontinued immediately and normal saline should be infused. Blood unit, patient's identity and compatibility report form should be checked. Patient should be promptly resuscitated with adequate crystalloid or colloid. Blood bank physician should be notified. Blood bags and transfusion set should be sent to blood bank immediately. Patient's urine output and ECG should be monitored.

- Infective shock due to bacterial contamination of red cells or platelets
- *Anaphylaxis:* Reaction to a protein (commonly IgA) deficient in the patient.
- *Transfusion-associated acute lung injury (TRALI):* Caused by donor plasma that contains antibodies against the patient's leukocytes.
- *Transfusion-associated circulatory overload (TACO):* TACO is a recognized transfusion reaction in critically ill patients. Occurs when the circulatory

system becomes overwhelmed by additional volumes of blood component, or a high infusion rate of such component. Clinically, patients present with sudden dyspnea, orthopnea, tachycardia and a wide pulse pressure, often associated with hypertension and hypoxemia developing within 1–2 hours of transfusion. Patients over 60 years of age, infants and severely anemic patients are particularly susceptible. Differentiating TACO from TRALI is difficult; however, hypotension seen with TRALI and the hypertension seen with TACO provides a clinical differentiation of the two. TACO patients usually respond well to diuretics and oxygen supplementation.

Delayed Transfusion Reaction

- *Delayed hemolysis* of transfused red cells occurring due to prior alloimmunization.
- *Transfusion-associated graft-versus-host disease (TA-GVHD)* occurs as a result of immune reaction of donor T-cells against the recipient who is either immunodeficient or of close HLA type to the donor.
- *Iron overload* occurs in patients who have received multiple transfusions.
- *Post-transfusion purpura* is an immune-mediated thrombocytopenia, which usually occurs in multi-parous women.

Management of Adverse Reaction due to Transfusion of Blood/Blood Components

Blood Sampling and Documentation

- For laboratory work-up in blood bank, patient's blood sample 2 mL in EDTA vial and 5 mL in plain vial should be taken.
- The blood samples should be labelled with name of the patient and registration/specific identification number.
- Details of reaction (signs and symptoms) should be documented.
- Postreaction blood sample, implicated blood/component unit with administration set and reaction report should be sent to the blood center immediately for evaluation.
- After completion of investigation, the blood center physician will notify the clinical services about the results and offer advice for further transfusion and suggestions for management.

Approach to Category I (Mild Transfusion Reactions)

Immediately stop the transfusion procedure
↓
Oral or parenteral antihistamine such as Avil
↓
Patient should be under observation at least for 30 minutes, if there is no progression of symptoms restart the transfusion at the normal rate
↓
In cases where there is no clinical improvement within 30 minutes, or if signs and symptoms worsen, management should be done as a category II reaction.

Prevention of category I transfusion reaction: If there is history of repeated transfusion reaction of similar kind, the implicated patient should be premedicated with oral antihistamines before giving transfusion of blood or blood components.

Approach to Category II (Moderate Reactions)

Immediately stop the transfusion procedure

↓

Replace the BT set and keep the IV line patent with infusion of normal saline

↓

Inform the BT service immediately

↓

Send the blood unit along with transfusion set, and following to the blood bank for investigations:
• Freshly collected urine and
• New blood samples (clotted and anticoagulated) from the vein opposite the infusion site
• Documentation of reaction observed

↓

Start management using administration of antihistamine and an antipyretic

↓

Give IV corticosteroids and bronchodilators, if there are anaphylactoid features (e.g. bronchospasm, stridor).

Note:
• If there is a clinical improvement during the line of management, transfusion may be restarted slowly with a new unit of blood under careful observation.
• If there is no clinical improvement within 15 minutes or the patient's condition deteriorates, shift the management considering the reaction as a category III reaction.
• Febrile reactions are quite common among all type of transfusion reactions, but fever is associated with other adverse reactions to transfusion and it is important to rule out the other causes, especially acute hemolysis and bacterial contamination, before arriving at a diagnosis of a febrile reaction. Fever may also be due to an unrelated cause, e.g. malaria.

Prevention of category II transfusion reaction: If the patient is a regular transfusion recipient such as thalassemics or has experienced two or more febrile nonhemolytic reactions in the previous transfusions, the patient should be subjected for following management to prevent recurrence of category II transfusion reaction:
• Premedicate with antipyretic 1 hour before starting the transfusion.
• Aspirin should be avoided in patient with thrombocytopenia.
• Repeat the antipyretic 3 hours after the start of transfusion.
• Rate of transfusion should be kept at slow rate.
• Use modified blood components such as buffy coat removed blood components or leuko-filtered blood components in cases where above-mentioned management has failed to control the febrile reaction and further transfusion is required.

Approach to Category III (Severe Reactions)

Stop the transfusion. Replace the BT set and keep IV line open with normal saline.
↓

Infuse normal saline 20–30 mL/kg (ensure cardiac and renal sufficiency), maintain systolic BP.
↓

If hypotensive, give over 5 minutes and elevate foot end of bed.
↓

Maintain airway and give high flow oxygen by mask.
↓

Give 1:1000 adrenaline 0.01 mg/kg body weight by intramuscular injection.
↓

Give IV corticosteroids and bronchodilators, if there are anaphylactoid features (e.g. bronchospasm, stridor).
↓

Consider to give diuretic.
↓

Notify the blood bank immediately.
↓

Send blood unit with BT set, fresh urine sample and new blood samples (clotted and anticoagulated) from vein opposite infusion site with appropriate request form to blood bank and laboratory for investigations.
↓

Check a fresh urine specimen visually for signs of hemoglobinuria (red or pink urine).
↓

Start a 24-hour urine collection and fluid balance chart and record all intake and output. Maintain fluid balance.
↓

Assess for bleeding from puncture sites or wounds.

If there is clinical or laboratory evidence of DIC with bleeding, give:

> RDP (*adult:* 5–6 units or 1 unit/10 kg) and
> Either cryoprecipitate (*adult:* 12 units) or FFP (*adult:* 3 units or 10–15 mL/kg).

SUGGESTED READING

1. Brecher ME (Ed). American Association of Blood Banks Technical Manual, 14th edn. Bethesda, MD: AABB Press, 2002.
2. Directive 2002/98/EC of the European Parliament and of the Council of the European Union. Setting standards of quality and safety for the collection, testing, processing, storage and distribution of human blood and blood components and amending Directive 2001/83/EC. Official Journal L033 08/02/2003.
3. Guidelines for the Administration of Blood and Blood Components. National Blood Users Group. January 2004.
4. McClelland DBL (Ed). Handbook of Transfusion Medicine, 3rd edn. London: The Stationery Office, 2001.

5. Stainsby D, MacLennan S, Thomas D, Isaac J, Hamilton PJ. British Committee for Standards in Haematology. Guidelines on the management of massive blood loss. Br J Haematol. 2006;135(5):634-41.

6. The administration of blood and blood components and the management of transfused patients. British Committee for Standards in Haematology, Blood Transfusion Task Force. Royal College of Nursing and the Royal College of Surgeons of England. Transfus Med. 1999;9(3):227-38.

7. The clinical use of blood, Handbook. World Health Organization. Blood Transfusion Safety. Geneva.

8. Voak D, Chapman JF, Phillips P. Quality of transfusion practice beyond the blood transfusion laboratory is essential to prevent ABO-incompatible death. Transfus Med. 2000;10(2):95-6.

61

Managing Needle-Stick Injury

Puja Srivastava, Anupam Wakhlu, Vikas Agarwal

INTRODUCTION

Needle-stick injury (NSI) and inadvertent exposure to blood products is perhaps the most common professional hazards in the field of medicine and health care. Health care workers (HCWs) are at risk of contracting transmissible blood-borne viruses, like human immunodeficiency virus (HIV), hepatitis B virus (HBV), hepatitis C virus (HCV) and others while performing routine hospital activities. The frequency of such incidents depends on the work load, use of universal precautions, safety devices and medical discipline.

Worldwide, every year, more than 35 million HCWs are at risk of sustaining sharp injuries at work place.[1] There is scarcity of data on actual incidence of occupation-related needle-stick and sharp injuries from India,[2,3] but according to data from the EPInet system, in a typical health care facility, HCWs incur roughly 27 needle-stick injuries per 100 beds per year.[4] Also, such injuries are associated with considerable health care expenditure. According to a study from tertiary care hospital in western India, approximate short-term cost is ₹ 9,000/HCW/episode of needle-stick injury.[5]

Accidental occupational exposures can lead to infections with blood-borne viruses like HBV, HCV, and HIV. In an unvaccinated person, the risk of transmission is highest for HBV infection, and varies between 6% and 30%.[1,6] The estimated risk of transmission of HCV is between 3% and 10%.[7,8] Transmission rate of HIV following NSI is 0.3%[9] and 0.1%[10] (Fig. 1) following mucous membrane exposure. However, if the source has very high viral load, transmission risk increased by greater than tenfold.[11] Although the transmission risk for HIV is 100 times less than HBV and 10 times less than HCV, it is associated with significant psychological trauma, social stigma and may adversely affect quality of life and functioning of the individual.

DEFINITIONS

Needle-stick Injury

The accidental puncture of the skin by a needle or sharps contaminated with blood and/or blood contaminated body fluids, during a diagnostic or therapeutic procedure.[12]

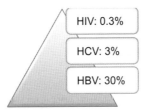

Fig. 1 Transmission risk pyramid due to different viruses

Abbreviations: HIV, human immunodeficiency virus; HBV, hepatitis B virus; HCV, hepatitis C virus.

Inadvertent Occupational Exposure

The unintended contact of eyes or mucous membranes with blood and or with body fluids contaminated with blood during a medical intervention.[13]

Health Care Worker

This term includes all paid and unpaid staff (e.g. physicians, nurses, medical and nursing students, sanitation staff, dieticians, physiotherapist and other allied staff) working in health care facility who are at risk of exposure to infectious materials (e.g. blood, tissue, and specific body fluids), contaminated medical paraphernalia. All categories of HCWs should undergo training for prevention of such injuries, and should be eligible for similar post-exposure prophylactic treatment program.[14,15]

PREVENTION FROM NEEDLE-STICK INJURY

Prevention is the Best Strategy

Prevention of occupational exposures should be the primary strategy. All HCWs should practice Universal precautions, which include:
- Washing hands before and after care of each patient.
- Appropriate use of protective equipment and devices—gloves, masks, gowns, boots, shoe covers, eyewear, etc.
- Any arterial or venous cannulation should not be performed without wearing protective gloves.
- Needles and sharps should be used with caution:
  - Sharp disposal container must be on the procedure trolley itself.
  - Sharps should be disposed in puncture proof containers immediately after use.
  - Needles should never be recapped (Fig. 2).

Vaccination

Among the three potential blood-borne infections, vaccination is available only for HBV. All HCWs should receive HBV vaccine and response to vaccination should be documented by measuring anti-HBs titers one month after completion of vaccination.

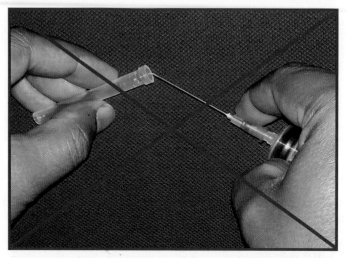

Fig. 2 Needle recapping is a medical sin

Periodic Training

All HCWs should undergo periodic training to minimize occupational exposures. All HCWs should have 24 × 7 access to post-exposure prophylaxis (PEP) in case of an inadvertent occupational exposure.

POST-EXPOSURE PROPHYLAXIS

Post-exposure prophylaxis refers to the comprehensive management program to minimize the risk of transmission of blood-borne pathogens (HIV, HBV and HCV), following potential exposure.[14,15] It includes counseling, risk assessment, relevant laboratory investigations based on informed consent of the source and exposed person and first aid. Depending on the risk assessment, there is provision of short-term (4 weeks) of antiretroviral drugs for potential HIV exposure and/or vaccination and immunoglobulin against HBV for potential HBV exposure, with 6 months follow-up and support.

Steps Involved in Post-exposure Prophylaxis

- First-aid measures for exposure site
- Document baseline information and report the incident
- Evaluate the exposure
- Evaluate the exposure source and exposed person at baseline
- Disease specific PEP management
- Follow-up care and testing.

Step 1: First-aid Measures for Exposure Site (Flow Chart 1)

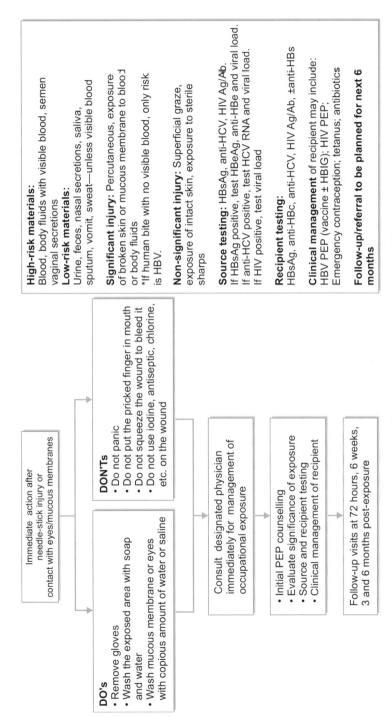

Flow chart 1 Immediate action after occupational needle-stick injury

Immediate action after needle-stick injury or contact with eyes/mucous membranes

DO's
- Remove gloves
- Wash the exposed area with soap and water
- Wash mucous membrane or eyes with copious amount of water or saline

DON'Ts
- Do not panic
- Do not put the pricked finger in mouth
- Do not squeeze the wound to bleed it
- Do not use iodine, antiseptic, chlorine, etc. on the wound

Consult designated physician immediately for management of occupational exposure

- Initial PEP counselling
- Evaluate significance of exposure
- Source and recipient testing
- Clinical management of recipient

Follow-up visits at 72 hours, 6 weeks, 3 and 6 months post-exposure

High-risk materials:
Blood, body fluids with visible blood, semen vaginal secretions
Low-risk materials:
Urine, feces, nasal secretions, saliva, sputum, vomit, sweat—unless visible blood

Significant injury: Percutaneous, exposure of broken skin or mucous membrane to blood or body fluids
*If human bite with no visible blood, only risk is HBV.

Non-significant injury: Superficial graze, exposure of intact skin, exposure to sterile sharps

Source testing: HBsAg, anti-HCV, HIV Ag/Ab.
If HBsAg positive, test HBeAg, anti-HBe and viral load.
If anti-HCV positive, test HCV RNA and viral load.
If HIV positive, test viral load

Recipient testing:
HBsAg, anti-HBc, anti-HCV, HIV Ag/Ab, ±anti-HBs

Clinical management of recipient may include:
HBV PEP (vaccine ± HBIG); HIV PEP; Emergency contraception; tetanus; antibiotics

Follow-up/referral to be planned for next 6 months

Abbreviations: PEP, post-exposure prophylaxis; HCV, hepatitis C virus; HBV, hepatitis B virus; HBIG, hepatitis B immune globulin

Step 2: Document Baseline Information and Report the Incident

Following first aid measures, such exposures should be reported immediately to designated hospital authorities, responsible for managing such occupational exposures. The report should include:

- *Circumstances in which the incident occurred:* Exact time and date of incident, procedure details and exposure type (mucosal/percutaneous).
- *Source information:* Whether infected with HIV, HBV or HCV? If yes, determine disease severity, viral load, CD4 count, history of antiviral therapy and drug resistance information, if any.
- *Baseline information about exposed HCW:* Baseline serology for HIV, HBV and anti-HCV, vaccination status for hepatitis B and anti-HBs titers, pregnancy or breastfeeding status, details of other medical conditions if any. Details of PEP plan for the exposed HCW, according to baseline information and future follow-up plan.

Step 3: Evaluate the Exposure

Each exposure should be assessed for its potential to transmit HBV, HCV or HIV, based on the route and severity of exposure, and the type of body fluid involved. To consider an exposure as significant, injured person should come in contact of potentially infectious body fluid in one of the following ways:

- *Percutaneous injury:* Needle stick or puncture/cut with a sharp object.
- *Contact with mucous membranes:* Splash to eyes, nose or mouth.
- Contact with non-intact skin.
- Human bites resulting in blood exposure to either person involved.

Various body fluids capable of transmitting blood-borne viral pathogens are listed in Table 1 whereas categories of exposure and their severity are listed in Table 2.

If a significant exposure has occurred, both source and injured person should be tested.

Determining the category of exposure helps in deciding dual versus triple drug PEP regimen, for potential exposure to HIV contaminated source. However, according to latest US Public Health Service guidelines,[16] in most cases it is

Table 1 Body fluids capable of transmitting blood-borne viral pathogens

Potentially infectious body fluids	Non-infectious body fluids (Unless evidently contaminated with blood)
• Blood, serum, plasma	• Feces
• Amniotic, pleural, peritoneal, pericardial, synovial, and cerebrospinal fluids	• Nasal secretions
	• Sputum
• Semen and vaginal fluids	• Tears
• Saliva (if it is contaminated with blood and for HBV even if it is not contaminated with blood)	• Urine
	• Vomitus
• Cultures of HIV, HBV or HCV in special labs, or pathology specimens that contain concentrated viruses	

Abbreviations: HIV, human immunodeficiency virus; HBV, hepatitis B virus; HCV, hepatitis C virus.

Table 2 Categories of exposure

Category	Definition and examples
Insignificant exposure	Contact with intact skin
Mild exposure	Contact with non-intact skin or mucous membrane with small volumes of blood
	For example, superficial skin abrasion with thin bore needles used for subcutaneous injections or contact with eyes or mucous membranes
Moderate exposure	Percutaneous superficial exposure with solid needle
	Contact with non-intact skin or mucous membrane with large volumes of blood
	For example, needle stick injury or cut penetrating gloved finger
Severe exposure	Percutaneous deep exposure with large volume of blood, e.g.
	• NSI with > 18-gauge needle contaminated with blood
	• Transfusion of significant amount of contaminated blood
	• Injury with used intra-venous/intra-arterial cannulas
	• Formation of a deep and painful wound

Wearing gloves serves as one of the protective factors against such injuries

Note: For NSI with sharps/needles contaminated for more than 48 hours prior to exposure, risk becomes negligible for HIV, and remains for HBV

(*Source:* CDC 2005; NACO 2007 Guidelines)
Abbreviations: HIV, human immunodeficiency virus; HBV, hepatitis B virus; NSI, needle-stick injury.

difficult to correctly determine the level of risk following individual exposures. It recommends considering all significant occupational exposure to HIV as severe exposure, and recommends uniform PEP for all.

Step 4: Evaluate the Exposure Source and Exposed Person at Baseline

If the viral status of the source is known (HIV/HBV positive or is high-risk candidate for these infections), then PEP should be initiated. However, if the status is unknown, serologic testing should be performed for HBV, HCV and HIV, both source person and the exposed person.

- *For the source person*
  - *Known source:* Serologic testing should be performed in the source person, after informed consent. If the source refuses to testing, the Mandatory Blood Testing Act, 2006 should be followed.
  - *Unknown source:* The likelihood of high-risk exposure to potential blood-borne pathogen should be assessed based on the number of HIV, HBV, or HCV-infected or at-risk patients in the medical unit, where the exposure occurred, and community prevalence rate, etc. Discarded needles should not be tested for blood-borne pathogens; as the reliability of these findings is not known.
- *For the exposed person*
  - Baseline blood sample to check antibodies against HBV, HIV and HCV; irrespective of whether PEP is initiated (Baseline testing is essential for the

purpose of any future claim for compensation for occupationally acquired blood-borne diseases).
- Baseline liver function test (LFT), if PEP is being planned for HIV.
- Repeat HIV, HBV or HCV serology at 3 and 6 months (if negative at baseline).

Step 5: Disease Specific PEP Management

This section will focus on specific PEP regimens recommended for exposure to HIV, HBV and HCV.

Post-exposure prophylaxis for HIV
Use of antiretroviral medicines was first introduced in guidelines for management of PEP in 1990, for occupational exposure to HIV, by the Centers for Disease Control and Prevention (CDC).[17] Subsequently in 1996, first US Public Health Service (PHS) recommendation for use of PEP after occupational exposure to HIV was published.[18] Since then, these recommendations have been updated 4 times.[19,14-16] Latest guidelines published in September 2013,[16] address several issues in interpretation and implementation of 2005 Guidelines. These include difficulty in determining the level of risk associated with individual exposures and thus, decision regarding two versus three drugs in PEP regimen. To resolve this issue, it recommends use of three (or more) drugs for management of all significant exposure to HIV infected source. It also recommends use of newer antiretrovirals with better side effect profile in PEP regimens, to improve compliance and thus, decrease the risk of transmission.
- *While initiating PEP, following points should be stressed:*
  - All HCWs receiving PEP, should complete a full 4-week regimen.
  - Few common side effects should be informed along with measures to control them.
  - HCWs should be informed about potential interaction of PEP drugs with other medications or herbals, which they might be taking.
- The first dose of PEP should be administered within the first 72 hours of exposure, preferably within first 2 hours. If the source person is tested negative for HIV, PEP should be discontinued, if already commenced (Flow chart 2).
- According to latest US-PHS recommendations,[16] all HCWs should receive a regimen containing three (or more) anti-retroviral drugs, following occupational exposures to HIV. An ideal regimen would be: Dual-NRTI (nucleoside reverse transcriptase inhibitor) backbone plus an INSTI (integrase strand transfer inhibitor), or a PI (protease inhibitor boosted with ritonavir), or a NNRTI (non-nucleoside reverse transcriptase inhibitor).
- *Preferred HIV-PEP regimen:* Raltegravir (RAL) 400 mg PO twice daily plus combination of tenofovir DF (TDF) 300 mg + emtricitabine (FTC) 200 mg once a day.
      Alternative PEP regimen and PEP regimen if exposed to drug resistant virus are mentioned in Tables 3 and 4, respectively.
- *Special considerations (pregnancy and lactation):* Efavirenz (EFV) based regimens are contraindicated in pregnant women, especially during the first trimester.[20] A pregnancy test must be done to rule out early pregnancy, before starting EFV-based PEP, for women in childbearing age group. All patients on EFV-based PEP should be advised contraception until PEP is completed.

Flow chart 2 Management of an exposed person by an HIV infected source or suspected high-risk exposure

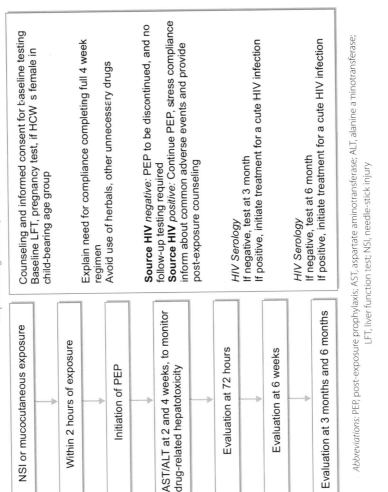

| NSI or mucocutaneous exposure | → | Within 2 hours of exposure | → | Initiation of PEP | → | AST/ALT at 2 and 4 weeks, to monitor drug-related hepatotoxicity | → | Evaluation at 72 hours | → | Evaluation at 6 weeks | → | Evaluation at 3 months and 6 months |

Counseling and informed consent for baseline testing
Baseline LFT, pregnancy test, if HCW's female in child-bearing age group

Explain need for compliance completing full 4 week regimen
Avoid use of herbals, other unnecessary drugs

Source HIV negative: PEP to be discontinued, and no follow-up testing required
Source HIV positive: Continue PEP, stress compliance inform about common adverse events and provide post-exposure counseling

HIV Serology
If negative, test at 3 month
If positive, initiate treatment for a cute HIV infection

HIV Serology
If negative, test at 6 month
If positive, initiate treatment for a cute HIV infection

Abbreviations: PEP, post-exposure prophylaxis; AST, aspartate aminotransferase; ALT, alanine aminotransferase; LFT, liver function test; NSI, needle-stick injury

Table 3 Alternative HIV-PEP regimens

Combine one drug or drug pair from the left column with one pair of nucleoside/nucleotide reverse-transcriptase inhibitors from the right column (according to local availability and institute protocols[16]

Choice of INSTI, NNRTI or boosted protease inhibitors	Dual NRTI backbones
• Raltegravir (RAL) • Atazanavir (ATV) + ritonavir (RTV) • Lopinavir/ritonavir (LPV/RTV) • Darunavir (DRV) + ritonavir (RTV) • Etravirine (ETR) • Rilpivirine (RPV)	• Tenofovir DF (TDF) + emtricitabine (FTC); available as Truvada • Tenofovir DF (TDF) + lamivudine (3TC) • Zidovudine (AZT) + lamivudine (3TC); available as Combivir • Zidovudine (AZT) + emtricitabine (FTC)

Abbreviations: PEP, post-exposure prophylaxis; INSTI, integrase strand transfer inhibitor; NNRTI, non-nucleoside reverse transcriptase inhibitor; NRTI, nucleoside reverse transcriptase inhibitor.

Table 4 Alternative options, if exposure occurred to drug resistant virus (HIV)

Antiretroviral agents for use as PEP only with expert consultation	Antiretroviral agents generally not recommended for use as PEP	Antiretroviral agents contraindicated as PEP
• Abacavir (ABC)	• Didanosine (ddl)	Nevirapine (NVP)
• Efavirenz (EFV)	• Nelfinavir (NFV)	
• Enfuvirtide (T20)	• Tipranavir (TPV)	
• Fosamprenavir (FOSAPV)		
• Maraviroc (MVC)		
• Saquinavir (SQV)		
• Stavudine (d4T)		

- *Expert consultation should be sought in following cases:[16]*
    - When the source person is unknown, decision regarding PEP should be decided on individual case to case basis.
    - When the source person is antiretroviral treatment experienced and is likely to harbor drug-resistant virus.
    - Exposed person is either pregnant or lactating.
    - *HCW reporting after 24–36 hours of exposure:* The interval after which benefit from PEP is undefined.
    - Persons with serious drug toxicity to initial PEP regimen.
- Follow-up of HCWs exposed to known or suspected HIV-positive sources.
- Counseling at the time of exposure and at follow-up appointments.
- *HCWs should be given adequate information about PEP drugs:*
    - Possible drug-related toxicities (e.g. rash and hypersensitivity reactions that could imitate acute HIV seroconversion and the need for monitoring).
    - Possible drug interactions.
    - The need for strict adherence to PEP regimens.
- Exposed HCWs should be advised to use precautions to avoid secondary transmission, especially during first 6–12 weeks of exposure (e.g. use of barrier contraception, avoid pregnancy and if possible breastfeeding and to avoid any blood or organ donations).
- *Re-evaluation at 72 hours after the exposure:* A follow-up visit at 72 hours is highly recommended, regardless of whether PEP is prescribed or not. By this time, baseline testing of exposed person and the source person would be available. If source patient is found to be HIV-negative, PEP should be discontinued. At this visit, importance of drug compliance should be emphasized, and early therapy-related adverse effects can be managed.
    - A HCW, who is detected to have HIV infection at any point of time during follow-up period, should be referred to a specialist for treatment of HIV and counseling.

Postexposure prophylaxis for hepatitis B
- Management of HCW exposed to HBV infected source depends on his or her vaccination status (Flow chart 3).[12] HBV-PEP should be initiated as soon as possible (*preferably in first 24 hours and at least within first 7 days*).

- If the HCW has completed HB vaccination, and his or her anti-HBs titers are more than 10 IU/L (i.e. exposed person is vaccine responder), the person is fully protected and no further vaccination is required. However, if the exposed person is unvaccinated or if vaccination or response to vaccine is incomplete (i.e. anti-HBs titer < 10 IU/L),[13] further management can be planned according to Flow chart 3.
- After initial treatment, HBsAg, AST (aspartate aminotransferase) or ALT (alanine aminotransferase) should be tested at 3 and 6 months, to detect HBV seroconversion or hepatitis. If during any follow-up testing, exposed person is found to be HBsAg positive, he or she should be referred to specialist for management of HBV infection.

Post-exposure prophylaxis for hepatitis C
- Till date, no prophylaxis is available for prevention of HCV infection. Hence, post-exposure management for HCV is primarily based on early identification of chronic HCV disease and referral to a specialist for management.[12] Exposed person should be tested at baseline, 3 and 6 months to monitor for seroconversion. If the exposed person is tested positive for HCV at any point of time during follow-up, he or she should be referred to a specialist for treatment. Pegylated interferon alpha and ribavirin is the current treatment of choice.

Step 6: Follow-up Care and Testing

Follow-up testing schedule for all occupational exposure, whether or not prescribed PEP regimen is 6 months (details listed in Table 5). At baseline, 2 and 4 weeks, complete blood counts, renal and hepatic function tests should be performed to check for any drug toxicities, for HCWs receiving PEP, and further testing may be indicated if abnormalities are detected. Testing for seroconversion should be performed at 6 weeks for HIV and at 3 and 6 months for HIV, HBV and HCV. Hardly any cases of seroconversion are reported after 6 months of exposure, hence no further testing is recommended if above mentioned tests are negative at 6 months.

POST-EXPOSURE COUNSELING

- Counseling should start from the very first visit at emergency department, and continued in small sessions on every visit.
- Initial counseling should concentrate on initiating antiretroviral therapy and on methods for reducing the risk of secondary transmission from the exposed person to others.
- Second counseling session at 48–72 hours is critical, as anxiety may limit understanding at first visit in the emergency department. Overall low-risk of transmission for all blood-borne pathogens (especially HIV) should be emphasized at each visit. The following are general guidelines,[13] for follow-up counseling to be advised at second counseling (Table 6).

Flow chart 3 Management of an exposed health care worker by an infected source (HBsAg+) or high-risk exposure

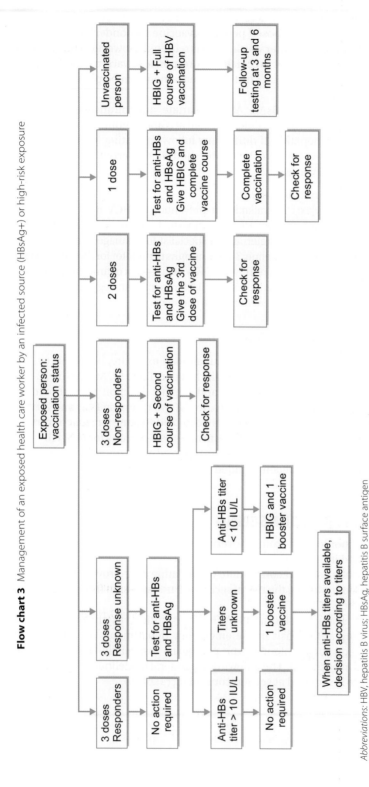

Abbreviations: HBV, hepatitis B virus; HBsAg, hepatitis B surface antigen

An accelerated vaccine course consists of doses at 0, 1 and 2 months. A booster dose is given at 12 months to those at continuing risk. The standard course is 0, 1 and 6 months

Hepatitis B immunoglobulin (HBIG) is only indicated where the source is known HBsAg positive, or where the recipient is a known non-responder to HBV vaccine and the source is known to be high-risk. HBIG should ideally be given within 48 hours but not later than 7 days after exposure.

Table 5 Summary of follow-up visits, and tests to be performed at each visit
(CDC/NACO 2007 Guidelines)

	HCWs on PEP regimen	HCWs not taking PEP
Week 2 and 4	Complete blood count$, AST/ALT*	--
Week 6	HIV-Ab	HIV-Ab
Month 3	HIV-Ab, Anti-HCV, HBsAg, AST/ALT*	HIV-Ab, Anti-HCV, HBsAg
Month 6	HIV-Ab, Anti-HCV, HBsAg, AST/ALT*	HIV-Ab, Anti-HCV, HBsAg

*AST/ALT should be checked at week 2 and 4 to detect PEP drugs toxicity, and at 3 and 6 months, for persons who contracted HBV/HCV from occupational exposure.
$For persons started on Zidovudine-based regimens

Abbreviations: HCW, health care worker; PEP, post-exposure prophylaxis; AST, aspartate aminotransferase; ALT, alanine aminotransferase; HCV, hepatitis C virus.

Table 6 Counseling recommendations blood-borne pathogen

HIV	• Do not share razors, toothbrushes, or needles • Do not donate blood, semen, organs or tissues for 6 months • Use barrier contraception for next 6 months to avoid the potential risk of secondary transmission to sexual partner • Avoid pregnancy for next 6 months • Avoid (if possible stop) breastfeeding
HBV	• Do not share razors, toothbrushes, or needles • Do not donate blood, semen, organs or tissues for 6 months • Consider using barrier contraception (Although exact risk of HBV transmission to sexual partner(s) of persons recently exposed who were non-immune and subsequently received hepatitis B immune globulin (HBIG) and/or the HBV vaccine is unknown)
HCV	• Do not share razors, toothbrushes, or needles • Do not donate blood, semen, organs or tissues for 6 months • Consider using barrier contraception, although the risk of sexual transmission is very low (0.1%) • Transmission from mother to infant is rare

REFERENCES

1. Deisenhammer S, Radon K, Nowak D, Reichert J. Needle stick injuries during medical training. J Hosp Infect. 2006;63(3):263-7.
2. Jayanth ST, Kirupakaran H, Brahmadatan KN, Gnanaraj L, Kang G. Needle stick injuries in a tertiary care hospital. Indian J Med Microbiol. 2009;27(1):44-7.
3. Rele M, Mathur M, Turbadkar D. Risk of needle stick injuries in health care workers – a report. Indian J Med Microbiol. 2002;20(4):206-7.
4. Pery J, Parker G, Jagger J. EPINET report: 2003 percutaneous injury rates. Adv Exposure Prev. 2005;7:42-3.
5. Mehta A, Rodrigues C, Ghag S, Bavi P, Shenai S, Dastur F. Needle stick injuries in a tertiary care centre in Mumbai, India. J Hosp Infect. 2005;60(4):368-73.
6. Rogers B, Goodno L. Evaluation of interventions to prevent needle stick injuries in health care occupations. Am J Prev Med. 2000;18(4 Suppl):90-8.

7. Trim JC, Elliot TS. A review of sharps injuries and preventative strategies. J Hosp Infect. 2003;53(4):237-42.
8. Hanrahan A, Reutter L. A critical review of the literature on sharps injuries: epidemiology, management of exposures and preventions. J Adv Nus. 1997;25(1):144-54.
9. Bell DM. Occupational risk of human immunodeficiency virus infection in healthcare workers: an overview. Am J Med. 1997;102(5B):9-15.
10. Ippolito G, Puro V, De Carli G. The risk of occupational human immunodeficiency virus infection in health care workers. Italian Multicenter Study. Arch Intern Med. 1993;153(12):1451-8.
11. Yazdanpanah Y, De Carli G, Migueres B, Lot F, Campins M, Colombo C, et al. Risk factors for hepatitis C virus transmission to health care workers after occupational exposure: a European case-control study. Clin Infect Dis. 2005;41(10):1423-30.
12. WGO Practice Guideline: Needle Stick Injury and Accidental Exposure to Blood. [online] Available from http://www.worldgastroenterology.org/assets/downloads/en/pdf/guidelines/16_needlestick_en.pdf. [Accessed March 2015].
13. Blood Borne Diseases Surveillance Protocol for Ontario Hospital. OHA/OMA October. 2010.
14. US Public Health Service. Updated U.S. Public Health Service guidelines for the management of occupational exposures to HBV, HCV, and HIV and Recommendations for Postexposure Prophylaxis. MMWR Recomm Rep. 2001;50(RR-11):1-52.
15. Panlilio AL, Cardo DM, Grohskopf LA, Heneine W, Ross CS. US Public Health Service. Updated US Public Health Service guidelines for the management of occupational exposures to HIV and recommendations for postexposure prophylaxis. MMWR Recomm Rep. 2005;54(RR-9):1-17.
16. Kuhar DT, Henderson DK, Struble KA, Heneine W, Thomas V, Cheever LW, et al. Updated US Public Health Service guidelines for the management of occupational exposures to human immunodeficiency virus and recommendations for postexposure prophylaxis. Infect Control Hosp Epidemiol. 2013;34(9):875-92.
17. Public Health Service statement on management of occupational exposure to human immunodeficiency virus, including considerations regarding zidovudine post exposure use. MMWR Recomm Rep. 1990;39(RR-1):1-14.
18. Centers for Disease Control and Prevention (CDC). Update: provisional Public Health Service recommendations for chemoprophylaxis after occupational exposure to HIV. MMWR Morb Mortal Wkly Rep. 1996;45(22):468-80.
19. Public Health Service guidelines for the management of health-care worker exposures to HIV and recommendations for postexposure prophylaxis. Centers for Disease Control and Prevention. MMWR Recomm Rep. 1998;47(RR-7):1-33.
20. Recommendations for Use of Antiretroviral Drugs in Pregnant HIV-1-Infected Women for Maternal Health and Interventions to Reduce Perinatal HIV Transmission in the United States. [online] Available from http://aidsinfo.nih.gov/contentfiles/lvguidelines/PerinatalGL.pdf. Published 2012. [Accessed March 2015].

Index